AMERICAN NURSING
Volume II

GARLAND REFERENCE LIBRARY
OF THE SOCIAL SCIENCES
(Vol. 684)

AMERICAN NURSING

A BIOGRAPHICAL DICTIONARY
Volume II

Edited by Vern L. Bullough
     Lilli Sentz
     Alice P. Stein

Contributing Editors
     Bonnie Bullough
     Olga Maranjian Church
     Signe S. Cooper
     Linda Sabin

GARLAND PUBLISHING, INC.
New York & London   1992

Library of Congress Cataloging-in-Publication Data
(Revised for volume 2)

American nursing.

(Garland reference library of social science ;
vol. 368–   )
   Includes bibliographies and indexes.
   1. Nurses—United States—Biography—Dictionaries.
I. Bullough, Vern L.   II. Church, Olga Maranjian,
1937–   .   III. Stein, Alice P.   IV. Series: Garland
reference library of social science ; v. 368, etc.
[DNLM: 1. History of Nursing—United States.
2. Nurses—United States—Biography.   WZ 112.5.N8 A512]
RT34.A44   1988   610.73′092′2 [B]   87-29076
ISBN 0-8240-8540-X (v. 1 : alk. paper)
ISBN 0-8240-7201-4 (v. 2 : alk. paper)

Photo Credits:

A. Beckwith—By permission of the Montana Historical Society,
Helena. M. Chase—Courtesy of Marjorie Bradshaw. C. Denni-
son—Courtesy of the Edward G. Miner Library, University of
Rochester. A. Fisher—By permission of the National Library of
Medicine. H. Fulmer—Courtesy of the Midwest Nursing History
Resource Center, Chicago, Illinois. R. Hubbard—By permission
of the Temple University Libraries Photojournalism Collection.
E. Johns—Courtesy of the Vancouver General Hospital.
M. Keller—Copyright by Bachrach. E. Lewis—Courtesy of Pach
Bros., N.Y. M. McPherson—Courtesy of Ellis Hospital School of
Nursing, Schenectady, N.Y. E. Odegard—By permission of the
State Historical Society of Wisconsin. A. Ohlson—Courtesy of
Agnes K. Ohlson. M. Riddle—By permission of the National
Library of Medicine.

Printed on acid-free, 250-year-life paper

MANUFACTURED IN THE UNITED STATES OF AMERICA

To those nurses who established
the profession for us

CONTENTS

..

LIST OF CONTRIBUTORS

Linda T. Anglin
R.N.C., D.A.

JoAnn Appleyard
R.N., Ph.D.

Sue Barkley
R.N., M.S.

Marianne Bankert
M.A.

Polly Belcher
B.S.N.

Nettie Birnbach
R.N., Ed.D.

Mary Brey-Schneider
B.S.N.

Marianne Brook
R.N., M.S.

Lillian Brunner
R.N., M.S.N., Litt.D., F.A.A.N.

Karen L. Buchinger
R.N., M.L.S.

Bonnie Bullough
R.N., Ph.D., F.A.A.N.

Vern L. Bullough
R.N., Ph.D., F.A.A.N.

Wendy Kent Burgess
R.N.C., Ph.D.

Linda M. Calley
R.N., Ph.D.

David Carson
Ph.D.

Olga Maranjian Church
R.N., Ph.D., F.A.A.N.

Stephanie Cleveland
R.N., M.N.

Anne E. Clifford
M.L.S.

Kathleen F. Cohen
M.L.S.

Signe S. Cooper
R.N., M.Ed., F.A.A.N.

Susan N. Craft
M.L.S.

Eleanor L. M. Crowder
R.N., Ph.D.

Carol A. Daisy
R.N., U.S.N.

Althea T. Davis
R.N., Ed.D.

Susan M. Davis
Ph.D.

Mary K. Delmont
M.L.S.

Janna L. Dieckman
R.N., M.S.N.

Susan Dudas
R.N., M.S.N.

Gerhard Falk
Ed.D.

Janet L. Fickeissen
R.N., M.S.N.

Laverne Gallman
R.N., Ph.D.

Laurie K. Glass
R.N., Ph.D., F.A.A.N.

Brother Roy Godwin
C.V.A.

Enid Goldberg
R.N., Ph.D.

Ellen Greenblatt
M.L.S.

Gayle J. Hardy
M.L.S.

Dolores J. Haritos
R.N., Ed.D.

Valerie Hart-Smith
R.N., M.S., C.S.

Judith C. Hays
R.N., M.S.N.

Eleanor Krohn Hermann
R.N., Ed.D., F.A.A.N.

Judith E. Hertz
R.N., M.S.N.

Mary Van Hulle Jones
R.N., M.A.

Ann-Marie Hurley
R.N., B.S.

Linda Karch
M.L.S.

Marilyn C. Kihl
M.L.S., M.A.

Lee Kraft
R.N., Ph.D.

Mary Ann Krol
R.N., M.S.N.

P.J. Ledbetter
R.N., Ed.D.

Sandra Lewenson
R.N., Ed.D.

Rosemary T. McCarthy
R.N., D.N.Sc., F.A.A.N.

A. Gretchen McNeely
R.N.C., M.S.N.

Michaeline P. Mirr
R.N., Ph.D., C.C.R.N.

Sharon Murphy
R.N., M.L.S.

Sandra A. Nagy
R.N., M.S.N.

Roberta M. Orne
R.N., M.S.

Robert V. Piemonte
R.N., Ed.D., F.A.A.N.

Patricia Pothier
R.N., M.S., F.A.A.N.

Alice Redland
R.N., Ph.D.

Linda Sabin
R.N., M.S.W.

Nancy Warren Schneckloth
R.N., M.S.N., C.N.O.R.

Lilli Sentz
M.L.S.

Judith Allen Shelly
R.N., B.S.N.

Judith Stanley
Ph.D.

Alice P. Stein
M.A.

Linda K. Strodtman
R.N., M.S.

Patricia Struckman
J.D.

Margretta M. Styles
R.N., Ed.D., F.A.A.N.

Jean Marie Symonds
R.N., Ed.D.

Dorothy Tao
M.L.S.

Leslie M. Thom
R.N., Ed.D.

Elizabeth M.B. Visone
R.N., B.S.

Francine Wallace
R.N., M.S.N.

Margaret R. Wells
M.L.S.

Mary Therese Whalen
M.A.L.S.

Hannah Williamson
R.N., Ph.D.

Alma S. Wooley
R.N., Ed.D., F.A.A.N.

Rosalee C. Yeaworth
R.N., Ph.D., F.A.A.N.

Paul A. Zadner
M.L.S.

Jacqueline C. Zalumas
R.N., Ph.D.

INTRODUCTION

This is the second volume of biographies of American nurses. Criteria for inclusion is essentially the same as for the first volume except for one basic change, that is, the date of birth. To be included in the first volume, the person had to be either born before 1890 or deceased. Only one nurse, Staupers, was still alive at the time Volume I went to press, and she has since died. Her biography is updated in this volume. To be included in this volume, the person had to be born in 1915 or before or be deceased. This allowed us to include several nurses, all retired from active nursing, who made significant contributions to nursing.

In other aspects, there is considerable overlap with Volume I since it was not possible to include all the significant American nurses in the first volume. The two volumes together make a far more comprehensive listing of the American nursing profession. Some important nurses might have been overlooked. This oversight is probably due to our inability to find any information about them. Readers are urged to suggest further names of significant nurses and provide information about them so that they can be included in Volume III, which hopefully will appear in 1997 or 1998. That volume will cover many of the present leaders of the profession who were too young to appear in Volume II.

To gather the list of nurses comprising Volume I and II, a search was made of various nursing journals, particularly the *American Journal of Nursing* and the *Trained Nurse and Hospital Review*. Published biographies of nurses either as individuals or as part of a collection were also studied and evaluated. Members of the American Association for the History of Nursing were urged to suggest those whom they regarded as significant figures in nursing because they had written important books and articles, made innovations in clinical care or in nursing theory, were significant leaders in nursing education or in nursing organizations, were barrier breakers or nurse heroines or role models, had major responsibilities in administration in the civilian or military setting, or had in some way achieved fame on either the national or international level. We also contacted individuals in various regions of the United States and asked them to suggest the names of nurses who had made significant regional contributions and who might not have been in the "inner circle" of the national nursing organizations. The total number of individuals gathered from such sources numbered well over 600, but as names were checked by our various nurse historian experts (both professional and amateur) and exploratory research was begun, many were removed from consideration. A major reason for not making the final list was that the individuals were too young (born after 1915 and still alive). Occasionally, also, individuals (both nurses and nonnurses) who were listed in other biographical collections for their contributions to nursing were eliminated because they were not judged significant enough to be included. Some nurses who made reputations outside of nursing have been included because they regarded their nursing preparation as significant or the fact that they were nurses was regarded as important by others. Lillian Carter, the mother of President Jimmy Carter, is an example. The end result is the biographies of 391 individuals, 177 in the first volume and the rest in this volume.

Nursing obviously was dominated by women; only nine of the biographies in the two volumes are of men, two in Volume I and seven in Volume II. Generally, the nurses in both volumes were born in rural areas. They came primarily from seaboard states of the East and from the Midwest, although there is a trend for more nurses to come from the southern and western areas of the United States, particularly for those born after 1880 and even more so for those born after 1900. Canadian-born nurses played an important role in nursing before World War I and less of a role afterward. In general, the earlier generation of nurses were older when they entered nursing school than were those born after 1900, when increasing numbers of nurses entered the nursing schools before the age of 20. Before World War I the Johns Hopkins nursing school was the dominant undergraduate school, but no one undergraduate school was that important afterward. Instead, there were groupings of important schools in such cities as Philadelphia, Boston, and New York. Teachers College, Columbia University, was the leading center for graduate studies until the end of World War II, and about a quarter of the individuals in both volumes either received an advanced degree there or attended it for a period of time. One of the surprising findings in a survey of the nurses in both volumes is how many of them had earned advanced degrees. In this the nursing leaders of the

past foreshadowed what is the current trend in nursing. The first generation of nurses to achieve doctorates in any number were those born between 1881 and 1900, and the number doubled for those born between 1901 and 1920. In both volumes the largest number of nurses were in nursing education with a total of 99 (25.1 percent), but clinical practice areas were also important. The second largest number were in public-health nursing, 69 (17.5 percent); 20 (5.1 percent) were in other areas of clinical practice. The two latter categories were more prevalent (and increasing) for those born between 1890 and 1920 than for the older generation.

One of the more obvious findings in a survey of the biographies is that the eminent nurses were not likely to marry. In the first volume 57.6 percent never married; in the two volumes 56 percent were never married. This indicates that there was a slight trend for those nurses born after 1881 and especially after 1900 to marry, but it was not until after World War II that a career and marriage became possible for larger numbers of women. The number of unmarried is probably larger than these figures indicate since many of those whose marital status is unknown were also probably unmarried. Moreover, some of the nurses who did marry, did so rather late in life. In fact, two married for the first time in their 60s, or as they were about to retire. Perhaps the lack of spouse and family obligations allowed the eminent nurses to be very mobile, and most of them did considerable moving around. Only 37 (9.4 percent) spent their lives in the same geographical area where they were born, while 165 (41.9 percent) lived in at least five different areas.

Nurses were also long-lived. Only 4 died before they were 40, one of them Clara Maas, a nurse heroine, while most lived well into their 70s (the median age at death was between 71 and 80), 96 (24.4 percent) lived to be past 80, 40 (10 percent) lived to be past 90, and 1 lived past 100; another included in the volume is approaching that mark.

The purpose of the biographies is to present the human side of nursing, emphasizing what it was like to be a nurse, the difficulties one encountered, and how nurses achieved success. It is hoped this volume will, like its predecessor, prove helpful to those who want to find out something about nursing in America and about a group of people, mostly women, who were the leaders in the development of American nursing.

Vern L. Bullough

ACKNOWLEDGMENTS

The editors would like to acknowledge with thanks the volunteer work of the many contributors. Obviously contributing to this volume was a labor of love. We would also like to acknowledge and give thanks to the professional assistance and advice of the Garland staff: Gary Kuris, Phyllis Korper, Kevin Bradley, and Shirley M. Cobert without whose efforts this volume would never have been published.

AMERICAN NURSING
Volume II

THE NURSES

Ellen Gertrude Ainsworth

1919–1944

Ellen Ainsworth died as a result of injuries sustained from enemy action near Anzio, Italy, during World War II. For her courage under fire and her selfless devotion to duty, she was awarded posthumously the Silver Star and the Purple Heart Citation.

Ainsworth was born on March 9, 1919, at Downsville (Dunn County), Wisconsin, the youngest of three children of Guy Henry and Emma Mathilda Moyle Ainsworth. Her siblings were Lyda Henrietta and William Moyle Ainsworth. The family belonged to the Methodist Church.

A fun-loving child, she spent much time engaged in antics with her two cousins. She had a delightful sense of humor and could find humor in her work, about which she was serious. Her sister remembers her as sensitive and kind.

Ainsworth attended grade school and high school in Glenwood City and then enrolled in the Eitel Hospital School of Nursing, Minneapolis. She completed her nursing program in 1941.

She was assistant supervisor on a medical-surgical unit at the Eitel Hospital before entering the U.S. Army Nurse Corps as a second lieutenant on March 9, 1942. She served at the Station Hospital at Camp Chaffee, Arkansas, until the end of that year and then was assigned to the 56th Evacuation Hospital, Brooke General Hospital, Fort Sam Houston, Texas. The hospital was sent to Bizerte, Tunisia, in North Africa; after several weeks it was relocated to Anzio, Italy.

While caring for patients in a hospital tent at the Anzio base, Ainsworth was hit by enemy fire on February 10, 1944. She died six days later.

Her citation for the Silver Star describes her gallantry: "Second Lieutenant Ainsworth was on duty in a hospital ward while the area was being subjected to heavy enemy artillery shelling. One shell dropped within a few feet of the ward, its fragments piercing the tent in numerous places. Despite the extreme danger, Second Lieutenant Ainsworth calmly directed the placing of surgical patients upon the ground to lessen the danger of further injury. By her disregard of her own safety and her calm assurance she instilled confidence in the assistants and her patients, thereby preventing serious panic and injury. Her courage under fire and her selfless devotion to duty was an inspiration to all who witnessed her actions, and reflect the highest traditions of the Army of the United States."

Ainsworth was awarded posthumously the Purple Heart and the Red Cross bronze medal, awarded for high meritorious service in time of war.

Ainsworth is buried at the U.S. Military Sicily-Rome Cemetery, Nettuna, Italy. The inscription on the headstone reads, "She Lies Among the Men She Served." A memorial marker is located in the family plot at Glenwood City.

In 1977 American Legion Post No. 168 in Glenwood City was renamed the Curry-Ainsworth Post in her honor. The next year the Ft. Hamilton, New York, Dispensary was named the Ainsworth U.S. Army Health Clinic, and in 1980 the Ainsworth Conference Room in the Pentagon was dedicated.

BIBLIOGRAPHY

Ainsworth, E.G. Military Personnel Records. National Personnel Records Center, St. Louis.

Ainsworth, L. Letters to author, November 14, 1988, and December 5, 1988.

"Army and Navy Nurses Tell Us." *American Journal of Nursing* 45 (January 1945): 65.

"Ellen G. Ainsworth." Obituary. *American Journal of Nursing* 44 (May 1955): 520.

"Enemy Fire Killed 1 Servicewoman from Wisconsin." *Milwaukee Sentinel*, May 26, 1986.

"More Awards to Army Nurses." *American Journal of Nursing* 44 (December 1944): 1179.

"Red Cross Bronze Medal Awarded Posthumously." *American Journal of Nursing* 46 (July 1946): 496.

"World War II Veteran's Heroism Remembered." *St. Paul Sunday Pioneer Press*, November 5, 1978.

Signe S. Cooper

Marian Alford

1904–1989

The major developments and interests of twentieth-century American nursing are mirrored in the life and career of Marian Alford, a prominent California nursing administrator and leader. A member of the California State Nurses' Association Board of Directors when it introduced collective bargaining to nursing in 1943, Alford was executive director of the organization when it abrogated the no-strike pledge 23 years later. An active participant in the movement to reorganize the national nursing associations at mid-century, Alford served as first director of the new National League for Nursing's Department of Hospital Nursing from 1952–56. A longtime director of nursing, Alford made patient care the central concern of modern nursing practice the focus of her professional career.

Marian Alford was born in Humboldt County, California, on August 17, 1904, into a family whose ancestors had come west in covered wagons. A family member (an aunt who loved her profession as a nurse) inspired Alford to choose nursing. She graduated from the University of California School of Nursing in 1926, received a B.S. from that institution in 1936, and an M.A. from Teachers College, Columbia University in 1948. Before beginning her career as a nursing administrator, Alford practiced briefly as a private- and general-duty nurse. Her clinical specialty was obstetrics, and, she later recollected, she "stayed pretty close to that."

From bedside nursing Alford moved to administration: she was a night supervisor at the University of California and Stanford hospitals, then assistant director of nursing at Stanford. In 1936 she was appointed director of nursing at Peralta Hospital in Oakland, a position she held until 1952.

During her years at Peralta Alford was very active in the Alameda County Nurses' Association (CSNA District 1) and in state association affairs: she was a District 1 president and board member, a CSNA board member and vice-president, and once admitted "to serving on nearly every district or state committee of the organization at one time or another." Among Alford's important assignments were chairing the committee that developed the first CSNA Minimum Employment Standards (Salaries and Personnel Practices) for Nurses in 1941, serving, also as chair, on the joint CSNA, California League of Nursing Education, and California State Organization for Public-Health Nursing Committee on the ANA Structure Study in the late 1940s, and chairing the Citizens Advisory Committee for CSNA's pioneering research study of nursing functions in the early 1950s. Alford won appointment to national committees as well: she was a member of the national Joint Committee on the Structure of National Nursing Organizations and the American Nurses'

Association Committee on Employment Conditions of Registered Nurses.

Alford's leadership years in her state professional organization were the years in which CSNA undertook to improve nurses' employment conditions and stabilize nursing services through collective bargaining and the Economic Security Program. In light of the refusal of the California Hospital Association to adopt CSNA's proposed minimum employment standards in 1942, the board of CSNA, under the leadership of Executive Director Shirley C. Titus, determined to embark upon collective bargaining. In 1943 it requested and received approval from its members to act as their bargaining agent; it was so recognized by the War Labor Board, which also authorized a 15 percent increase in nursing salaries sought by CSNA. A new era in nursing had begun.

Alford was a strong supporter of CSNA's pioneering use of the professional organization to represent the economic interests of its membership, and she stood firmly with the board in 1944 when ANA-proposed revisions to CSNA by-laws appeared to compromise its ability to engage in collective bargaining. Observing that "we do not want to give this [collective bargaining and the Economic Security Program] up," she counseled fellow board members to "say what we will do and what we will not do, and then we are through." Alford's commitment to CSNA as a bargaining agent was also evident in her spirited opposition to the 1945–46 attempt of the Alameda County Nurses' Guild, a CIO affiliate, to represent nurses in her home district.

A major objective of CSNA's collective bargaining and Economic Security programs was maintenance of an adequate nursing service for the public. As a director of nursing, Alford was immediately and professionally concerned with nursing service and the quality of patient care. Throughout her career she worked in a variety of ways through nursing organizations to improve the quality of care, e.g., through the CSNA study of nursing functions and as ANA representative on the National Commission for the Improvement of the Care of the Patient. In 1952

Alford's work in the area was recognized by her appointment as first director of the NLN Department of Hospital Nursing.

Alford saw that department as "a unique development, for there never has been before a national organization or a department in a national organization given over entirely to the improvement of nursing services in hospitals." Eager to take advantage of a new and special opportunity to improve nursing services, she set out to build understanding and alliances, to initiate "a cooperative movement," between and among the sometimes hostile groups involved with hospital nursing—administrators, doctors, directors of nursing, nursing supervisors, and those giving direct care to patients. "I see the urgent need for nurses to work with all others so nothing pertaining to nursing will go on without our participation," she observed. Under Alford's leadership nursing participation was assured.

"It was a pioneering and uphill job and Miss Alford did it," the director of the NLN Division of Nursing Services reported. "She cemented relationships among dissident groups, always with complete charm, and in a captivating way." The American Hospital Association, Alford was proud to report to delegates to the CSNA Annual Convention in April 1956, shortly before she assumed her new position as CSNA executive director, "has increasingly turned over all inquiries pertaining to hospital nursing service to this department [Hospital Nursing] of the League." Because it had been prepared to take the initiative, she added, nursing had retained "a responsibility for guidance in hospital nursing that might well have been taken over by the AHA alone."

Alford's successful experience with the AHA and her proven ability as a conciliator and mediator had very much to do with her selection by the CSNA Board of Directors to succeed Shirley C. Titus as CSNA executive director in 1956. After a decade of increasingly contentious relationships with hospital administrators and hospital associations in the state, responsibility for which the board attributed to the belligerent tactics of the Titus years, the board wished to develop "congenial relationships with allied organizations." It wanted "fences mended" and "rapport . . . established." In light of her experience of "good working relationships" with the hospital industry, Alford was the ideal candidate for the job.

As CSNA executive director from 1956–66 (the organization became CNA in 1961—California Nurses' Association) Alford made "increased cooperative relationships" with the California Hospital Association and regional hospital organizations a major priority. To promote cooperation, liaison committees composed of nursing and hospital representatives were established: they provided a forum in which nursing and mutual interests in patient care could be "frankly and firmly" discussed.

The most prominent of the committees was that organized in 1961 with the 200-member Hospital Council of Southern California (HCSC). Relations between CNA and HCSC flourished: CNA was eventually given the opportunity to comment on nursing salaries and personnel practices proposed for implementation by council members. This was a great breakthrough, for Southern California hospitals had long resisted CNA's efforts to represent the economic interests of their nurses. The director of CNA's Economic Security Program described the CNA/HCSC liaison committee as "a third method of representation of nurses," adding that "the importance of opening communications in such an influential Hospital Council area far outweighed any reasons for holding back on this approach."

At Alford's direction, and consonant with her desire to improve relations with the hospital industry, CNA undertook a different approach toward collective bargaining and the Economic Security Program as well. The director was instructed to strive "to remove the belligerency with which the program was surrounded," and Economic Security Program staff members were advised to consider "how to establish working relationships with hospital administrators." Local districts were also given more responsibility for Economic Security activities.

To assist with these activities and to assure a high quality of patient care, always a central concern of the Economic Security Program, local districts were encouraged to promote the organization of hospital-based professional performance committees (PPCs). In the committees nurses discussed such things as general welfare, practice conditions, salaries, and employment conditions, and through them they communicated their concerns about the quality of patient care in their institutions. The nursing shortage of the 1960s made patient care a critical issue, and the PPCs were increasingly vocal and influential advocates of needed reform.

Patient care and PPCs, in fact, were directly involved with what many consider the most dramatic "reform" in Alford's term as CNA executive director and in the history of nursing, i.e., the August 1966 decision of the CNA board to abrogate the no-strike pledge. The board's decision was prompted by the mass resignations of thousands of nurses in the San Francisco Bay area protesting against low wages and the unprofessional patient-care conditions identified by PPCs in their hospitals.

Alford strongly supported the board's decision. As she saw it, nurses in the state had been forced to act because of "the gradual deterioration over the past 25 years in the quality of patient care." She applauded the emergence of "a new generation of nurses" who "see themselves as a profession" and "refuse to compromise their ideals" to accept "a pattern in which the motives of industry are smothering the basic human ideal of giving quality nursing care."

Quality nursing care was the major preoccupation, the central focus of Marian Alford's career. It is fitting that one of her last official acts should be endorsement of a policy that her professional organization, to which she had given decades of distinguished service and leadership, deemed essential to assuring that care.

Marian Alford retired as executive director of the California Nurses' Association in September 1966. Her decade of leadership had clearly produced improved relationships with the hospital industry and, a colleague commented, "active and thoughtful, participation" by the membership in association affairs. The hallmark of her administration, the colleague continued, was "involvement" by and with a host of individuals and groups to the end of serving and "caring for their fellowman." Sad to say, Alford's personal involvement with the world during her retirement years was seriously limited by a profound hearing loss. She died in Oakland, California, on October 14, 1989.

PUBLICATIONS BY MARIAN ALFORD

"Speech to House of Delegates By Marian Alford. *Bulletin of the California State Nurses' Association* 52 (June 1956): 182–86.

BIBLIOGRAPHY

Alford, M. Papers of Marian Alford. California Nurses' Association Archives, San Francisco.

"Marian Alford Accepts NLN Position." *Bulletin of the California State Nurses' Association* 48 (September 1952): 256.

"Marian Alford Appointed New CSNA Executive Director." *CNA Bulletin* 52 (March 1956): 71.

"Meet Marian Alford, Our Executive Director." *CNA Bulletin* 57 (November 1961): 171–72.

"Minimum Employment Practices and How They Grew." *Bulletin of the California State Nurses' Association* 54 (April 1958): 91–94.

Minutes of the meetings of the Board of Directors of the California State Nurses' Association, 1941–56, *passim.* California Nurses' Association Archives, San Francisco.

Pross, E. "A Decade of Progress." *CNA Bulletin* 62 (July–August 1966): 1, 7.

Judith Stanley

Lydia E. Anderson

1863–1939

Lydia E. Anderson spent her entire adult life in the cause of nursing education. She was born on January 16, 1863, in New York City, the daughter of Lucy Spence Anderson and the Rev. Thomas D. Anderson, a Baptist minister. She lived 76 years. She was never married. For her lifetime she achieved a great deal. Her early education was in private schools. She then entered the Rutgers Female College in New Brunswick, New Jersey, and thereafter attended the New York Hospital Training School for Nurses, graduating in 1897. When she was 46 years old, she returned to school and took a postgraduate course at Columbia Teachers College, New York City, in 1909–10. Throughout her early career Lydia Anderson worked as a hospital administrator. Later, for a period of 26 years, she devoted herself to teaching.

She became superintendent of the Homeopathic Hospital in Providence, R.I., in 1897, that same year she became associate superintendent of Sloane Maternity Hospital in New York City, where she remained until 1902.

The years 1902–03 were spent in private nursing, but then Lydia Anderson returned to nursing administration. In 1905 she became assistant superintendent at the Long Island Hospital. The next four years she held the same position at Mt. Sinai Hospital in New York City and thereafter began her astonishing teaching career during which she taught or lectured occasionally at 32 schools in New York State and New Jersey. Her principal task, however, was to serve as nursing instructor at both the Mt. Sinai School of Nursing and the New York Hospital Training School, which she did until 1936.

During those many teaching years, Anderson devoted all of her extra time to nursing organizations. She served on the board of the New York Hospital School of Nursing Alumni Association, participated actively in the work of the Red Cross, the American Nurses Association, the National League of Nursing Educators, and the History of Nursing Society. For one year she was secretary and for seven years president of the New York State Board of Nurses Examiners, possibly signing as many as 27,000 certificates in those years.

Throughout her career she was viewed as an excellent teacher by her many students. She inspired her students to learn. She taught with humor and wit and exuded a feeling of security and relaxation, all of which created an atmosphere conducive to learning.

In honor of her 30 years of service to the nursing profession, Anderson was feted by her colleagues at a special dinner. At this dinner sufficient funds were roused to establish the Lydia Anderson Loan Fund. Administered by the New York League of Nurses Education, the fund enables nurses to continue their studies in order to become a nursing instructor.

Anderson was always devoted to the New York Hospital School of Nursing, where she had learned the profession. In 1927 she published the *History of the New York Hospital School of Nursing.* In recognition of her service, New York Hospital in 1941, on the forty-fourth anniversary of her graduation and two years after her death, named the library after her.

PUBLICATIONS BY
LYDIA E. ANDERSON

History of the New York Hospital School of Nursing. New York: New York Hospital, 1952.

BIBLIOGRAPHY

American Journal of Nursing 27 (June 1927,) 29 (February 1929), 39 (May 1939,) 41 (June 1941).

Dictionary of American Nursing Biography. M. Kaufman, ed. Pp. 7–9. Westport, Conn.: Greenwood, 1988.

Jordan, H. Jamieson. *Cornell University-New York Hospital School of Nursing, 1877–1952.* New York: New York Hospital, 1952.

Lehmkuhl, Bertha H. "Lydia E. Anderson, R.N., B.S." *American Journal of Nursing* 29 (February 1929): 201–02.

National League of Nursing Education Biographical Sketches. 1937–1940. New York: The League, 1940.

Gerhard Falk

Mother Angela
(Eliza Maria Gillespie)

1824–1887

Mother Angela provided significant nursing leadership during the Civil War as Mother Superior of the Sisters of the Holy Cross. Sixty nuns served thousands of war victims in crude converted warehouses in Mound City, Illinois. Although prepared as an educator, Mother Angela used her leadership abilities and common sense to provide nursing services and the necessities of life to sick and wounded men. After the war she returned to teaching and administration but strongly supported the need for nursing preparation as the result of her wartime experiences.

Eliza Maria Gillespie was born in Brownville, Pennsylvania, to John P. and Mary (Myers) Gillespie. Her father, a lawyer, died while she was still very young; her mother then moved to Lancaster, Ohio. Eliza studied in a school run by the Dominican sisters in Somerset, Ohio, and then went to Washington, D.C., to complete her studies with the Sisters of Visitation. She graduated with highest honors in 1842.

Eliza sought areas of parish service after returning home to her mother and stepfather in Ohio. She participated in programs to relieve the sufferings of refugees of the Irish potato famine and served as a volunteer nurse during a disastrous cholera outbreak in 1849. She also helped to establish a parish school, where she taught from 1847–51.

In 1852 Eliza moved to St. Mary's Seminary, St. Mary's City, Maryland, to serve as a lay teacher. A year later she entered the Congregation of the Holy Cross, taking the name of St. Angela. She completed her novitiate in France and returned to America in 1855. Sister Angela was sent to the Academy of St. Mary in Bertrand, Michigan, which later relocated to South Bend, Indiana. This academy eventually became St. Mary's College, and it developed adjacent to Notre Dame University.

During the Civil War, Mother Angela served primarily at the hospital at Mound City, Illinois. She directed the conversion of warehouses and a pork house into a hospital that served 1,500 patients. Mother Angela and her sisters also served on evacuation riverboats carrying wounded to hospitals. In addition, sisters under Mother Angela's direction served patients in hospitals at Paducah and Louisville, Kentucky, Memphis, Tennessee, and Cairo, Illinois. By the end of the war over 80 nuns had served in the hospitals directed by Mother Angela. These sisters provided a disciplined corps of hard workers who kept hospitals functioning under the worst conditions. The courage, strength, and dedication of these religious sisters won the admiration and appreciation of many in the war effort, including Mary Livermore, a U.S. Sanitary Commission worker.

After the war, like many other volunteer nurses, Mother Angela resumed her educational and administrative duties at St. Mary's. She died on March 4, 1887, of heart disease at St. Mary's Convent at Notre Dame, Indiana. Nearly 40 institutions, schools, academies, asylums, and hospitals had been established under her direction after 1855.

BIBLIOGRAPHY

Barton, G. *Angels of the Battlefield: A History of the Labors of the Catholic Sisterhoods in the late Civil War.* Philadelphia: Catholic Publishing, 1908.

Livermore, M. *My Story of the War: A Woman's Narrative of Four Years Personal Experiences.* Hartford: Worthington, 1889.

Medeleva, Sister. *Notable American Women 1607–1950.* Vol. II, pp. 34–35. E.T. James, ed. Cambridge: Belknap Press of Harvard University, 1971.

Walsh, T. "Mother Angela and the Sisters of the Civil War." In *Those Splendid Sisters.* New York: Harper, 1932.

Willard, I., and M. Livermore. *American Women: 1500 Biographies.* Vol. I, pp. 321–22. Kirkpatrick, N.Y.: Mast Crowel, 1897.

Linda Sabin

Edith Augusta Ariss

1878(?)–1952

E. Augusta Ariss came from Toronto, Canada, to Great Falls, Montana, on June 6, 1902. She was the first Montana deaconess matron. She is best known for establishing 8 of the 15 deaconess hospitals and training schools in that state. She was also instrumental in founding the Montana hospitals. She organized and was superintendent and director of the

Montana Deaconess Hospital and Training School in Great Falls, but also was the instructor of the school for many years. Four of these hospitals and schools later formed the foundation for the largest baccalaureate-nursing program and the only graduate-nurse program in Montana. Her contributions toward patient care, nursing education, and nursing service are reflected through her role in organizing graduate nurse alumni associations, the state nurses' association, and the state licensing board. At various times Ariss was the president for all three organizations that she helped found.

Although no date of Ariss's birth has been found, records estimate the year to be 1878. She was born in Guelph, Ontario, the third girl in a family of six girls and one boy. Little is known of her family or childhood except that her father was a farmer near Guelph, and she grew up on the family farm. It is likely that her primary and secondary education was gained in Guelph. After Ariss moved to Montana, her immediate and extended families were very important to her, and she maintained close ties with them throughout her life. Throughout the years of her career and retirement she consistently drove from Montana, and later from California, to spend vacations with her family. Since she considered the nursing students and graduates of the Great Falls program as "hospital" family, she included the annual alumni meetings in her route to and from Canada after her retirement. The last alumni convention she attended was in 1948, four years before her death.

Ariss was 17 years old when she graduated from a two-year nursing program at Guelph General Hospital Training School in 1895 and shortly after graduation entered the Chicago Training School for Deaconesses, completing the program in 1897. The Chicago school was founded in 1890 by Mrs. Lucy Rider Meyer. She and her husband Reverend Meyer had visited the school run by the Fliedners in Kaiserwerth, Germany, and were inspired to carry on a similar school in Chicago. Ariss's nursing education was complimented by the Christian and social-work aspects of this school.

In Montana the deaconesses were associated with the Methodist Church. The deaconess philosophy of caring and being charitable resulted in semicharitable hospitals being built and run by such deaconesses as Ariss who worked free of charge in the hospital and community and received only a little more than their room and board.

It was five years after Ariss completed her Deaconess program there that Mrs. Meyer recommended that Ariss, RN, Deaconess, be brought from Toronto to Montana to be superintendent of a bankrupt hospital in Great Falls. Through her dedication, managership, and organization this hospital became the Montana Deaconess Hospital and remains the major clinical teaching site for nursing students in the present Montana State University College of Nursing.

Ariss continued her education in Montana by visits to Johns Hopkins in Baltimore and hospitals in Toronto, St. Paul, Cincinnati, Chicago, and New York to keep informed about nursing and nursing schools.

Ariss devoted herself to the needs of others. A frequent comment from her was that folks, including students, were her first love. She loved children and in many of her annual hospital reports she would include a picture of babies in the nursery. Frequently, she would be holding some of the babies. She never married. Her total commitment was transmitted to students through rules she had set as hospital administrator and teacher. For example, students were not permitted to have dates because the nursing shortage was acute, and she did not want the students to marry and leave nursing. Her life centered around her hospital and nursing school as well as the deaconess responsibilities for herself and for other deaconesses.

Ariss retired with her colleague Edith Long, a deaconess too, from the hospital in 1931. Although the pair had a home in Long Beach, California, Ariss continued to perform volunteer hospital work and served on professional organizations through 1933 in Montana. They did not move permanently to Long Beach until 1940. The last time Ariss came to the annual Great Falls alumni meeting was in 1948, at which she was honored. At the same meeting a hospital room was also dedicated to her colleague and friend Edith Long in memory of her years of service. Long had died in Long Beach in 1946. Following Long's death, a sister of Ariss moved to Long Beach and lived with Ariss.

Ariss's first position as a registered nurse and deaconess was with the Fred Victor Rescue Mission, Toronto, Canada, as a visiting nurse in 1897. She found this work ideal, for she used her nursing, Christian philosophy, and interpersonal skills in working with patients. In 1902 Rev. W. Van Orsdel, following the recommendation by Meyer, called on Ariss to reorganize the Great Falls Hospital, which had closed in 1901 due to financial difficulties. He was looking for a good manager, and the progress Ariss made through the years thereafter indicated that his choice had been excellent. Ariss was loaned for only two years by the Canadian Rescue Mission to the northern Montana mission for work at Great Falls. However, she remained for 33 years.

She arrived on June 16, 1902, accompanied by three other deaconesses. After Ariss and her "team" cleaned up the hospital, it was reopened on July 1, 1902. Ariss also started a nurse training school the first year with two students. As with many early schools of nursing, for several years patient care was learned at the bedside from Ariss's lectures, doctors' discussions, and nurses and older students on the wards. The nursing principles identified by Florence Nightingale were used in setting up the curriculum. Ariss was responsible for founding 8 of the 15 Montana Deaconess Hospitals and Training Schools from 1902 through 1927. Ariss gave overall direction to the deaconess movement in Montana as it related to hospital work. (Through her and the Methodist Church, Montana Deaconess Hospital in Great Falls became the "Mother Hospital" for the seven other deaconess hospitals that she set up.) Although she devoted herself mainly to Great Falls after 1911, Ariss remained the overseer of the deaconess-nursing programs until her retirement. During the influenza epidemic of 1918 she requested the deaconess training schools be closed for three months. During this time students were expected to serve whenever and wherever they were needed. Even prior to 1918 students were assigned home care with pay. This payment was then given to the school to help offset expenses. By 1913 the students did three months of home nursing as a part of their training program.

Ariss strove to upgrade the deaconess-nursing programs and worked with the university system in Great Falls and Bozeman to enable students to take some courses at the colleges and apply them to their nursing program. As superintendent and general overseer of the 15 deaconess hospitals in Montana, she used principles of nursing care, management, and community relationships to upgrade patient nursing care. In 1919 Ariss announced that only graduate RNs of Montana Deaconess Training School would be charge nurses. She insisted on the establishment of a State Board of Nursing (1913) that must be run by nurses—not doctors. She was elected president of the board from 1920-33.

World War I influenced her life greatly, and she encouraged nurses to join the armed services through the Red Cross Nursing Service.

Ariss received many awards and honors. Before her retirement, the Methodist Church and the doctors with whom she worked gave her a mountain cabin near Great Falls. Students and nurses enjoyed using this cabin as well. The Montana Deaconess Alumni Association furnished a hospital room in her honor, naming it E. Augusta Ariss Alumnae Room. The association also honored her at their 1937 meeting, at which she was toastmistress, and again in 1942. In 1937 the nursing students dedicated their annual to her and requested that she write her perception of the school for this annual.

As has been noted, Ariss was active in establishing the Association of Montana State Graduate Nurses in 1912. She served as president of the Montana Nurses' Association in 1915 and 1920. She was able to meet her 1920 goal of

hiring an executive secretary for the association. Work with the State Board of Nursing began in 1913, and on May 10, 1913, the first examinations were given. Ariss served as president of the State Board of Nursing from 1921-33. She organized the Montana Deaconess Hospital Training School Alumni Association in 1914 and was made an honorary life member. In 1932 the Montana State Nurses' Association sent Ariss and Long to the International Convention of Nurses in Paris and Brussels in recognition of their contributions to nursing.

Ariss died of a heart attack at her home in Long Beach on January 9, 1952. Students in uniform and registered nurses in uniform and wearing the deaconess caps formed the honor guard for the funeral services held in the First Methodist Church in Great Falls, Montana. In her obituary Ariss was referred to as "the Florence Nightingale of the Northwest."

PUBLICATIONS BY EDITH AUGUSTA ARISS

BOOKS

Historical Sketch of the Montana State Association of Registered Nurses and Related Organizations. 1937. (Printer unknown.)

ARTICLES

"Why I Remain a Deaconess." Montana Methodist Conference Report of August 21, 1928. Methodist Church, Great Falls, Montana.

"A History of the Montana Deaconess Hospital School of Nursing." Class of 1937: *White Caps* (Montana Deaconess Hospital School of Nursing) (1937): 4-11.

PAMPHLETS

"Annual Report of the Montana Deaconess Hospital, Superintendent's Report, 1910-11, 1915-16, 1919-20, 1920-21, 1921-22." Great Falls, Mont.: Tribune Printing and Supply Co.

"Annual Report of the Bozeman Deaconess Hospital, Superintendent's Report, 1912-13, 1913-14." Bozeman, Mont.: Bozeman Daily Chronicle.

"First Annual Report of the Bozeman Deaconess Hospital, Superintendent's Report, 1911-12." Bozeman, Mont.: Bozeman Daily Chronicle.

Letter by Ariss to Anna Pearl Sherrick. Montana State University College of Nursing Collection, Bozeman, December 14, 1944.

BIBLIOGRAPHY

Ackerman, E.R. "Annual Report of the Bozeman Deaconess Hospital Superintendent's Report 1914–15, 1915–16, 1916–18." *Bozeman Daily Chronicle* (Mont.)

"Deaconess Hospital Observes 50th Anniversary." *Gallatin County Tribune and Belgrade Journal*, May 11, 1961, 4.

"The Deaconess Hospital to be Re-opened." *Great Falls Daily Tribune*, June 3, 1908, 8.

"Dewey Street Recounts Hospital History." *Gallatin County Tribune and Belgrade Journal*, February 17, 1972, 6.

"E. Augusta Ariss." Obituary. *Great Falls Tribune*, January 11, 1952, 2.

"Ex-Deaconess Hospital Head Dies (1/9/52): Funeral Rites Pending." *Great Falls Tribune*, January 10, 1952, 7.

Hamm, J. "The Montana Deaconess Hospital Nurses Alumni Association, History, Constitution and By-Laws." Great Falls, Mont.: Electric City Printing, 1947.

McCullough, R.S. "Development of Four Pioneer Deaconess Hospital Training Schools for Nurses in Montana—1902–1937." Master's thesis, Montana State College School of Nursing, Bozeman, 1968–70.

McDonnell, C.L. "Study of the Development of the Montana State College School of Nursing." Master's thesis, Montana State University College of Nursing, Bozeman, July 1961.

Rubens, M.W. "Miss Ariss in Love with her Task" (Poem). Montana Deaconess Alumnae Association (Class of 1920), 1927.

Sherrick, A.P. Interview with author, 1987, 1989. (Professor Emeritus, Montana State University College of Nursering.)

Sherrick, A.P., S.R. Davison, and M.D. Munger. "Deaconess Hospitals"; "International Council of Nurses"; "Presidents of Montana Nurses Association—1912–1960"; "Schools of Nursing." In *Nursing in Montana.* Great Falls, Mont.: Tribune Printing, 1962.

Simpson, H. Interview with author, 1989, 1990. (Member of Montana Nurses Association.)

"Two Honored at Reception Given Here." *Great Falls Tribune*, August 24, 1942.

Sue Barkley

Lois Marintha Austin

1903–1985

Lois Austin was a nurse educator who held positions at several universities including Boston, the University of Virginia, Loyola, the University of Pennsylvania, and the University of Pittsburgh. She was the national president of Sigma Theta Tau from 1955–58 and of the National League for Nursing from 1963–67.

Austin was born on May 8, 1903, at Hinsboro, Illinois. Her parents were Homer Moon and Lenora Anne (Clipson) Austin. She studied at Iowa State Teachers College, Cedar Falls, from 1921–22. She taught in elementary schools in Illinois and Iowa from 1922–29 before resuming her college education. She received a bachelor of science degree in liberal arts and nursing from the State University of Iowa in 1931. She studied nursing education at Teachers College, Columbia University, in 1940 and received an M.A. in education from Ohio State University in 1949. In 1956 she was a National League of Nursing doctoral fellow and the following year received her Ph.D. degree in curriculum and instruction from the University of Chicago.

Austin was an instructor in nursing arts at the Minnequa School of Nursing, Corwin Hospital, Pueblo, Colorado, from 1931–33 and at the Ohio State University School of Nursing from 1933–36. She joined the faculty of the University of Pittsburgh as a lecturer in nursing in 1937. Between 1939 and 1958 she taught nursing and directed education programs at the University of Texas School of Nursing, Galveston; Tacoma General Hospital School of Nursing, Washington; Boston University School of Nursing, Boston; the Extension Division and Cabaniss Memorial School of Nursing at the University of Virginia, Charlottesville; the Loyola University School of Nursing, Chicago; and the University of Pennsylvania School of Nursing, Philadelphia.

She returned to the University of Pittsburgh in 1958 as an associate professor in the graduate program of nursing education and became a full professor in 1961. From 1959–73 she held the title of acting chairman of the Department of Nursing Education as well. In the later years of her career there, she also was assistant to the dean. She retired in 1973.

Beginning in 1954, Austin served as a

consultant on curricular problems of nursing schools for more than two decades. In 1964 she was a member of the women's advisory committee to the New York World's Fair.

During the years she was president of the NLN, she also served on its Executive Committee and its task-force Committee on Organizational Structure.

She was a fellow of the NLN, a member of the American and Virginia District nurses associations, the Virginia League of Nursing, the Virginia League of Nursing Education, Pi Lambda Theta, and Kappa Delta Pi.

Her awards included the Ethel Smith–Josephine McLeod Memorial Award of the Virginia Nursing Association in 1949 and the Key Award of Alpha Tau Delta.

She died on June 10, 1985, at her retirement home in Pittsburgh.

BIBLIOGRAPHY

"Austin, Lois Marintha." *Who's Who of American Women, 1974–75.* Chicago: Marquis, 1975.

"Austin, Lois M., Individual Faculty Information." Typescript. University of Pittsburgh School of Nursing, updated.

"Lois Austin Dies." Typescript. International Nursing Library. Sigma Theta Tau International, Indianapolis.

Alice P. Stein

Lucy C. Ayers

1865–1940

Lucy C. Ayers was an organizer of the Rhode Island State Nurses' Association and served as the first secretary-treasurer of the Rhode Island State Board of Nurse Examiners.

She was born in Canterbury, New Hampshire, in 1865, attended local schools, and graduated from the Connecticut Training School for Nurses in 1891.

After doing private-duty nursing, she became superintendent of nurses at the Women's Hospital in Chicago, and the Women's Hospital in Sioux City, Iowa. She left nursing for several months around the turn of the century to travel abroad.

She was appointed as the first director of nursing at Rhode Island Hospital in Providence in 1900 and served until 1910. The state had a new law for professional registration of nurses, and she worked to upgrade both the school's program and nursing service throughout the state. During her tenure, the hospital's nursing school affiliated with Providence Lying-in Hospital in 1903 so that students could get training in obstetrics. In 1906 it affiliated with the Providence District Nursing Association to provide experience in home care. The school gained additional residence facilities and its first classrooms, and, by 1910, when she left to spend a year in California, it had a teaching staff of 13 and 126 students.

Ayers became superintendent of nurses at Woonsocket (Rhode Island) Hospital in 1911 and performed similar functions there. Throughout her tenure at the two hospitals, she served on the Rhode Island State Board of Nurse Examiners, leaving that post in 1935. After retiring from Woonsocket Hospital in 1926, she returned briefly the next year in an interim capacity.

Ayers was an organizer of the Rhode Island State League of Nursing Education and was second vice-president of the Rhode Island State Nurses Association. She was a member of the National League of Nursing Education from its inception as the American Society of Superintendents of Training Schools for Nurses. She was one of the original members of the Central Directory for Nurses. For many years she served on various committees of the state and local American Red Cross organizations.

She created the Lucy C. Ayers Fund in 1926 to establish and maintain a home for aged, convalescent, and disabled nurses. She continued to be active professionally with the Woonsocket Public Health Nursing Association, the Woonsocket Day Nursery and Children's Home, the volunteer service committee of the Woonsocket Red Cross, the Woonsocket Hospital Aides Association, and the YWCA.

BIBLIOGRAPHY

Garland, J.E. *To Meet These Wants.* Providence: Rhode Island Hospital, 1963.

"Lucy C. Ayers." Obituary. *American Journal of Nursing* 40 (April 1940): 482.

Pennock, M.R., ed. *Makers of Nursing History.* New York: Lakeside, 1940

Alice P. Stein

Edith Annette Aynes

1909–1980

Edith Aynes was an army nurse, a writer, and an administrator. She wrote extensively about nursing for nurses and for the public, advocating broader-based education for nurses and efficient utilization of nursing personnel. Her writings have contributed to an understanding of some of the issues facing the profession, especially during the World War II years.

Aynes was born in Atwood, Kansas, on April 2, 1909. Her father, Andrew Festus Aynes, died when she was 13 years old, and her mother, Marion Pearl McIrvin Aynes, raised her and her two brothers. She was influenced to enter nursing by stories of her physician-grandfather, a pioneer in Rawlins County, Kansas, and by her own experiences as a patient in her youth. During her high-school years she wrote high-school news for a local weekly newspaper, was active in school theatrical productions, and played violin with her older brother's dance orchestra. After her graduation from high school her mother opposed her becoming a nurse and arranged a scholarship for her to learn typing and shorthand in order to become a court reporter. She first made use of her skills to write by completing applications for nursing schools.

Aynes finally entered Presbyterian Hospital School of Nursing, Denver, Colorado, graduating from there in 1932. She continued her formal education throughout her career. She was awarded a B.S. from the University of California, Berkeley, in 1950 and an M.A. from Kean College, Union, New Jersey, in 1963.

When she graduated as a nurse, it was at the depth of the Depression and there were few civilian jobs for nurses. Thus after a few months at the end of 1932, as night nurse and surgical nurse at a small rural hospital, she joined the Army Nurse Corps as a "reserve" nurse. She served first at Fitzsimmons General Hospital in Denver. In the Army Nurse Corps she was able to realize her ambition to work as a surgical scrub nurse and then, in 1939, completed training and certification as a nurse-anesthetist at Philadelphia Jewish Hospital. Following this, she was appointed operating-room supervisor and anesthetist at Ft. Bragg, North Carolina. During her next tour of duty, at Tripler General Hospital, Honolulu, she began to communicate about the hospital world to the public in a column in the *Honolulu Advertiser,* "Speaking of Operations," written under the pseudonym Pat Eleanor Pierce.

After the Japanese attack on Pearl Harbor, Aynes volunteered for overseas duty and was assigned to the 148th General Hospital, San Francisco as chief nurse. During the next five months of the "waiting war," Aynes drew on her early writing, musical, and theatrical experience to address the problems of morale among her staff by instituting an "Amateur Night" show and a nurses' glee club. She wrote lyrics for an army nurse version of "Army Blue" for the nurses to sing. The "waiting war" continued for 14 months more after her unit was moved in June 1943 to Hawaii. The need for activity prompted her to arrange for lessons in Hawaiian culture (language and hula lessons!) for the nurses in addition to the glee club and nurses' participation in a dramatic group formed by the soldiers. At this time she wrote the column "Operation on the Hill" for an army insert in the *Hilo Tribune.* She endeavored to include as many names of personnel as possible (with the Army's approval). The *Hilo Tribune* was often mailed home by the G.I.s and nurses because they were not allowed to write home themselves about activities or locale because of security. Aynes continued to be concerned about the nurses' morale and wrote in "The Waiting War" that the narrowness of a nurse's education little prepared her to cope with the boredom of few patients to care for or helped her to fit as a professional into social situations. In September 1943 she was promoted to captain and assigned to the office of the chief of the Army Nurse Corps, Colonel Florence Blanchfield, as a public relations officer.

The effort to recruit nurses for military service was at its peak, and competition with the other women's services was high. In this post Aynes worked with the author and producer of "One Man's Family," a popular radio serial to create the character Teddy who joined the Cadet Nurse Corps and took part of her training at an army hospital. Aynes supplied the details of army and hospital life and Teddy "lived" until 1956. "Nurse's Prayer," a poem written when Aynes was a student nurse, and subsequently set to music by her, and "Song of the Army Nurse" were sung on nationwide radio by popular singer Jo Stafford to aid the recruitment effort.

At the end of World War II Aynes requested leave to attend the University of California to work on a bachelor's degree. In 1947, one semester and one summer session short of her degree, she returned to Washington under Colonel Blanchfield's successor, Colonel Mary G. Phillips, to publicize the newly established Organized Reserve Corps, for which 50,000 recruits were sought. This was a difficult undertaking because at the end of the war more than 27,000 nurses had been discharged because successful recruiting had generated an "oversupply." Part of the publicity campaign to recruit reserve nurses involved offering an honorary reserve commission to a female celebrity who could then include remarks about the reserve in her radio program. Singer Kate Smith agreed to do this, and in February 1949—the forty-eighth anniversary of the Army Nurse Corps—nurses across the country took their oaths of office, which was written by Aynes, while Smith read the oath to two nurses in the New York studio on live radio. This first group of nurses became known as the Kate Smith Class. During this time Aynes was editor of *Army Nurse,* the official monthly of the Army Nurse Corps (no longer published).

Having completed an army course in hospital administration since her three semesters at Berkeley, Aynes returned to the University of California and completed her degree, receiving her B.S. in nursing education in 1950. Following this, she was assigned to the 279th General Hospital, Osaka, Japan, and then transferred to Medical Section Headquarters, Japan Logistical Command, as chief nurse.

At the end of the Korean conflict, Major Aynes was assigned to 5th Army Headquarters, Chicago, and then to Brooke Army Medical Center, Fort Sam Houston, Texas as instructor at the Medical Field Service School. She retired from the army in 1956.

Following her retirement, Aynes became coordinator of information and public education for the National Foundation of the March of Dimes in New York City. In 1961 she was appointed executive director of the Cerebral Palsy School and Treatment Center, Belleville, New Jersey. From February 1964 until the end of her life, she was administrator of the Andrew Freedman Home in the Bronx, New York.

Aynes continued to write about nursing for professional and popular publications. Her book, *From Nightingale to Eagle: An Army Nurse's History* was published in 1973.

Aynes was decorated twice by the army for her service. In 1945 she recieved the Commendation Ribbon with Medal Pendant for her recruitment and publicity work for the Army Nurse Corps. In 1952 she was awarded the Legion of Merit for her service in Japan.

Aynes was a member of the American Nurses' Association, the National League for Nursing, Gerontology Society, the National Council for Aging, the American Guild for Authors and Composers, the American Society of Composers, Authors and Publishers, the Retired Officers Association, the Retired Army Nurses' Association, the National Writers' Club, and the International Platform Association. In addition, she was a 53-year member of the Order of the Eastern Star.

Edith Aynes died in the Bronx, New York, on December 31, 1980. She was a multifaceted nurse: operating-room nurse, nurse-anesthetist, writer, administrator. She utilized her talents in creative and professional writing to inspire nurses' confidence in their own competence and to explain nursing and nurses to the public. She spoke out about the need for nurses to have a broad education for the enrichment of their professional and personal lives and relationships. She urged the public to be knowledgeable about the health-care system.

PUBLICATIONS BY EDITH ANNETTE AYNES

BOOKS

From Nightingale to Eagle. Englewood Cliffs, N.J.: Prentice-Hall, 1973.

ARTICLES (Selected)

"Army Nursing." *American Journal of Nursing* 40 (May 1940): 539–42.

"This Waiting War." *American Journal of Nursing* 43 (June 1943): 542–45.

"The Hospital Ship 'Acadia.'" *American Journal of Nursing* 44 (February 1944): 98–100.

"The Registered Nurse-Anesthetist." *RN* (December 1947): 7, 72, 74, 76–77.

"Army Nursing: Then and Now." *American Journal of Nursing* 49 (April 1949): 205–06.

"The Nation Sometimes Remembers." *Trained Nurse* 122 (May 1949): 220–21.

With O.W. Snyder. "A Receiving Ward for Air Evacs from Korea." *Hospitals* 25 (October 1951): 61–63.

"Hospital Trains in Korea." *American Journal of Nursing* 52 (February 1952): 166–67.

"The Army Area Chief Nurse." *Nursing Outlook* 2 (March 1954): 136–39.

"Toward Professional Competence." *Nursing Outlook* 5 (January 1957): 38–40.

"Colonel Florence Blanchfield." *Nursing Outlook* 7 (February 1959): 78–81.

"The Coming Scandal in Nursing." *McCall's* (March 1964): 100–01, 134, 136.

"Military Nursing—1950 Style." Washington, D.C.: U.S. Center of Military History, n.d.

BIBLIOGRAPHY

"Army Nurse Corps Officers in Far East Win Decorations." News release. Washington, D.C.: U.S. Army Center of Military History, 1953.

"Citation for the Legion of Merit." Unpublished.

Washington, D.C.: U.S. Army Center of Military History.

"Edith A. Aynes." Obituary. *New York Times,* January 10, 1981.

"Edith A. Aynes." Obituary. *The Citizen-Patriot* n.d. Rawlins County (Kans.) Historical Society.

"Major Aynes, Army Nurse Corps, Returns to States After Receiving Citation for Work in Far East." News release. Washington, D.C.: U.S. Center of Military History, 1953.

"Major Edith Aynes Assigned to Medical Field Service School." News release. Washington, D.C.: U.S. Army Center of Military History, 1954.

"Mansion-Like Home for Aged in the Bronx Solaces Only the Once-Wealthy." *New York Times,* May 17, 1974.

News clippings, miscellaneous, undated. Rawlins County (Kans.) Historical Society.

Marianne Brook

Bessie Baker

1875–1942

Bessie Baker was a nursing administrator. She was the first superintendent of nurses at the Charles Miller Hospital at the University of Minnesota and the first dean of the Duke University School of Nursing, serving at Duke from 1930–38.

Baker was born in Maryland in 1875, the daughter of William Henry and Elizabeth Vickers Baker. She studied under a scholarship at the Johns Hopkins Hospital Training School in Baltimore, graduating in 1902.

In 1910 she was named assistant to the director of the Hospital of the Women of Baltimore and its associated training school. She was named first assistant to the director of the nurses' home of Johns Hopkins Hospital in 1912. The following year she became one of four assistant superintendents of the Johns Hopkins Training School.

During World War I she was asked to head the nursing staff of Base Hospital 18, known as the Johns Hopkins Base Hospital Unit. The unit arrived in France June 28, 1916, and was established at Ba-zoilles-sur-Meuse on July 24. After her war service she was reappointed to her former post at Johns Hopkins.

She later undertook studies at Columbia University and during the summer of 1920 spent a month of intensive observation of public-health work in New York City. In February 1922 she received a bachelor's degree from Columbia and a diploma in administration from the Department of Nursing and Health at Columbia's Teachers College.

She then spent eight years as superintendent of the new training school for nurses at the Charles Miller Hospital, University of Minnesota, St. Paul, and an assistant professor of nursing at the university. Baker was instrumental in establishing a five-year course in arts and nursing that lead to a bachelor of science degree and a diploma in nursing. She believed that taking university courses for a couple of years immediately following high school gave students a chance to mature more fully before finally choosing a profession.

On April 29, 1929, she was named dean and professor of nursing education at the school of nursing that opened in October 1930 at Duke University in Durham, North Carolina. Baker's plan was to set the same standards of admission that applied to other university students and to offer a bachelor of science degree to students who completed 60 semester hours at Duke or another institution. Once the nursing school and related divisions of the university were fully organized, she envisioned specialized courses in such areas as teaching, administration, and public-health nursing.

Because of failing health, she left Duke on July 1, 1938, and returned to Baltimore. The June of the following year a portrait of her was presented to Duke University by the alumnae association of the School of Nursing.

Baker was run over by a car in Baltimore and died at Johns Hopkins Hospital on June 24, 1942. In September 1943 the nurses' home at Duke University was renamed Baker House in her honor.

PUBLICATIONS BY BESSIE BAKER

ARTICLES

"An Outline of the Work of Our Nursing Unit." *Johns Hopkins Nurses Alumnae Magazine* 18 (May 1919): 58–61.

"Observation Work with the Public Health Service of New York City." *Johns Hopkins Nurses Alumnae Magazine* 17 (August 1920): 98–99.

"The Appeal of the Five-Year Course in Nursing." *Johns Hopkins Nurses Alumnae Magazine* 22 (August 1923): 81–82.

"The Duke University School of Nursing." *Johns Hopkins Nurses Alumnae Magazine* 29 (May 1930): 59–60

BIBLIOGRAPHY

"Bessie Baker." Obituary in unidentified newspaper. Historical section, Talbot County, Maryland, Public Library.

Notices of Baker's appointments. *Johns Hopkins Nurses Alumnae Magazine* 9 (September 1910): 122; 11 (September 1912): 108; 12 (November 1913): 237; 15 (August 1916): 127–29; 15 (November 1916): 282; 17 (May 1918): 77; 20 (November 1921): 264; 21 (February 1922): 21; 29 (February 1930): 25.

Pennock, M.R., ed. *Makers of Nursing History.* New York: Lakeside, 1940.

Alice P. Stein

Emma Maud Banfield

ca. 1870–1931

Emma Banfield, born in South Wales, Great Britain, about 1870, was a leader in British and American nursing during the first part of the twentieth century, not only because of her considerable contribution to nursing education, but also because she exhibited the kind of courage in World War I that earlier had made Florence Nightingale the epitome of the nursing profession.

Banfield was, in fact, a very "international" nursing leader. She was educated in Bruges, Belgium, where she attended a convent school and converted to Catholicism. There she also learned to speak French. At the age of 18 she returned to

England and entered the St. Bartholomew Hospital School of Nursing in London for the customary two-year course of study.

By 1895 she had become director of nursing of the St. Agnes Hospital in London, thus giving her an opportunity to modernize the nursing service there. She stayed until 1897, when she first came to the United States as superintendent of nurses and assistant superintendent of the Polyclinical Hospital of Philadelphia. For 13 years, until 1910, Banfield remained in Philadelphia and distinguished herself by organizing help for soldiers wounded in the Spanish-American War of 1898 and by improving and lengthening the course of study for nurses from two years to three years. In addition, she developed the first nurses "alumni association" thus giving additional support to those entering the profession after her. She also developed the first "postgraduate" course for nurses.

In 1897 Banfield became one of the first women ever to serve as superintendent of a hospital when she was appointed to that position at the Polyclinical Hospital. Her annual reports to the board of trustees indicate a great concern not only with nursing the sick, but also with the prevention of illness. Banfield proposed the use of visiting nurses for tuberculosis patients, a concept then both innovative and revolutionary. Her efforts to remove tuberculosis and OBS patients from the wards met with considerable opposition, but in the end she succeeded.

During her tenure as superintendent, Banfield supervised the construction of a residence for the superintendent, a home she occupied in 1903. From there she used her skill and energy in yet other endeavors of benefit to her profession. She chaired the Hospital Economic Committee of the Society of American Superintendents, became active in the Association of Hospital Superintendents, and succeeded in combining the Polyclinical Hospital postgraduate course in nursing with the University of Pennsylvania, thus making that course the foundation for the postgraduate department of nursing at that university.

By the time she "retired" from her position as superintendent in 1910, she had promoted the cause of nursing in the United States and Canada as well as increased the number of nursing students and the number of patients at the Polyclinical Hospital.

Banfield had also been active in founding the Department of Nursing at Teachers College of Columbia University in New York City, in 1899, where she was also among those who taught a course on nursing. The founding of that department was indeed one of the most significant events in the history of nursing in the United States. This, however, was not at once apparent to those who enrolled in that first course or who witnessed its beginnings. On the contrary, the editor of the new *American Journal of Nursing*, Sophia Palmer, severely criticized the course and claimed that the work required was beyond the comprehension of the nurse-students. There is some evidence that this dissatisfaction by the editor was caused by the complaints of her sister who was one of the students in the course. In a letter on that subject, dated, March 12, 1901, Banfield wrote: "It also seems to me that although Miss Palmer has expressed herself in an unfortunate way, we should be careful not to give any loophole for the impression that we, the Executive Committee, resent criticism, whatever we may privately feel as to the justice of it." Ever the diplomat, Banfield then suggested that Palmer be invited to explain her idea of a better course of study and that "it would be both polite and politic of us to notice." Other members of the committee that had organized the course did not agree with Banfield and saw no reason to ask the advice of Palmer. A good deal of correspondence developed in regard to this controversy including a considerable amount of worry about the financial aspects of teaching a course at Columbia Teachers' College.

Banfield had been elected the chair of the Hospital Economics Committee in 1901 and made this report at the 1902 convention of the Society of Superintendents: "We simply live from hand to mouth so that our finances are easily told." She explained that the society owed Columbia College $900 in order to use Columbia's facilities to teach the course again the next year and yet only $189 was available. Said Banfield: "Unless the ladies this morning will all promise me $10 each, we shall have only $130 with which to pay the $900 (to the College) the next year." Evidently, Banfield and her friends were successful as nursing education at Columbia became firmly rooted there and then spread to other colleges and universities in the ensuing years.

Emma Banfield also wrote for the *Ladies Home Journal.* She published a number of articles on nursing and even conducted a column of advice for readers of the *Journal.*

In 1910, after her return to England, Banfield was called upon once more to provide leadership in the nursing field, for when World War I broke out in 1914, the (British) Royal Red Cross recruited her. She served in France in 1918 and was decorated for "gallant and distinguished conduct in the field." Previously she had participated in the war effort as a staff nurse at the Lord Darby Hospital in London and as "matron" at the hospital in Warrington. Her only injury came as a result of a bicycle accident in 1919.

In 1923 Emma Maud Banfield married a childhood friend, attorney A.R. Atkinson. They moved to New Zealand, and she died of cancer there at Wadestown on September 22, 1931, at the age of 61. It was said of her that even in her last days she faced death with that "quiet heroism" that had marked the achievements of her fruitful life.

BIBLIOGRAPHY

Christy, T.E. *Cornerstone for Nursing Education.* New York: Teachers College Press, Columbia University, 1969.

Higgins, L.P. "Emma Maud Banfield." *Dictionary of American Nursing Biography.* M. Kaufman, ed. Westport, Conn.: Greenwood, 1988.

M. Adelarde Nutting Collection, Teachers College, Columbia University, New York City.

Gerhard Falk

Mary Rose Batterham
1858–1927

In 1903 Mary Rose Batterham became the first U.S. nurse to be awarded a certificate of registration.

Batterham was born in England in 1858, the daughter of William and Mary Rose Batterham. She came to the United States at about age 20 and was graduated from the nursing program of Brooklyn City Hospital, Brooklyn, N.Y., in 1893. She also did postgraduate work there.

She then went to Asheville, North Carolina, where she spent her career mostly in private-duty and public-health nursing. Among the positions she held were head nurse at Oakland Heights Sanitarium and a Metropolitan Life nurse. She received her certificate of registration in Buncombe County, on June 5, 1903.

After attending a meeting in Raleigh in 1901 to discuss formation of a state nurses' organization, Batterham became an organizer, charter member, and the first vice-president of the North Carolina State Nurses' Association in 1902. In 1916, when a public-health section of the association was formed, she was elected chairman.

Batterham was a member of the North Carolina State Red Cross Nursing Committee and in 1895 became a charter member of her alumnae association. She wrote for professional journals and had a special interest in the history of her profession in North Carolina.

As a leader and writer, Batterham was an outspoken advocate of shorter hours and improved living and working conditions for nurses. She urged the broadening of nursing curricula to provide a superior cultural background. She urged graduating nurses to donate their services occasionally to charity and to go where they were needed rather than choosing their cases.

Batterham died of acute appendicitis and acute chronic myocarditis at the French Broad Hospital, Asheville, on April 4, 1927. At her funeral in Trinity Episcopal Church the pall bearers were nurses.

BIBLIOGRAPHY

Death certificate. North Carolina State Board of Health, Raleigh.

"Mary Rose Batterham." *American Journal of Nursing* 27 (May 1927): 410.

"Nursing: First R.N." *Southern Hospital* (January 1938): 11.

"Who's Who in the Nursing World: LXII, Mary Rose Batterham, RN." *American Journal of Nursing* 26 (September 1926): 700.

Wyche, M.L. *The History of Nursing in North Carolina.* Chapel Hill: University of North Carolina Press, 1938.

Alice P. Stein

Anna Totman Beckwith

1903–1984

From her appointment in 1941 to her retirement on July 1, 1968, Anna Totman Beckwith provided outstanding nursing leadership during her 27 years as the executive secretary of the Montana State Board of Nursing. Through her many years of work with the Montana Nurses' Association's committee on legislation and her persuasive activity with the Montana legislators and governors, she was best known for her ability to interpret the Nursing Practice Acts to the public as well as to members of the profession.

Anna Totman Beckwith, named after her maternal grandmother, was born at St. Patrick Hospital in Missoula, Montana, on March 31, 1903. She was the eldest child and only daughter of Eva Elizabeth Totman and George Henry Beckwith. Her brothers, Philip Henry and John (Jack) Keith Beckwith, were born on July 5, 1904 and June 10, 1906. A fourth child, known only as "Baby Beckwith" was a stillborn on June 17, 1913.

Her father, a merchant of English descent, was one of 16 children who was raised in St. Leonard, New Brunswick, Canada, before moving to Missoula. Anna's mother was born and raised in Wisconsin. She moved to Missoula, in 1898, following her graduation from a Normal School in Wisconsin. There she met and married George.

They lived for a short while in Missoula before moving to the St. Ignatius Mission area of the Flathead Indian Reservation.

All of Anna Beckwith's childhood was spent in Saint Ignatius where her parents owned and operated the Beckwith Mercantile, a family restaurant, grocery, grain, and lumber business. Because the business was operated on the Indian Reservation, her father was required by the federal government to procure a credential as a "licensed trader."

In an effort to make friends with others who spoke English in the predominantly Indian population of the Flathead Reservation, Anna's mother became acquainted with the Ursuline Sisters, who operated a nursery school and kindergarten for the tribal orphans at the Saint Ignatius Mission Church. She often took Anna as an infant and toddler in a "baby buggy" to the mission to visit the sisters. Because she was a very beautiful blond, rosy-cheeked child, Anna was used by the well-known artist, Brother Joseph Carignano, as the model for the angels and cherubs in the 58 frescoes he painted on the ceiling of the Saint Ignatius Mission Church during a seven-month period in 1904 and another seven-month period in 1905.

Both of Anna's parents were very civic-minded and religious individuals. Her father was a member of the St. Ingatius District #28 school board in 1912. When the Women's Club was organized in 1924, Eva was elected as its first president. Beckwith's father became the first mayor of St. Ignatius when the town was incorporated in 1938.

When Anna Beckwith was about 5 or 6 years of age, she and her brother Philip contracted infantile paralysis. Both carried the effects of the illness with them throughout their lives: Beckwith with a scoliosis and her brother with a hand deformity. Because of this experience as a youngster, Anna Beckwith worked tirelessly with the Montana Rehabilitation Association during her adult years in Helena, especially for the children crippled from polio.

She attended the public schools in

Saint Ignatius, graduating from St. Ignatius High School in May 1921. She then enrolled at the State University of Montana in Missoula. She majored in biology with a minor in chemistry, graduating with honors upon the completion of a B.A. degree on June 15, 1925.

Since she had contracted polio as a child, her mother was sure that her daughter was too frail for the strenuous work required of nurses. But in the autumn of 1925, Beckwith entered the Johns Hopkins Hospital School of Nursing in Baltimore, more than 2,000 miles from home. The Johns Hopkins nursing program was highly regarded and was very selective of the students accepted for the programs. It offered the young Montanan the opportunity for a "thorough and varied experience" as well as a chance to get away from home for a while.

Upon Beckwith's graduation in 1928, it was noted that she was one of 10 graduates in a class of 70 who held a baccalaureate degree and she was classified as a woman of "superior education and culture." Beckwith passed the state board examination and received her certificate of licensure as a registered nurse in Maryland, dated June 17, 1929. Her qualifications led to her appointment in various capacities at Johns Hopkins Hospital between 1928 and 1934: first as the head nurse of the women's medical ward, then as an assistant instructor of practical nursing, and finally as the assistant supervisor of the new medical clinic, a position that carried with it teaching responsibilities and follow-up of students. She also was in charge of the building when the supervisor was off duty and during vacation periods. When the hospital received funding for a ward instructor, Beckwith was given that responsibility as well.

One of the head nurses who came under her tutelage during that period was K. Virginia Betsold, who later became the associate director of Johns Hopkins Hospital School of Nursing. In writing to the Montana Nurses' Association in 1962, when Beckwith was being honored for her many years of nursing service and her contributions to the profession, Betsold

wrote that Beckwith was a "gracious, understanding, good-humored, tolerant and helpful" person and that "she typified for us the kind of nurse that we were all striving to become."

In 1934 Beckwith chose to return to her home state of Montana and accepted the position of superintendent at St. Peter's Hospital in Helena, becoming both the director of nursing and the hospital administrator. St. Peter's was founded in 1884 by the Rev. F.T. Wells of the Episcopalian Church. Its training school was begun in 1909 and closed in 1933, just a year before Beckwith's arrival.

In 1935 a series of devastating earthquakes destroyed St. John's Catholic Hospital in Helena, placing an added responsibility on St. Peter's. Beckwith effectively coordinated emergency nursing services in the city, managing the crisis and extra patient load until St. John's reopened in 1939. She held her position at St. Peter's until 1941, when she assumed the responsibilities of executive secretary of the Montana State Board of Examiners for Nurses. She was the second full-time paid executive, succeeding Edith Lucille Brown, who filled the position from 1932 to 1941.

Beckwith was first appointed as a member to the State Board of Examiners by Governor Roy E. Ayres on May 28, 1940. Mary D. Munger, former executive director of the Montana Nurses' Association, noted that during Anna Beckwith's 28-year tenure with the board, she not only witnessed, but encouraged, the closure of most of Montana's remaining diploma schools of nursing. She additionally sought the development of several practical-nursing programs within the vocational educational system of the state, and two associate-degree nursing programs in community colleges were established during that time as well. Beckwith worked diligently for legislation that provided initial licensure for practical nurses in 1953 and mandatory licensure for both registered and practical nurses in 1967. According to Dr. Laura Copple Walker, former director of the Montana State University College of Nursing and president of the State Board of Nursing, Anna Beckwith's leadership and direction to the faculties of the schools of nursing and their supportive agencies provided tremendous improvement in both Montana's professional and practical schools of nursing.

Beckwith also provided leadership on a national level as a member of the American Nurses' Association (ANA) Blueprint Committee, which was appointed by the executive committee of ANA's Special Committee of State Boards of Nursing. In addition to developing test construction policies and objectives for state board test pool examinations, the Blueprint Committee prepared the second draft of test items for the examinations following the first draft prepared by the National League of Nursing (NLN) item writers.

At the state level, she served as a member of the Montana Nurses' Association from 1934 until her retirement. She held the office of treasurer from 1936 to 1938, chaired the Legislative and By-Laws committee in 1937 and again in 1952, served on the Red Cross State Committee from 1935 to 1937, the State Nursing Council for War Service in 1942, the Recruitment Council in 1944, and the Professional Counseling and Placement Service Committee in 1945. She was appointed the chair of the MNA's P and A Committee in May 1945 to study organization structure during 1945–46 and was the secretary of MNA's Educational Administrators, Consultants, and Teachers section (EACT) in 1946. She also served on and was a consultant to the Committee on Nursing Practice in 1959.

Beckwith took responsibility for leadership at the local level by serving as the president of District #4 (Helena). In October 1962 she was honored at the Montana Nurses' Association's fiftieth-anniversary celebration and was presented with a special jeweled pin provided by the American Nurses' Association.

As a member of the Montana League for Nursing, Beckwith held the office of secretary from 1946 to 1950. In 1962 she served as the treasurer and at other times was on the board of directors. She was president of the Montana Public Health Association in 1951 and again in 1961. She was one of seven who received distin-

guished service awards in public health from that organization at its annual meeting in Missoula on April 17 and 18, 1962. She served on the board of directors of the Montana Tuberculosis Association for 10 years and was active in the Montana Rehabilitation Association and the Montana Health Planning Council.

Her activities outside of nursing included membership in the American Association of University Women, serving as the president of the state division from 1956 to 1958, and the president of the national organization in 1960. At that time, to her delight, Beckwith experienced her first flight in a small airplane, which carried her to Boston for the annual convention. She actively participated in Kappa Kappa Gamma and was a member of a national women's sorority (PEO sisterhood) that supported the education of women.

Though she had been baptized on April 30, 1903, in the Holy Spirit Episcopal Church in Missoula and confirmed in the St. Ignatius Episcopalian Church as a child, Beckwith apparently did not remain active in the church as an adult. She never married but maintained close personal relationships with the many friends she cultivated through the years as well as her numerous colleagues both at Johns Hopkins and in Montana.

Beckwith spent many weekends and vacations with her relatives at the McLeod cabin at Seeley Lake, Montana. Because of her close family ties and her love for the Mission mountains, she also spent a number of holidays with her family in Saint Ignatius until the death of her parents. Her mother died on December 11, 1949, and her father on June 30, 1952.

Upon her retirement from the Montana State Board of Nursing in 1968, Beckwith was again honored by the MNA for the many years she had devoted to the nursing profession.

Following her recovery from a fractured hip in 1977, Beckwith moved from Helena to Missoula. She lived at the Missoula Manor Retirement Home, where she remained until May 1983, when her emphysema and cardiac conditions required the care provided in Hillside Manor, a nursing home. Though she had been bedridden for some time, she managed to be up in a wheelchair for a party given in honor of her eightieth birthday at the Maclay residence.

After a brief stay of several days, she died in Missoula Community Hospital on February 5, 1984, at the age of 80. Sunset Memorial Park Crematory in Missoula, Montana, the town of her birth, carried out her wishes that her body be cremated and her ashes scattered over Lake McDonald (now St. Mary's).

PUBLICATIONS BY ANNA TOTMAN BECKWITH

ARTICLES

"Montana Law and the Practice of Nursing." Helena: Montana State Board of Nursing, March 1960.

"That Licensing Examination." *The Pulse* (Spring 1960): 13, 15.

ADDRESSES

"Legislation for Nursing." Paper presented at the 23rd Annual Convention of Montana State Nurses' Association, June 11–12, 1935, in Missoula.

"What is a Nurse?" Address to the first graduating class of practical nurses in Great Falls, Montana, June 1962. Montana Nurses' Association Manuscript Collection #170, Box 1, Folder 2. Montana Historical Society, Helena.

BIBLIOGRAPHY

"About People You Know—Anna T. Beckwith." *American Journal of Nursing* 42 (1942): 95.

"Biographical Sketches: Anna T. Beckwith." Montana Nurses' Association Manuscript Collection #170, Box 1, Folder 2. Montana Historical Society, Helena.

Dudley, J. "St. Ignatius Community Methodist Church." *St. Ignatius Post*, September 23, 1954, 2.

"Honoring the Past ... Challenging the Future." *Pulse* (Winter 1962): 8–9.

Logan, S.R. "Some early recollections of School District #28." *St. Ignatius Post and the Ronan Pioneer* (Mission Centennial Edition), September 23, 1954, 16.

Maclay, Mrs. D.J. (Frances Hughes). Interview with author in Missoula, Montana, April 28, 1989.

Montana Nurses' Association. Official minutes, 1934–68. Montana Nurses' Association Manuscript Collection #170, Box 3, Folders 3, 4, 5; Box 4, Folders 1, 2, 3, 4. Montana Historical Society, Helena.

Munger, M.D. "Nursing Leader Dies in Missoula." *Pulse* 20, no. 3 (1984): 3.

"Nurses Honored for Public Health Service." *Pulse* (Winter 1962): 14.

Obersinner, Rev. Joseph L., and Judy Gritzmacher. *St. Ignatius Mission: National Historic Site*. Missoula, Mont.: Gateway Printing and Litho, 1977.

"Obituaries: Anna T. Beckwith." *Missoulian*, February 7, 1984, 12, col. 1.

Pitch, M.M. Personal correspondence from Helena, Montana, May 10 and May 21, 1989.

Reisig, W. "Biographical Sketch: Anna T. Beckwith." Address to the Montana Nurses' Association's 50th anniversary celebration banquet, October 1962. Montana Nurses' Association Manuscript Collection #170, Box 1, Folder 2. Montana Historical Society, Helena.

Schoenberg, W.P. *Jesuits in Montana (1840–1960)*. Portland: Oregon Jesuits, 1960.

Wehr, O. C., ed. *The Heritage of Mission Valley*. St. Ignatius, Mont.: Mission Valley News, 1975.

Wehr, O.C., ed. *To Live on a Reservation: 1854–1976*. Bicentennial edition. St. Ignatius, Mont.: Mission Valley News, 1976.

A. Gretchen McNeely

Edna Behrens
1897–1990

A long-time nurse activist and leader, Edna Behrens played a central role in the development and growth of collective bargaining in nursing. President of the California State Nurses' Association when it introduced the tactic to the profession in 1943, and a strong advocate of CSNA's companion Economic Security Program, she worked closely with CSNA Executive Director Shirley C. Titus to educate nurses about collective bargaining and about "what could be done if they got together, worked together, increased the membership of the organization and began to get their working conditions down in writing." Described as "the instrument which assured the survival" of CSNA's collective bargaining program, Behrens received the ANA's Shirley C.

Titus Award in 1976: the award honors individuals who make significant contributions to the economic and general welfare of nurses.

Edna Behrens was born in Petaluma, California, on January 4, 1897, one of four children of a family of Danish immigrants. A 1917 graduate of the School of Nursing at Franklin Hospital in San Francisco, Behrens practiced there for 18 years as an operating-room supervisor; she subsequently served as director of nursing for three years. In 1937 she was appointed director of nurses at Sonoma County Hospital in Santa Rosa. With the exception of a year's leave in 1949 to help organize the nursing service at a new hospital in Glenn County, Behrens remained at Santa Rosa until 1951, when, CSNA associates suggest, she was terminated because of her efforts in behalf of collective bargaining and the Economic Security Program.

"Edna was fired as Director of Nursing at Sonoma County Hospital in a stormy way just before coming to the CNA staff," former CNA Executive Director A. Lionne Conta recalls. "We always felt it was due to her Economic Security Program activities as a Director of Nursing." Behrens herself once ruefully reminded nurses that they must stick together and not expect the director of nursing to do things for them. "She's an employee and can lose her job just like I did." After losing her job at Santa Rosa, Behrens joined the CSNA staff and served as an assistant director and field representative, acting director of the Economic Security Program, and associate executive director and RN consultant to the Economic Security Program until her retirement in 1963.

Behrens' association with CSNA began early in her career. Active at the district level—she was president of both District 9 (San Francisco) and District 15 (Sonoma)—she won her first election to the CSNA board of directors in 1937 and remained on the board until she was elected CSNA president in 1943. Behrens served six years as president, the maximum term allowed, and was then reelected to the board in 1949. Her electoral successes, including an unprecedented landslide victory in her third presidential election, re-

flect her widespread popularity among California's nurses. She was recognized as someone who understood and cared about nurses and worked well with them. Behrens enjoyed the respect and admiration of her colleagues throughout her life: the high regard in which she was held made her an especially effective advocate of CSNA's collective bargaining and Economic Security programs.

Behrens's years as a CSNA board member and president were years in which the organization was working to improve wages and practice conditions for nurses—and patient care as well—by developing, promulgating, and seeking hospital acceptance of minimum employment standards for nurses. The need for such standards became acute after the United States entered World War II: hospital practice conditions deteriorated rapidly as staff left for military service for more lucrative civilian employment; nurses' salaries, at the same time, failed to keep pace with wartime inflation. When the California Hospital Association refused to accept CSNA's proposed standards in 1942, the CSNA board, at the suggestion of Executive Director Shirley C. Titus, voted to embrace collective bargaining and seek authorization from the membership to represent them in negotiating their employment conditions.

Behrens strongly supported the board action and was instrumental in securing membership approval of the use of their professional organization in collective bargaining. "Human beings," she once explained, "should have a voice in determining the conditions under which they work." With membership recognition, CSNA made a successful appeal to the War Labor Board in 1943 for a 15 percent increase in nurses' salaries; three years later it negotiated its first contracts, signed by President Edna Behrens. That same year the American Nurses' Association at its 1946 Biennial Convention endorsed "greater development of nurses' professional associations as exclusive spokesmen for nurses in all questions affecting their employment and economic security."

Acceptance of collective bargaining by nurses, and by ANA, did not come about easily. There were continuing struggles within and outside CSNA: some nurses believed the tactic was "unprofessional," and others objected to the centralization of authority in the board and executive director that accompanied the expansion of collective bargaining activity. ANA was also initially unsympathetic: in 1944 it sought to compromise CSNA's collective bargaining activity through by-law revisions. Behrens's commitment did not waver throughout; she traveled with Titus to CSNA district meetings and ANA national meetings to explain the program and its importance to nurses and the future of the profession.

Behrens displayed the same stalwart spirit in CSNA contract negotiations with hospitals, which, it should be added, became increasingly difficult after the Taft-Hartley Act exempted nonprofit hospitals from the provisions of the National Labor Relations Act in 1947. "Continuous, intensive, and at times single-minded effort has been required to bring about an effective implementation of this program," Behrens reminded delegates to CSNA's 1948 Annual Convention. Colleagues who worked with Behrens in her years as a CSNA staff member report that she went through "hundreds and hundreds of *agonizing* negotiating sessions without losing her drive and faith." All of her negotiating was done, furthermore, before CSNA abrogated the no-strike pledge it had taken when it commenced collective bargaining.

Absent the strike weapon, Behrens employed a variety of strategies, including "concerted action," or the threat of mass resignations by nurses, in attempts to secure CSNA recognition by hospitals and improved wages and personnel practices. Concerted action did not always work—at Sutter Hospital in Sacramento in 1951–52, for example, threatened nurse resignations, which came after an unsuccessful ten month struggle to persuade the hospital to negotiate with CSNA, failed to produce either CSNA recognition or a contract, although the hospital eventually increased wages. Undaunted, Behrens continued the struggle for nurses' economic security: "I guess I've always been a fighter, haven't I?," she observed in 1976.

Behrens's fighting qualities and her ability and persistence as a negotiator were sometimes acknowledged by hospital administrators. In 1953 a hospital spokesman admitted that the CSNA negotiating team, with Behrens on it, was the "sharpest" yet mounted by the organization. There was ample testimony to her skill and verve from CSNA associates as well. Perhaps the most widely recounted incident concerns Behrens's representation of a group of nurses employed by San Luis Obispo County Hospital.

On this occasion Behrens flew from Northern California to speak before the San Luis Obispo County Board of Supervisors in behalf of a recommended pay increase for the nurses. Her small plane landed in a hayfield, and she was rushed to the supervisors' meeting where she learned that she must produce evidence of the nurses' support for the pay increase. Assured that the increase would be approved if she secured the signatures of all the nurses involved, Behrens spent the next two days in the linen closet of the county hospital collecting them one by one! The nurses got their raise.

Increases in nurses' wages were important to Behrens; she pledged not to quit her work with CSNA, in fact, "until nurses are earning $400 a month." Nurses in California achieved that salary by 1963, the year in which Behrens retired. By then, thanks to collective bargaining by their professional organization, nurses had achieved much more besides, e.g., the 40-hour week (1947); statewide fees for private-duty nurses; overtime, on-call, and call-back pay; shift differentials; tenure increases; paid vacation and sick leave; health insurance; retirement plans; and hospital-based professional performance committees. The improvements in nurses' personnel policies and practice conditions were historic and would not have been possible without the work of Edna Behrens, which, *California Nurse* observed in its obituary for her, "is part of the history of nursing in California and the nation."

In 1941, shortly before she and CSNA began to make nursing history, Edna Behrens described for CSNA's *Pacific*

Coast Journal of Nursing the kind of leaders and attitudes she believed contemporary nursing and its associations required. It is by far the best description of Behrens herself one could hope to find.

"You know," she reminded her readers, "we too frequently elect officers because of their charm and personality. What we need now is not charm but achievement, not personality but perseverance, not glamor but gumption." Give us governing boards, she continued, that are "hardworking," "progressive," "open and eager for new ideas," "willing to try innovation." And let them, she concluded, be characterized by "originality, vision, and courage."

Edna Behrens spent her retirement years at her home in Mill Valley, California. She enjoyed gardening: "50 years of unwavering tending and composting," a visitor commented, had produced a "lush, expansive flower garden that miraculously bursts out of the rocky mountainside." She died on June 9, 1990, at Hillhaven Convalescent Center in Mill Valley.

PUBLICATIONS BY EDNA BEHRENS

"Effective Board Meetings, New Problems: New Answers." *Pacific Coast Journal of Nursing* 37 (October 1941): 592–93.

"Edna Behrens, Past President, CNA, Sketches a History of Nursing Legislation in California." *CNA Bulletin* 59 (March 1963): 12–19.

BIBLIOGRAPHY

Draft Manuscript of CNA Region 9's nomination of Edna Behrens for the ANA Shirley Titus Award, n.d.

"Early Strategist Never Took 'No' for an Answer." *California Nurse* 86 (July/August 1990): 3.

"Edna H. Behrens, National Award-Winning Nurse." Obituary. *Independent Journal* (San Rafael, Calif.), June 12, 1990.

"Marin Nurse Takes National Honor." *Nurses' Notes, Newsletter of the North Bay Coastal Region 9, CNA* III (June 1976).

Mason, R.S. "Aspects of Collective Bargaining with the California State Nurses' Association with Emphasis on the East Bay." Research paper, May 15, 1953. California Nurses' Association Archives, San Francisco.

"Meet Edna Behrens." *CNA Bulletin* 57 (December 1961): 198–99.

Minutes of the meetings of the Board of Directors of the California State Nurses' Association, 1937–49, 1951–52, *passim.* California Nurses' Association Archives, San Francisco.

"Report of the President to the House of Delegates, Forty-Third Annual Convention, CSNA." *Bulletin of the California State Nurses' Association* 44 (November 1948): 336–37.

"Resolution of Appreciation to Edna H. Behrens." *Bulletin of the California State Nurses' Association* 46 (January 1950): 11.

Judith Stanley

Eleanor Robson Belmont
1879–1979

Although better known as the mother of New York's Metropolitan Opera Guild, Eleanor Robson Belmont had enough careers in her long life for four women. Renowned actress, millionaire's wife, and opera doyenne, she devoted more than 30 years to the American Red Cross as a fund raiser and administrator.

Eleanor Elise Robson Belmont was born in Wigan, Lancashire, England, on December 13, 1879, the only child of Madge Carr Robson and Charles Robson. Both her mother and grandmother, Evelyn Cameron, were well-known English actresses, and her father, who died shortly after her birth, was an orchestra conductor. Her stepfather, Augustus Cook, was also an actor. In 1886, at the age of 7, Eleanor Robson was brought to the United States and attended St. Peter's Academy, Staten Island, New York. Upon graduation she joined her mother and stepfather in San Francisco, and began acting in small parts with her mother's company. The role of Bonita Canby in Augustus Thomas's play *Arizona* provided her first success, followed in 1903 by *Merely Mary Ann*, dramatized by Israel Zangwill, a play that catapulted her to fame. Eleanor Robson was so well known that George Bernard Shaw wrote his play *Major Barbara* for her, although she never performed in it. On February 26, 1910, Miss Robson, 30, married the millionaire August Belmont, 57, banker, founder of the Rapid Transit Subway Construction Co., New York, owner of Belmont Racing Stables, and retired from the stage. As Mrs. Belmont, she devoted the rest of her life to philanthropic and charitable activities.

Although a participant in the social milieu of the elite of New York, Belmont, with the wealth, prestige, and leisure to promote social welfare causes, became personally involved in the successful operation of them, supporting them not only with her name and money, but also with her time. Fortunately, she displayed energetic and formidable administrative abilities. She founded the Society for the Prevention of Useless Giving in order to direct money from contributors toward worthy causes. She organized a benefit for Belgian Relief in the early days of World War I. Upon the entrance of the United States into the war in 1917, President Woodrow Wilson formed the War Council to direct the operations of the American Red Cross, with Henry P. Davison as chairman of the council. The Red Cross established a goal of raising $100 million in 1917, and Mrs. E.H. Harriman, who headed the New York team, asked Eleanor Belmont to assist in the fund raising. In the first three months of the war, Belmont made 45 speeches in 38 cities. With her commanding stage presence and beautiful voice, she energized audiences and inspired them to contribute toward the final total of $114 million. So successful were her speeches that a Red Cross official described just one of them as "worth $500,000." Indeed, Pierre du Pont challenged the Wilmington, Delaware, community to double its quota of $500,000 to thank Eleanor Belmont for her address. The community raised $2,155,000.

Traveling to Europe in the fall of 1917 to inspect U.S. Army camps for the Red Cross, Belmont carried a letter of introduction from former President Theodore Roosevelt, which read that she had "a man's understanding, a woman's sympathy, and a sense of honor and gift of expression such as are expressed by very, very few, either among men or women." While in England, she visited military hospitals and greatly admired the British Volunteer Aid Detachment (VAD). She recommended to Surgeon General Bradley of the American Expeditionary Forces that American nurses be allowed nearer the front lines, and that the U.S. Army make use of available Red Cross hospital supplies rather than waiting for its own supplies.

Upon her return to the United States in February 1918, Belmont was appointed an assistant to the War Council, ostensibly "to represent the woman's point of view," on August 21, 1918. She concerned herself with Red Cross programs devoted to women in general, but most particularly with nurses. She is credited with creating the Home Service, which, combined with the Department of Military Relief, served American troops in training camps, on active duty overseas, and with their families. She participated in the founding of the Junior Red Cross, the design of Red Cross service badges and medals, the founding of a Red Cross museum whose curator was Irene Givenwilson, and supported the development of the League of Red Cross societies. She served on a committee of the War Council whose purpose was to discuss the future of the Red Cross after the war. Well-known to Red Cross workers across the country due to her fund-raising speeches, she was appointed to a subcommittee to ascertain the opinions of Red Cross workers regarding the future of the organization. The survey of the chapters resulted in recommendations for a peacetime program that provided services to veterans, public-health nursing service (supported by Jane Delano), educational activities, first-aid instruction, home care of the sick, and Braille service. Although the War Council had seriously considered disbanding the American Red Cross at the conclusion of the war, it decided to approve the peacetime program.

Elected to the Central Committee of the American Red Cross in 1919, Eleanor Belmont continued to participate in innovative programs and services. She was a signer of the 1920 charter of the Institute for the Crippled and Disabled, which was founded in 1917 as a Red Cross project. She was a member of the Delano Memorial Committee in 1921. Although she was widowed in 1924, she did not cease her philanthropic activities during the years of the Great Depression and World War II. She served as chairwoman of the Nurses' House Committee of the Association for Improving the Condition of the Poor in New York City during the Depression, and from 1931 until 1934 she was chairwoman of the Women's Division of the Emergency Unemployment Relief Commission of New York and was vice-chairwoman of the Community Service Center. She also was a member of the board of directors of the New York City Chapter of the Red Cross.

During this period Belmont maintained contact with the nursing community. She was the commencement speaker at Presbyterian Hospital nursing graduation ceremonies in New York on May 28, 1929. At the 1934 Biennial Convention in Washington, D.C., she delivered an address on the nurse's influence in the community; the *American Journal of Nursing* described her as "a good friend to many nurses." For the anniversary session of the National League of Nursing Education in June 1935, she ghosted a letter from Florence Nightingale to Adelaide Nutting. In the unsettled world situation of 1940, she pointed out to the 500 nurse members of the New York State League of Nursing Education convention in October that they were all potential Red Cross nurses.

The beginning of World War II increased her role in the Red Cross. As chairwoman of the National Council on Red Cross Home Nursing, Belmont led recruitment drives for nurses, giving teas at her home on Fifth Avenue to recruit student nurses from New York area nursing schools. In 1943 she resigned from the Red Cross's Central Committee after 25 years of service, remaining as an honorary member; in October 1944 she was elected to the board of directors of the New York City chapter of the Red Cross.

Belmont's years of service did not go unrecognized. She was the first woman to deliver the commencement address at New York University on June 7, 1933, and received a doctor of letters. She also received honorary degrees from the University of Rochester in 1934 for relief activities as well as from Moravian Seminary and College for Women (1936), Yale University (1948), and Columbia University (1950). The Red Cross in 1934 awarded her a gold medal for service. That same year the National Institute of Social Sciences awarded her a gold medal for her social work activities, and in her acceptance speech she advocated the adoption of federal unemployment insurance. On April 12, 1936, she received a medal for outstanding civil service from New York's One Hundred Year Association, the first woman so honored, because of "far-reaching contributions to the theater, to music, and to the cultural life of the city . . . [and] . . . for distinction as a Red Cross executive in this country and abroad." The American Woman's Association voted her its annual achievement award for "stage, in the fields of opera, social work, and philanthropy" in November 1940. She received the Roosevelt Medal for distinguished public service in October 1943, and on May 8, 1956, the American Red Cross presented her with a Distinguished Service citation for 40 years of service.

Eleanor Belmont died in her sleep on October 24, 1979, at her home in New York City. She was 100 years old.

Belmont was an extraordinary woman. Her activities with the Red Cross, significant as they were, represented only a small portion of her life's work. She is best known as the woman who almost singlehandedly saved the New York Metropolitan Opera from extinction through the unceasing and creative efforts of the Opera Guild. Her contemporaries described her as forthright, dogged, with a brilliant mind for organization and administration, coupled with an understanding of human relations and awesome powers of persuasion. Although never a nurse, she strove to provide nursing services to needy Americans through the auspices of the Red Cross.

PUBLICATIONS BY ELEANOR ROBSON BELMONT

BOOKS

The Fabric of Memory. New York: Farrar, Straus and Cudahy, 1957.

ARTICLES

"American Nurses Lead the World in Healing Its War-Worn Races." *New York Times*, April 22, 1923, VII, 14, col. 1.

"The Nurse as Interpreter of the Hospital to the Community." *American Journal of Nursing* 34 (June 1934): 611.

"'Letter' from Florence Nightingale to Adelaide Nutting, presented for the National League of Nursing Education Convention, New York, June 3–8, 1935, Anniversary Session." *American Journal of Nursing* 35 (July 1935): 680.

BIBLIOGRAPHY

"Belmont, Mrs. August." In *Current Biography, 1944*. New York: Wilson, 1945.

"Belmont Nurses." *Trained Nurse and Hospital Review* 88 (June, 1932): 748–49.

Birmingham, S. *The Grandes Dames*. New York: Simon & Schuster, 1982.

Coleman, E. "Woman Behind the Met." *New York Times Magazine*, December 18, 1960, 20.

Dock, L., et al. *History of American Red Cross Nursing*. American National Red Cross Nursing Service. New York: Macmillan, 1922.

"Eleanor Robson Belmont." Obituary. *New York Times Biographical Service*. New York: Arno Press, 1979.

Kolodin, I. "Mother of the Met Family." *Saturday Review* 39 (October 27, 1956): 33–35.

Lovett, L.D. "A Word of Gratitude." *Opera News* 43 (December 9, 1978): 31.

Merkling, F. "The Grand Manner." *Opera News* 43 (December 9, 1978): 23–30.

"Mrs. Belmont Honored." *New York Times*, May 9, 1956, 30, col. 3.

Pennock, M.R., ed. *Makers of Nursing History*. New York: Lakeside, 1940.

Woolf, S.J. "From the Stage to the Drama of Life." *New York Times Magazine*, November 29, 1931, 9.

Woolf, S.J. "A Medal for an Outstanding Role." *New York Times Magazine*. October 24, 1943, 13.

Kathleen F. Cohen

Jeanne Saylor Berthold

1924–1983

Jeanne Saylor Berthold was a highly respected educator, nurse, and administrator. During her career she earned three degrees from the University of California at Berkeley (a B.S. in 1953, an M.S. in psychiatric nursing in 1955, and a Ph.D. in counseling psychology in 1961), and she worked her way from positions of health-staff nurse and public-school nurse in Los Angeles to director of nursing research and education at Downey's Rancho Los Amigos Hospital in Downey, California.

Berthold was born on June 4, 1924, She decided early in life on a nursing career, holding her first nursing position at age 21. Within two years she became staff assistant and evening supervisor at Sonoma County Hospital in Santa Rosa, California, and she remained there from 1947 to 1951. From Santa Rosa she moved to San Francisco, where she worked as a psychiatric nurse at Langeley Porter Neuropsychiatric Institute while also completing her master's work in psychiatric nursing. After receiving that degree in 1955, Berthold began a career as an educator and became an instructor at the School of Nursing, University of California Medical Center in San Francisco. An accomplished and effective teacher, she moved to the Francis Payne Bolton School of Nursing at Case Western Reserve University in Cleveland in 1961 and rose through the academic ranks from assistant professor to full professor—the position she held when she left Case Western in 1971.

After teaching for 16 years, Berthold essentially began her third career. While maintaining her ties to academe (she was adjutant professor in the University of Colorado School of Nursing), she became principal investigator and program director of the Western Interstate Commission for Higher Education. During the last decade of her life Berthold won wide acclaim for her work in nursing research while directing nursing education and research at Downey's Rancho Amigos Hospital in Downey, California.

Berthold published extensively in nursing and educational journals. As her reputation grew she became a research consultant for the McGraw-Hill Book Company and for the Veterans' Administration and served as an educational consultant for the National Commission for the Study of Nursing. She chaired the American Nurses Association Commission on Nursing Research from 1970 to 1975, served as president of the American Nurses Foundation from 1969 to 1971, and also chaired the *Nursing Research* editorial board from 1972 to 1973. She held memberships in numerous professional societies.

Berthold died of cancer at the age of 59 in Downey, California, on July 6, 1983.

PUBLICATIONS BY JEANNE SAYLOR BERTHOLD

Creating a Climate for Educational Technology in Nursing. Cleveland, Ohio: Case Western University, Frances Payne Bolton School of Nursing, 1971.

Educational Technology and the Teaching-Learning Process; A Selected Bibliography. Washington, D.C.: U.S. Department of Health, Education, and Welfare, 1968.

Human Rights Guidelines for Nurses in Clinical and other Research. Kansas City, Mo: American Nurses' Association, 1975.

Nursing Service in a Specialty, a Rural, and an Urban Hospital. New York: National League for Nursing, 1979.

BIBLIOGRAPHY

"Berthold, Jeanne Saylor." *American Men and Women of Science,* 12th ed. *Social and Behavioral Science.* Vol. 1. New York: Cattel Press, 1973.

"Berthold, Jeanne Saylor." *Who's Who of American Women, 1977–1978.* Chicago: Marquis, 1978.

"Berthold, Jeanne Saylor." *Who's Who in the West, 1978–1979.* Chicago: Marquis, 1978.

"Jeanne Saylor Berthold." Obituary. *American Journal of Nursing* 83 (October 1983): 1490.

David Carson

Ella Best

1892–1991

Executive secretary of the American Nurses' Association, Ella Best served the organization in various capacities for 28 years, and her leadership was in large measure responsible for the progress of the association during that period.

Best was born in Williamsfields, Illinois, on November 2, 1892, the daughter of John and Anna Carolyn (Millen) Best. She graduated from St. Luke's Hospital School of Nursing in Chicago in 1915 and did postgraduate work at Teachers College, Columbia University and at the University of Chicago. After completing her training, she taught nursing and served as administrator at a number of schools, including her alma mater, until 1930 when she became field secretary for the American Nurses Association and secretary of the important Registry Committee. As secretary, she worked on a revision of the minimum standards for professional sponsored registries for the purpose of coordinating the nursing needs of entire communities with other agencies. In 1935 she became associate director of the ANA after having served as acting director since 1933, and in 1946 she was appointed executive secretary.

When Best retired on June 15, 1958, she could look back upon a period of great progress for the ANA. In 1930 headquarters had a professional and clerical staff of 10, and the association numbered about 84,000 members. By 1958 there were close to 200,000 members, and headquarters consisted of eight sections with a combined staff of 100, each representing a major field of nursing. Best viewed research, economic security, and legislation, as well as relationships with allied professions and the general public as major activities of the ANA. The structure and programs of the organization as developed under Best's leadership during those years have been recognized as fundamental to the development of the nursing profession in the United States.

Between 1948 and 1958 the ANA expanded its international relations. In her capacity as executive secretary, Best participated in meetings with the Board of Directors of the International Council of Nurses, serving as chair of the Public Relations Committee and traveling to conferences in Rio de Janeiro, Rome, and Stockholm. She was also a participant at the first postwar meeting of the International Hospital Federation Congress in the Netherlands in 1949. The ANA supported the United Nations actively and was granted observer status with the objective of furthering peaceful and healthful conditions. In addition, Best acted as consultant to the surgeon general of the United States Air Force and as civilian consultant to the Army Nurse Corps. Energetic and efficient, she guided the ANA with objectivity, sensitivity, fairness, and vision.

A member of the Illinois State Nurses Association, Best served as president of the first district from 1927 to 1930. After her retirement she moved to Florida, where she maintained an active interest in the ANA, served as secretary for the Audubon Society, and taught Sunday school. She died in 1991. An account by Pearl McIver published on the occasion of Best's retirement in the *American Journal of Nursing* captures her absorbing interest in birds.

PUBLICATIONS BY ELLA BEST

ARTICLES

"A Summer Course in the Oxford of the West." *American Journal of Nursing* 26 (February 1926): 129.

"Nursing Service—How to Balance Supply and Demand?" *Modern Hospital* 39 (August 1932): 97–102.

"The American Nurses' Association Economic Security Program." *Hospital Management* 84 (July 1957): 28–30.

"The International Council of Nurses." *Nursing Outlook* 5 (August 1957): 457.

"ICN Congress: Public Relations." *International Nursing Review* 8 (July–August 1961): 32.

PAMPHLETS

The Use of the Graduate Nurse on a Staff Basis. New York: American Nurses' Association, 1931. 25pp.

Survey of Nursing Facilities in California. San Francisco: California State Nurses' Association, 1934. 30pp.

Brief Historical Review and Information About Current Activities of the A.N.A. New York: American Nurses' Association, 1940. 88p.

BIBLIOGRAPHY

"Addition to Staff." *American Journal of Nursing* 30 (August 1930): 1077.

"A.N.A. Field Secretary Chosen." *Pacific Coast Journal of Nursing* 27 (January 1931): 33.

"Best, Ella." *Who's Who of American Women, 1958–59.* Chicago: Marquis, 1959.

Bridges, D.C. *A History of the International Council of Nurses 1899–1964. The First Sixty-five Years.* London: Pitman Medical, 1967.

"Ella Best, R.N." Death Notice. *American Nurse* 23 (March 1991): 28.

Flanagan, L. *One Strong Voice. The Story of the American Nurses' Association.* Kansas City: American Nurses' Association, 1976.

McIver, P. "A Job Well Done." *American Journal of Nursing* 58 (July 1958): 965.

Roberts, M.M. *American Nursing. History and Interpretation.* New York: Macmillan, 1954.

Lilli Sentz

Josephine Beatrice Bowman
1881–1971

Josephine Beatrice Bowman was the third superintendent of the United States Navy Nurse Corps, serving from 1922 until 1934. She was recognized widely for her administrative skills and her efforts to encourage nurses to continue their education.

Bowman was born in Des Moines, Iowa, on December 19, 1881. Seafaring, military service, and medical practice had been traditional occupations in her family. She attended public schools in Des Moines and did her nurse's training at the Medico-Chirurgical Hospital Training School for Nurses in Philadelphia, graduating in 1904.

She enrolled in the American Red Cross Nursing Service, and in the spring of 1908 she assisted in the first Red Cross disaster relief effort that followed a tornado in Hattiesburg, Mississippi. In the fall of that year she was one of 20 members of the first class to pass the rigorous examinations for the Navy Nurse Corps.

Bowman became one of the first 20 nurses named to the new Navy Nurse Corps on October 3, 1908. She was promoted to the rank of chief nurse, effective February 23, 1911.

On October 31, 1914, she was granted a leave to join the nursing unit on the S.S. *Red Cross*, a medical relief ship dubbed the "Mercy Ship" by President Woodrow Wilson. She first served as supervising nurse of Unit D at the Hassler Royal Naval Hospital near Portsmouth, England. After six weeks, she was named general night matron of Unit F at Paignton.

She returned to the Navy Nurse Corps on May 7, 1915, and was named chief nurse on May 10. On duty in the Orient when the United States entered World War I in 1917, she was recalled to become chief nurse of the U.S. Naval Hospital in Great Lakes, Illinois. The post called for extraordinary executive and nursing skills because the hospital had grown suddenly from 100 to 2,800 beds. In 1918 she also provided nurses for an additional 1,000 beds in a nearby detention camp that had been converted to serve during the influenza epidemic. Although the day-to-day pressures were heavy, Bowman encouraged professional excellence among her nurses by offering them special postgraduate courses. Her handling of her myriad responsibilities during this period brought her lasting recognition and respect.

Bowman entered upon a unique adventure in nursing on August 5, 1920, when she was named chief nurse on the U.S.S. *Relief*, a newly commissioned navy hospital ship. The idea of assigning women to regular sea duty was new and controversial, but the performance of navy nurses on transports during the war emergency encouraged the trial effort. Nurses have been serving on navy hospital ships ever since.

On the recommendation of Surgeon General E.R. Stitt, Bowman was appointed superintendent of the Navy Nurse Corps on December 1, 1922. During her tenure, she drew further praise by appointing regional supervisors who would have a better understanding of local needs. She also established postgraduate courses for specially selected navy nurses.

While serving as navy superintendent, she held several posts in professional organizations. She was a member of the National Committee on the American Red Cross Nursing Service, the advisory committee of nurses to the medical director and the Medical Council of the U.S. Veterans' Bureau, the American Public Health Association, and the American Association for the Advancement of Science. She was chairperson of the government section of the American Nurses' Association from 1930–32 and president of the Graduate Nurses' Association of the District of Columbia from 1931–34. In April 1934 she was a member of the central arrangements committee for the convention of the American Nurses' Association in Washington, D.C.

She retired from the navy effective January 1, 1935, and was succeeded as superintendent of nurses by Myn M. Hoffman. She made her retirement home in Hanover, Pennsylvania, and died at the Golden Age Home there on January 3, 1971.

PUBLICATIONS BY JOSEPHINE BEATRICE BOWMAN

"The History and Development of the Navy Nurse Corps." *American Journal of Nursing* 25 (May 1925): 356–60.

"Disability Bill for Army and Navy Nurses." *American Journal of Nursing* 30 (August 1930): 1016.

BIBLIOGRAPHY

"Josephine Beatrice Bowman." Undated biographical typescript. U.S. Navy Historical Center.

"News, Mainly About People." *American Journal of Nursing* 35 (February 1935): 185.

Pennock, M.R., ed. *Makers of Nursing History.* New York: Lakeside, 1940.

Report of Casualty, March 22, 1971, U.S. Navy Historical Center, Washington, D.C.

"Who's Who in the Nursing World." *American Journal of Nursing* 24 (November 1924): 1122.

Alice P. Stein

Rena E. Boyle

b. 1914

Rena E. Boyle influenced nursing education both regionally and nationally. Through her role as a teacher at the University of Minnesota, as a consultant and administrator in the United States Public Health Service and at the National League for Nursing, she was an outstanding educator and leader in nursing. She later served as dean at the University of Nebraska, where the innovative programs developed under her leadership were accorded national recognition.

Boyle was born on September 9, 1914, in Chicago, the daughter of Thompson S. and Claire Rena (Green) Boyle. Although always desirous of being a teacher, she was unable to afford college and instead enrolled in the Methodist Hospital School of Nursing in Peoria, Illinois, from which she received a diploma in 1938. She earned a B.S. in nursing in 1941, an M.A. in educational psychology in 1946, and a Ph.D. in higher education in 1953 from the University of Minnesota. While pursuing her advanced degrees, she first served as instructor and later as associate professor and director of student teaching in nursing at the University of Minnesota, thus combining her interests in teaching and nursing.

From 1954 to 1956 Boyle was a consultant with the International Cooperative Administration (ICA) in Haiti and Guatemala. She later was consultant to the University of Panama, where she assisted with the establishment of a baccalaureate program in nursing.

In 1956 she was appointed chief of the newly created Nursing Research and Consultant Branch of the Division of Nursing of the United States Public Health Service. Four years later she became director of the Department of Baccalaureate and Higher Degree Programs at the National League for Nursing. During this period she also served as consultant to various collegiate programs and to the surgeon general of the army. In 1957 she left the league to become dean at the University of Nebraska and pursue her long-term interests with students and faculty.

During her tenure as dean, Boyle was instrumental in effecting various changes within the university structure. The School of Nursing became an autonomous college in 1968, and student enrollment increased from 79 in 1967 to 722 in 1979.

A master's program was developed, and students were admitted in the fall of 1969. In the fall of 1971 students entered the newly developed associate degree program, the only such program in Nebraska. Still something was lacking since each of the three programs was complete in itself. After major curriculum changes the associate, baccalaureate, and master programs were articulated into a career ladder and qualified students could move from one to the other without loss of time or credit. Responding to the statewide demand for collegiate programs, the College of Nursing extended its associate and baccalaureate programs to Lincoln and still later offered off-campus programs in nursing to enable registered nurses to continue working while earning their baccalaureate degrees in nursing.

Boyle is the author of numerous articles on nursing education, nursing research, and the preparation of teachers. Her honors include the Outstanding Achievement Awards from the University of Minnesota in 1959, the Nebraska Nurses' Association in 1978, and the National League for Nursing in 1979. Also in 1979 she received the Mary Adelaide Nutting Award, the highest award given by the National League for Nursing.

Upon her retirement in July 1979, Boyle was named professor emerita. She moved to Mesa, Arizona, and since then has been active as a consultant in nursing education and a volunteer in community services and in church-related activities. On May 25, 1980, she was honored with the Distinguished Service to Nursing Award from the University of Nebraska College of Nursing and in June 1987 received an honorary doctor of science from the University of Nebraska for her legacy of innovation.

PUBLICATIONS BY RENA E. BOYLE

BOOK

Selected Writings of Rena E. Boyle. Omaha: University of Nebraska, 1987.

ARTICLES AND REPORTS

"A Study of Programs of Professional Education for Teachers of Nursing in Nineteen Selected

Universities." *Nursing Research* 2 (February 1954): 100–25.

With G.M. Inlow. "Common Problems in the Preparation of Nursing and Public School Teachers." *Educational Administration and Supervision* 41 (March 1955): 142–53.

"How Well Do We Know the Patients We Know Best?" *American Journal of Nursing* 58 (November 1958): 1540–543.

"A Study of Student Nurse Perception of Patient Attitudes." Public Health Service Publication No. 769. Washington, D.C.: U.S.G.P.O., 1960.

"Introduction to Areas and Methods of Research in Nursing." *Report of an International Seminar on Research in Nursing*, Florence Nightingale Foundation, International Council of Nurses, London, 1960.

"Evaluating and Writing the Research Proposal." *Report of an International Seminar on Research in Nursing*, Florence Nightingale Foundation, International Council of Nurses, London, 1960.

"The International Seminar in Delhi." *Nursing Research* 9 (Fall 1960): 196–97.

"The Hospital Setting and Nursing Research." *Pennsylvania Nurse* 16 (April 1961): 20–26; (May 1961): 8–13.

"Critical Issues in Collegiate Education in Nursing." *Nursing Outlook* 10 (March 1962): 165–67.

With F.K. Peterson. "The Registered Nurse Seeks a College." *Nursing Outlook* 10 (October 1962): 652–54.

"Implications of Study of Current Status of Baccalaureate Programs for Registered Nurse Students." Report of the Council of Member Agencies of the Department of Baccalaureate and Higher Degree Programs of the National League for Nursing, November 1962, pp. 74–77.

"Federal Legislation: Its Impact on NLN's Accrediting Programs." *Nursing Outlook* 13 (March 1965): 34–39.

"National Health Insurance: Implications for Nursing." Challenge to Nursing Education, NLN Council of Member Agencies Report, November 1971.

"Articulation from Associate Degree Through Masters." *Nursing Outlook* 20 (October 1972): 670–72.

BIBLIOGRAPHY

Boyle, R.E. Interview with the author. March 1989.

"Boyle, Rena E." *Who's Who of American Women.* Chicago: Marquis, 1966, 1970, 1972.

"Dr. Boyle to Head Research Branch." *Nursing Research* 8 (Summer 1959): 180–81.

Rena E. Boyle Honorary Doctor of Science Degree. Citation. University of Nebraska Medical Center, College of Nursing and Alumni Association, June 13, 1987.

Schneckloth, N.W. *The University of Nebraska College of Nursing 1917–1987.* Omaha: University of Nebraska Medical Center, 1987.

Yeaworth, R.C. Interview with the author. February 1989.

Lilli Sentz

Annie M. Brainard

1864–1942

Founding member of the Visiting Nurse Association in Cleveland and editor of the *Visiting Nurse Quarterly of Cleveland* from 1911 to 1923, Annie Maria Brainard was a leader in public-health nursing and the author of an influential textbook on the subject.

Brainard was born on March 14, 1864, the daughter of Silas and Emily C. (Mold) Brainard. Her father, an early Cleveland settler, was a piano dealer and music publisher who was said to be the owner of the first piano store west of the Allegheny Mountains. Her mother was one of the original members of the Trinity Episcopal Church in Cleveland.

Nothing is known about Brainard's education and training, except that she had traveled widely. In 1904 Brainard became a member of the Board of Trustees of the Cleveland Visiting Nurse Association under the tutelage of Isabel Hampton Robb and Mathilda L. Johnson. Nine years later she was elected president of the association.

In January 1909 the trustees decided to issue a quarterly report to bring associate members in closer contact with the work of the public-health nurses; shortly thereafter the first issue of the *Visiting Nurse Quarterly* was published with Brainard as editor and Isabel Wetmore Lowman as associate editor. Before long the subscription list included individuals from the entire country, and when the National Organization for Public Health Nursing was founded in 1912, the *Quarterly* was accepted as its official organ and the name changed to the *Public Health Nurse Quarterly*. In 1918 it became a monthly publication, the *Public Health Nurse*. The journal continued to be published in Cleveland until 1923, when Brainard retired as editor, and it was turned over to the national organization office in New York City.

Interested in nursing education, Brainard became lecturer on the administration of public-health nursing at Western Reserve University in 1916 and continued on the faculty until 1926. When the University School of Nursing was established in 1923, she became a member of the Advisory Committee, an office she held until her death, and she also served on the Committee on Nursing Education at Flora Stone Mather College. She was a member of the original Board of Governors of the Nursing Center, an organization devoted to the centralization of nursing efforts throughout the city.

A prolific author, Brainard's book *The Evolution of Public Health Nursing* published in 1922 traced the development of organized visiting of the sick in their homes since the Christian era. The book was reprinted by Garland Publishing in 1985.

Brainard had a long association with St. Barnabas Guild, one of the oldest nursing organizations in the country and founded the Opportunity Shop, which raised scholarship funds for the guild. This organization concerned with linking the nursing profession to its foundation in the early Christian church brought missionary nurses from many parts of the world to Cleveland for training. Like her mother, Brainard was a member of Trinity Episcopal Cathedral and was active in the woman's auxiliary, serving as president.

Highly respected for her leadership qualities and sense of fairness, Brainard influenced the growth of public-health nursing not only in Cleveland, but throughout the country. She died suddenly from a cerebral hemorrhage on April 4, 1942, at the age of 79 in Cleveland.

PUBLICATIONS BY ANNIE M. BRAINARD

BOOKS

Organization of Public Health Nursing. New York: Macmillan, 1919.

The Evolution of Public Health Nursing. Philadelphia: Saunders, 1911; New York: Garland, rept. 1985.

ARTICLES

Editorials. *The Visiting Nurse Quarterly* 1909–23.

"The Extra-Cantonment Zones." *Public Health Nurse Quarterly* 10 (January 1918): 7.

"Why the Visiting Nurse Is a Public Health Nurse." *Public Health Nurse* 11 (July 1919): 448–90.

BIBLIOGRAPHY

"Annie M. Brainard." *Public Health Nursing* 34 (June 1942): 322–4, 9.

"Annie M. Brainard." Obituary. *Cleveland Plain Dealer*, April 5, 1942, 17–A.

Bower, I.M. *Public Health Nursing in Cleveland 1895–1928*. Cleveland: Western Reserve University, 1930.

Fitzpatrick, M.L. *The National Organization for Public Health Nursing, 1912–1952: Development of a Practice Fields*. New York: National League for Nursing, 1975.

Lilli Sentz

Mary Williams Brinton
1895–after 1950

Mary Williams Brinton was a nurse and author whose career was described in her autobiography *My Cap and My Cape*, which was published in 1950. She was not a nursing "leader" in the sense that she was nationally involved in the profession or achieved great renown. Her contribution is her delightful account in her book of nursing and the various experiences she had from the 1920s until shortly after World War II. Brinton's book gives one a feel for the life of an "ordinary" nurse who was bright, articulate, and eager to nurse in a variety of settings.

Brinton was born at home in Bala, Pennsylvania, in 1895. She had one older brother, David Evans Williams, and two younger sisters, Elizabeth Good and Emilie Duval Williams. As a child, Brinton had been impressed by both the family physician, "Dockety" [Dr.] Service, and Miss Daisy, the graduate nurse who was called whenever illness occurred in the family. Brinton, her brother and sisters, and the neighbor children often played nurse and doctor with the toys in the nursery. Her autobiography indicated that she came from a socially prominent family; she attended Miss Irwin's school in Philadelphia and was a debutante. Memorial Hospital in Roxborough, Pennsylvania, had been founded by her Merrick grandparents.

At the time of her debut, Brinton still held to her childhood dream of someday becoming a nurse. She felt that her education at Miss Irwin's had broadened her knowledge but had not prepared her for the role she envisioned for herself. Brinton was traveling abroad with her family when World War I broke out. In England she offered her services as a nurse to the Queen's Needlework Guild. She was told that she could not serve in either England or France without training.

On her return to the United States, Brinton and a friend entered a course for "trained attendants" sponsored by the YWCA. She decided that this was not sufficient preparation and enrolled in the Presbyterian Hospital of Philadelphia training school in 1917. Her mother was supportive of that effort and encouraged her action by writing her a note that said "Mary has chosen the better part." She graduated in 1920.

Brinton's first employment was with the Visiting Nurse Society of Philadelphia. She was then offered an industrial-nursing position at the Philadelphia Electric Company—the first company nurse. She left that job because it had become "humdrum" and the "idealism I had found in other branches of nursing was entirely lacking" (*My Cap and My Cape*, p. 73). Brinton decided to take a position with the Grenfall Mission but first spent six months as a private-duty nurse in Philadelphia.

Graduate nurses had been serving with the Grenfall Mission since 1892. Many were American nurses, some of whom came in the summer and worked without pay. Brinton's experiences with the Grenfall Mission included a stint at the Grenfall Mission Hospital in Battle Harbor, Labrador, and at St. Anthony's Hospital in Newfoundland.

These assignments were a challenge as the nurses not only provided general-nursing care and assisted in surgery, but also "taught the maids their various duties, and sometimes did the cooking" (Nevitt, 1978, p. 71). "Among the health problems . . . were gun-shot wounds . . . hernias, mastoiditis, tubercular glands, beri-beri, pneumonia, and phtisis" (Nevitt, 1978, p. 71).

Brinton, after leaving the Grenfall Mission assignment, traveled in Alaska. She worked for a time at Wrangell, Alaska. She then returned to Philadelphia and took classes in the administration of anesthesia. She also took additional anesthesia training at Memorial Hospital in Roxborough, Pennsylvania. She worked as office nurse and anesthetist for Dr. Piper at the Piper Clinics.

Brinton herself needed surgery for appendicitis and traveled abroad to facilitate a full recovery. During her travels she visited hospitals in England and in Austria. On her return home, she met Clarence Brinton of Philadelphia, whom she married on June 20, 1936.

Brinton retired from nursing after her marriage, but the coming of World War II and the nursing shortage caused her to volunteer her services at a Philadelphia Hospital. She found at that time there were many changes in the profession, but she still believed that "nursing was the better part" (*My Cap and My Cape*, p. 262).

Brinton's autobiography, *My Cap and My Cape*, provided an interesting view of nursing by discussing various opportunities available to nurses between the World Wars. Its informal narrative style and personal perspective give readers the opportunity to visualize nursing's appeal to an adventurous upper-class young woman. The time period covered is an interesting one as it is late enough to see elements of nursing as it exists today but early enough to provide a glimpse of the "quaint" and pioneer period of nursing practice.

PUBLICATION BY MARY WILLIAMS BRINTON

My Cap and My Cape. Philadelphia: Dorrence, 1950.

BIBLIOGRAPHY

Nevitt, J. *White Caps and Black Bands: Nursing in Newfoundland to 1934.* St. John's, Newfoundland: Jesperson, 1978.

Southcott, M. "Nursing in Newfoundland." *Canadian Nurse* 11 (June 1915): 309–13.

Leslie M. Thom

Marion Turner Brockway
1863–1940

Marion Turner Brockway was an early leader in industrial nursing and the first graduate of the Johns Hopkins Hospital Nurses Training School.

Brockway spent her childhood in Mt. Savage, Maryland. As a young adult, she went to Baltimore daily for piano lessons. She first became interested in nursing when she stopped on the way home at the city hospital to read to patients.

On June 5, 1889, she became the first probationer at Johns Hopkins. During her training, she met Dr. Frederick John Brockway, the house physician. They were married in 1891, soon after her graduation, and had two daughters. He died in 1901.

Brockway took a position in social service at the American Museum of Natural History in New York City. From 1908–13 she was executive secretary of the New York office of Stony Wold Sanitarium and then became director of vacation lodgings in New York City. At the outbreak of World War I she was placed in charge of nurses at the Government Debarkation Hospital No 3 in New York City.

From 1919–31 she was an industrial nurse and "housemother" for the Metro-politan Life Insurance Company in New York, which, at the time, had 11,000 employees. She retired from the company with the rank of director of social services.

She was a founder of the Central Club for Nurses, established in New York City in 1916 under the auspices of the YWCA. In 1920 she became the founder and first president of the Industrial Nurses' Club of New York. After it was organized, the National Organization of Public Health Nurses (NOPHN) established a section for industrial nurses, and the National Safety Council set up a committee on industrial nursing in its industrial health section. Brockway was instrumental in organizing the Association of Graduate Nurses of Manhattan and the Bronx.

She also served as a director of the St. Barnabas Guild in New York, which was the first organization for nurses, president of the New York State Federation of Business and Professional Women's Clubs, president of the New York State Organization for Public Health Nursing, and president of the Zonta Club.

She died suddenly of a stroke on June 2, 1940, at the home of a friend in Baltimore.

BIBLIOGRAPHY

"Industrial Nurses Honor Mrs. Brockway." *Trained Nurse and Hospital Review* 84 (March 1930): 414.

"Mrs. Frederick Brockway." Obituary. *New York Times,* June 4, 1940.

"Mrs. Marion Turner Brockway." Obituary. *American Journal of Nursing* 40 (July 1940): 845.

Pennock, M.R., ed. *Makers of Nursing History.* New York: Lakeside, 1940.

Alice P. Stein

Brother Sebastian Brogan
1883–?

Brother Sebastian Brogan served as director of the Alexian Brothers School of Nurses from 1924–29. As director, he helped reorganize the School of Nurses, and his progressive changes in the nursing curriculum led to the school's accreditation in 1932 by the Illinois Department of Registration and Education. He staunchly believed the future of nursing depended on the quality of education.

Brother Sebastian was born on December 9, 1883, in Newark, New Jersey. Prior to joining the Alexian Brothers, he was a brother of the Christian Schools in Baltimore, from 1897–1914. He became an Alexian Brother on December 12, 1919, and took his last vows on March 3, 1927. He served in Chicago, and St. Louis before leaving the order on May 2, 1930.

Brother Sebastian began his nursing education in 1920. In his diary Brother Sebastian describes the School of Nurses before 1920 as being "a name only for many years. The lectures were given haphazardly, once a week, and mostly attended, not for enlightenment, but out of curiosity." In 1920 a brother would study nursing procedures, taught by a Dr. Klein, and nursing ethics, taught by a Dr. Murphy. These courses were complemented by the brother's daily duties in the hospital, but the nursing program was not state certified. However, when Brother Sebastian became the director in 1924, getting the students certified as registered nurses became the focus. In 1925, after a thorough tour of the Alexian Brother's nursing facility, the state Board of Nurses agreed to let the graduates sit for the State Board Examination. Brother Sebastian took the state board examination in May, 1925 and passed. He then taught nursing courses while serving as director until 1929.

Brother Sebastian was dedicated and proud of the Alexian Brothers' efforts to care for the sick and poor. He kept a detailed diary of all the meetings and activities of the nursing school. This diary begins with a brief history of the Alexian order and recounts how the brotherhood built hospitals by soliciting help from the best physicians and not being afraid to face change.

This progressive spirit is one Brother Sebastian brought to the School of Nurses.

Many laymen felt one only needed a general education in order to be a nurse, but Brother Sebastian felt this view was not only dated but "reprehensible." Physicians in America and Europe agreed that trained nurses were indispensable but, as with all newly formed professions, the public was slow to see the need. This may be one reason why Brother Sebastian was reticent about allowing laymen to enroll in the School of Nurses. The nursing profession needed dedicated men devoted to caring for the sick and genuinely interested in medicine. The nursing program needed time to grow and the brothers' patience was important to the growth of the Alexian Brothers School of Nurses and to the nursing profession. Still, this process was not without its problems. Hard feelings were voiced by the brothers and laymen about the nursing program. Disdain about the number of hours needed to pass a subject caused many young laymen to leave the Alexian Brothers to work at other hospitals where the standards were not as strict. Despite this, Brother Sebastian stuck to his goal of a professional education for Alexian's nursing students.

> To me there seems to be only one danger, and that is that we will consider the school good enough for our young men. This idea would be a big mistake. There is nothing too good for these young men in the educational line, for on them the future of nursing depends.

The curriculum did tighten. Mistakes were pointed out to the novices and explanations were given to them to help them along. Schedules were reworked to an orderly fashion and "pep" talks given every week by brothers in charge. Brother Sebastian's dedication became so focused that he read on technical subjects during supper on Sundays.

Although the school's accreditation in 1925 was a positive event, this did leave the order with fewer teachers because of the stiffer requirements needed to teach. A high school education was now required before anyone could take the exam to be an accredited registered nurse. After

Brother Sebastian and Brother Camillus passed their state board examinations, 18 other Brothers took and passed their examinations between July 1925 and February 1927. By early 1927, then, the qualified staff of registered nurses was not only an accredited staff but formidable in size as well; and this accomplishment was done in just two years. It is no wonder that the reputation of the Alexian Brothers spread as fast as it did.

An example of this is an October 1926 entry in Brother Sebastian's diary that a school "down state" asked to affiliate with the Alexian Brothers and allow their second-year students to study at the hospital. Brother Sebastian regretfully declined because his supervisors decided that equipment and facilities were not up-to-date.

Orderliness and attention to detail came naturally to Brother Sebastian, and this resonated to his staff. As a consequence, the atmosphere at Alexian only got better.

During Brother Sebastian's administration at the hospital more equipment was purchased. This was partly due to the staff doctors who not only recommended what they needed, but also personally took the time to make sure the hospital got what it needed. The roster of trained brothers grew as did, slowly, the layforce. There was always a steady stream of laymen ready to work for the Alexian Brothers, and Brother Sebastian surmised that they would be most important in the future. On January 13, 1929, four years into it's life, the School of Nurses had 33 registered nurses working outside the hospital and had not lost a single brother who registered. Brother Sebastian's pride of these nurses resounds in his entry of 1929 when he says of his nurses: "They would be a credit to any school of nursing, and I think I am voicing the sentiments of all the teachers when I say that the novices are doing exceptionally well and show a very good spirit."

The year 1929 also marks the end of Brother Sebastian's tenure as director. He hints to his state of mind when he bears out that another is needed to "bring pep and vigor to the position than the present incumbent." He goes on to say that the School of Nurses is the backbone to the life of the hospital and the morale of the hospital will be measured by the nurses the school turns out.

Before Brother Sebastian left his post, he had one last wish to the supervisors of Alexian Brothers for the betterment of their hospital. It was for the future affiliation with Loyola University. This, in Brother Sebastian's mind, would only enhance the quality of the order's excellent nurses as well as raise the quality of the community at large and "rebound to the honor and glory of God." Brother Anthony Wessel replaced Brother Sebastian as director of the School of Nurses on January 17, 1929.

BIBLIOGRAPHY

Archives. PRO-7.C SS 133.1. Alexian Brothers Immaculate Conception Province. Elk Grove Village, Illinois.

Brother Roy Godwin

Amy Frances Brown

1908–1984

Amy Frances Brown was an educator and writer, influencing nursing students and nursing education through her many articles and books.

She was born in Alexis, Illinois, on December 5, 1908. In 1930 she received a bachelor of education degree from Western Illinois State Teachers' College, Macomb, and pursued graduate studies in English at the University of Iowa, Iowa City, in 1932 and 1933. Brown then changed careers and graduated from the University of Iowa, School of Nursing at Iowa City in 1936. After working as a staff nurse at Lutheran Hospital, Fort Dodge, Iowa, for a brief time, she took a position as instructor in the Good Samaritan Hospital, Lexington, Kentucky, and during this same time, 1937–38, enrolled in public-health nursing postgraduate studies at the University of Kentucky. In 1940 she received a master of nursing degree from Western Reserve University, Cleveland, Ohio. Between 1940 and 1944 Brown was instructor of pharmacology and medical and psychiatric nursing at the Vanderbilt University School of Nursing; clinical instructor and supervisor of medical nursing, the Medical College of Virginia; and director of nursing education, Kentucky State Board of Nurse Examiners.

Her writings at this time paralleled her experience. Her first articles, published by the *American Journal of Nursing* (*AJN*) in 1940, stressed the need for student nurses to learn to use communication skills effectively in speaking, teaching, and writing and outlined ways for teachers of nursing to incorporate this learning in clinical classes. Articles appearing in AJN in 1943 (March) and 1944 (January) represented clinical approaches to specific medical problems. In 1945 the first edition of her book *Medical Nursing* was published. Her writings emphasized clinical information that the nursing student could relate to the care of patients.

Brown returned to Western Reserve University as assistant professor of nursing in 1945, remaining until 1947. From 1948–55 Brown was assistant and associate professor of medical nursing at State University of Iowa College of Nursing. She earned a Ph.D. in education from the University of Chicago in 1955. Her dissertation title was "A Method of Case Analysis for Inferring Learning Needs in Medical Nursing."

Brown taught at Loyola University, Chicago, from 1955–57 as associate professor of nursing. After 1957 she was instructor of medical nursing and in-service educator at Moline Public Hospital, Moline, Illinois. Following this, she was a visiting professor at Nazareth College (now Spalding University), Lexington, Kentucky, for an undetermined period of time.

Medical Nursing (3rd edition) was published in 1957. *Medical and Surgical Nursing* and *Medical and Surgical Nursing II* were published in 1958 and 1959, respectively. Also in the late fifties, Brown was one of the first nurses to write a research text. In 1976 she became a member of the American Academy of Nursing. She died in December 1984.

Throughout her career as a nurse educator, Brown sought to bring principles of education to the teaching of nursing students and to stress the preparation of nurses as teachers in clinical, community, and classroom settings.

PUBLICATIONS BY AMY FRANCES BROWN

BOOKS

Clinical Instruction. Philadelphia: Saunders, 1949.

Medical Nursing, (3rd ed.) Philadelphia: Saunders, 1957.

Research in Nursing. Philadelphia: Saunders, 1958.

Medical and Surgical Nursing. Philadelphia: Saunders, 1958.

Medical and Surgical Nursing II. Philadelphia: Saunders, 1959.

Curriculum Development. Philadelphia: Saunders, 1960.

ARTICLES

"Teaching Drugs and Solutions." *American Journal of Nursing* 39 (May 1939): 509–12.

"What Supervision Isn't!" *Trained Nurse* 103 (October 1939): 354–57.

"Guided Practice in Speech: Suggestions for the Course in Professional Adjustments II." *American Journal of Nursing* 40 (April 1940): 431–34.

"Learning to Write Effectively." *American Journal of Nursing* 40 (November 1940): 1256–60.

"Coronary Occlusion-Nursing Care." *American Journal of Nursing* 42 (March 1942): 248–51.

"Subacute Bacterial Endocarditis." *American Journal of Nursing* 44 (January 1944): 9–12.

"Medical Nursing in the Basic Curriculum." *Nursing Outlook* 4 (June 1956): 347–49.

"Organization of Clinical Learning Experiences." *Nursing Outlook* 5 (February 1957): 95–97.

"Ability Grouping." *Nursing Outlook* 5 (March 1957): 168–69.

BIBLIOGRAPHY

American Journal of Nursing (April 1940): 415; (March 1942): 297; (August 1943): 777; (December 1944): 1184; (November 1945): 966; (November 1955): 1320.

Marianne Brook

Martha Marie Montgomery Brown

1918–1987

Martha Marie Montgomery Brown was an outstanding nurse scientist and educator. Her early work in developing a psychodynamic approach to nursing fashioned a conceptualization of nursing as a psychodynamic process of interaction and biosocial intervention. The textbook which she coauthored with Grace R. Fowler, *Psychodynamic Nursing—A Biosocial Orientation*, had four editions over a 17-year period. It was a major influence not only on psychiatric nursing, but on nursing generally. During the 1960s Brown conducted research investigating the effect of skilled nursing upon "psychosocial atrophy" of institutionalized elderly patients. This research was notable not only for its innovative methodology and significant findings, but also for the fact that a nurse researcher served as project director of a multidisciplinary team that included a psychiatrist, psychologists, a cultural anthropologist, and other nurses. Brown's research and writing had national influence and contributed to national health policy and delivery system models. Brown was an advocate for research and education on care of the elderly. She was also a facilitator of research and a role model for scores of faculty and graduate students.

Brown was born on November 22, 1918, in Alexandria, Indiana, the oldest of four daughters of Floyd Montgomery and Esther Mehling Montgomery. Her father was a factory worker and self-employed welder. Her mother spent most of her life as a homemaker, but she did work some in a factory and in a small hospital. A sister, Helen Louise, died in infancy, but her other two sisters, Genevieve Grace Balser and Clara M. Murray survived her. Brown grew up in Alexandria and attended public schools. She loved school, excelled in her school work, and was encouraged by teachers to go to college. During high school Brown worked as an assistant librarian in the Alexandria library to earn money for college. As a youngster, she took violin lessons and became an accom-

plished violinist. She also had artistic talent, doing charcoal sketches and oil paintings, which she gave to her friends. She was an accomplished gourmet cook.

When it came time to choose college, Brown decided on the nursing school at the University of Michigan, Ann Arbor. There she earned a nursing diploma in 1941. Her first job was as a staff nurse at University Hospital in Ann Arbor. She also worked as a private-duty nurse, supervisor in industrial nursing, and as a part-time student counselor at Wayne State University in Detroit before she moved to Cleveland, Ohio, in 1947. There, she enrolled in the bachelor of science in nursing program at Case Western Reserve University (CWRU) and worked as a head nurse at University Hospitals in Cleveland. She continued at CWRU to earn an M.A. in nursing with minors in psychology and education.

Brown spent one year as an instructor at State Hospital, Jacksonville, Illinois, before going in 1949, to Washington University School of Nursing, St. Louis, as instructor and assistant director of the school. She taught psychiatric nursing and progressed through the academic ranks until, in 1961, she was promoted to full professor and assumed the deanship of the school, a position she held until 1968. When Washington University announced its intent to close the School of Nursing, Brown left. During the seven years she served as dean, she also was a nursing consultant to the Medical Care Research Center of the Washington University Social Science Institute and the Jewish Hospital of St. Louis.

Ever true to her love of learning, Brown took advantage of the educational opportunities in St. Louis and became one of the first nursing scientists to graduate from the prestigious Ph.D. program in health organization research and sociology at St. Louis University. This background aided her research in conceptualizing the influence of the social system in nurse-patient interaction and functioning. Brown served as principal investigator and project director of a study of nursing interventions to prevent the social systems of institutional settings from hastening the deterioration of patients' social attributes and functions. This large multidisciplinary study extended from 1957 through 1966 and was reported in the book *Nurses, Patients, and Social Systems. The Effects of Skilled Nursing Intervention Upon Institutionalized Older Patients.* From 1957 through 1962, Research Grant GN-5535 from the National Institutes of Health (NIH), USPHS provided funding for this research. Brown also received other NIH funding (GN5226) for research on institutionalized elderly. Her dissertation, which was completed in 1968, dealt with role strain in hospital nurses. Thus, her research topics have remained relevant over time.

Dr. Faye G. Abdellah, assistant surgeon general, U.S. Public Health Service, wrote a letter supporting the nomination of Brown for the Elizabeth McWilliams Miller Award for Excellence in Research for the 1981 Sigma Theta Tau Founders awards. Abdellah stated:

> The Mental Health Systems Act signed by former President Carter in 1980 for the first time addressed the special needs of the elderly in relation to mental health problems. Dr. Brown's research contributed extensively to the drafters of this bill. Again at the national level, Dr. Brown's research, "Nurse Patient Interchange in the Arrestment of Psychosocial Atrophy of the Aged, Institutionalized Patients" (1970), was an influential resource in my own research with long-term care patients and confirmed the findings of our national study published in 1974–75.

Brown did postdoctoral study in epidemiology at the University of Minnesota. While serving on St. Louis University's original committee for defining nursing diagnoses, she used epidemiological concepts in developing these diagnoses and advanced the work by emphasizing the use of a taxonomy. In her graduate nursing course in gerontological nursing, she used an inductive research approach to promote the identification and description of nursing diagnoses in elderly patients. Brown also served as research consultant to the Visiting Nurses Association

of Omaha in their seminal work on developing nursing problem classifications for community and home-health nursing.

In 1968 Brown went to the University of Nebraska College of Nursing as professor of nursing and chairman of the graduate nursing programs. She aided in moving the master's program in psychiatric nursing from the Department of Psychiatry to the College of Nursing, and was the major determiner of the philosophy of the graduate programs and of the development of the curriculum. Brown was given the charge of establishing a Nursing Care Research Center, one of the first nonfederally funded centers in the nation (established in 1968). Brown had the task not only of teaching research to students, but also of developing faculty in research. By teaching, by continuous individual assistance, by the use of outside consultants, she assisted faculty in developing research cores in their clinical areas and in developing teams of faculty and students. She also assisted them in joint publications. Brown emphasized the need for nursing students to participate in the all-campus student research forums held annually. While teaching and mentoring students and faculty, Brown worked with an outside consultant and an architect to plan and develop the physical space for a nursing research center in the College of Nursing building that was dedicated in 1976.

Brown's contributions have been acknowledged by a variety of awards and honors bestowed upon her. In 1962 she was the St. Louis Bicentennial Honoree of the American Association of University Women. Her book *Nurses, Patients and Social Systems* was nominated for the 1968 Socio-Psychological Prize of the American Association for the Advancement of Science. The University of Michigan School of Nursing recognized her as a distinguished alumni in 1972. The Second District Nebraska Nurses' Association presented her with a professional achievement award in 1976, and the state association presented her with a Distinguished Service Award in 1977. In 1981 Sigma Theta Tau honored her with the Elizabeth McWilliams Miller Award for Excellence in Research. The University of Nebraska Medical Center recognized her contributions to the College of Nursing and nursing generally with a Distinguished Service to Nursing Award in 1982.

Brown retired from the University of Nebraska in 1981. She moved to Glendale, Arizona, where she did some private-duty nursing. Her health began to fail rapidly from complications of diabetes, and so she moved back to Indiana to be near her family. On October 28, 1987, Brown died in Mercy Hospital in Elwood, Indiana.

Selected Publications by Martha Marie Montgomery Brown

BOOKS

With E. Cardew (ed.), L. Brunner, J. DeClue, J. Torrance, and G. Wilkins. *Study Guide for Clinical Nursing—A Co-Ordinated Survey.* Philadelphia: Lippincott, 1953; 2nd ed., 1961.

With G.R. Fowler. *Psychodynamic Nursing.* Philadelphia: Saunders, 1954; 2nd, 3rd, and 4th ed, 1961, 1966, and 1971.

With P.R. Brown, J.C. Glidewell, R.G. Hunt, and J.M.A. Weiss. *Nursing, Patients and Social Systems.* Columbia: University of Missouri Press, 1968.

MONOGRAPHS

"Personalization of the Aged Institutionalized Patient." In *ANA Clinical Conferences.* New York: Appleton-Century-Crofts, 1969.

With G. Fowler and C. Gilchrist. "Report on the Conference on Advanced Programs in Psychiatric Nursing." New York: National League for Nursing, 1951.

With P.R. Brown. "Nurse Patient Interchange in the Arrestment of Psychosocial Atrophy of Aged, Institutionalized Patients." In *Sixth Annual Research Conference of the American Nurses' Association.* New York: ANA, 1970.

ARTICLES

"The Epidemiologic Approach to the Study of Clinical Nursing Diagnoses." *Nursing Forum* XIII (1974): 348–50.

"The Need for Reallocation of Health Resources." *Nursing Homes* (January–February 1980): 12–15.

With J. Boosinger, M. Henderson, J. Kubat, S. Rife, O. Taylor, and W.W. Young. "Drug-Drug Interaction Among Residents in Homes for the Elderly." *Nursing Research* XXVI (1977): 47–52.

With J. Cornwell, E. Kelleher, and J. Weist. "Learned Helplessness Among the Institu-

tionalized Elderly: A Pilot Study." *Issues in Mental Health Nursing* No. 3 (1981): 293–303.

With J. Boosinger, J. Black, and T. Gasper. "Nursing Innovations for Prevention of Decubitus Ulcers in Long-Term Care Facilities." *Journal of Plastic and Reconstructive Surgical Nursing* 1, (May 1981): 51–55.

With J. Weist and J. Cornwell. "Reducing the Risks to the Institutionalized Elderly (Part I and Part II)" *Journal of Gerontological Nursing* 7 (July 1981): 401–07.

BIBLIOGRAPHY

Abdellah F.G. Letter to chairperson, Sigma Theta Tau Awards Committee, April 17, 1981.

Boyle, R.E. Letter to author, February 23, 1989.

Boyle, R.E. Letter to Sigma Theta Tau Awards Committee, May 11, 1981.

Weiss, J.M.A. Preface. *Nurses, Patients and Social Systems.* Columbia: University of Missouri Press, 1968.

Rosalee C. Yeaworth

Sadie Johnson Metz Brown

b. 1904

Sadie Brown's major contributions to nursing in Texas came partially through her numerous activities and offices held in professional nursing organizations throughout Texas, the southern region of the American Nurses' Association, and the Texas League for Nursing. Her intense involvement in nursing organizations gave her a vision for nursing that she took to a larger arena. Her overriding goal was a "determination to make everyone with whom she was associated understand that nursing was a part of the entire community, not something one only thought about when one was ill." Through active membership and holding offices in the San Antonio City Federation of Women's Clubs, she was able to bring nurses and the larger community of women together.

Brown was born at the home of her parents Lydia Marguerite Collett and Arthur Thomas Johnson on September 3, 1904. At the time the family resided in El

Dara, Pike County, Illinois. A sister Gertrude was born in January 1906. A sister Merle was stillborn about 1911, and another sister Pauline (Polly) was born in 1916. Because of her father's employment as well as family pressures, the family moved frequently. At various times they lived in Washington State, New Mexico, Colorado, and New Mexico.

Brown attended public school in Leadville, Colorado, through eleventh grade. Her mother's ill health forced the family to move to San Angelo, Texas, in 1919, where a maternal grandmother and uncle lived. Brown started her senior year of high school in San Angelo, but because she was the eldest of the children, she had to drop out of school to provide continuous care for her ill mother. She credited the ability to give her mother nursing care to a Red Cross home-nursing course she had taken while in high school.

A combination of factors led her to choose nursing as a career. As a teenager during World War I, she "fell in love with nursing." She had enjoyed her school course in home nursing and derived considerable personal satisfaction nursing her mother. The family physician recognized Brown's nursing ability and suggested that she enter nurses' training. Although her father wanted her to be a teacher, he recognized his inability to finance a college education and acquiesced to her attending nursing school.

The training school for nurses of St. Johns Hospital in San Angelo had a good reputation among the local medical community. Because the family's religion was Protestant, Brown's father had concerns about her attending St. Johns, a hospital and training school that was owned and operated by a Roman Catholic order. Nevertheless, he agreed to her applying for admission. He accompanied her to her admission interview to get his questions answered regarding the issue of religion. He was assured by the director of the school that no effort would be made to try to convert his daughter to Catholicism. Satisfied with the answer, Sadie Brown enrolled in the school in 1920. The school's administration went so far as to send her to the First Methodist Church every Sunday in the hospital-owned car.

The hospital with approximately 50 beds, was the only hospital with a school of nursing between Fort Worth and El Paso. Students worked 12-hour shifts, and those students working days had classes between 7:30 and 9:00 P.M. The teachers were a nun pharmacist and physicians on the staff.

Shortly after Brown graduated from St. Johns in 1923, she was offered a position as director of nursing for a hospital that was just being organized. Two physicians, Drs. Rush and Chambers, had bought the Findlater mansion in San Angelo with accompanying servants' quarters and converted the buildings to a private surgical hospital with 16 beds. Brown saw the job offer as a challenge and accepted the position. She soon realized the magnitude of the position. The physicians purchased the instruments to be used in the operating room, but the new graduate nurse was responsible for purchasing all other supplies and equipment with which to run the hospital. Shortly after the hospital opened, Brown hired a dietitian. This relieved her of the responsibilities of planning diets and supervising food-service activities but still left her with too many other responsibilities to accomplish alone. She saw opening a training school for nurses as a potential solution to her staffing problems and initiated actions to do so. Her professional naivete kept her from recognizing both her lack of qualifications to teach and the problems that she would encounter with the Board of Nurse Examiners for the state.

A. Louise Dietrich, the newly appointed education secretary of the Texas Board of Nurse Examiners, counseled her about the peril in undertaking such an endeavor, but Brown proceeded with her plans, complying, as best she could, with the board's regulations. Six students were admitted. Thus not only was she responsible for supervising the functioning of the operating room and overseeing the general operations of the hospital, but she was also responsible for the education of the students. Her salary of $75 a month hardly compensated for the burden of the responsibilities.

A year and a half after embarking on her first employment endeavor, Brown realized that she was not prepared for what she had undertaken and resigned with the hope of returning to school. She explored the options available to her for post-graduate courses, but none that she could afford were of the quality that would substantially advance her knowledge base. She then turned to private-duty nursing for employment.

On February 21, 1925, she married Metz Bishop and stopped working outside the home. Their first son was born in 1926 and died before he was a year old. A second son, Louis, was born three years later. The Depression caused the firm for which Metz worked to close, forcing him to seek other employment. He leased a ranch and was raising sheep when he died of a coronary occlusion in 1930 at the age of 43. His premature death left the family in dire straits. Brown and her son moved in with her in-laws whose financial status was not much better than her own. That household consisted of her father-in-law, who was a retired pharmacist, a "pampered mother-in-law," and a "spinster" sister-in-law.

Brown returned to work as a public-health nurse in San Angelo, Texas. Simultaneously, she hired a man to be responsible for operating the ranch, and she found a good market for the ranch's sheep and wool. With astute management skills and ongoing advise from a local banker, Brown gradually retired the debt against the estate.

Brown came to believe that the demands of the public-health nursing position necessitated that she have more education in the field of public health. During the summer of 1931 she went to Vanderbilt University to attend a summer course for public-health nurses.

In 1934, she married Ed Brown, a Border Patrol officer, and continued working as a public-health nurse for about eight months prior to moving to Del Rio, Texas in 1935. A son Mike was born in 1938.

Her husband was assigned to the newly opened immigration office in Dallas in 1941, and the family moved there. An influx of illegal aliens had necessitated opening of an immigration office in that city. Because of the shortage of nurses caused by World War II, and the opportunity to improve the family's financial status, Brown accepted a position at Methodist Hospital in Dallas in the outpatient department. Her employment was facilitated by the presence of a child-care center within two blocks of the hospital that only accepted children whose mothers were engaged in work essential to the war effort. Nursing fell within that category.

In 1943 Ed Brown was transferred again, this time to San Antonio. In 1950, because of a continuing nursing shortage, Brown accepted a "temporary" position as the director of nurses at the Robert B. Green Hospital in San Antonio. At the time the hospital was in dire financial straits. With the assistance of many local organizations the hospital survived, and in 1951 it became a component of the San Antonio/Bexar County Hospital System.

Brown's numerous community activities played a hand in saving the hospital. Sixteen years after assuming the "temporary" position as director of nursing (1966) she was promoted to the newly created position of special assistant administrator of the Bexar County Hospital District. She retired from active nursing in 1970. She credits much of her success in nursing to nurse mentors and colleagues such as A. Louise Dietrich, Mildred Garrett Primer, and Olga Breihan.

While still in nursing school, Brown had heard A. Louise Dietrich, then executive secretary of the Texas Graduate Nurses' Association, speak about the importance of nurses belonging to, and being active in, the professional organization. Brown internalized the admonition and applied for membership in the American Nurses' Association (ANA) shortly after becoming a registered nurse. Later in her life she lamented, "We believed if we were not accepted for membership in the ANA, our RN would do us no good in the nursing world."

Brown held numerous offices at the district and state level of the professional organization throughout her career and even after her retirement from active nursing. She was president of District 16 of the Texas Graduate Nurses' Association (TGNA) early in her career and of District 8 TGNA considerably later. She also served in the offices of president, first and second vice-president and director of the state-level TGNA. In addition, she was active in the San Antonio League for Nursing and served a term as vice-president of that organization.

During World War II, with the exception of two university schools, the majority of nursing schools in the South were of such poor quality that the graduates of those schools were unable to join the American Red Cross. At the time Red Cross membership was requisite to entering military service as a nurse. Nurses in leadership positions in the South were incensed at the large number of graduate nurses who found themselves victims of the proliferation of schools with inadequate educational programs for their students. The state associations of Alabama, Arkansas, Virginia, North and South Carolina, Louisiana, Georgia, Mississippi, Florida, and Texas banned together to form an organization called the Southern Region of the ANA to take action against the educational inadequacies. The organization's major thrust was to help nurses, in the states affected, to develop and pass legislation forcing the elevation of educational standards within the states. Brown served as president of that organization in 1955; that year it disbanded because other organizations were then able to serve as monitors of educational standards.

Brown also took a keen interest in matters outside of nursing. She served as president in both San Angelo and San Antonio of the Business and Professional Women's clubs as well as state health chairman and district director for the San Antonio organization. In San Antonio 300 groups of women had banded together to form a City Federation of Woman's Clubs for many years. Brown served as president, first vice-president, and health chairperson of that federation. Collec-

tively, the organizations did such things as conduct a massive chest x-ray program, force the use of voting machines rather than hand-written ballots, and conduct a speakers' bureau. Brown was president of the federation when the Robert B. Green Hospital was in financial difficulty. Through the efforts of various individual organizations, sections of the hospital were able to remain open, for example, the cancer ward, which was financed by the Junior League.

Brown's numerous civic activities did not go unnoticed. In addition to being listed in *Who's Who of American Women*, she received the Rosicrucian Humanist Award in 1964 for dedication to serving the community. In 1967 she received station KBAT's Texas Star Award for community service, and in 1969 she was chosen as "Headliner" by the women's editor of the San Antonio *Express-News*.

Even after retirement, Brown has remained active in nursing and civic organizations. She served on TNA's Bicentennial Committee, serves as parliamentarian for local women's groups, and is an officer in Zonta. She resides in San Antonio, Texas.

BIBLIOGRAPHY

Brown, S.J. Interview with the author, March 14, 1989.

Eleanor L.M. Crowder

Helen Edith Browne
1911–1987

Helen E. Browne was a leader in the development and expansion of nurse-midwifery services in this country and abroad. Known affectionately as "Brownie," she was widely recognized for her contributions to health care for large numbers of people in rural Kentucky, as well as for being a caring and patient administrator who dedicated her life to the continued development of the Frontier Nursing Service (FNS). As an early advocate of the concept of caring, she spoke often on the subject, saying "Nurses care, doctors cure."

Born on February 3, 1911, at Bury, St. Edmonds, England to Phil and Agnes Browne, Helen Browne graduated from Ipswich High School in Suffolk, England. She graduated from St. Bartholomews Hospital School of Nursing in 1934 to become a state registered nurse. She then completed a one-year course at the British Hospital for Mothers and Babies in London and was appointed the nurse in charge at St. Bartholomews Hospital. In 1937, she became the midwifery supervisor for the British Hospital for Mothers and Babies.

Browne left England in 1938 in response to a request from Mary Breckinridge, founder of the Frontier Nursing Service, for a nurse midwife who would be willing to work in Kentucky. While many other British nurse midwives left the states to return to England when World War II broke out in 1939, Browne remained in Kentucky, where she served as district nurse midwife caring for families both at home and in hospital under difficult wartime conditions compounded by the culture of rural Kentucky.

District nurse midwives in Kentucky in their work had to contend with gas rationing, reaching patients by horseback over swollen mountain streams, and helping mothers in labor at the barrel end of a shotgun held by a distrustful man of the mountains. Even under these conditions, the maternal and infant death rate for patients cared for by these nurse midwives was lower than for patients in more modern facilities.

Browne spent 38 years as a member of the Frontier Nursing Service, moving from district nurse midwife to assistant director and then to associate director of FNS. During this time she also served as midwifery supervisor and superintendent to Hyden (Kentucky) Hospital as well as director of the Southeastern Kentucky Health Demonstration Corporation. When Mary Breckinridge (the founder of the Frontier Nursing Service) died in 1965, Browne was unanimously elected director of the service. She served in that capacity and as director emeritus until her retirement in 1975.

During her tenure as FNS director Browne was the driving force and major capital fund raiser for the Mary Breckinridge Hospital, led the initiative to combine the family nursing and nurse midwife components of the FNS educational program into an integrated curriculum, and worked to merge the American Association of Midwives with the American College of Nurses Midwifery to form the American College of Nurse Midwives. In addition, she worked with visitors from many foreign countries to help them adapt the practices of the FNS to their cultures.

In retirement, Browne was an active volunteer for the Frontier Nursing Service, both as a fund raiser and a speaker. For her many accomplishments in the field of nurse midwifery, she received the Distinguished Service Award from Berea College, an honorary doctorate degree in nursing from Eastern Kentucky University, the Order of the British Empire, and the Commander of the Most Excellent Order of the British Empire.

Browne died at her home in Milford, Pennsylvania, on January 20, 1987. She is remembered as "the ulitmate midwife—strong, sure, sensitive."

PUBLICATIONS BY HELEN E. BROWNE

"American Congress on Obstetrics and Gynecology, 4th, New York (City)." *Frontier Nursing Service Quarterly Bulletin* 25 (Spring 1950): 55–56.

"The Frontier Nursing Service Celebrates Its Silver Anniversary." *Trained Nurse* 124 (May 1950): 224–25.

"A Tribute to Mary Breckinridge." *Nursing Outlook* 14 (May 1966): 54–55.

"Family Nurse Practitioner Project." *Frontier Nursing Service Quarterly Bulletin* 46 (Summer 1970): 23.

"International Congress of Midwives." *Frontier Nursing Service Quarterly Bulletin* 48 (Autumn 1972): 3–5.

With G. Isaacs. "Primary Care Nurse in Community Health." *American Journal of Obstetrics and Gynecology* 124 (January 1976): 14–17.

BIBLIOGRAPHY

Dock, L., and I. Stewart. *A Short History of Nursing.* New York: Putnam, 1938.

"A Life of Service." *Frontier Nursing Service Quarterly Bulletin* 62 (Winter 1987): 1–4.

Powell, J. "A Friend Remembered." *Frontier Nursing Service Quarterly Bulletin* 62 (Spring 1987): 9–12.

Who's Who of American Women, 1974–75. Chicago: Marquis, 1974.

Linda M. Calley

Mother de Sales Browne (Frances Browne)

1826–1910

Mother de Sales Browne led the first group of Irish Sisters of Mercy to Vicksburg, Mississippi, on the eve of the American Civil War. The sisters' location in downtown Vicksburg enabled them to provide seriously needed nursing services to injured soldiers and to citizens suffering from communicable diseases. Mother de Sales Browne led her sisters throughout the war years and directed them in nursing activities in the community for over 30 years. The sisters provided emergency assistance in times of crisis for the remainder of the century, including a disastrous yellow fever epidemic in 1878. Her followers credit her ability to assess needs, improvise nursing care, and meet human needs in times of disaster as the reason her leadership was so lasting and effective.

Frances, known to her family as Fannie, was born to Michael and Mary Browne in Westmoreland, Pennsylvania, on July 3, 1826. She was the eldest of five children in a close-knit Roman Catholic family. The Browne family could observe mass on rare occasions when a missionary priest would come to their rural neighborhood. Because of this isolation, Mary Browne had to educate her children about the history, teachings, and mysteries of their faith.

In 1845 Fannie left home to enter the Convent of Mercy established in Pittsburgh. Then she moved to Washington, D.C., to take charge of a new infirmary for the sick poor. In the summer of 1860,

Mother de Sales became ill and went to Baltimore to recover. Soon after beginning her convalescence, an urgent request for help came to the order from the Natchez diocese in Mississippi. A school for Catholic children was desperately needed in Vicksburg.

Late in the summer of 1860 Mother de Sales led a group of four sisters and two postulants southward to establish a school in Vicksburg. The school opened on October 22, 1860, and soon the sisters had organized the parishioners of the nearby parish to visit and care for the sick and poor.

The outbreak of the Civil War did not immediately affect the sisters in rural Vicksburg, but their spiritual advisor, Father LeRay, reminded the sisters of their responsibility to care for the sick and wounded if the need should arise. By spring 1862 the war reached Vicksburg via the Mississippi River, and the sisters were evacuated from the city due to its vulnerability from military action. Just a few days after evacuating, however, Mother de Sales and two of her sisters returned to their convent, which had been converted into a hospital. Many of the men hospitalized were suffering from measles and typhoid fever as well as wounds from conflict. Mother de Sales and the sisters gave as much care and comfort as possible under the primitive conditions in the hospital.

The Confederate government soon moved the patients to a larger hospital set up at Mississippi Springs, and the sisters followed. Once in the new hospital, they were joined by other Catholic sisters from New Orleans, but within two weeks the patient population grew to over 700, overwhelming the sisters and their limited resources in the field hospital. Without adequate numbers of workers or supplies, the death rate was high.

In October 1862 the sisters moved to Jackson, to prepare a hospital for 300 patients at the Deaf and Dumb Institute, but they were soon called to Oxford to serve the more than 1,000 patients dispersed in the twelve buildings then known as Oxford College. The conditions there were crude, and hygiene was very poor. The worst problem facing the sisters was the task of providing adequate nourishment, for food supplies were very scarce. The sisters cared for patients until late November 1862, when Federal troops overran Oxford. They escaped by train, returning to Jackson. Soon, they were caring for patients in another military hospital.

In May 1863 General Sherman occupied Jackson, then moved to Vicksburg. After Vicksburg surrendered in July, the sisters were ordered to evacuate to Alabama to care for patients in Shelby Springs. They remained at the hospital there until May 1864. During the closing months of their service, Mother de Sales and her sisters experienced severe deprivations due to the failing supply system of the Confederacy. Everything necessary to run a hospital, but especially food, became scarce and finally unobtainable. Half of the group returned with Mother de Sales to Vicksburg in late 1864; the rest remained in Alabama until the end of the war.

In the years after the war, Mother de Sales led her sisterhood through many changes, which included much growth in the number of postulants, convents, and service institutions including hospitals in Mississippi. She served the order as Mother Superior for over 30 years. On July 19, 1910, Mother de Sales died of complications of a fractured hip.

BIBLIOGRAPHY

Archives of the Sisters of Mercy, St. Frances Xavier Academy, Vicksburg, Mississippi. *Annals* of the Sisters of Mercy (1860–65).

Bernard, Mother M. *The Story of the Sisters of Mercy in Mississippi, 1860–1930.* New York: Kennedy, 1931.

Bettersworth, J. *Mississippi: A History.* Austin, Texas: Steck, 1959.

Cabaniss, Frances and Cabaniss, James Allen. "Religion in Antebellum Mississippi." *Journal of Mississippi History* 1 (October 1944): 191–224.

Pillar, Thomas. *The Catholic Church in Mississippi, 1837–65.* New Orleans: Hanser Press, 1964.

Linda Sabin

Helen Lathrop Bunge
1906–1970

Helen L. Bunge was instrumental in promoting research in nursing during its development in the early 1950s. She also was dean of two major schools of nursing, influencing both undergraduate and graduate nursing education.

Bunge was born on October 11, 1906, in La Crosse, Wisconsin, to George William and Sarah Wheeler Bunge. She grew up in LaCrosse with three brothers: George, William and Jonathon. A sister, Mary Dorthea, died in childhood. Both of her parents were college graduates; education was important to the family. Bunge's great-grandfather, Stephen Pearl Lathrop, was a professor of chemistry and natural history at the University of Wisconsin beginning in 1854.

Bunge earned a B.A. in sociology from the University of Wisconsin in 1928, after attending the Connecticut College for Women in New London for the first two years of her college education (1924–26). She was elected to Phi Beta Kappa prior to graduation. Remaining at Wisconsin, Bunge entered the nursing program and received her certificate of graduate nurse in 1930. Bunge took her postgraduate education at Teachers College, Columbia University, New York, where she earned an M.A. in 1936 and an Ed.D. in 1950. Her dissertation was titled "Changing the Basic Curriculum of the Frances Payne Bolton School of Nursing, Western Reserve University."

Helen Bunge had extensive experience in nursing education and research. Her first job was as head nurse at Wisconsin General Hospital, Madison. Her career in nursing education began in 1931 when she taught nursing arts and ward management at the University of Wisconsin School of Nursing. She also served as an assistant to the director of the school. In 1940 she left Wisconsin to pursue her doctorate in New York City. While a student at Teachers College, Bunge worked as an assistant to Isabel M. Stewart (the director of the Department of Nursing Education) and lived with M. Adelaide Nutting. In 1942 Bunge moved to Cleveland to serve as the coordinator of the Basic Program at the Frances Payne Bolton School of Nursing, Western Reserve University. She became the dean of that program in 1946 and remained in the position until 1953.

From 1953 until 1959 Bunge was the executive officer of the Institute of Research and Service in Nursing Education at Teachers College, Columbia University. This was one of the first organized efforts to facilitate research in nursing. Simultaneously, Bunge was chair of the Association of Collegiate Schools of Nursing Committee on Research, thus was asked to serve as the volunteer editor of *Nursing Research* (the first research journal for nurses) when it was initiated in 1952.

In 1959, although she really enjoyed living in New York City, Bunge decided to return to her native Wisconsin. She was recruited to lead her alma mater, thus served as director (later dean) of the University of Wisconsin School of Nursing from 1959 until 1969.

Helen Bunge is best known for her involvement in the growth of nursing research. She described her work as being "the study of nursing education and the business of helping other people with their research." Indeed, these areas are the main topics of her publications, mainly journal articles. As the first editor of *Nursing Research* (1952–57) Bunge was instrumental in its success as a journal and was described as the "principal guiding hand and spirit." She remained on the editorial board and advisory committee until 1966. As the executive officer of the Institute of Research and Service in Nursing Education, Bunge assisted others with research and became a spokesperson for "how research can best be worked into the structure and function of the university." Bunge also promoted nursing research by giving speeches across the country and internationally to nursing and other groups and by advocating research content in baccalaureate curriculums and research courses in the master's programs.

Nursing education was another area of influence for Bunge. Her presence was felt most at Western Reserve University and the University of Wisconsin. As dean at Western Reserve University's Frances Payne Bolton School of Nursing following World War II, Bunge is remembered for three important changes: admitting men to the school, implementing a 44-hour work week for the basic baccalaureate program, and, in 1948, requiring a research course in the master's program. During Bunge's leadership at the University of Wisconsin, nursing enrollment doubled, a graduate program was started, the school became an autonomous unit (was previously part of the medical school), and a second school of nursing was created at the University of Wisconsin–Milwaukee.

During her career Bunge gave generous service to the profession. Her major committments included the American Nurses' Association, serving on numerous committees and the Board of Directors (1946–50); various NLNE/NLN committees including the Board of Review; chair of the ACSN Committee on Research (1946–53); vice-chair of the Council of the Florence Nightingale International Foundation (1956–57); member of the first Nursing Research Study Section of the USPHS Division of Research Grants (1955–59); chair of the Nursing Service Advisory Committee, American National Red Cross (1954–62); American Nurses' Foundation Board of Director Member (1963–65); member of the Special Medical Advisory Group, Veterans Administration (1961–66); the fifth United States Army civilian consultant in nursing (1964–69); and member and officer of many state and local nursing organizations. At the national level Bunge was elected or appointed to leadership positions in all the major organizations.

During her lifetime, Bunge was honored for her contributions. These honors culminated with the receipt of the NLN M. Adelaide Nutting Award in 1969. She had received an Achievement Award in Research and Scholarship from the Teachers College Nursing Education Alumni Association (1967) and a Distinguished Service Award (science) from the University of Wisconsin Alumni Association (1969). In 1970 both schools of nursing at Western Reserve University and the University of Wisconsin established Helen L. Bunge Scholarships/Awards in her honor. After her death, her achievements were recognized by induction in the American Nurses Association Hall of Fame.

Bunge had many friends. She was known not only for her intellectual abilities, but also for her sense of humor and fun, as well as for playing the piano. Her hobbies were travel and music. She had traveled to many countries but claimed Ireland was her favorite place.

Helen Lathrop Bunge died April 12, 1970 in Madison, Wisconsin. The majority of her papers are in the University of Wisconsin Archives in Madison.

PUBLICATIONS BY
HELEN LATHROP BUNGE

Numerous editorials. *Nursing Research* 1–6 (1952–57).

"An Experiment in the Use of Problem Solving Methods." *Nursing Outlook* 1 (1953): 446–47.

"The Meaning and Importance of Research in Nursing." *Canadian Nurse* 51 (1955): 945–48.

"Research in Nursing in the United States; Some Reflections on its Development." *Teachers College Record* 58 (April 1957): 371–76.

"Research is Every Professional Nurse's Business." *American Journal of Nursing* 58 (June 1958): 816–19.

"The Institute of Research and Service in Nursing Education, Teachers College, Columbia University." *Nursing Research* 7 (October 1958): 113–15.

"Research in Nursing: Is There a Need." *International Nursing Review*, 6 (1959): 33–37.

"The First Decade of Nursing Research." *Nursing Research* 11 (Summer 1962): 132–37.

With Jean A. Curran. *Better Nursing—A Study of Nursing Care and Education in Washington.* Seattle: University of Washington Press, 1951.

Major author of *A Guide for Studying the Utilization of Nursing Service Personnel in Veterans Administration Hospitals.* Washington, D.C.: Veterans Administration, 1961.

BIBLIOGRAPHY

"ANA Hall of Fame Nomination–Helen Lathrop Bunge." Madison: School of Nursing, University of Wisconsin.

Cooper, S.S. "Nursing in Transition: Breaking Barriers of Tradition, the School of Nursing, 1924–74." In *A Resourceful University: The University of Wisconsin-Madison in its 125th Year.* Pp. 235–44. Madison: University of Wisconsin Press, 1975.

Curriculum Vitae–Helen Lathrop Bunge. Madison: School of Nursing, University of Wisconsin, February 1, 1968.

Faddis, M.O. *A School of Nursing Comes of Age.* Cleveland: Alumni Association of Frances Payne Bolton School of Nursing, 1973.

Hilbert, H. "Five Years of Leadership." *Nursing Research* 6 (October 1957): 51.

Notter, L.E. "Helen L. Bunge, First Editor of Nursing Research." *Nursing Research* 19 (July–Aug 1970): 291.

Personal communication with Susan Bunge-Quigley (great-niece), September 7, 1990. Madison, Wisc.

Smith, L.C. *Helen L. Bunge: Nurse, Teacher, Scholar.* Madison: University of Wisconsin School of Nursing, 1979.

"Your Madisonian: Helen L. Bunge." *Wisconsin State Journal*, June 30, 1968, Sec. 5, 4.

Laurie K. Glass

Charlotte Burgess
1865–1949

Charlotte Burgess was an outstanding nursing leader in Nebraska for 29 years. She organized the University of Nebraska School of Nursing in 1917 and served as the director of the school and the Nursing Service Department of University Hospital until her retirement in 1946.

Burgess was born on October 22, 1865, on a homestead near Vermillion, South Dakota. Little is known about her family except that her parents had settled in Clay County before the Civil War. She was one of eight children. Following her secondary education, Burgess attended the University of South Dakota and in 1892 received a bachelor of philosophy degree from the University of Wisconsin. After teaching for several years in South Dakota, she entered the Illinois Training School for Nurses in Chicago, graduating in 1904. She served as the director of nursing education at the Illinois Training School from 1908–14.

Burgess was extremely patriotic throughout her life; this was apparent during World War I when she enlisted in the American Red Cross Nursing Service even before the United States entered the war. She served as chief nurse of the Chicago unit in Kiev, Russia, from 1914–15.

Burgess then became a student at Teachers College, Columbia University, New York City during 1916–17; it was from here that her career as founder and director of the Nebraska school was launched. Adelaide Nutting, then director of the postgraduate nursing program at Teachers College, was asked to recommend a nurse for the position of superintendent of nurses for the soon to be opened University of Nebraska Hospital and School for Nurses. Nutting advised Burgess to accept the position.

Burgess was reluctant to "undertake so important a piece of work" since she had no experience with a university school of nursing. She accepted the challenge, however, and spent a full day with Louise Powell at the University of Minnesota. The Minnesota nursing school had been organized in 1909 as an integral part of that university, and Powell was very helpful in giving suggestions for organizing a university school.

On August 4, 1917, Burgess arrived in Omaha. She was shocked to find that the hospital was still under construction, the furniture was still in the packing crates, and there was "not one nurse in sight." On September 3 the hospital and school opened as scheduled. Burgess recruited 4 graduate nurses to staff the hospital and by September 12 had recruited 16 postgraduate and affiliation students. On October 16, the new nursing program opened with 13 beginning students.

It was the standard of this era to provide women with an education in nursing in return for their service to the hospital. The Nebraska program was unusual, however, in that there were few schools that offered a combined liberal arts and basic nursing curriculum leading to a bachelor's degree. Schools associated with a university were the exception rather than the rule.

Burgess designed the curriculum based on *A Standard Curriculum for Schools of Nursing*, published by the National League for Nursing Education (NLNE) in 1917. Students could earn the nursing diploma in three years and continue for two more years to earn a bachelor of science or bachelor of arts degree. The program reflected many of the tenets suggested by Florence Nightingale. Admission requirements were high—a four-year high-school education was required; the majority of U.S. nursing schools required only one year of high school for admission. Burgess said it was incorrect to assume that *anyone* could be a nurse. "Ice-men can be found at 42nd & Leavenworth-what I want are nurses with brains!"

Throughout her early years at the school, Burgess implemented the recommendations of the NLNE, published in the Goldmark Report (1923) and the revised Curriculum Guide (1927). The school was ranked with the best nursing schools in the final report of the Committee on the Grading of Nursing Schools in the early 1930s. In 1939 the school was one of the original 51 that was used by the Committee on Accrediting of the NLNE to determine criteria for national accreditation.

Despite the rigors of running the school and the nursing-service department of the hospital, Burgess was active in local, state, and national nursing organizations. She helped to organize the State League of Nursing Education in 1920 and served as its president in 1922. She was appointed to the State Board of Nurse Examiners in 1921 and served until 1927. She served on committees of the district and state nurses' associations and attended the national NLNE and ANA conventions regularly. The Red Cross and Altrusa Club also benefited from her membership and committee work.

While Burgess never became a nationally known nursing leader, her influence on nursing and nursing education in Nebraska was immeasurable. Despite several serious illnesses and accidents, she strengthened the nursing education program at the university and provided strong support for nursing throughout the state.

In 1940 Burgess resigned her position as director of nursing, but no replacement could be found. Although she was now 75 years old, she agreed to stay and guided the hospital and school through another world war. On April 1, 1946, she ended her 29-year tenure at the age of 80; she retired to her family home in Vermillion, South Dakota, and enjoyed relatively good health for three years. Following a fall early in 1949, her health began to fail; she then suffered a stroke and died on July 31, 1949.

Burgess is remembered as a woman of limitless vision; a stern, formidable woman, yet a warm, fun-loving friend; a truly dedicated nurse educator; and a woman with high ideals for the profession of nursing. She encouraged all around her to do their best and often reminded her students that "university nurses have no equals."

BIBLIOGRAPHY

"Educator Dies at Vermillion." Obituary. *Sioux City Journal*, August 2, 1949.

"Miss Charlotte Burgess." *Nurse Reporter* (Official Publication of the University of Nebraska College of Nursing Alumni Association) XXII, No. 7 (October 1949): 1–4.

Schneckloth, N.W. *The University of Nebraska College of Nursing, 1917–1987.* Omaha: University of Nebraska Medical Center, 1987.

Schryver, G.F. *A History of the Illinois Training School for Nurses, 1880–1929.* p. 134. Chicago: Illinois Training School for Nurses, 1930.

Nancy Warren Schneckloth

Saint Frances Xavier (Mother) Cabrini

1850–1917

Frances Xavier Cabrini, foundress of the Missionnary Sisters of the Sacred Heart, established schools, orphanages, and hospitals for the relief of Italian immigrants in the United States.

On July 15, 1850, Maria Francesca Cabrini was born to Agostino and Stella Oldini Cabrini. She was the youngest of 13 children, of whom only three girls and a boy survived to adulthood. She was educated by her sister Rosa and in nearby Arluno by the Daughters of the Sacred Heart. In 1868 she received her teacher's license.

From an early age, Cabrini wanted to become a missionary in China, but because of her poor health, she was refused admission to the Daughters of the Sacred Heart. She taught for two years in the village school in Vidardo and then went to work in the House of Providence, an orphanage in Codogno. It was here that she started her religious vocation and, without joining a formal order, took her vows on September 14, 1877.

In November 1880 Bishop Gelmini of Lodi instructed Francesca to form a missionary order. With seven orphan daughters, Francesca found an abandoned convent in Codogno, and there founded the Missionary Sisters of the Sacred Heart on November 14, 1880.

Over the next few years, the order grew quickly. Convents were established in Grumello, Milan Casalpusterlengo, Borghetto Lodigiano, and Rome. On March 12, 1888, the order received papal approval by a Decretum Laudis (Decree of Praise).

Mother Cabrini met Bishop Giovanni Battista Scalbrini, founder of the Order of Missionaries for the Italian Immigrants and of the Congregation of St. Charles Borromeo of New York City. He encouraged her to send her missionary sisters to the United States to work with Italian immigrants who needed spiritual guidance, schools, orphanages, and medical care. Though sympathetic, she at first refused; she still felt her missionaries were to travel to China. Pope Leo XIII, however, informed her that it was his wish that she establish her missionaries among the Italians in the United States. Mother Cabrini and six nuns arrived in New York City on March 31, 1889. Financial assistance from Liugi Palma di Cesnola, director of the Metropolitan Museum of Art, allowed her to establish the American motherhouse and orphanage on East 59th Street.

In the spring of 1890 she acquired a 450-acre Jesuit farm in West Park, New York, and moved the orphanage to the country.

The order continued to grow. Convents and schools were established in New Orleans, London, Paris, Madrid, Nicaragua, Panama, Brazil, and Argentina.

Appalled by the lack of medical care for the poor, Mother Cabrini, in 1892, founded Columbus Hospital in New York City with 10 beds and little in the way of medical supplies or staff. By 1895 the institution had grown to a modern, 100-bed facility and was certified by the State of New York.

In 1905 she established a second Columbus Hospital in Chicago, and in 1916 the doors to Columbus Hospital in Seattle were opened.

Mother Frances Xavier Cabrini became a naturalized citizen of the United States in Seattle in 1909. In 1910 she was named Superior General for life. By the time of death on December 22, 1917, the Missionary Sisters of the Sacred Heart had 67 houses in Europe and the Americas and more than 1,500 members of the order. She was buried in West Park, New York at the order's cemetery on January 2, 1918. Her remains were later moved to the chapel of Mother Frances Xavier Cabrini High School in Fort Washington, New York City.

On November 13, 1938, Mother Frances Xavier Cabrini was beatified. She was canonized and became the first United States citizen to become a saint on July 7, 1946.

PUBLICATIONS BY SAINT FRANCES XAVIER CABRINI

BOOKS

Parole Sparse della Beata Cabrini. Compiled and edited by Giussepe de Lucca. Rome: Istituto Grafico Tiberino, 1938.

A Visit to Santa Catalina. Foreword by Francis J. Webster. Monterey, Calif.: Hilleary and Petko, 1979.

BIBLIOGRAPHY

Border, L.P. *Francesca Cabrini: Without Staff or Scrip.* New York: Macmillan, 1945.

Daughters of St. Paul. *Mother Cabrini.* Boston: St. Paul Editions, 1977.

Di Donato, P. *Immigrant Saint: The Life of Mother Cabrini.* New York: McGraw-Hill, 1960.

Martindale, C.C. *Mother Francesca Saverio Cabrini, Foundress of the Missionary Sisters of the Sacred Heart.* London: Burns Oates and Washbourne, 1931.

Maynard, T. *Too Small a World: The Life of Francesca Cabrini.* Milwaukee: Bruce, 1945.

Melville, A.M. "Cabrini, Saint Frances Xavier." In *Notable American Women 1607–1950,* Vol. 1, edited by E.T. James. Cambridge: Belknap Press of Harvard University Press, 1971.

Saveio de Maria, Madre, M.S.C. *Mother Frances Xavier Cabrini,* translated and edited by R.B. Green. Chicago: Missionary Sisters of the Sacred Heart of Jesus, 1984.

Sullivan, M.L. *Mother Cabrini: Italian Immigrant of the Century.* New York: Center for Migration Studies of New York, 1991.

Anne E. Clifford

Lillian (Bessie) Carter
1898–1983

Lillian Carter, better known as "Miss Lillian" was a registered nurse, a peace activist, and the outspoken mother of President Jimmy Carter. Always independent, Miss Lillian usually spoke her mind and followed her heart, sometimes to the delight of friends and well-wishers and the embarrassment of her son. With her bright blue eyes and toothy smile, she possessed the same combination of folksiness and strong moral principle that played such a large role in her son's early appeal.

Lillian Carter was born Bessie Lillian Gordy in the southwest Georgia town of Richland on August 15, 1898, the fourth of nine children of James Jackson Gordy and Mary Ida (Nicholson) Gordy. She asserted her independence soon after the Gordy family moved to nearby Plains in 1921. Depite her parents' objections, she began nurses training at Wise Hospital. She later explained, "I always wanted to be a nurse. I guess if I had my life to live over, I would realise that what I really wanted was to be a doctor." While working at the hospital, she met and became engaged to farmer-businessman James Earl Carter. With his encouragement, she went to Atlanta to complete her nurses training at Grady Memorial Hospital before the two were married on September 25, 1923. Their first child, Jimmy, was born in 1924, then Gloria in 1926, Ruth in 1929, and Billy in 1937.

Long before she earned international celebrity as First Mother of the White House, she was known in Georgia as a champion of civil rights. Throughout the 1920s and 1930s she continued to work as a nurse, often among the black population of Plains and nearby Archery. This astonished her neighbors and dismayed her conservative husband, who silently disapproved of his wife's violations of segregation's code of conduct. She regularly nursed the Carter's black farmhands and routinely received black visitors in her parlor. She later told an interviewer, "I've always had a feeling for the underdog, right or wrong. And I guess it's a fact that I'm just different. I'm not in the same mold as some of the people I know. I'm just different."

In the late 1940s the Carters moved from Archery back to Plains, where they became that town's premier family—active in church, community and politics. James Earl Carter, Senior, was elected to the state legislature in the early 1950s but died during his first term. Miss Lillian was shocked and lost. Her husband deceased, her children grown, and the peanut business in the hands of her eldest son, she decided on a mid-life career change. She moved to Alabama and for eight years served as housemother to the Kappa Alpha fraternity at Auburn University. She resigned in 1961 because she was "getting nervous over things," and she returned to Plains. Within months she was working again, managing a nursing and convalescent home in Blakely, Georgia. But she left that post two years later, complaining that most of the patients were younger than she was.

In 1966, while son Jimmy was making his first, unsuccessful try for the Georgia governorship, Lillian Carter, at age 67, began a project that symbolized her independence, her humanitarianism, and her indomitable spirit. Intrigued by a televised public service message for the Peace Corps, and taking seriously the claim that age was no barrier, she volunteered for the corps and requested assignment to India. Despite her children's misgivings, she was delighted to learn that she had been accepted. After several months of study and orientation in Chicago, she left for Vikroli, India, in December 1966 to begin work in the family-planning clinic of Godrej Industries, a complex of factories and mills about thirty miles from Bombay. She later explained her reasons for joining the corps and requesting assignment in India. "I was frustrated in the South. I wanted to go and work with people who were underdogs, and I realized why I had asked for India. I wanted a dark country with a warm climate."

The poverty and disease Carter encountered at the family-planning clinic at first overwhelmed her, especially because she was forbidden to treat anyone not associated with the factories. She became more and more despondent, hitting her lowest point after being prevented from helping a woman with terminal infectious leprosy who had been left to die at the side of a road. Reflecting on these days, she later told the Washington *Post*, "India was killing me. I just couldn't bear it. I couldn't touch the dirt, the blood, the lice, the leprosy. I hadn't the strength to bear the horrible cruelty and indifference." But one day, she climbed a nearby hill to pray for strength. "And Christ let something come into me, and I knew I could do anything. I could wipe up blood—and blood had always appalled me—and I could touch leprosy without running to scrub my hands. . . . I could stay in India."

She was later transferred to the factory complex's treatment clinic, where she set about trying to clean up the deplorable unsanitary conditions while also treating as many as 300 people a day. She gave injections, administered intravenous feedings, treated lepers, and even performed minor surgery. Galled by the rules preventing treatment of anyone not employed at the factory complex, she secretely gave bandages and drugs to the poor. She appealed to the factory owners, who finally allowed her to dispense medical supplies at her own expense. She persuaded friends back home to send contributions, and by pretending to know the presidents of several major pharmaceutical houses, she convinced them to donate drug supplies. Within a year, Miss Lillian, as she was known, was operating a well-stocked free clinic.

When her two-year tour of duty ended in 1968, Miss Lillian returned home weakened by her work and her virtually vegetarian diet. She had lost nearly 20 pounds. But she maintained till the end of her life that her work in India, "meant more to me than any other thing in my life. It strengthened my faith in God, and my relationship with minorities. Whether I did anything for the Indian people, they did so much for me."

In 1977 she returned to India as the official American representative to the funeral of Indian president Fukhruddin Ali Ahmed. After the ceremony she revisited Vikhroli, where she was greeted by the governor of Maharashtra and 7,000 cheering Indians. "I never knew you thought so much of me," she told the crowd. "But I give you my word, I was happier here than I am now in the President's place."

Miss Lillian was a good-will ambassador for the United States during her son's presidency, visiting India, Italy, West Africa, and Israel. For her efforts to heal the sick, feed the poor, and fight for peace, she became the first woman to receive the Covenant of Peace Award from the Synagogue Council of America in 1977. She also received the Ceres Medal from the Food and Agriculture Organization in 1978.

An inspiration to the nation's widowed and elderly, Lillian Carter continued to champion civil rights issues, women's causes, and senior citizens programs until the end of her life. At the age of 85 she died of cancer on October 30, 1983, in Americus, Georgia, and was buried in Plains, Georgia.

PUBLICATIONS BY LILLIAN CARTER

BOOKS

Away from Home: Letters to My Family. New York: Simon & Schuster, 1977.

In a Mirror Darkly. New York: Vantage Press, 1973.

Miss Lillian and Friends: The Plains, Georgia, Family Philosophy and Recipe Book. New York: A & W Publishers, 1977.

ARTICLES

With Mary Ostendorf. "The Awakening of Adolescent Femininity." *Journal of School Health* 40 (April 1970): 203–05.

BIBLIOGRAPHY

"Lillian Carter," *Contemporary Authors*, H. May ed., Detroit: Gale Research Co., 111: 96, 118: 81–83. 1984, 1986.

"Lillian Carter," *The Annual Obituary*, 1983, ed. by Elizabeth Devine. Chicago: St. James Press, 1984.

"Lillian Carter," *Current Biography*, ed. by Charles Mortiz. New York: H.W. Wilson Co., 1978.

"Lillian Carter," Obituary, Washington *Post*, Oct. 31, 1983.

Neyland, J. "Carter Family Scrapbook," *Good Housekeeping* 185 (July 1977): 100–05.

Stroud, K. *How Jimmy Won: The Victory Campaign from Plains to the White House.* New York: William Morrow, 1977.

Who's Who of American Women, 1981–82, Chicago: Marquis, 1982.

The Woman's Book of World Records and Achievements, ed. by Lois O. O'Neill, New York: Anchor Press, 1979.

David Curson

Martha Jenks Wheaton Chase

1851–1925

Martha J.W. Chase never studied nursing and never served as a volunteer nurse, yet she strongly influenced health care with the "sanitary" and "hospital" dolls that she designed and made for the purposes of demonstrating and practicing proper hygiene and basic nursing procedures.

Her influence was worldwide and prevailed long after her death.

Chase was born to Dr. James L. and Anna Maria (Jenks) Wheaton on February 12, 1851, in Pawtucket, Rhode Island, a city founded by one of her ancestors nine generations earlier. Both parents were community leaders. Her father, a prominent physician, was politically active, served as chairperson of the Pawtucket Committee on Education, was captain of the state's Bicycle Club, and was president of the Rhode Island Automobile Association. Her mother, who had organized aid projects during the Civil War, later further distinguished herself as a founder of the Homeopathic Hospital in Providence, founder of a girls club and president of several civic organizations in Pawtucket. The charitable activities of the Wheatons significantly influenced their daughter's developmental years.

At the age of 19, Martha was widowed by the death of her husband, Dr. William P. White. Four years later, in 1874, she married Dr. Julian A. Chase, who was associated with her father. After her new husband completed additional medical training in Vienna and Berlin, the couple settled in Pawtucket, where he established himself as a general practitioner. The Chases had seven children; a set of twins died young, but two sons and three daughters reached maturity.

As was customary for Victorian women, Chase devoted most of her early married years to domestic concerns and child rearing. Observations of her children at play led Chase to note that the then popular European dolls were usually too heavy or too fragile for their small hands. Consequently, she decided to make soft, lightweight fabric dolls. She added movable joints and realistic facial features, made them hygienically safe, and appropriate for both girls and boys. The results were so satisfactory that soon Chase was making the dolls for friends, relatives, and neighbors as well. On a trip to Boston's Jordan Marsh department store in 1891, where Chase had gone to outfit one of her dolls with clothes, an astute clerk asked Chase to make dolls that could be sold in the store. Chase's agreement to do so began a cottage industry that was set up in the family garage that eventually became known as the Doll's House. The dolls produced by Chase, however, were more than toys. They also were symbolic of emerging middle-class ideologies of motherhood and childhood—values that were at odds with industrialism and the culture of bourgeois luxury that it had created.

Further, Chase was keenly aware that industrialization had brought large numbers of young families into crowded cities where they, along with recent immigrants, experienced poverty, poor sanitation, and cramped tenement living. For both groups, the transition usually had separated them from the advice of more experienced family members who otherwise might have taught them mothering and child-rearing skills. Chase's concern for the health of the women and children in those settings, coupled with her commitment to the tenets of social reform, gave her work new direction. Consequently, in 1913, she introduced infant and child-size "sanitary" dolls for use in public demonstrations where such aspects of infant hygiene as feeding, dressing, and bathing were taught. The underlying social objective was to convey middle-class values of the home that would ultimately decrease child morbidity and mortality among the poor.

The "sanitary" dolls, however, were not the first that Chase made for educational purposes. In 1910, chiefly at the urging of Lauder Sutherland, then principal of the Hartford (Connecticut) Hospital Training School for Nurses, Chase made an adult-size mannequin on which basic nursing procedures could be demonstrated and practiced. The doll, which was based on Chase's personal body height and proportions, was tested at Pawtucket's Memorial Hospital and then sent to the Hartford Hospital Training School in 1911. There it served the many students who became the future's health-care providers, just as succeeding models of the mannequin became standard equipment for individuals in state health departments, the American

Red Cross, and schools of nursing around the world.

Indicative of the affectionate regard that the student nurses had for the adult-size mannequin are the names that they gave it. Examples are Josephine, Sally, and Arabella. More commonly, however, the mannequin was referred to as Mrs. Chase, though few knew why. The significance of the mannequin is also reflected in poems like the following, written by a Hartford Hospital School of Nursing graduate, Marguerite Manfreda, who had practiced nursing procedures on the original mannequin during her student nurse days.

MY DEAR MRS CHASE
(To the Chase Doll)

My dear Mrs. Chase of the cameo face
My dear Mrs. Chase you deserve this grace.

In the classroom you've been our faithful guide
So your fame in nursing will ever abide
Your history is one we can no longer hide
For we're destined to spread it far and wide.

Though we've bathed and pummelled you with treatments galore
And turned you until you must have been sore
You never once spoke or an angry look wore
As we practiced the nursing you made us adore.

You've been touched and observed to teach detection
Of the signs and symptoms of mankind's infections
You've had purposeful ails and many injections
That we gave to you with heart torn affection.

You are dearly beloved by all those in white
And students speak of you day and night
As they tell the Chase stories with girlish delight
You're a dear who will reach historical height.

My dear Mrs. Chase of the cameo face
My dear Mrs. Chase you deserve this grace.

Martha Jenks Wheaton Chase died in Pawtucket, Rhode Island, in August 1925. That her doll business, carried on by family members, survived until 1981 is a testament to the values that gave impetus and sustenance to her progressive era work.

BIBLIOGRAPHY

Bradshaw, M. *The Doll House: Story of the Chase Doll.* Privately published by the author, 1986.

Bourcier, P., and Formanek-Brunell, M. *Dolls and Duty: Martha Chase and the Progressive Agenda.* Providence: Rhode Island Historical Society, 1989.

Chase, R.D. Personal correspondence with author, January 30, 1978.

Herrmann, E.K. "The Chase Exhibition." *American Association for the History of Nursing Bulletin* (Winter 1990): 3.

Herrmann, E.K. "Mrs. Chase: A Noble and Enduring Figure." *American Journal of Nursing* 81 (October 1981): 1836.

Manfreda, M. "My Dear Mrs. Chase." Unpublished private papers. Wallingford, Conn., 1948.

Smith, L. "A Patient Patient." *American Journal of Nursing* 39 (January 1939): 27.

Eleanor Krohn Herrmann

Luther P. Christman
b. 1915

Luther P. Christman, the oldest of six children of Elmer and Elizabeth (Barincott) Christman, was born February 26, 1915, in Summit Hill, Pennsylvania. Christman grew up in a small town surrounded by mountains, thereby, he said, inspiring a lifelong love of nature. As a child, he was expected to do many household chores, and his free time was spent reading and taking long walks through the mountains. His walks and various readings helped develop his sense for poetry and art. As a youth of the Great Depression years, he was discouraged from pursuing a career in the arts by his family and friends. He realized the need for a profession that would provide well for his future in times of economic uncertainty.

On December 5, 1939, Christman married his high-school sweetheart Dorothy Mary Black. In the years to follow, they became parents of three children: Gary James Christman (also a nurse), Judith Ann Christman Kinney, and Lillian Jane Christman Blakely. Christman's reasons for becoming a nurse were clearly not part of a childhood fantasy. He wanted a profession that he and Dorothy could enjoy together. Both enrolled in nursing schools in Philadelphia. He graduated from the Pennsylvania School of Nursing in 1939, from the School of Nursing for Men, and Dorothy from the School of Nursing at the Methodist Hospital. Early in his nursing experience, Christman realized that men were a minority in the nursing profession and his training was jeopardized as a result of being part of this minority group. For example, he was unable to attend a rotation in maternity nursing due to his gender. As a result, Christman decided that a diploma from a hospital school was insufficient for him, and he subsequently enrolled in a collegiate program to advance his education and future opportunities.

Christman was a young graduate when World War II broke out. He deliberately confronted the fact that men in nursing who volunteered for the armed services would not be commissioned. At the time well over 1,200 male nurses had been drafted and yet were not allowed to serve in their professional capacity; rather they were delegated to nonnursing positions.

Christman volunteered his services requesting immediate and permanent assignment as a nurse to the front lines for the balance of the war. After receiving a condescending letter of rejection, Christman distributed copies of the letter to every U.S. senator as evidence of the inappropriate and inconsistent policy with regard to the nation's needs for nurses. Christman spent the remainder of the war

years (1943–45) as a pharmacist mate in the U.S. Maritime Service.

Except for his wartime duty, Christman spent from 1939–48 at Pennsylvania Hospital in Philadelphia working as a private-duty nurse and as an assistant head nurse. In 1948 he received his bachelor of science degree in nursing from Temple University, Philadelphia. He continued his education at Temple and in 1952 received a master of education in clinical psychology. Upon completion of his master's degree, he was offered a position as assistant dean of the School of Nursing at the University of Pittsburgh. However, he declined the opportunity, feeling he should be doctorally prepared for such a position. Christman later believed he should have taken the position, which would have greatly enhanced his career.

Upon completion of his bachelor's degree in nursing, Christman spent 1948–53 at Cooper Hospital School of Nursing, Camden, New Jersey, as an instructor of nursing, during which time he completed his graduate studies. He was firm in his beliefs of the need for an advanced educational program base for the profession. Nursing instructors were being taught at teacher's institutions, where they learned how to teach, but what should be taught was not emphasized. Nursing as a science was in danger of being overlooked.

Christman brought these ideas with him to his next appointment as director of nursing in Yankton State Hospital, Yankton, South Dakota. He spent from 1953–56 in this position. There he was involved in reorganizing the state mental health programs to enhance the quality of patient care. He also developed the "nurse-physician team" arrangement similar to what is now referred to as "primary nursing." Providing not only service, but also education, is a large part of his theory. Christman was appointed to the first national committee to study clinical practice funded by the National Institute of Mental Health at the graduate level.

In 1956 Christman left South Dakota to take a position as a nurse consultant for Michigan's Department of Mental Health in Lansing. His primary responsibility was to change the mental-health system of the state. He focused on the local state hospitals, training nurses for leadership and encouraging them to examine their own concepts of structure in order to improve the quality of nursing care. He became very active in the National League of Nurses (NLN) and the American Nurses' Association (ANA) and was elected president of the Michigan Nurses' Association (MNA). While president of MNA, he examined the economic status of nursing. At this same time, he enrolled in a doctoral program in sociology and anthropology at Michigan State University.

Christman left his nurse-consultant position with the Michigan Department of Mental Health in 1963 and moved on to the University of Michigan, Ann Arbor, as an associate professor of psychiatric nursing. He remained there from 1963–67. His main concentration of study was in examining the role of the nurse specialist. Between 1964 and 1967 Christman also held appointments while at the University of Michigan as a research associate for both the Institute of Social Research and Bureau of Hospital Administration. Here Christman developed his "Laws of Behavior." He completed his Ph.D. in sociology and anthropology in 1965.

During this period one of his ideas gained national recognition and support—the establishment of the American Academy of Nursing. At the 1964 ANA convention his resolution to set up the academy was overwhelmingly approved and passed by the House of Delegates. However, the American Academy of Nursing was not formally initiated until January 31, 1973, with the adoption of a resolution by the ANA Board of Directors designating 36 charter fellows as pro-tem officers. Christman, however, was not inducted into the academy until 1974.

In 1967 Christman had accepted a position at Vanderbilt University, Nashville, Tennessee. There between 1967 and 1972 he served as dean of nursing, professor of nursing, professor of sociology for the College of Arts and Science, and also the director of nursing at Vanderbilt University Hospital. His appointment at Vanderbilt was the first time a man had been named dean of a university school of nursing.

While at Vanderbilt, Christman continued to expand his practitioner-teacher model, developing nursing as an applied science.

Also, he was nominated for president of the American Nurses' Association. Though well qualified, Luther P. Christman was not elected ANA president. This was one of a series of disappointments that were clearly perceived to be gender-related experiences in a female-dominated profession.

In 1972 Christman accepted a position at Rush University, Chicago, as vice-president of nursing affairs and the John L. and Helen Kellogg dean of the College of Nursing. Other appointments included professor of sociology in the College of Medicine and in 1976, professor of sociology in the College of Health Sciences. It was at Rush that his ideas could be realized at last. Christman was very influential in placing the practitioner-teacher role model into effect. The emphasis was on higher education from the undergraduate level to doctorally prepared nurses. Clinical practice, teaching, research, consultation were all elements of the program. While at Rush, Christman and Michael Counte published two books: *Interpersonal Behavior and Health Care* and *Hospital Organization and Health Care Delivery.*

Christman's main contribution to the profession has been his consistent emphasis on clinical competence as the raison d'être for the nursing profession. He speaks of the "reluctant dragon theory," the slow but steady acceptance of the baccalaureate as the basic degree— and the need for master's level specialization.

Christman's faith in clinical competence is guided by his inclusive definition of the term: "Clinical practice is not just being a scientist; it's the empirical management of issues and workloads and delivery of care that are as important as anything else."

Luther P. Christman's pioneering contributions to nursing have not gone unnoticed. He has received numerous awards and honors and has contributed a generous amount of time to many different organizations. He was instrumental in establishing the American Assembly for Men in Nursing in 1971, and he served as its "permanent chairman" while at Rush. However, even though Christman worked his way through the ranks, much of his work has only recently been appreciated. His visibility and controversial challenges to the nursing profession has provoked reactions and responses that have touched on every aspect of his career.

He considers himself to be a "minority member" of a female-dominated profession and as such can readily cite examples of discrimination suffered because he is a man who happens to be a nurse, such as being refused a daytime position as an administrator because the patients were not to know there was a male on staff. He feels his educational training suffered by being limited, i.e., unable to care for certain female patients.

Christman has accomplished much in spite of negative reactions from some peers who do not feel comfortable with nursing as a gender-free profession. The artificial constraints of being a man in a woman's profession has only strengthened his resolve to be a "free agent." His persistence over the years and his productivity has served him well. A select list of some of the numerous awards and honors received by him include:

Fellow of the American Academy of Nursing, 1974

Fellow of Institute of Medicine of Chicago, 1974–

Named outstanding male nurse in the nation by the National Association of Male Nurses, 1975

Visiting fellow of New Zealand Nurses Educational and Research Foundation, 1978

Certificate of appreciation from the Veterans Administration, 1980

D.H.L. from Thomas Jefferson University, 1980

Nursing award from the Council of Specialists in Psychiatric and Mental Health, 1980

Edith Moore Copeland Founders Award for Creativity Sigma Theta Tau, 1981

Named distinguished practitioner by the National Academics of Practice, 1985

Old Master Award from Purdue University, 1985

Jesse M. Scott Award from American Nurses' Association, 1988

Trustees medal, Rush-Presbyterian-St. Luke's Medical Center, 1990

In 1991 Luther Christman resided in Chapel Hill, Tennessee, with his family.

PUBLICATIONS BY LUTHER P. CHRISTMAN

BOOKS

With Michael Counte. *Hospital Organization and Health Care Delivery.* Boulder, Col.: Westview, 1981.

With Michael Counte. *Interpersonal Behavior and Health Care.* Boulder, Col.: Westview, 1981.

ARTICLES (SELECTED)

"The Nursing Team in a Psychiatric Setting." *Nursing Outlook* 4 (January 1956): 53–54.

"Nurse-Physician Communications in the Hospital." *Journal of the American Medical Association* 194 (November 1, 1965): 539–44. Reprinted in *International Nursing Review* 13 (July–August 1966): 48–57.

"Knowledge, Change and Nursing Care." *American Journal of Nursing* 66 (September 1966): 2627–29.

"What the Future Holds for Nursing." *Nursing Forum* 9 (1970): 12–18.

"Education of the Health Team." *Journal of the American Medical Association* 213 (July 13, 1970): 284–85. Reprinted in *Selected Papers from the 66th Annual Congress on Medical Education,* Chicago, February 8–9 (published January 1971).

"Men in Nursing—One Means to Efficiency in Patient Care." *Pennsylvania Nurse.* 25 (September 1970): 6.

"The Nurse Specialist as a Professional Activist." *Nursing Clinics of North America* 6 (June 1971): 231–35.

"The Autonomous Nursing Staff in the Hospital." *National Joint Practice Commission Bulletin* 2 (October 1976). Reprinted in *Nursing Administration Quarterly* 1 (Fall 1976): 37–44.

"On the Scene: Uniting Service and Education at Rush-Presbyterian-St. Luke's Medical Center, the Division of Nursing and the College of Nursing: An Overview." *Nursing Administration Quarterly* 3 (Spring 1979): 7–13.

With Robert L. Bracken. "An Incentive Program Designed to Develop and Reward Clinical Competence." *Journal of Nursing Administration* 8 (October 1978): 8–18.

With Ralph Kirkman. "A Significant Innovation in Nursing Education." *Peabody Journal of Education* 50 (October 1972).

BIBLIOGRAPHY

Contemporary Authors. Vol. 24. H. May and S.M. Trosky, eds. Detroit: Gale, 1988.

Lysaught, J.P. *A Luther Christman Anthology. Nursing Digest* 6, No. 2 (Summer 1978).

Schoor, T.M., and A. Zimmerman. *Making Choices, Taking Chances: Nurse Leaders Tell Their Stories.* St. Louis: Mosby, 1988.

Who's Who in American Nursing, 1988–1989. J. Franz, ed. Society of Nursing Professionals. Owings Mills, Md.: National Reference Press, 1989.

Ann-Marie Hurley

Ellen Evalyn Church (Marshall)

1904–1965

Ellen Evalyn Church Marshall conceived the idea of nurses serving as airline stewardesses and was the first nurse to be employed in this capacity. She also served as one of the early flight nurses during World War II.

Church was born on September 22, 1904, at Vernon Springs, Iowa, to Gaius Windsor and Isabella Johnstone Church. She had one brother, Frank.

She was graduated from Cresco (Iowa) High School and entered the University of Minnesota School of Nursing in Minneapolis in September 1923. At the time the school offered a three-year nursing program, and she graduated in June 1926. Church later returned to the university and earned her B.S. degree in 1936.

After completing the nursing program in Minneapolis, she returned to her hometown of Cresco and served for a short time as a school nurse and later as an office nurse. In 1927 she went to Tucson, Arizona, where she worked for a year as a staff nurse in the Desert Sanatorium.

She then moved to San Francisco, where she was an instructor at the French Hospital. She also took flying lessons, and her interest in flying led her to explore ways of combining flying with nursing. She learned that Boeing Air Transport (predecessor to United Airlines) was considering the employment of men as flight attendants. She discussed her idea of women in this position with Steve Stimson, head of Boeing's San Francisco office, and convinced him that having nurses on board would reassure nervous passengers. In the early days of flying, most passengers fit this category.

Simpson got in touch with William Boeing, a company director, and eventually the company agreed to a three-month trial. On the first flight, May 15, 1930, Church was the stewardess on a three-engine plane that carried 11 passengers. Flights were rough in unpressurized cabins with frequent stopovers at barren airstrips.

Church was responsible for finding the first eight stewardesses employed by the company, not an easy task when most people were afraid to fly. And the early stewardesses were not always welcomed by the other airline employees. But they soon proved their worth, and passengers liked the service. The stewardesses were expected to help load and unload baggage, check tickets, serve food, and aid air-sick passengers, but they did not have to serve alcoholic beverages in early days of flying; prohibition was still in force.

Church also helped establish requirements for the stewardesses. They were to be unmarried registered nurses, under 25 years of age, weigh no more than 115 pounds, and no taller than 5 feet 4 inches.

At first the stewardesses wore their nursing caps and white smocks. Church helped select the first stewardess uniform: a tailored green suit with a grey blouse, a green tam, and a matching full-length cape (planes were unheated).

After 18 months as a stewardess, Church was grounded as the result of injuries that she received in an automobile accident. She then did a brief stint of psychiatric nursing at Livermore Sanitarium, Livermore, California, before returning to Minneapolis for a postgraduate course in pediatric nursing at the Eustis Children's Hospital of the University of Minnesota.

While completing requirements for her degree, she worked as nurse in the nursery school and kindergarten of the university's Institute of Child Welfare.

In 1936 she accepted a position as pediatric nursing supervisor at the Milwaukee County General Hospital in Milwaukee, Wisconsin. In this position she was responsible for teaching student nurses. Available records indicate that she was a respected, effective teacher, one with considerable leadership ability. After four years, she left Milwaukee to become director of nursing at the Children's Free Hospital in Louisville, Kentucky.

Church joined the U.S. Army Nurse Corps on December 5, 1942, and was one of the first 25 nurses trained at a special school for flight nurses at Bowman Field, Kentucky. She served with a troop carrier command, evacuating the wounded from North Africa, Sicily, France, and Belgium to military hospitals elsewhere. For her outstanding service she was awarded the Air Medal. During the last 20 months of her military career, she taught at the air evacuation school at Randolph Field, Texas. She attained the rank of captain and was released from military duty on June 18, 1946.

She returned to Children's Hospital in Louisville for a short time, then was employed at the Sherman Hospital, Elgin, Illinois. In 1951 she was awarded a master's degree in nursing administration from the University of Chicago. That year she went to Union Hospital in Terre Haute, Indiana, as director of nursing and the following year was named hospital administrator, a position she held until 1965. Here her accomplishments included improving working conditions for employees, increasing the nursing staff, and planning and having built a new psychiatric wing.

She and Leonard Briggs Marshall, president of the First National Bank, Terre Haute, were married at the Irvington Presbyterian Church in Indianapolis September 11, 1964. Less than a year later, on August 27, 1965, Church died during surgery, after a severe head injury sustained in a horseback riding accident.

In 1965 Church received the Amelia Earhart Award for her contributions to aviation. Two years after her death United Airlines dedicated an addition to its stewardess-management training center in Chicago as the Ellen Church Marshall Memorial Wing. A bronze statue of her is prominently displayed in the lobby. The company also had a bronze plaque made recognizing her as "humanitarian, war heroine, and aviation pioneer." A copy of the plaque was sent to 25 airlines in various parts of the world for their flight-attendant training centers and to the Union Hospital, Terre Haute, where it hangs on the wall of the reception room. The bust and plaque were the work of New York artist Rene Shapshak. And the airport in her hometown of Cresco, Iowa, bears her name.

Church was a creative person who made many contributions to nursing. She will be best remembered for her innovative idea for airline stewardesses, opening a new career for nurses and eventually for other women.

PUBLICATIONS BY ELLEN EVALYN CHURCH (MARSHALL)

"Air-Minded Nursing." University of Minnesota School of Nursing *Alumnae Quarterly* 13:3, in *Remembering Things Past: An Heritage of Excellence*, edited by B. Canedy. Minneapolis: University of Minnesota, 1983.

"Nursing Up in the Air." *Public Health Nursing* 23 (February 1931): 73–74.

BIBLIOGRAPHY

"Awards to Army Nurses." *American Journal of Nursing* 46 (May 1946): 345

"Building Named in Honor of First Air Stewardess." *Terre Haute Tribune*, October 25, 1967.

Church, E. File. University of Minnesota School of Nursing, Minneapolis, Minnesota.

Church, E. Personnel record. Milwaukee County Medical Complex, Milwaukee, Wisconsin.

"Church, Ellen E." *Who's Who of American Women, 1961–62*. Chicago: Marquis, 1961.

"Flying—A New Field For Nurses." *Trained Nurse and Hospital Review* LXXVII (August 1931): 195.

Marshall, E.C. File. Union Hospital, Terre Haute, Indiana.

"They were the First (Airline Stewardesses)." *American Journal of Nursing* 75 (September 1975): 1550.

"This is the Army." *Bulletin of the Wisconsin State Nurses' Association* 12 (September 1944): 15.

"Whatever became of . . . (Ellen Church)." *Hospitals* 31 (August 16, 1957): 16.

Signe S. Cooper

Martha Jane Clement

1888–1959

Martha Jane Clement was an army nurse who spent more than 28 years in the service, rising through the Army Nurses Corps to the rank of lieutenant colonel and the position of director of the Army Nurses Corps in the Southwest Pacific during World War II.

Born June 11, 1888, she attended the Southern Illinois Hospital School of Nursing in Anna. After her graduation she did private-duty nursing and then joined the staff of Pacific Hospital, Missoula, Montana. In 1918 she received an appointment in the Army Nurses Corps and was first assigned as an army nurse at Base Hospital, Camp MacArthur, Waco, Texas. This was followed by tours of duty at General Hospital No. 31, Carlisle, Pennsylvania; Base Hospital, Fort Sam Houston, Texas; and Army and Navy General Hospital, Hot Springs, Arkansas. She briefly resigned from the corps to be married, but after her husband's death in 1924, she was back in the army and on duty at Walter Reed General Hospital in Washington, D.C. She remained in Washington until 1929, when she was transferred to the Philippines and served at Sternberg General Hospital, Manila, and at Station Hospital, Fort Mills. Returning to the United States in 1931, she reported once again to Walter Reed Hospital, where she remained until 1938, when she was transferred to Langley Field, Virginia. There she was promoted to chief nurse, first lieutenant, and charged with opening the Air Force Hospital at Langley Field. She remained in Virginia until 1942.

Sent to the Pacific in October 1942, Clement was promoted to captain and assigned to the headquarters of the U.S. forces in Australia as director of the Army Nurses Corps Southwest Pacific Theater of Operations. Her duties expanded so that she eventually commanded 4,000 nurses operating in 87 hospitals. New hospitals were set up as troops occupied island after island. In March 1943 she was promoted to the rank of lieutenant colonel. Clement shuttled by plane to each of the island outpost hospitals and affectionately became known as "Ma" Clement to thousands of soldiers wounded in combat.

The nurses that arrived in Australia with Lieutenant Colonel Clement in 1942 were the first nurses in that theater. The hospital they set up went into operation one week after their landing and provided care to American and Australian troops who returned from the Middle East. Late in 1942 the hospital was ordered to New Guinea. This unit of doctors, nurses, enlisted men, and Red Cross social workers—the first on that island—set up their tent hospital, and in less than a week the wards were filled. During the first few months Clement and her nurses coped with torrential rain that rushed through their tents washing their shoes away and leaving them knee-deep in mud as they each tended 250 to 300 patients. General Douglas MacArthur cited the unit for its treatment of casualties from the Battle of Buna, and the chief surgeon's office reported that Clement's unit had the highest morale of any unit in New Guinea. The nurses who served under Clement were nearly unanimous in their desire to remain in the Southwest Pacific as long as there was still combat nursing to be done.

Lieutenant Colonel Martha Jane Clement retired in 1946 after more than 28 years of service. She died on October 10, 1959, and was buried in Arlington National Cemetery with full military honors.

BIBLIOGRAPHY

"Captain Clement in Australia." *American Journal of Nursing* 42 (1942): 1081.

"Directors of Nursing Service in Five War Areas." *American Journal of Nursing* 43 (1943): 684.

"I'd Take Combat Duty Again." *American Journal of Nursing* 44 (1944): 676.

"Martha Jane Clement." Obituary. *New York Times*, October 11, 1959.

"Nurse Dietitians in the Southwest Pacific." *American Journal of Nursing* 44 (1944): 601.

"With Army and Navy Nurses." *American Journal of Nursing* 43 (1943): 505.

David Carson

Anna Laura Cole

b. 1909

Anna Laura Cole was a significant figure in Texas nursing as director of nursing in a hospital, as a teacher, as a member of the Board of Nurse Examiners, and as a Texas voice on various national nursing committees.

Born in Turney (Cherokee County), Texas, on October 27, 1909, to Laura Priestly and Thomas Lewis Cole, Anna Laura Cole was the youngest of eight children—five boys and three girls. She first became interested in nursing as a career when as a teenager she became a patient at Baylor Hospital. After graduating from high school in Gallatin, Cole enrolled in Lon Morris Junior College in Jacksonville. She attended the community college for a year before enrolling in the Scott and White Hospital Training Program in Temple, from which she received her diploma in 1931. Among her teachers was Helen Nahm. Upon graduation she was appointed assistant director of nurses at the Scott and White Hospital and in 1933 director, a position she held for some 36 years.

Cole continually upgraded her education, and in 1941 she was the first person to be awarded a bachelor of science in nursing education from the University of Texas at Austin. Technically, there were two nurses in the first class, but since her name was first alphabetically, she claimed the right to be first. Cole then went on to attend several summer sessions at the University of Chicago program in nursing although she never completed the master's degree there.

Cole served for eight years as a member of the Texas Board of Nurse Examiners, and when vocational nurses began to be licensed in Texas, she was also appointed to the first Board of Vocational Nurse Examiners. She was elected secretary of the Texas League for Nursing and served on the national committee of the National League for Nursing. She was also active in the district, state, and national affairs of the American Nurses' Association. Under her leadership the Scott and White Hospital School of Nursing became a part of a college system of nursing shortly before her retirement. Among her many honors was being named the Outstanding Citizen in Temple in the early 1960s and recognition as a distinguished alumna of the Scott and White Hospital School of Nursing. In 1989 the Anna Laura Cole Lectureship in Nursing was established at the Scott and White Memorial Hospital. In June 1990 the Texas Senate passed a resolution in her honor, and in Temple the mayor designated June 23, 1990, as Anna Laura Cole Day. After her retirement Cole worked with a committee of alumnae to prepare a history of the school of nursing.

PUBLICATIONS BY ANNA LAURA COLE

And others. *Sixty-Six Years Remembered.* Waco, Texas: Texian Press, 1976.

BIBLIOGRAPHY

Cole, A.L. Interviews with the author.

Laverne Gallman

Charity E. Collins

1882–?

Charity E. Collins was a public-health nurse and school nurse in Atlanta, Georgia. She was the first black nurse appointed to the Atlanta Health Department.

Collins, who was probably born in Atlanta, was educated in Atlanta at Spelman Seminary and the MacVicar Hospital Nurse-Training School, from which she graduated in 1906. At some time she was married to a Mr. Miles. Until 1911 she worked as a private-duty nurse and then was appointed to the Atlanta Health Department as a public-school nurse. At that time there was one doctor, nine schools, and 4,000 children in the public-school system. She served the Health Department for her entire career, contributing to the growth of community health programs, such as school oral hygiene and health education, prenatal clinics, and child-health clinics. In addition, she gave special service during the influenza epidemic of 1918, for which she received a certificate of commendation from Surgeon-General Rupert Blue.

In 1919 she sought and was granted registration without examination by the Georgia State Board of Nurse Examiners.

Collins was active in nursing during a time of national interest in public health, particularly in the areas of maternal, infant, and child health.

BIBLIOGRAPHY

Bullough, V. and B. Bullough. *The Emergence of Modern Nursing.* Toronto: Macmillan, 1969.

Dock, L. *A History of Nursing, Vol. III.* New York: Putnam, 1912.

Thoms, A.B. *Pathfinders: A History of the Progress of Colored Graduate Nurses.* New York: Garland, 1985.

Marianne Brook

Hazel Corbin

1895–1988

Hazel Corbin was a pioneer in maternal- and infant-health care. She was noted for her efforts to upgrade such care through demonstration projects, education of parents, and research. She had a special concern for the role of the father and, in 1939,

published a popular book, *Getting Ready to Be a Father.* She was general director of the Maternity Care Association of New York City from 1923–65, during which time the association published many teaching aids that were used worldwide. Corbin was an advocate of natural child-birth and of nurse midwifery, and she shepherded the development of a certification program for this profession. She also assisted in founding the International Childbirth Education Association.

Corbin was born in Nova Scotia and spent her early life there. At the onset of World War I, she decided to become a nurse and went to New York City to seek training. She studied nursing at Brooklyn Hospital. At that time the Women's City Club of New York City was becoming actively concerned about high rates of infant and maternal mortality in certain parts of the city. The organization established its first maternity center in 1917, and Corbin became its first field nurse and later also trained other nurses. She served for a time as nurse in charge at the Brooklyn Maternity Center.

In January 1918 two more centers were organized, and in April the Maternity Nursing Center Association (MCA) was founded to set up more centers in Manhattan. Corbin became assistant director in 1922 and director in 1923. At that time President Calvin Coolidge had withdrawn funds for child-welfare programs. The MCA offered a range of services designed to fill that gap partially. It published instructional materials, loaned exhibits, sent press releases, held classes for prospective parents, and trained nurses and nurse midwives. One of its clinics prepared nurse midwives for service in isolated places. In cooperation with New York Hospital and Columbia University Teachers College, MCA presented courses that would help nurses organize maternal-care programs in their own communities.

During 1939 and 1940 the MCA worked with two food manufacturers to present an exhibit on safe maternity in the Hall of Man at the New York World's Fair. Life-size sculptures of a developing fetus were shown, and over 1.4 million pamphlets were distributed to over 1 million visitors. Afterward, a book of photographs of the sculptures became one of the association's most popular publications.

Corbin also helped to develop nurse-midwife certification programs at Columbia University, Yale University, the Johns Hopkins University, and the State University of New York Downstate Medical Center. Corbin was part of a group who founded the Association for the Promotion and Standardization of Midwifery in 1934 and affiliated it with the MCA.

Outside the field of maternal and infant nursing care, Corbin also had wide influence. In 1936 she was an organizer of the Public Health Association in New York City and during World War II she recruited nurses in New York for the American Red Cross.

After Corbin retired in 1965, the MCA established the Hazel Corbin Fund to assist nurses aspiring to careers in nurse midwifery. In 1966 she received the American Public Health Association Martha May Eliot Award and in 1968 the MCA Medal for Distinguished Service, the organization's highest award.

Corbin died on May 18, 1988, of cardiac failure, at her retirement home in New Smyrna Beach, Florida.

PUBLICATIONS BY HAZEL CORBIN

BOOKS

Getting Ready to Be a Father. New York: Macmillan, 1939.

ARTICLES

"Maternity Nursing." *Trained Nurse* 82 (March 1929): 345–48.

"What Result—Maternity Nursing?" *Public Health Nursing* 28 (September 1936): 730–31.

"Safe Maternity for All." *Public Health Nursing* 37 (June 1945): 289–93.

"A Nurse Looks Ahead." *American Journal of Obstetrical Gynecology* 51 (June 1946): 811–18.

"Modern Obstetrical Nursing." *American Journal of Nursing* 46 (August 1946): 535–37.

"Nurse Midwives—the Torch Bearers." *Public Health Nursing* 44 (September 1952): 499–501.

"Maternity Nursing Education—Yesterday, Today and Tomorrow." *Nursing Outlook* 7 (February 1959): 82–84.

BIBLIOGRAPHY

"Hazel Corbin, Health Expert, Is Dead at 93." *New York Times*, May 20, 1988.

Log 1915–1980. New York: Maternity Center Association, n.d.

Pennock, M.R. *Makers of Nursing History.* New York: Lakeside, 1940.

Alice P. Stein

Pearl Parvin Coulter
b. 1902

In 1962 Pearl Parvin Coulter was awarded the Pearl McIver Public Health Nurse Award from the American Nurses' Association for her contributions to public-health nursing. She was born in Almyra, Arkansas, on August 19, 1902, to Isaac Newton and Joye (Lehman) Parvin. She attended the University of Denver in Denver, Colorado, where she majored in biology, psychology, and education, receiving her A.B. in 1926 and her M.S. in 1927. She taught in a small rural school in Idaho for a year and then accepted a position in an elementary school in Canon City, Colorado, where she remained for one year. Coulter married Samuel Monds Coulter on May 29, 1929. After teaching sciences in the public schools in Idaho and Colorado, she returned to the university setting as a graduate assistant in botany at the University of Denver.

Because of Coulter's strong science background and her interest in community health, she entered nursing and received her diploma in 1935 from the University of Colorado in Boulder. She then attended George Peabody College for Teachers in Nashville, Tennessee, in 1936 to become a certified public-health nurse. She began her career as a staff nurse for the Colorado Visiting Nurse Association and left this job to accept an appointment as assistant professor at George Peabody

College in a demonstration project involving a public-health nurse and a nursery school. She later was promoted to the rank of associate professor. The George Peabody program was for nurses who wanted their certificate in public-health nursing.

Coulter was also responsible for the health of a twelve-grade facility and a nursery school where education majors did practice teaching under master's prepared teachers.

Coulter next took a position as educational director of public-health nursing at the Nashville Health Department. She remained in this position where she was responsible for black students enrolled in a five-year degree nursing program at the Hubbard School of Nursing, associated with Fisk University in Nashville. Coulter also supervised these students at the Health Department, and in her spare time continued to teach nursing courses on the Peabody campus.

From 1943 to 1957 she directed and taught in the public-health nursing program at the University of Colorado, where she demonstrated her talent and insight as a public-health nurse educator by developing a new educational model for teaching public-health nursing. Coulter described the program in a letter to a former student as follows: "The unique thing about our field teaching program was the assignment of a full-time faculty member to the field unit to assume responsibility of teaching Public-Health Nursing students." In the late 1940s this was considered futuristic and innovative for nursing education.

As a full professor of nursing, in 1957 she accepted an invitation to start a new baccalaureate nursing program at the University of Arizona, Tucson, where she served until 1973, when she retired as dean emeritus. The Arizona nursing program was housed in the basement of the home-economics building, and from that early beginning, under Coulter's careful guidance, grew into a nationally recognized baccalaureate nursing program, as a college with its own building and for which Coulter served as dean from 1964 to 1967. The program included Coulter's

model for teaching public-health nursing, with a large block of practicum time devoted to community-health nursing and centered on the family in the community. Coulter's book, *The Nurse in the Public Health Program*, published in 1954, explained her model and set a new standard for collegiate nursing education in public-health nursing. This model was adopted by many programs throughout the United States and Canada. As the program grew, Coulter had the vision to "mentor" an extremely talented young faculty member, Gladys Sorensen, for the dean's position. When Coulter retired, Sorensen assumed leadership for the College of Nursing.

Coulter was not only committed to collegiate nursing education, but also to establishing high standards of nursing practice. When she discussed professional practice and responsibility, she demonstrated her beliefs through her participation in the state nurses' associations in Colorado and Arizona, in which she held numerous offices on the executive committees. Coulter was also active in the National Organization for Public Health Nursing prior to its merger with the American Nurses' Association. She maintained her professional involvement within the American Nurses' Association by serving as second vice-chairman of the Public Health Nurses Section. In May 1970 she was recognized by the American Nurses' Association for her outstanding contributions to nursing and received the Honorary Membership Award. She also served on the board of directors of the American Journal of Nursing Company and was a member of the Executive Committee for the Council on Higher Education for Nursing of the Western Interstate Commission for Higher Education. Her expertise in public-health nursing gained her positions on the National Advisory Committee on Public Health Training and on the Nursing Advisory Panel on Vocational Rehabilitation for the Public Health Service. Because of her commitment to maintain nursing standards and the respect of her colleagues, she served as a board member for ten years and as President of the Arizona State Board of Nurse Registration and Nursing Education from 1963 to 1964. Coulter worked within the National League for Nursing as a board member and as a member of the Task Force on Organizational Structure. Her colleagues within the profession and within academia recognized her outstanding contributions. She was the recipient of two honorary doctor of science degrees, one from the University of Colorado in May 1970 and the other from the University of Arizona in May 1983.

Pearl Parvin Coulter, with her piercing blue eyes, unwavering demeanor, and silver-gray hair, demonstrated her commitment to excellence in professional nursing. From 1956 to 1967 she published 13 articles, a monograph, a pamphlet, and a book. On one occasion she was asked by a prospective nursing student what she would do if she did not like "hospital nursing." Coulter replied, "Why public-health nursing is my first choice anyway. I never considered anything else." She served as a mentor, educator, and, above all, a public-health nurse. Coulter challenged her faculty and students to strive for excellence and personally set the standard. She retired to Sun City, Arizona, where she is currently writing a history of the College of Nursing at the University of Arizona. Her legacy is the students who learned from her, the colleagues who worked with her, and the results of her efforts to promote the education of nurses and the health of the community.

PUBLICATIONS BY PEARL PARVIN COULTER

BOOKS

The Nurse in the Public Health Program. New York: Putnam, 1954.

MONOGRAPHS

The Winds of Change: A Progress Report of Regional Cooperation in Collegiate Nursing Education in the West, 1956–1961. Western Interstate Commission for Higher Education, 1963.

With Anelia Leino. *Validation of the Collegiate Nursing Curriculum through Use of the Critical Incident.* Laramie: Publication Section, Division of Adult Education and Community Service, University of Wyoming, December 1965.

ARTICLES

"Newer Trends in Nursing Education." *The Florida Nurse* (March–April 1958): 9–11.

"The Value of the Health Council in Program Development." *Military Medicine* (November 1958).

"New Ways in Patient Care—Implications for Nursing Education." Proceedings, Third Annual Conference, Western Council on Higher Education for Nursing. *Conference Proceedings.* March 1960.

"The Teaching-Learning Process in Nursing Education." *Nursing Outlook* (October 1960): 575–578.

"Continuing Education Program for Nurses in the West." *Nursing Outlook* (February 1962): 113–117.

"Know All Things—Serve All People." *Arizona Medicine* (February 1962): 3.

"Inservice and Continuing Education for Nurses." *Hospital Progress* (December 1963): 72–82.

"Watch Them Grow." *Arizona Nurse* (September–October 1964): 13–15.

"Research and Education—A Symbiotic Relationship." *Arizona Nurse* (September–October 1965): 15–17.

"Recruitment in an Age of Change." In "This I Believe" section, *Nursing Outlook* (April 1966): 31–33.

"An Experiment in Preparation for the University of Arizona's Nursing College." *Arizona Nurse* (November–December 1966): 16–17.

"Programming for Nursing Service." *Nursing Outlook* (September 1967): 33–38.

With H. Erikson. "New Patterns for Field Instruction in Public Health Nursing." *Nursing Outlook* (February 1956): 76–79.

BIBLIOGRAPHY

Anglin, L.T. Material collections and personal reminiscence of a former student (Linda T. Anglin), Bradley University, Peoria, Illinois.

Coulter, Pearl. Personal communication, October 20, 1989; January 10, 1991.

Curriculum Vita, College of Nursing, University of Arizona, Tucson, Arizona.

"Mrs. Pearl Coulter Receives Nurse Award." *Tucson Daily Citizen*, June 27, 1962.

Unruh, J. Telephone interview with author, November 1, 1988; October 10, 1989.

Van Ort, S. Telephone interview with author, October 10, 1989.

Who's Who of American Women, Vol. 1, p. 279. Chicago: Marquis, 1958.

Linda T. Anglin

LeRoy N. Craig
1887–1976

Throughout his nursing career, LeRoy Nathaniel Craig was in the vanguard of political and educational activities promoting professional recognition and opportunity for men in nursing. He was instrumental in lobbying for, and ultimately obtaining, the passage of federal legislation that for the first time allowed male nurses to be commissioned as officers in the armed services at parity with female nurses. As a member of the National League of Nurses' Committee on Careers and as chairman of the Men Nurses' Section of the American Nurses' Association, he also championed unprecedented educational experiences and employment opportunities for men in the nursing profession.

Craig was born in Dixmont, Maine, in 1887, only 12 miles from the birthplace of another renowned American leader, Dorthea Dix. He completed a high-school education at Hampden Academy, Hampden, Maine, and at age 21 was accepted into the McLean Hospital Training School for Nurses, Waverley, Massachusetts. At McLean, which he attended from July 1909 to 1912, he was known as Roy. After graduating on January 4, 1912, he worked for approximately one year as a private-duty nurse and later as a head nurse at McLean Hospital, a private psychiatric hospital associated with the training school.

In 1914 he was appointed as the founding director and superintendent of nurses of the Men's Nursing Department of the Pennsylvania Hospital for Mental and Nervous Diseases, Philadelphia. He concurrently served as the first director of nurses at the Pennsylvania Hospital School of Nursing for Men and remained active in both of these positions until his retirement in 1956. While serving in these positions, Craig made a number of academic and political contributions to the nursing profession on both the local and national levels. His contributions were especially notable in issues related to recognition of the nursing needs of male psychiatric patients and in issues related to the education, recruitment, and retention of male nurses in the nursing profession.

During the 1940s and 1950s Craig wrote several journal articles that skillfully noted the contributions of male nurses.

Craig was concerned about the impact that a nursing shortage would have on the quality of patient care. The shortage of qualified nurses needed to meet patient needs, especially noticeable in urologic and psychiatric nursing practice at that time, was he felt, due both to an inability to attract men in adequate numbers to the nursing profession and to the attrition of male nurses who were not offered parity of professional status with their female counterparts in many areas of employment.

Craig was responsible for initially interesting Congresswoman Frances P. Bolton (Ohio) in the plight of male nurses in the armed services. These men were not allowed to receive an officer's commission, as did their female counterparts. Craig recognized that male nurses provided equal service and accepted equal responsibility yet were not given equal status and official recognition in the armed services. Almost 15 years of continued political activism was required to obtain passage of what became known as the Bolton Bill (H.R. 2559). This legislation authorized the appointment of qualified male nurses as commissioned officers. It was an amendment to the Army-Navy Nurse Act of 1947. Craig tirelessly lobbied on behalf of this legislation and was elated when the Bolton Bill was finally signed into law by President Eisenhower on August 9, 1955. Winifred Stanley, who became Craig's wife, was serving as a nurse recruiter for the Army Nurse Corps in Philadelphia during this period. Both she and Craig attended the swearing-in ceremony of one of the first men to be commissioned in the Army Nurse Corps as a result of the Bolton Bill.

During his 42-year tenure as director of nurses at the Pennsylvania Hospital School of Nursing for Men, Craig established innovations in the curriculum that reflected his belief that nursing educators should provide their students with a broad-based education within the recommended standards of the educational guidelines of the National League of Nurses. He also ensured that male nursing students were offered specialized courses that placed particular emphasis on psychiatric and urologic nursing. He believed that men nurses were particularly suited to provide genito-urinary and psychiatric nursing care to male patients, and such specialized curriculum would provide male nurses with expertise in these clinical areas. He consistently urged male nurse graduates to enter specialized areas of nursing practice and stressed opportunities in industrial, military, private-duty, psychiatric, and urologic nursing, which he felt provided the greatest employment opportunities for men nurses.

During World War II his prominence as a proponent for the inclusion of psychiatric nursing courses in nursing-school curriculum resulted in the selection of the Pennsylvania Hospital School for Men Nurses as one of the few schools of nursing to provide an intensive 12-week course of instruction in neuropsychiatry to navy corpsmen serving in naval hospitals. This was an early recognition that such psychiatric training would be invaluable for hospital personnel involved in treating war casualties.

Craig was held in high regard by the over 300 men nurses who graduated from the Pennsylvania Hospital School during his directorship. He was cited by his students for his skilled leadership in maintaining high standards of student selection and for his insistence on an academic program at the Pennsylvania Hospital School that promoted the personal and professional growth of his students.

In 1956 a citation from the Pennsylvania State Nurses' Association was presented to Craig in recognition of his numerous contributions to psychiatric nursing and for his efforts in introducing significant legislation that affected the status of men in nursing.

On October 27, 1976, Craig died at age 89 in the Lake Wood Nursing Home, in Pemberton, New Jersey.

Although Craig was most often involved with issues related to men nurses, his numerous professional activities ultimately enhanced equity in the professional recognition, education, and employment of all within the nursing profession.

PUBLICATIONS BY LEROY N. CRAIG

"History of the Pennsylvania Hospital School of Nursing for Men." *Asclepiad* (Pennsylvania Hospital School of Nursing for Men, Philadelphia) (1928): 46–47.

"Opportunities for Men Nurses." *American Journal of Nursing* 40 (June 1940): 666–70.

"The Man Nurse: II His Contribution in One Community." *Modern Hospital* 58 (January 1942): 63–64.

"Psychiatric Nursing for the Navy Hospital Corpsmen." *American Journal of Nursing* 44 (May 1944): 459–60.

"Men Nurses in Our National Planning." *Nursing Outlook* 2 (April 1954): 193–94.

"Another Goal Achieved." *Nursing Outlook* 4 (March 1956): 175–76.

BIBLIOGRAPHY

Archives of Pennsylvania Hospital. Philadelphia.

"LeRoy N. Craig, Pioneer Male Nurse." Obituary. *Philadelphia Inquirer*, November 26, 1976.

McLean Hospital Archives. Belmont, Massachusetts.

"More History in the Making." *Pennsylvania Hospital Bulletin* 12(3).

"Mr. Craig: Leader and Man." *Asclepiad* (Pennsylvania Hospital School of Nursing for Men, Philadelphia) (1928): 45.

Personal correspondence with Patricia O'Brien D'Antonio, Ph.D. candidate. University of Pennsylvania School of Nursing, Philadelphia.

"Testimonial Dinner." *Pennsylvania Hospital Bulletin* 13(5). (1957).

Karen L. Buchinger

Namahyoke Gertrude (Sockum) Curtis

1861–1935

Namahyoke Curtis served as a contract nurse during the Spanish-American War of 1898. She, like many other nurses who provided nursing care to American troops during the war, was not formally trained in nursing but was asked to provide such care due to the difficulty of recruiting adequate numbers of graduate nurses who could be presumed to have immunity to yellow fever and the many additional tropical diseases that were decimating American troops fighting in the war. Not only did Curtis render care to the troops during the conflict, but she also demonstrated the ability to recruit, organize, and lead over 30 additional black women whom she recruited as "immune nurses."

Namahyoke was descended from a family of mixed racial heritage. Her maternal grandmother was German, and her maternal grandfather was Afro-American. They met and married in California during the California Gold Rush of 1849. Namahyoke's mother married Hamilton Sockum, a Native American of the Aucome tribe. Namahyoke was the first of seven offspring. She was raised by an aunt, educated in the public-school system in San Francisco, and furthered her studies in Oakland, California where she attended Phelps Institute and graduated from Snell Seminary in 1888.

After graduation, Namahyoke went East to visit Native American relatives in Philadelphia, and met Austin Maurice Curtis, who was then a senior at Lincoln University. They were secretly married on May 5, 1888, when Namahyoke was 18 and Austin was 20. After their marriage, Namahyoke returned to California, and Austin started medical school at Northwestern University Medical School. The couple remained apart until their families discovered that the marriage had taken place and sent Namahyoke to rejoin her husband in Chicago.

While living in Chicago, Namahyoke displayed a keen interest in civic and charitable activities, especially those that were related to improvement in the welfare of the black community. Her social activism and natural political acumen were put to frequent use during the years the Curtises lived in Chicago. She was an instrumental figure in the successful efforts to found Provident Hospital in 1891 through her ability to interest Philip D. Armour, a prominent Chicago business-

man, in the movement to construct the hospital. Through his and other local contributions, adequate financial backing was achieved. This hospital was able to provide a high standard of medical care to the Chicago black community and served as an outstanding training facility for black nurses and physicians.

Namahyoke also became active in local, state, and national politics, including William McKinley's campaign for the Presidency. She held a number of politically appointed government positions while the Curtises lived in Chicago and Washington, D.C. She appeared to have a natural skill in the political arena. This was invaluable in generating support for the civic projects that she promoted.

Her husband, Austin Curtis, earned an M.D. from Northwestern University in 1891 and subsequently trained at Provident Hospital under the renowned black surgeon Dr. Daniel Hale Williams. He was also house physician at Provident from 1897–98. He served as the surgeon-in-chief and administrator of Freedmen's Hospital for four years, necessitating the relocation of the Curtis family from Chicago to Washington, D.C., in 1898. In succeeding years he was appointed as professor of surgery at Howard University and held that appointment for the remaining 40 years of his life.

Namahyoke and Austin Curtis were the parents of four children—Arthur L., Austin M., Jr., Merrill H., and Gertrude E. (Norris). All three sons became physicians.

In 1898, during the period immediately following Dr. Curtis's appointment as chief administrative officer at Freedmen's Hospital in Washington, D.C., Namahyoke Curtis was contacted by Dr. Anita Newcomb McGee, a public-health physician, to organize and lead a group of "immune nurses." These nurses were to assist in the care of American troops fighting in the Spanish-American War who had become ill with yellow fever and other tropical diseases. Namahyoke had already had yellow fever at an earlier point in her life, and she and the other black women she recruited were presumed to be immune to this disease.

Beginning on July 13, 1898, she was commissioned by the War Department as a contract nurse and sent by the surgeon general of the U.S. Army to several southern states, including Louisiana, Florida, and Alabama. Her initial task was to recruit the services of blacks living in those states who were immune to yellow fever and willing to work as contract nurses for the established rate of $30 a month plus a daily ration. Thirty-two black women were registered by Namahyoke Curtis for this service, a substantial proportion of the 80 black nurses who served as contract nurses during the Spanish-American War.

Namahyoke was given high official commendation for her work as a nurse during the war and for her leadership of the "immune nurses" she had recruited. The indispensable medical support that she and the other contract nurses provided contributed directly to the eventual acceptance of women as nurses in the armed services.

At the conclusion of the war, Namahyoke applied for, and later received, a lifetime government pension for the nursing service that she had rendered to the army under contract.

In 1900, during the Galveston Flood in Texas, she worked under the direction of Clara Barton as a Red Cross volunteer. In 1906 she carried another commission, from then Secretary of War William A. Taft, to provide assistance to victims in the San Francisco earthquake. She remained active in public service during World War I and was involved in obtaining military approval for a black officers' training camp at Fort Des Moines. After the Armistice she continued to promote numerous public projects.

Namahyoke Curtis died on November 25, 1935, and was buried in Arlington Cemetery with the nation's honored military dead in recognition of her service as a contract nurse in the Spanish-American War and her other government service.

During her funeral service, which took place in her home in Washington, D.C., on November 28, 1935, she was eulogized for her "unconquerable patriotism" as an American and for her lifelong activism in endeavors that enhanced the lives of black Americans.

BIBLIOGRAPHY

Carnegie, M.E. "Black Nurses at the Front." *American Journal of Nursing* 84 (October 1984): 1250–52.

Carnegie, M.E. *The Path We Tread: Blacks in Nursing, 1854–1984.* Philadelphia: Lippincott, 1986.

Dannett, S.G.L. *Profiles of Negro Womanhood.* Vol. II. Negro Heritage Library. Yonkers, N.Y.: Educational Heritage, 1966.

Elmore, J.A. "Black Nurses: Their Service and Their Struggle." *American Journal of Nursing* 76 (March 1976): 435–37.

Hine, D.C. *Black Women in White: Racial Conflict and Cooperation in the Nursing Profession 1890–1950.* Bloomington: Indiana University Press, 1989.

Leffall, L.D., Jr. "Austin Maurice Curtis." In *Encyclopedia of Black America.* W. A. Low, ed. New York: McGraw-Hill, 1981.

Mather, F.L. *Who's Who of the Colored Race.* Vol. I. New York: Gale, 1976.

Karen L. Buchinger

Emma D. Cushman

1860–1930

Emma D. Cushman was an American missionary nurse whose practice and exploits in the Near East during World War I earned her the designation of "humanitarian" by the *New York Times* as well as decorations from the Near East Foundation and the governments of France and Greece.

Cushman was born in Exeter, New York, and educated in New Berlin, New York. She was descended from an old American family; among her ancestors was Robert Cushman, who had chartered the *Mayflower.* She was a Congregationalist. Prior to becoming a nurse, Cushman worked as a school teacher in New York State. She graduated from the School of Nursing of the Paterson, New Jersey General Hospital in 1892. Cushman also took postgraduate training in pharmaceutics and the care of women.

Cushman worked in Missouri as superintendent of Scarritt Hospital in Kansas City. Her responsibilities included the nurses' training school.

While in Kansas City, Cushman took a course in missionary work. In 1899 she was given an assignment to serve in Asia Minor by the American Board of Commissioners of Foreign Missions—the youngest nurse ever to be sent. Except for short visits to the United States, Cushman spent most of the rest of her life abroad "too busy to go home to America to lecture and to be interviewed and to be written and talked about."

Cushman's initial assignment was on the medical staff of the American Board of Foreign Missions in Konia, Turkey. She established a school of nursing at the American Hospital there and, having learned Turkish, translated nursing texts for the students. Later, after Cushman had left, the school was discontinued for lack of qualified students. Cushman left the Board of Missions and affiliated herself with the Near East Relief Foundation.

Missionaries and foreigners were ordered out of Turkey when World War I began. All left except Cushman, who refused to go. In his book *Bible Lands Today*, W. Ellis noted: "There was nothing in the experience of the Turkish officials that taught them how to deal with this kind of woman; especially since their country was not at war with America, and they could not well resort to extreme measures."

During this time Konia was a central prison camp with no liaison between the city and the outside world. Cushman was appointed the acting consul for 17 allied and neutral nations. She became the intermediary for the supply of funds and other forms of relief to the groups of prisoners representing 46 races and nationalities. Cushman's reputation among the local bankers and merchants enabled her to procure over $1 million worth of bank drafts, all of which were later honored by governments and relief agencies.

When the war ended, Cushman had not only adult refugees under her care but at least 1,000 orphans. She continued her relief work and was put in charge of three orphanages and 2,000 orphans in Turkey. In addition, she worked with trachoma patients in Istanbul.

The "Smyrna disaster" occurred in 1922 when the Greek and Christian areas of the city were burned. The Turkish government did not offer assistance, and Christians and Greeks fled Turkey. Cushman helped to evacuate 22,000 orphans and personally escorted 1,700 children to Greece. After her arrival in Corinth, Cushman continued her work with the orphans.

Cushman took the responsibility of caring for the 3,000 children who had been evacuated to Greece. The orphanage housing these children was under the auspices of the Near East Relief Foundation and one of Cushman's staff members was Alice Griffith Carr, a Johns Hopkins Nurses Training School graduate who had been doing extensive health-care work in Greece.

Malaria was responsible for the poor health and debilitation of not only the orphans but others in Corinth. The orphan boys, under Carr's direction, were responsible for digging 100 miles of trenches to help drain the stagnant water from the city. In addition, residents were encouraged to cover cisterns and wells. The work of the orphanage was successful enough for the civil authorities to become involved in malaria eradication efforts which improved the health of the population. Carr was later recognized for her efforts in malaria control throughout the Near East.

Cushman, believing that inequality of the sexes hindered progress, introduced the concept of coeducation at the orphanage school. This was an unheard-of innovation in that part of the world. She allowed boys and girls to sit in the same classroom and encouraged coeducational competition in sports. She also introduced a form of self-governance for students.

In the spring of 1925 a short revolution in Greece resulted in the presence of warplanes near the vicinity of the orphanage as well as some shelling from a warship. Cushman sent word to the commanders of both factions to pursue their battle elsewhere. She had some orphan boys roll the enemy planes about one-half mile away. *The New York Times* in her obituary noted: "It has been suggested that her acts had something to do with the termination of the revolution in three days."

Cushman's educational efforts resulted in her charges becoming self-supporting. She had taught her orphans to be among the "best farmers, most skillful artisans, and tidiest housewifes to be found." As soon as the majority of the orphans had reached an age to be on their own, Cushman retired and sent her remaining charges to another Near East Relief Foundation orphanage.

Cushman's health had deteriorated from the climate and unsanitary conditions under which she had been working. She retired to St. Theodore's, a village near Corinth, to live as a chicken farmer. Her home had been built for her by some of the orphans.

In 1930 she left home to spend Christmas in Cairo with some of her orphans who had been relocated there. Cushman died in Egypt of malignant malaria and anemia on December 31 of that year. The funeral service was conducted by the president of the American University in Cairo and attended by representatives from the American and Greek governments as well as officials from various humanitarian and religious organizations located in Egypt. Five hundred of the orphans she had assisted also attended.

Cushman's honors included the Cross of the Legion of Honor from France for her work with French prisoners of war; the Gold Cross of the Saviour, Greece's highest civilian honor, for leadership and training of women in the Near East (1926); the Blessing of the Greek Orthodox Church by the Patriarch of Constantinople; and the Distinguished Service Medal of the Near East Relief Foundation for "bravery under fire" (1925).

Cushman provided nurses of the past and of the present with a magnificent role model. Her determination, bravery, and obvious talent directly benefited those she served. Her legacy is also a challenge to other nurses to meet those same standards of caring and competence. This author regrets that Cushman's accomplishments are not better known both to nurses and to the public at large.

BIBLIOGRAPHY

Dock, L., and I. Stewart. *A Short History of Nursing*, 3rd ed. P. 234. New York: Putnam, 1931.

Ellis, W. *Bible Lands To-Day*. New York: Appleton, 1927.

"Emma D. Cushman." Obituary. *American Journal of Nursing* 31 (April 1931): 417–18.

"Emma D. Cushman, Humanitarian, Dies." Obituary. *New York Times*, January 3, 1931.

Goodnow, M. *Nursing History*, 7th ed. Pp. 425–26. Philadelphia: Saunders, 1944.

Goodnow, M. *Nursing History*, 9th ed. Philadelphia: Saunders, 1953. 388.

Smith, M. "Keeping Her Hand In." *American Journal of Nursing* 28 (November 1928): 1101–02.

Leslie M. Thom

Louise M. Darche
1852–1899

Louise M. Darche's major accomplishments in nursing were in the fields of administration and education. As superintendent of the Training School for Nurses, Blackwell's Island, New York City, she was responsible for reforming and reorganizing the school at a time when standardized criteria for nurses' training schools did not exist. She also formulated a comprehensive plan for a New York City nursing department. In addition, she was a strong voice in urging nurses to organize and to establish a voice for themselves via an official publication for their organization. She became the first secretary of the American Society of Superintendents of Training Schools for Nurses, which later became the National League for Nursing.

Darche was born on August 20, 1852, in Lambton Mills, Ontario, now part of the city of Toronto. Her father died when she was 18. After his death, Darche became a teacher. By 1871 she was living in St.

Catharines, Ontario, where she became the teacher-in-charge of St. George's Ward Primary School, a public school. She is listed in the St. Catharines census of 1871 as a Methodist. In 1882 Darche resigned from her position for health reasons. The following year she entered the Bellevue Training School for Nurses in New York City, from which she graduated in 1885. From 1886 to 1888 Darche was a private-duty nurse in Chicago, first for a young boy, the son of a Chicago millionaire, and after the young boy died, for a young girl with double hip disease.

In 1888 Darche returned to New York City, where she became the superintendent of the Training School for Nurses on Blackwell's Island. Darche had been recommended for the job when Mrs. Cadwalader Jones of State Charities Aid asked Miss Perkins, the superintendent of the Training School for Nurses at Bellevue, to suggest someone possessing the tact and skill to manage the difficult job. As a condition of employment, Darche was permitted to choose her own assistant, and she chose her good friend Diana C. Kimber.

Previous to Darche's appointment at Blackwell's Island, the hospital was under the control of the New York City political machine Tammany Hall. The hospital was corrupt, squalid, and disorganized. Women prisoners did the housework. There was no systematic course of study and no lectures. Student nurses at the training school worked only in the Maternity Hospital and in Charity Hospital and received no general nursing experience. Darche upgraded the school of nursing. She established criteria required for an effective school; expanded clinical experience to include general nursing; increased the number of hospitals in which the student nurses rotated to five, including Gouverneur, Harlem, and Fordham hospitals; installed a board of physicians and surgeons to teach the students. She advocated a standardized curriculum and management and provided such amenities for the students as libraries and parlors in the nurses' residence so that they could be rejuvenated when not at work. Another one of her innovations was the training of male nurses, who had pre-

viously not had organized instruction or supervision.

It was Darche's idea that a city nursing department should be established under a city charter. It should be supervised by one head, a trained nurse. The nursing department would manage all of the nursing, housekeeping, and domestic service of the city hospitals. A training school would train nurses who would rotate through the hospitals for general experience. Those hospitals requiring specialized nursing care, such as Babies Hospital, should have permanent trained staff, graduates also of the training school. In addition, Darche advocated graded salaries and opportunities for promotion.

Because of her managerial talent, Darche eventually oversaw five hospitals—Maternity, Charity, Gouverneur, Harlem, and Fordham—including 100 nurses and over 800 patients daily. In 1893, speaking at the Chicago World's Fair, she urged nurses to organize to promote improved standards for their profession. In 1896 she proposed publishing a nursing journal, to express the concerns of the profession. She later became the first secretary of the American Society of Superintendents of Training Schools for Nurses, which later became the National League for Nursing.

Darche's work took its toll. She had had to fight daily against the New York political machine to effect her plans. Eventually, her health broke under the strain. She resigned on February 1, 1898. After spending six months resting with her sister in Canada, Darche went to England to travel and, according to some reports, to study medicine.

On June 1, 1899, the day before she was scheduled to return to the United States, Darche shot herself with a pistol in the Metropole Hotel in London. The inquest that appeared in the *Times* of London reported that a Mrs. Tausig was with her at the time of the shooting. She was said to have been depressed from overwork. Darche died the next day, June 2, 1899, at a nursing home run by Alice Kimber, the sister of Diana Kimber. Darche left a note asking to be buried in England. A funeral service was held on June 6, 1899, in St. Savior Church, St. George's Square, London.

Darche was eulogized by Lavinia Dock for her achievements at the New York Training School, Blackwell's Island, for her plans for a city nursing department, and for her personal sacrifice and struggle against political corruption for the public good. She will also be remembered for her pioneer effort in professional nursing organization.

The 1916 graduating class of the City Hospital School of Nursing, formerly Blackwell's Island, established a scholarship fund called the Darche and Kimber Scholarship fund to honor the work of the two women who were instrumental in the establishment of their school and who were leaders in nursing education and administration. Darche was also selected to become an honorary member of the Matrons' Council of Great Britain and Ireland.

PUBLICATIONS BY
LOUISE M. DARCHE

"Improved Methods of Nursing," *Lend a Hand* (August 1895): 122–25.

BIBLIOGRAPHY

American Journal of Nursing 20 (October 1919): 39–43.

"Darche, Louise." *Dictionary of American Nursing Biography.* M. Kaufman, ed. Westport, Conn.: Greenwood, 1988.

Dock, L.L. *Louise Darche. A Reformer in Nursing and in the Civil Service.* New York: The author, n.d. (*Pamphlets in American History.* Biography; B 554.)

"Inquest." *Times* (London), June 6, 1899.

M. Adelaide Nutting Collection, Teachers College, Columbia University, New York City.

Mottus, J.E. *New York Nightingales: The Emergence of the Nursing Profession at Bellevue and New York Hospital 1850–1920.* Ann Arbor, Mich.: University Microfilms International, 1981.

National League of Nursing Education. *Early Leader of American Nursing Calendar.* New York: The League, 1922.

St. Catharines Historical Museum records, St. Catharines, Ontario, Canada.

Stewart, I.M. "Darche-Kimber Scholarship Fund." *American Journal of Nursing* 20 (October 1919): 39–43.

"Suicide of Miss D'Arche." *New York Times*, June 2, 1899.

Dorothy Tao

Sue Sophia Dauser
1888–1972

Sue Sophia Dauser, the first woman captain in the U.S. Navy, directed the nursing services of the U.S. Navy during World War II as superintendent of the Navy Nurse Corps.

Born in Anaheim, California, on September 20, 1888, the daughter of Francis X. and Mary Anna Steuckle Dauser, Sue Dauser graduated from Fullerton High School in 1907 and attended Stanford University from 1907 until 1909. She entered the California Hospital School of Nursing in Los Angeles in 1911, and after graduation in 1914 she worked there as surgical supervisor until 1917. Dauser became a nurse in the navy in 1917 and remained in the service until her retirement in 1946. During her career she served overseas during World War I, on hospital ships in the Pacific, at naval installations on the West Coast of the United States, and directed more than 11,000 navy nurses during her tenure as superintendent of the Navy Nurse Corps from 1939 until 1945. She was the first woman to wear the four gold stripes of a U.S. Navy captain. After retirement from the navy in 1946, she resided in La Mesa, California, until her death in Anaheim on March 8, 1972, at the age of 83.

The United States entered World War I on April 6, 1917, and in September of that year Dauser joined the naval reserve, going on active duty in October and training at the Naval Hospital in San Diego, California. She was appointed chief nurse, naval reserve, in charge of Base Hospital #3, which was organized by the Red Cross in Los Angeles and mobilized in Philadelphia, December 1917. Dauser entered the regular navy on July 10, 1918, and was promoted to chief nurse the following day. She and the nurses in her charge did temporary duty in Philadelphia until August 1, 1918, when they embarked for Liverpool, England, on the HMS *Mandingo*, landing on August 15, 1918. The next day the group arrived in Edinburgh, Scotland, by train, and proceeded to Seafield Leith, near Edinburgh, to convert the existing facility to the U.S. Navy Base Hospital #3.

For the previous four years the hospital had been under the jurisdiction of the British naval service to attend patients from the Grand Fleet in the North Sea. The American nurse contingent cared for sick and injured sailors and soldiers from both the British and American armed forces who came on convoy trains from the Channel ports.

At the end of the war, in late 1918, Dauser performed temporary duty in Brest, France, while awaiting transport to the United States. Upon her return, she was first stationed as chief nurse at the Naval Hospital, Brooklyn, New York, for a brief time and then sent to the San Diego Naval Hospital where she had first begun her naval career. Until 1939 her assignments took her to every naval station on the West Coast of the United States as well as to Guam and the Philippines.

Dauser served not only at shore hospitals, but also aboard ship. After a short tour at San Diego, she sailed with the SS *Relief* on its Pacific Fleet cruise to Australia, New Zealand, and Samoa and on the *Argonne* transport ship from the East to the West Coast of the United States. She accompanied President Warren G. Harding as night nurse on his Alaskan cruise on the *Henderson* in the summer of 1923 and was at the President's bedside when he died suddenly in San Francisco on August 2, 1923.

From 1926 to 1928 Dauser saw duty in naval hospitals in Guam and the Philippines, returning to San Diego Naval Hospital as principal chief nurse until 1931, when she was transferred to Puget Sound, Washington. In 1934 she was assigned to Mare Island, California, briefly; from 1935 to 1939 she directed nursing services at the U.S. Naval Dispensary at Long Beach, California.

After 22 years of providing nursing care and directing the activities of Red Cross volunteer nurses, naval reserve and regular navy staff nurses, and naval corpsmen on ships, stateside naval hospitals, and tropical island stations, Dauser succeeded Myn M. Hoffman as superintendent of the Navy Nurse Corps on January 30, 1939. As superintendent, she reported directly to the surgeon general of the United States, Ross T. McIntyre, rather than to a naval officer. Since the establishment of the Navy Nurse Corps in 1908, navy nurses, although legally members of the U.S. Navy, were neither officers nor enlisted personnel. They received the respect due an officer but enjoyed neither an officer's pay nor other benefits attached to an officer's rank. Thus Captain Dauser had two responsibilities upon her appointment to the superintendency: to prepare and enlarge the nursing corps to face coming war and to obtain equitable rank and privileges for the nurses in the Navy Nurse Corps.

During Superintendent Dauser's "watch," the Navy Nurse Corps increased from 600 nurses in the prewar period to over 11,000 commissioned officers, all volunteers, by 1945. In addition to overseeing and administering the activities of the corps, she worked closely with the nursing heads of the other services, including the army and the American Red Cross, as well as Allied armed services, to monitor the supply of nursing personnel on all fronts and to investigate ways to improve nursing care off the battlefield. She was instrumental in establishing postgraduate training programs for navy nurses and ensured the navy's participation in the Cadet Nurse Training Program. While she was superintendent, the first black woman nurse, Phyllis Daley, was sworn into the Navy Nurse Corps as an ensign on March 8, 1945.

One of Captain Dauser's most difficult tasks was to convince the navy and members of the United States Congress to give commissions and equivalent pay and privileges to the women in the Navy Nurse Corps. The low pay and ambivalent status of navy nurses acted as deterrents in recruiting nurses for navy service, especially in contrast to the army, which offered relative rank for its nurses. Congress slowly remedied this situation over the course of the war. On July 3, 1942, Congress granted relative rank to navy nurses, and Dauser obtained the relative rank of lieutenant commander. In December 1942 navy nurses were granted equivalent pay, and Dauser became a captain, relative rank. Thus, Sue Dauser wore four gold stripes on her uniform as the first woman captain, and highest ranking woman officer, in the U.S. Navy. Navy nurses received full military commissions in February 1944, and Captain Dauser was confirmed in her rank for the duration of the war plus six months.

Captain Dauser retired from the superintendency in November 1945. Secretary of the Navy James Forestal presented her with the Distinguished Service Medal in ceremonies at the Navy Department on December 14, 1945. She was the first navy nurse honored with this distinction. In his remarks, Forestal noted her "keen foresight and superb professional ability" in discharging "the heavy responsibilities of this vital assignment." Secretary Forestal praised "her constant devotion to duty [which] reflects the highest credit upon herself, her command, and the United States Naval Service."

Lieutenant Commander Nellie Jane DeWitt succeeded Captain Dauser as superintendent of the Navy Nurse Corps. Captain Dauser retired from the navy in April 1946. She lived in La Mesa, California, until her death in Anaheim, on March 8, 1972.

PUBLICATIONS BY
SUE SOPHIA DAUSER

Preface to *Navy Nurse*, by Page Cooper. New York: McGraw-Hill, 1946.

BIBLIOGRAPHY

"Appointment in the Navy Nurse Corps." *American Journal of Nursing* 39 (April 1939): 441–42.

Archives, Office of the Superintendent of the Navy Nurse Corps, Washington, D.C.

"Captain Dauser Awarded Distinguished Service Medal." *American Journal of Nursing* 46 (February 1946): 138–39.

"Captain Sue Dauser Retires from Navy Nurse Corps." *American Journal of Nursing* 45 (December 1945): 1064.

"Dauser, Sue Sophia." *Current Biography, 1944.* New York: Wilson, 1945.

"Dauser, Sue Sophia." *Webster's American Military Biographies.* Springfield, Mass.: Merriam, 1978.

"Dauser, Sue Sophia." *Liberty's Women.* Robert McHenry, ed. Springfield, Mass.: Merriam, 1980.

Dock, L., Sarah Pickett, Clara Noyes. *History of American Red Cross Nursing.* New York: Macmillan, 1922.

Pennock, M.R. *Makers of Nursing History.* New York: Lakeside, 1940.

"Sue Dauser." *Pacific Coast Journal of Nursing* 35 (March 1939): 150.

"World War II NNC Chief Dies." *American Journal of Nursing* 72 (August 1972): 1482.

Kathleen F. Cohen

Mabel Davies
?–1960

Mabel Davies, the administrator of the Beekman-Downtown Hospital in New York City from 1925–55, was noted for her professional administrative and humanitarian achievements.

Davies was born in London, England. The date of her birth is not known. She migrated to America and became a U.S. citizen. She attended the Presbyterian Hospital School for Nursing in New York City and was graduated in 1915. After a short period of private-duty nursing, she returned to Presbyterian Hospital to take charge of the wards.

She served at the American Ambulance Station at Juilly, France, in 1916 and later held various administrative nursing posts at wartime hospitals in Paris and Neufchateau.

After the United States entered World War I, Davies remained in Paris to minister to the wounded and to take part in organizing and equipping army, navy, and Red Cross nursing units. For these services, she was awarded the American Red Cross Medal for Foreign Service, the War and Victory medals of Great Britain, and the *Medaille des Epidemies* of France.

Returning to New York to Presbyterian Hospital in 1919, Davies became a charge nurse, assistant director, and then assistant superintendent of nurses. She remained there until her appointment as superintendent (later changed to "administrator") at Beekman Street Hospital in 1925. During her tenure, the hospital first changed its name to Beekman Hospital and finally to Beekman-Downtown Hospital. When the hospital moved to new quarters nearby in 1953, she oversaw the orderly transition of hospital services.

Davies had planned to retire when the hospital moved into its new $5.5-million facilities. However, she was so enchanted by what she called, "the house of a thousand windows, a lovely dream that came true," that she stayed on for another two years. At the time of the move, she was honored at a surprise presentation of a mural in the new hospital showing her as the central figure.

Davies served as assistant to the deputy administrator of the New York area Civil Works Administration during the 1930s. She was on the War Manpower Commission Procurement and Assignment Service for Nurses during World War II, and was a member of several professional organizations during her nursing career.

She died on December 20, 1960, at the Sky View Haven Nursing Home in Croton-on-Hudson, New York, after a long illness.

PUBLICATIONS OF MABEL DAVIES

BOOKS

Hygiene and Health Education for Training Colleges. London: Longmans, Green, 1932 (subsequent editions to 1954).

Physical Training, Games and Athletics in Elementary Schools. London: Allen and Unwin, 1927 (subsequent editions to 1951).

With L. Wilkes. *Some Methods in Health Education*. London: Longmans, Green, 1935.

BIBLIOGRAPHY

"Mabel Davies, Hospital Leader." Obituary. *New York Times*, December 21, 1960, 31.

"News Highlights." *American Journal of Nursing* 55 (July 1955): 784.

Alice P. Stein

Mary E.P. Davis

1840?–1924

One of the founders of the American Journal of Nursing Company and its first president, Mary E.P. Davis has been acknowledged as the driving force behind the successful launching of the *American Journal of Nursing (AJN)* in 1900. The early financial stability of the journal has been attributed to Davis's determination, business acumen, and organizational ability.

Davis was born in New Brunswick, Canada; her exact birth date remains unknown. It has been noted, however, that she was considerably older than her colleagues, and it is generally accepted that she was born in or around 1840 to John and Charlotte (McFarland) Davis. Her father was an officer in the British army, and religion was a significant component in her upbringing. Little else is known of her early years, her mother, or whether she had any siblings.

Davis graduated from the Massachusetts General Hospital School for Nurses in 1878 and remained on the staff as a graduate nurse until 1879. She subsequently gained experience in private-duty nursing and later worked in district nursing during its early development in the Boston area. From 1889–99 she held the position of superintendent of the University of Pennsylvania Hospital and Training School for Nurses. During her ten-year administration, the hospital underwent extensive reorganization and expansion and a three-year course of study was initiated for the nursing school.

At other times in her career, Davis held executive positions as superintendent of the Boston State Hospital in Dorchester, Massachusetts, where she implemented a training school for nurses, and as Superintendent of the Washington (D.C.) Training School for Nurses. She was the first registrar of the Central Directory for Nurses in Boston and organized central directories in Philadelphia and Washington, D.C., as well. During World War I she served as examiner for classes given by the American Red Cross.

Davis was committed to improving educational standards for nursing and viewed appropriately educated nurses as most qualified to assume the responsibilities of the superintendent's role. She recognized that lack of business knowledge was a deficiency in the preparation of nurses and strongly supported the post-graduate course in hospital economics begun at Teachers College, Columbia University in 1899 (the first course for nurses to be given in a school of higher education).

An active participant in the proceedings of the nursing congress held at the 1893 World's Columbian Exposition in Chicago, Davis presented a paper in which she described the role of superintendent as requiring: advanced education, ethical precepts, flexibility, collegiality, and decision-making ability. At the conclusion of the congress, Davis joined with 17 other superintendents to establish the American Society of Superintendents of Training Schools for Nurses, forerunner of the National League for Nursing. Davis was one of a committee of seven appointed to determine the direction of the society, the requirements for membership, and the duties involved. One of the society's principal goals was the development of an organization for the rank and file, and in 1897 the Nurses' Associated Alumnae of the United States and Canada was founded (Associated Alumnae). That organization later became the American Nurses' Association.

Davis was prominent in both organizations. She served as first vice-president of the Superintendents' Society from 1894 to 1895 and was elected president in 1896. During that year she presided at the third annual convention, where the major topic of debate was a uniform curriculum for training schools. The subject generated much discussion, including the kinds of textbooks that might be used for such a curriculum.

With respect to the Associated Alumnae, Davis served as chairman of the Committee on Periodicals from 1899 to 1902. It was the committee of 1900, comprised of Davis, Sophia Palmer, Isabel Hampton Robb, Lavinia Dock, Anna Maxwell, and Isabel Merritt, that established the guidelines for development of the *American Journal of Nursing* (*AJN*). The committee saw the dispersion of nurses as one of the reasons underlying the need for such a journal. The *AJN* was to be the voice of organized nursing, published by nurses for nurses, and was seen by Davis as a professional undertaking and responsibility. The journal would bring important news to scattered groups of nurses and would also help to increase public understanding of nursing.

A joint stock company was selected as the way to finance the project. Shares were sold at $100 each, and sales were limited to nurses and nursing organizations. By May 1900, 24 shares were sold; purchasers included some of the great names in nursing. J.B. Lippincott Company of Philadelphia offered the best financial arrangement and was selected as publisher. Davis was named president of the board of directors, and Sophia Palmer was designated editor-in-chief.

Announcements of the forthcoming journal elicited approximately 550 one-year subscriptions (at $2 each) prior to publication. The first issue published in October 1900 showed neither profit nor loss. Davis and Palmer, however, worked without salary for the first year in order to increase the journal's chances for survival.

By 1901, 1,800 subscriptions had been sold, and Davis was appointed business manager, a position she held until 1909. Davis was instrumental in establishing the Book Department section of the *AJN* as well as masterminding the financial solvency of the company. The journal became the official organ of the Associated Alumnae and set a standard for excellence in nursing publications.

Davis never forgot the school where she first received her training as a nurse. In 1895 she and Palmer (who also graduated from the Massachusetts General Hospital in 1878) helped organize the School of Nursing Alumnae Association, which became one of the first associations to join the Associated Alumnae in 1897. Davis served her alumnae association as corresponding secretary for a number of years beginning in 1917. In 1920 she was named an honorary member.

Davis also made a significant contribution to the founding of the Massachusetts State Nurses' Association (MSNA) in 1903. During its early years MSNA was one of the many state nurses' associations seeking legal regulation of nursing education and practice through the enactment of registration laws. Davis was chairman of MSNA's legislative committee, which presented a series of such bills to the Massachusetts legislature. Enactment of a registration law was finally achieved in 1910. Davis was elected president of MSNA from 1911–13.

Davis's health declined in the early 1920s, and she died on June 9, 1924, at Norwood, Massachusetts, where she made her home.

In 1982 Davis was selected for inclusion in the American Nurses' Association Hall of Fame, a fitting tribute to an outstanding pioneer in nursing.

PUBLICATIONS BY MARY E.P. DAVIS

ARTICLES

"Trained Nurses as Superintendents of Hospitals." in *Nursing of the Sick.* Proceedings of the papers and discussions of the International Congress of Charities, Correction and Philanthropy, Chicago, 1893. Reprint—New York: McGraw-Hill, 1949.

"Address of the President." *Third Annual Report of the American Society of Superintendents of Training Schools for Nurses.* Harrisburg, Pa.: Harrisburg Publishing, 1896.

"Hospital Diet from the Standpoint of the Hospital Superintendent." *Fifth Annual Convention of the American Society of Superintendents of Training Schools for Nurses.* Harrisburg, Pa.: Harrisburg Publishing, 1898.

"Preparatory Work for Nurses—The Central School Idea." *American Journal of Nursing* 3 (January 1903): 256–61.

"Short History of the Founding of the American Journal of Nursing." *Rapports de la Conference International of Nursing.* Paris, 1907.

"What We Are Overlooking of Fundamental Importance in the Training of the Modern Nurse." *American Journal of Nursing* 7 (July 1907): 764–66.

"Organization, or Why Belong?" *American Journal of Nursing* 12 (March 1912): 474–77.

"As Known by Her Friends." *American Journal of Nursing* 19 (June 1919): 695–97.

BIBLIOGRAPHY

American Journal of Nursing and Its Company. New York: American Journal of Nursing Co., 1975.

"The Central Directory." *American Journal of Nursing* 14 (April 1914): 568.

Dock, L.L. *A History of Nursing.* Vol. 3. New York: Putnam, 1912.

"Editorial." *American Journal of Nursing* 50 (October 1950): 584.

"Journal Directors Re-elected." *American Journal of Nursing* 6 (February 1906): 287.

Leaders of American Nursing. New York: National League of Nursing Education, 1923.

"Mary E.P. Davis." *American Journal of Nursing* 24 (July 1924): 811–12.

"Miss Davis' Retirement." *American Journal of Nursing* 10 (December 1909): 152–53.

"Miss Mary E.P. Davis." *American Journal of Nursing* 2 (October 1901): 74.

"Our Old-Young Member." *American Journal of Nursing* 20 (December 1919): 186.

Parsons, S. *History of the Massachusetts General Hospital Training School for Nurses.* Boston: Whitcomb and Barrows, 1922.

Perkins, S. *A Centennial Review 1873–1973 of the Massachusetts General Hospital School of Nursing.* Boston: School of Nursing Alumnae Association, 1975.

"Report of the Fourth Annual Convention of the Trained Nurses' Associated Alumnae of the United States." *American Journal of Nursing* 2 (January 1902): 321–22.

Riddle, M. "Twenty Years at the Journal." *American Journal of Nursing* 21 (October 1920): 6–12.

The Story of the American Journal of Nursing. New York: American Journal of Nursing, 1935.

Thirty Fruitful Years. New York: American Journal of Nursing, 1930.

Nettie Birnbach

Philip Edson Day

1916–1989

Philip Edson Day was president and publisher of the *American Journal of Nursing* (*AJN*) from 1964 to 1971, when he retired.

Day was born in Ripton, Vermont, the son of Milo Edson Day and Helen (Smith) Day, June 23, 1916. He was married to Agnes Nielson on November 27, 1937; the couple was divorced in February 1966. They had four children, two sons and two daughters. After service in the U.S. Army in World War II, Day entered the Pennsylvania Hospital School for Men. After receiving his R.N. he served as instructor at the school from 1950 to 1955 and at the same time the University of Pennsylvania School of Nursing from which he received his bachelor's degree in 1955. He then moved to Burlington, Vermont, where from 1956 to 1964 he was director of nursing service at the Mary Fletcher Hospital. In 1964 he received his master's degree in nursing service from Teacher's College, Columbia University, and in July of that year he was appointed to the *AJN* position. At the time of his appointment, three of the six members of his family were nurses—Day, his wife Agnes, and his daughter Carol.

Prior to joining the board of *AJN* he had served on the editorial board of *RN* and *Hospitals*. He had written articles for both publications. Day was the first man elected as president of a state nursing association, that of Vermont (1960–62), and he served as treasurer and board member of the organization as well. He was a member of the ANA committee, Promotion of Program, Public Relations, and Membership and also served as chairperson of the Division of Nursing Service. After retiring from his position with the *AJN* in the 1980's he moved to California. He died of a heart attack in Arnold, California, on May 9, 1989.

BIBLIOGRAPHY

"Former AJN Publisher Philip E. Day Dies." *American Journal of Nursing* 89 (July 1989): 18.

"Journal Company Has New Executive Director." *American Journal of Nursing* 64 (July 1964): 136.

Who's Who in America, 41st ed. Chicago: Marquis, 1980/Vol 1, p 823.

Vern L. Bullough

Agnes Gardiner Shearer Deans

1871–1948

Agnes Gardiner Shearer Deans, a pioneer in nursing throughout the first half of the twentieth century, was known for her work in the professional organizations, in the political struggle for nursing registration, and in the developing arena of public-health nursing. Additionally, she worked with the Red Cross and with A. L. Austin contributed to nursing literature with their historical account of the Farrand Training School for Nurses (Detroit). Deans's dedication to nursing was known and recognized in national and international nursing circles. It was her commitment, energy, and zeal, at a time of immense growth and change in nursing, that is most remembered.

Agnes G. Deans was born in St. Mary, Ontario, in 1871. Her parents, James and Mary Deans, were of Scottish descent. As a child, she moved with her family to London, Ontario. Other than the fact she had two sisters, little is known about her family life. She attended both the private and public schools of London. In the years following high school, Deans moved to Detroit, Michigan, where she first graduated from a business college and then in 1896 from Farrand Training School for Nurses, Harper Hospital in Detroit.

The Farrand Training School for Nurses, which had opened in 1883, was directed by Lystra Gretter. Under the influence of Gretter and the help of the early alumnae, the Farrand Training School Alumni Association was founded in 1893. Deans became an active member on graduation and over the years a leader of the association, one of the first nurses' associations in Michigan and among one of the fifteen alumni associations then in existence in the United States in the year of its founding. An invited delegate from the Farrand association participated at the founding convention of the Nurses' Associated Alumnae in 1896.

Deans's early exposure to Lystra Gretter's strong interests in the formation of nursing organizations, public-health nursing, and the Red Cross, seemed to have had its affect on her.

Deans's strong organizational and leadership abilities were demonstrated in her career by the many positions held in public-health nursing and in national nursing organizations. Her first position as head nurse of the Children's Free Hospital in Detroit began soon after graduation from nurse-training school. She worked in that position for about two and a half years and then moved on to become superintendent of the Woman's Hospital in Duluth, Minnesota for two years. After resigning as superintendent, Deans moved back to Detroit as head nurse in the Detroit Health Department and spent over two years in that position before becoming first superintendent of the Tuberculosis hospital in Detroit and then associate superintendent of the Visiting Nurses Association of Detroit. The dates of when she left one position for another is unclear, although it is known she was with the Visiting Nurses Association for over seven years.

In addition to Deans's work in public health, she worked closely with the developing city, county and state nurses' associations in Michigan. In October 1902 Deans had served on a committee of three to draft the tentative constitution and by-laws for the newly formed Detroit Graduate Nurses Association. In 1905 the Detroit Graduate Nurses Association became the Wayne County Graduate Nurses Association and Deans served in both of these associations as secretary. The Wayne County Graduate Nurse Association became known as the First District within the Michigan State Nurses Association begun in 1904, and Deans was a charter member. In 1908 under the sponsorship of the Wayne County Graduate Nurses Association, Deans helped establish a Central Directory for all nurses in Detroit and was appointed as its first registrar for one year.

On the state level, Deans played an instrumental role in drafting and enacting a Michigan state registration bill for nurses. Lavinia Dock remembered her as one of the "specially active workers" in campaigning for the bill. She worked with other members of Michigan's state association until the bill was finally passed in 1909.

From 1909–13, Deans moved into the national arena and served as the secretary of the American Nurses' Association (ANA). While filling this role, Deans kept abreast of the activities of the alumnae associations throughout the country and of the topics of the day affecting all women. At the 13th Annual Convention of the American Nurses' Association, she included an announcement about the suffrage activities of various nursing organizations, seemingly indicating her own awareness of the current topic of the period. Specifically, one of the lectures she reported about, "An argument for Equal Suffrage," was being offered at that time in the District of Columbia.

In addition to her work as secretary, Deans served for 12 years as a member of the board of directors of the American Nurses' Association. Between June 1917 and July 1920 she was an administrator in the Department of Nursing of the American Red Cross. In 1918 she became a member of the National Committee on Red Cross Nursing Service. She also held the post as director of the Social Service Department at the Washington University Dispensary in St. Louis for two years (1920–22).

An announcement appeared in November 1922 of the *American Journal of Nursing* that Agnes G. Deans had been appointed as representative at ANA's national headquarters in New York. While at national headquarters, Deans studied nursing care and administration in the country and made recommendations for the future. The delegates to the 1924 convention of the American Nurses' Association changed the title of the position from "representative of the board at headquarters" to "director at headquarters." Deans became chair of the Revisions Committee as well, served on the committee to which she had been appointed in 1914. During her tenure at ANA headquarters, Deans planned the trip for the nursing delegates who attended the International Conference held in Helsinki, Finland, in July 1925.

Deans resigned as secretary of ANA in January 1925. An editorial in the *American Journal of Nursing* referring to her resignation described her "indefatigable efforts and work" in the office of secretary from one which could be operated out of a trunk into a national office with a paid staff.

Although Deans resigned from one position, her work in the American Nurses' Association was not yet finished. She chaired the Program Committee for the 1926 convention held in Atlantic City, New Jersey. Additionally, she accepted the post as field secretary early in the summer of 1927. Her work in this new position was anticipated to be enriching to the profession. Some of the broad issues Deans was to address were those in areas affecting nursing registries, meeting public-health needs, collaborating with other health professionals, and strengthening the professional organization.

Aside from the official roles she played, Agnes Deans served the American Nurses' Association in other capacities too. She participated in the work of several standing committees, including those on publication, relief, revisions, finance, and program. Her service on so many varied ANA committees indicated both her in-depth knowledge of ANA and her dedication.

In 1930 Deans began work, in collaboration with her friend Anne L. Austin, on the history of their training school. The book, *The History of the Farrand Training School for Nurses*, was published in 1936. In 1938 Deans accepted the position of executive secretary for the Farrand alumnae association. Although she formally retired in 1938 she continued to advance the profession of nursing in her volunteer work in the alumnae association and in the national association.

Deans moved to Oswego, New York, in 1928. She had a sister who lived there, and another in Binghamton. She lived in Oswego until she died following a long hospitalization on March 16, 1948, at the age of 77.

She was remembered with affection by her contemporaries for the many hours she devoted to nursing. The following excerpt, from an editorial in the August 1926 issue of the *American Journal of Nursing*, aptly describes the appreciation of her colleagues through the years for her dedication to nursing:

> Few if any, members of the organization had both her comprehensive knowledge and her love of the detail work of the organization....

> The debt of the Association is one that can never be repaid except by the affection in which she is held by thousands of nurses.

PUBLICATIONS BY AGNES GARDINER SHEARER DEANS

BOOKS

With A.L. Austin. *The History of the Farrand Training School for Nurses*. Detroit: Alumnae Association of the Farrand Training School for Nurses, 1936.

ARTICLES

"Proceedings of the Thirteenth Annual Convention of the Nurses' Associated Alumnae: Report of the Interstate Secretary." *American Journal of Nursing* 12 (1912): 861.

"Lystra E. Gretter, Teacher, Counsellor, and Friend." *Leaders of American Nursing Calendar*. New York: Publications Committee of the National League of Nursing Education, 1923.

With E. Van Ness. "One Hundred Thousand and Up: The Story of the A.N.A. Nurses' Relief Fund." *American Journal of Nursing* 26 (December, 1926): 943–47.

REPORTS

"Proceedings of the Twenty-Fourth Convention of the American Nurses' Association: Secretary's Report." *American Nurses' Association—Proceedings: 1924–1932*, pp. 5–7.

"Proceedings of the Twenty-Fifth Convention of the American Nurses' Association: Report of the Program Committee." *American Nurses' Association—Proceedings: 1924–1932*, p. 10.

"Proceedings of the Twenty-Fifth Convention of the American Nurses' Association: Report of the Director at Headquarters." *American Nurses' Association—Proceedings: 1924–1932*, pp. 15–17.

BIBLIOGRAPHY

"An Announcement." *American Journal of Nursing* 23 (November 1922): 139.

"Books on Professional Subjects." *American Journal of Nursing* 36 (October 1936): 1066.

Dock, L. *A History of Nursing*. Vol. 3, pp. 180–82. New York: Putnam, 1912.

"Expansion at National Headquarters." Editorial. *American Journal of Nursing* 23 (February 1923): 377–88.

Francis, S. "Proceedings of the Twenty-Fifth Convention of the American Nurses' Association: Report of the Secretary." *American Nurses' Association—Proceedings: 1924–1932*, pp. 5–7.

"Harper Hospital School of Nursing 1883–

1983." Detroit: Harper Hospital School of Nursing Association, n.d.

"Miss Deans Resigns." Editorial. *American Journal of Nursing* 26 (August, 1926): 624–25.

"Miss Delano and Staff in her Office." Photograph. *American Journal of Nursing* 18 (May 1918): 711.

"News: The American Nurses' Association." *American Journal of Nursing* 26 (December 1926): 979.

"News: The American Nurses' Association." *American Journal of Nursing* 27 (July 1927): 597.

"News: Northwestern Division." *American Journal of Nursing* 27 (August 1927): 687.

"Obituaries." *American Journal of Nursing* 48 (May 1948): 44, 46.

"Obituary." *Oswego Palladium Times*, March 15, 1948, 4.

Roberts, M. *American Nursing: History: History and Interpretation.* New York: Macmillan, 1957. Pp. 202–05.

"Who's Who in the Nursing World." *American Journal of Nursing* 24 (June 1924): 736.

Woodford, F.B., and P.P. Mason. *Harper of Detroit: The Origin and Growth of a Great Metropolitan Hospital.* Detroit: Wayne State University Press, 1964. Pp. 372–73.

Sandra Lewenson

Clare Dennison

1891–1954

Nurse-educator Clare Dennison worked to improve the quality of education and to provide better academic preparation for nurses, to improve the working conditions of student and staff nurses in teaching hospitals, and to improve the status of nursing faculty in academia. She strengthened the educational backgrounds of both nursing faculty and students during her professional career, although hospital administrators and doctors frequently opposed her goals.

Dennison was born in Grand Pre, Nova Scotia, Canada, on July 21, 1891, the daughter of Lewis Palmer and Florence Calkin Dennison. She attended Acacia Villa Seminary, Nova Scotia, 1906–10.

After immigrating to the United States in 1915, she enrolled as a student nurse at Boston's Massachusetts General Hospital (MGH) School of Nursing. After her graduation in 1918, Dennison became a clinical instructor in medicine at the school, 1918–20, and then served as assistant superintendent of nursing and head nurse at MGH, 1921–28. She received her B.S. degree from Teachers College, Columbia University, New York City, in 1931. In that same year she assumed the position of superintendent of nurses and director of the School of Nursing at Strong Memorial Hospital, University of Rochester, Rochester, New York, where she remained until her retirement in 1951. Dennison lived in Hingham, Massachusetts, from 1951 to 1953. She died of cancer in Rochester, on February 15, 1954, at age 63.

Dennison's leadership qualities and executive abilities had been evident from the time she was a student nurse at MGH, where she worked as head nurse after graduation in 1918. In 1921 her promotion from head nurse to assistant superintendent of nurses required not only more management responsibilities but also involvement with the education of the student nurses at MGH. She assigned student nurses in the Training School to the wards and special areas of MGH, ensuring provision of patient care 24 hours a day, 7 days a week. In addition, she took care of the affiliations to and from MGH, planned electives and senior experiences, and kept track of each student's records. Under her complex direction of rotations, no student missed a single required assignment.

An interest in reconciling theory with practice led Dennison to take an active part in the development of ward teaching at MGH. In her plan clinical supervisors, rather than the head nurse, taught the students in the wards. The utilization of experts as teachers, supplemented by the provision of outside reading in the subject literature in each field, encouraged students to provide nursing care and to teach both prevention and health care to patients. Although this method placed a burden on the head nurse and ward helper, who had to care for patients while the students were being taught, the method achieved a deeper understanding of the health-care process and thus better nursing.

Dennison's personal characteristics of determination, perseverance, and hard-headed practicality, fully developed during her time at MGH, promoted the best aspects of nursing theory in spite of the realities of hospital staffing shortages and heavy patient loads. She had no use for activities that nurses traditionally did, but no longer had time to perform, such as bed making by a certain time in the morning. In her pragmatic realism, such things could fall by the wayside if they impeded the teaching process or nursing care.

In 1928 Dennison took a leave of absence from MGH to attend Columbia University. She resigned from Massachusetts General in September 1930, and upon graduation from Columbia with a B.S. in 1931, Dennison replaced Helen Wood as director of the Nursing School and superintendent of nurses at Strong Memorial Hospital, University of Rochester.

While at Rochester, Dennison devoted her energies to several diverse but related areas of nursing education. Her concerns centered around improving the quality of nursing education, lessening the work load of student nurses, and raising the nursing faculty to equal status with other professors in the university.

Under Dennison's direction, the diploma program increased to 30 months in 1932 and to 36 months in 1934. Continuing her interest in teaching prevention, she instituted two-month affiliations in public-health nursing and some experience in psychiatric nursing in the diploma program. She believed that a three-year program not only limited the supply of nurses, but also produced a nurse who was more mature and better educated. The baccalaureate program required three years of college and two years of classes in the nursing school, plus nursing in the hospital. Dennison revised the degree curriculum to require more study in the sciences. By 1946 a clinical course in public-health nursing was included in the baccalaureate program.

Dennison did not neglect the continu-

ing education of registered nurses. In 1941 the University of Rochester created a Department of Nursing Education within the College of Arts and Sciences; the department offered courses for RNs interested in improving their knowledge of ward management and their skills in teaching. These courses developed into a program offering a bachelor of science degree with a major in nursing education. By 1947 the Department of Nursing Education offered formal courses in public health, obstetrics, and operating-room nursing and expanded into continuing education by providing noncredit courses, institutes, workshops, and consultation services for registered nurses and area health agencies. The Department of Nursing Education became a division of the university's School of Liberal and Applied Studies in 1951, offering a master of science degree with a major in nursing education.

The health of nursing students, under the impact of a heavy course of study combined with nursing responsibilities, concerned Dennison greatly. At MGH she attributed a six-day work week to the rise in cases of tuberculosis among her student nurses. At Rochester she deplored the heavy work load demanded of nursing students, and in 1937 an advisory committee of the university agreed with her observations and recommended that student nurses carry a maximum of 48 hours a week, including class work. However, the advent of World War II prevented the improvement of work-load conditions.

Dennison's own nursing training at Massachusetts General Hospital took place during World War I, sharpening her awareness of the pressures war brought to the health-care system. The demands placed on health professionals in general, and nursing schools in particular, by World War II, brought her concerns to a head. From 1941 to 1945 enrollment in the Rochester School of Nursing increased from 137 to 325, but resignations of teaching and supervisory staff, who left to join the armed forces, forced even more responsibility on student nurses. Replacements for staff were almost impossible to find, and all nurses worked long hours and extra shifts. Student nurses provided almost 50 percent of nursing hours for patient care and sometimes were put in charge of a floor at Strong Memorial Hospital. In addition to their own students, the instructors at the School of Nursing trained Red Cross nurses' aides and volunteers.

Early in the war, in May 1942, Dennison presented a paper to the National League of Nursing, warning of the problems created by wartime conditions. She deplored the practice of nursing schools, under war-created pressures, to hurry ill-prepared students through programs to satisfy the demand for nurses. In addition, the draining away of staff nurses by the military services meant that student nurses had to perform duties and responsibilities usually done by staff, thus increasing the work load of the students, eventually affecting their health.

In her paper she drew a clear distinction between nursing services and nursing care. Vacancies created by war demands increased the burdens on depleted nursing staffs, who traditionally had to provide such nursing services as billing, keeping statistics and supply records, serving meals, admitting and discharging patients, and arranging for patient transportation. These services took the nurse away from her real responsibility of providing nursing care for patients. In Dennison's opinion, nurses could not continue to perform both functions satisfactorily. Dennison urged doctors and hospital administrators to realize that nursing education had raised nursing to the status of a profession, and they must cease trying to save money by requiring nursing professionals, at low salaries, to perform services that took time away from the nurse's real function—to provide nursing care. Dennison ended her speech by stating ". . . staff nurses in our hospitals [must] receive remuneration in proportion to the work they do and the responsibility they carry . . . [nursing must be] a career in which women can live normally and make provision for old age."

Despite Dennison's apprehensions, she did all in her power to provide nurses for the war effort. In 1942 the School of Nurs-

ing compressed the five-year degree program into just over four years. In 1943 the United States Government established a Cadet Nurse Corps at the University of Rochester and provided monthly allowances to each student. In spite of increased enrollments in the school during the war, sometimes resulting in classes of over 100 students, demand for nurses was so high that sections of Strong Memorial Hospital had to be closed at times due to a lack of nursing staff.

The position of nursing instructors at the University of Rochester was an anomaly, and during Dennison's tenure their status became an important issue in nursing education. Organizationally, the School of Nursing was attached to the Strong Memorial Hospital, not to the university. The College of Arts and Sciences controlled the admission of nursing students to both the diploma and degree programs and recommended the awarding of degrees, but the School of Nursing at Strong appointed the instructors and arranged the curriculum. With little coordination between the two units, academic standards for instructors were difficult to apply, and professors in the Medical School regarded the Nursing School as a nonacademic department. Because the nursing instructors did not have faculty status at the University of Rochester, the School of Nursing never held full membership in the Association of Collegiate Schools of Nursing. Indeed, until 1940, the nursing students did not receive their diplomas in the university's graduation ceremonies but graduated with the city's four nursing schools in a common graduation exercise, emphasizing the university's disregard of nursing as an academic discipline.

However, the increasing intellectual demands of nursing education and Dennison's unceasing efforts to maintain high academic standards for the School of Nursing necessitated a change in attitude at the university. After World War II nursing enrollments fell, although patient loads increased. Competition for students was great, and lack of faculty status for nursing instructors acted as a deterrent for recruitment of new students. In May

1950 Dennison requested the university president, Alan Valentine, to consider academic rank for nursing instructors, citing several benefits from such a move, including improved competition for students and accreditation. Some of the medical faculty strongly opposed the proposal, believing that too much emphasis was placed on nursing education, and the matter was dropped. However, the following year, in March 1951, the nursing educators at the University of Rochester gained nontenured-earning faculty rank. Academic rank for her faculty was Dennison's last major achievement before her retirement in 1953.

Dennison made a lasting impression not only on the academic development of nursing education, but also on the people she worked with. Known as Denny to her students, her insistence on high academic standards and excellent patient care was tempered with a sense of humor and kindliness. Her constant concern for the health and well-being of the student nurses under her care endeared her to all. Always personally interested in nursing education, as president of the Massachusetts General Hospital Alumnae Association in 1928 she was instrumental in the establishment of a loan fund for nursing students engaged in postgraduate study. Upon her retirement, the Alumnae Association of the University of Rochester School of Nursing honored her with a tea and presented the School of Nursing with a portrait of her.

During her short retirement in Hingham, Massachusetts, with a long-time friend, Ruth Adie, Dennison devoted herself to church work, the League of Women Voters, the Hingham Theatre for Children, and gardening. Illness forced her to return to the University of Rochester for treatment in late 1953, but she succumbed to cancer on February 15, 1954.

Recognizing her contributions to nursing education, Strong Memorial Hospital in 1954 sponsored an award in her memory for the student showing the greatest nursing proficiency, and in 1959 the University of Rochester, through the Department of Nursing, established a memorial lectureship in her name for the purpose of inviting distinguished nursing educators to come to the university each year.

PUBLICATIONS BY CLARE DENNISON

"Maintaining the Quality of Nursing Service in the Emergency." *American Journal of Nursing* 42 (July 1942): 774–84.

"Review of *Ethics: The Inner Realities*, by Phyllis A. Goodall." *American Journal of Nursing* 42 (September 1942): 1101.

With M.M. Ball. "Suggestions for Supervisors." *American Journal of Nursing* 40 (July 1940): 759–60.

With M. McKay. "Developments of Ward Teaching, Massachusetts General Hospital." *Massachusetts General Hospital Nurses Alumnae Association. The Quarterly Record* 16 (December 1926): 16.

BIBLIOGRAPHY

Archives. Edward G. Miner Library, University of Rochester Medical Center, Rochester, New York. Recollection of Margaret McGashan Ruch.

"Clare Dennison." *Massachusetts General Hospital Nurses Alumnae Association. The Quarterly Record* 56 (June 1954): 32–33.

"Dennison, Clare." *Who Was Who in America, 1951–1960*. Chicago: Marquis, 1966.

May, A.J. *A History of the University of Rochester, 1850–1962*. Rochester, N.Y.: The university, 1977.

"Obituary." *New York Times*, February 16, 1954, 25.

Perkins, S. *A Centennial Review: the Massachusetts General Hospital School of Nursing, 1873–1973*. Boston: School of Nursing Nurses' Alumnae Association, 1975.

To Each His Farthest Star: A Book of Essays Commemorating the Fiftieth Anniversary of the University Medical Center, 1925–1975. Rochester, N.Y.: The center, 1975.

Kathleen F. Cohen

Kezia Payne de Pelchin

1828–1893

Kezia Payne de Pelchin was a pioneer in the fields of teaching, nursing, and social work in Houston, Texas. With no formal education, but endless faith, energy, and courage, she endeavored to provide care and education to the young, the sick, and the homeless. Through her hard work and personal sacrifice she helped to elevate the status of the professions to which she devoted her life.

Kezia Payne was born on July 23, 1828, in Funchal, Madeira, which was then a part of Portugal. Her father, Abraham Payne, was an Englishman whose first wife had died, leaving him with four children: Abraham, Catherine, Sarah, and Hepzibah. It is believed he was a merchant, who met his second wife, Catherine Armstrong Cartwright, while in Funchal. Abraham and Catherine Payne had three children: Benjamin, Frances, and Kezia. After his wife Catherine's death in 1833, Abraham Payne began to make plans to move to America. It was decided that little Kezia would make the trip with her governess, Hannah Bainton, and that her father would join them in Galveston, Texas, as soon as he could complete his business transactions in Funchal. On December 12, 1836, eight-year-old Kezia arrived in New York City with her governess. They immediately proceeded to Galveston, where they arrived in January 1837. In 1839 Abraham Payne married Hannah Bainton. Unfortunately, a yellow-fever epidemic raged through Galveston that year, killing Kezia's brother Benjamin and half-sister Catherine. Her father also caught the fever, eventually succumbing to the disease. In 1841 Kezia and Hannah moved to Houston, where Hannah began teaching in order to support herself and her stepdaughter. On August 23, 1862, Kezia married Adolph de Pelchin. De Pelchin, born in Ostend, Belgium, in 1835, was rumored to be a drifter, and after only one year of marriage, the couple separated. Although she gave birth to no children of her own, Kezia grew very fond of her husband's young son, Stephen.

Throughout Kezia's life the three professions of teaching, nursing, and social work were intertwined. It was from her stepmother that Kezia received her education, including instruction in German, French, Latin, and piano. Beginning in her early teens, de Pelchin assisted her stepmother in teaching, thus beginning

her first career. As there were no public schools in Houston until after 1877, de Pelchin eventually opened her own academy, as well as teaching at various private schools. Her teaching career continued in the public-school system after its incorporation in 1877.

It was into nursing and social work that Kezia invested vast amounts of her energy, skill, and persistence. At the time, cholera and yellow fever were rampant, devastating families and entire towns. Perhaps the knowledge that yellow fever had killed her father, brother, and half-sister increased her determination to attend to the sick and help lessen their suffering. Her own recovery from yellow fever conferred upon her an immunity to the disease, and she was therefore able to bypass the quarantines that were set up to confine stricken towns. During the Civil War, she joined the nursing corps. Following the war, she continued her work as nurse and teacher. In 1883 she was appointed head nurse at Stuart and Boyles Infirmary, an almshouse, in Houston. In fact, she was often the *only* nurse in attendance at this institution. At that time the status of the nurse was often viewed as only one degree above that of the domestic servant. The dedication of Kezia Payne de Pelchin to the nursing profession is evident in her continued work to reform the conditions of the sick and the poor, often giving away her pay to the needy.

Following the Civil War, there was no organized social or relief work in the city of Houston. De Pelchin saw the need to improve the poor conditions that existed in the charity hospitals and, especially, the orphanages. It is during this phase of her life that she focused her attention on the plight of the orphan. In 1888 she became the matron of Bayland Orphans' Home in Houston. Recognizing the need to provide a home for infants and young children who could not be accommodated at Bayland, she opened Faith Home in 1892. De Pelchin died on January 13, 1893, at the Bayland Orphans' Home.

Her Faith Home continued for many years after her death. In 1893 the De Pelchin Faith Home Association was organized in her memory to provide an orphanage and day nursery for the care and protection of dependent, neglected, and homeless children. After 1929 the Faith Home was expanded into a general childcare agency, the De Pelchin Faith Home and Children's Bureau. By 1939 the Faith Home, which consisted of one permanent building in 1895, had grown to include nine buildings on 12 acres.

At the time of her death, de Pelchin's will stipulated that her niece, Martha Payne, receive all her worldly assets—a parcel of land worth $150 and $30.20 in the bank. Through her personal sacrifice, Kezia Payne de Pelchin left behind a rich legacy to the professions of teaching, nursing, and social work.

BIBLIOGRAPHY

Matthews, H.J. *Candle By Night: The Story of the Life and Times of Kezia Payne de Pelchin, Texas Pioneer Teacher, Social Worker, and Nurse.* Boston: Bruce Humphries, 1942.

Nursing Studies Index. Vol. II, 1930–49, p. 53. Philadelphia: Lippincott, 1970.

Linda Karch

Naomi Deutsch

1890–1983

Naomi Deutsch was a public-health executive and federal official who headed the Public-health Nursing Division of the U.S. Department of Labor Children's Bureau in the late 1930s and early 1940s. In that position, she tried to increase government and public awareness of the need for improved prenatal care.

Deutsch was born in Brux (Most), Czechoslovakia, on November 5, 1890. As a young girl, she moved to the United States with her parents, Gotthard and Hermine Bacher Deutsch. Her father was a history professor. She was graduated from the Walnut Hills preparatory high school in Cincinnati, Ohio, and in 1912 from the Jewish Hospital School of Nursing there. In 1921 she received a B.S. degree from Teachers College, Columbia University, where she was a member of the Delta Omega Society.

After college Deutsch worked with the Visiting Nurse Association in Cincinnati and the Jesse Kaufmann Settlement in Pittsburgh, Pennsylvania. From 1916–24 she served the Henry Street Nurse Service in New York successively as a supervisor, field director, and acting general director. She was director of the Visiting Nurse Service in San Francisco from 1925–33. The University of California appointed her a lecturer in public-health nursing in 1933, and in 1934 she received the rank of assistant professor.

From 1935–43 she was director of the public-health nursing unit of the Federal Children's Bureau. In 1941 she represented the Children's Bureau on the National Council on National Defense.

She was named principal nursing consultant for the Pan American Sanitary Bureau on March 1, 1943, and worked with Dr. John R. Murdock in developing health programs for Caribbean and Central American countries. From headquarters in Panama City, she visited Mexico City, Guatemala City, San Salvador, Tegucigalpa, Managua, and San Jose. At the time she was chairman of the Joint Committee on Inter-American Nursing of the American Nurses' Association, the National League of Nursing Education, and the National Organization of Public Health Nursing.

Deutsch was named president of the California State Organization for Public Health Nursing and a member of the board of directors of the California State Nurses' Association in April 1933. Other offices she held in professional organizations included the following: president, San Francisco Organization for Public Health Nursing, San Francisco Social Workers Alliance; member, board of directors, California Organization for Public Health Nursing; member, governing council, American Public Health Association; secretary, San Francisco County Nurses'

Association; chairman, nursing section, American Public Health Association.

She also was a member of the American Nurses' Association, the National League of Nursing Education, the American Association of Social Workers, the National Conference of Social Work, and the League of Women Voters.

She died in New Orleans on November 26, 1983.

PUBLICATIONS BY NAOMI DEUTSCH

ARTICLES

"Nursing the Community." *Pacific Coast Journal of Nursing* 22 (December 1926): 713–14.

"Generalized Public Health Nursing Services in Cities." *American Journal of Public Health* 25 (April 1935): 475–78.

"How Are the Goals of Tomorrow's Community Nursing Service to be Reached? Through Public Health Nursing." American Nurses' Association: *Proceedings of the 30th Convention (1936) of the American Nurses' Association.* New York: American Nurses' Association, 1936. Pp. 576–81.

"Public Health Nursing in Programs for Crippled Children and the Role of the Public Health Nurse." *Public Health Nurse* 29 (January 1937): 10–15.

"Economic Aspects of Maternal Care." *Public Health Nursing* 31 (November 1939): 619–24.

With H. Hilbert. "Public Health Nursing under the Social Security Act, Developments under the Children's Bureau." *Public Health Nursing* 28 (September 1936): 582–85.

With M.B. Willeford. "Promoting Maternal and Child Health." *American Journal of Nursing* 41 (August 1941): 894–99.

BIBLIOGRAPHY

American Women 1935–40: A Composite Biographical Dictionary. D. Howes, ed. Detroit: Gale, 1981.

"Changes in Children's Bureau Staff." *American Journal of Nursing* 43 (April 1943): 402.

"Naomi Deutsch." *Pacific Coast Journal of Nursing* 30 (September 1934): 487.

"Naomi Deutsch." *Pacific Coast Journal of Nursing* 32 (January 1936): 34–35.

"News." *American Journal of Nursing* 34 (March 1934): 285–86.

"News About Nursing." *American Journal of Nursing* 41 (January 1941): 94.

Women of the West. M. Benheim, ed. Los Angeles: Publishers Press, 1938.

Alice P. Stein

Josephine Aloyse Dolan
b. 1913

Josephine Aloyse Dolan, nursing historian, achieved a national reputation for her contributions to nursing education and nursing scholarship. Dolan is best known as the author of the history text *Nursing in Society.* In 1958 she succeeded Minnie Goodnow as author of the nursing history series, which had been continuously published since 1916 but with different titles.

Born July 27, 1913, in Cranston, Rhode Island, Josephine Dolan was the second of two daughters and a younger son born to Thomas and Josephine Tynan Dolan. She is a descendent of Irish ancestors who settled in this country early in the 1800s. She was a young child when the family relocated to Lawrence, Massachusetts, where her father was owner and partner in a wholesale meat company.

Her early education was attained in private schools where Dolan acknowledges she was mischievous and much more interested in having fun than being a student. Dolan was a high-school student when her 48-year-old father's sudden death drastically changed her life and her entire attitude toward education. Ironically, his untimely death proved to be the stimulus for her interest in nursing. Dolan recalls the lack of sophisticated medical knowledge and technology characteristic of that era. The experienced group of physicians summoned for consultation had few diagnostic tools and virtually no treatments or drugs to save her critically ill father. Their sole recommendation was that a highly qualified "trained nurse" was needed. The vivid recollection of how the nurse's comfort measures eased her father's dying left a profound impression on Dolan. But she knew little else about the profession of nursing. When she sought guidance from a high-school counselor, he was "horrified" that she would even consider pursuing a nursing education. Nevertheless, following her high-school graduation, she entered St. John's Hospital School of Nursing in nearby Lowell, Massachusetts.

Reminiscing about the St. John's diploma program, Dolan recalls she "never worked so hard in my life." She graduated in 1935 and was awarded a scholarship to continue her education. For a short time, however, she did private-duty nursing to help the family's now considerably reduced financial status. On one occasion she remembers "being in a home where there were five ill children and helping the mother to care for them. I was there a week and at the end of the week I decided I couldn't take money from this lady because she was having so much trouble. My mother said she didn't think that we were going to make out very well if this was what I was going to do on a regular basis."

After spending one semester at the Boston "in-town" campus of Boston College, she enrolled in the new nursing program at Boston University. At that time the nursing program was not an autonomous school but, patterned after the program at Teachers College, Columbia University, part of the School of Education. Dolan received a baccalaureate degree from Boston University in 1942 and taught for one year at St. Vincent's Hospital School of Nursing in Bridgeport, Connecticut. To better prepare herself for teaching, Dolan returned to Boston University in the fall of 1943 to begin work on her master's degree.

In June 1944 she began her long association with the University of Connecticut when she became the first instructor in the new School of Nursing, joining its only other faculty member and founder of the school, Dean Carolyn Ladd Widmer. Her initial teaching assignment included the history of nursing. Dolan recalls:

> I couldn't believe it. I hated nursing history. I had had the most boring, dull, horrible course in history of nursing. So I told Dean Widmer I didn't care for history of nursing, but she wasn't impressed and said, "Well, you will love it." She told me how her grandfather, who founded Robert College in Istanbul, offered his services to Florence Nightingale in the Crimean War and a number of interesting stories about Nightingale and I thought, my word, Florence Nightingale was a living person because

as far as I had been concerned she was some dead, dusty old lady.

This encounter proved to be the beginning of a metamorphosis for Dolan's interest in the history of nursing, the catalyst for her distinguished career as a nurse historian.

Continuing to teach full time at the University of Connecticut, she completed her master's degree at Boston University in 1950. To enrich and broaden her background and assist her in developing a sound historical research methodology, she also took most of the courses that the University of Connecticut's Department of History had to offer. Dolan rose through the professorial ranks to become a full professor of nursing in 1961. Throughout her tenure at the University of Connecticut (1944–76) she taught, in addition to other courses, the required undergraduate course for nurses that dealt with the historical and philosophical nature of the discipline. This popular survey course was open to and elected by students in other schools of the university. It provided a vehicle for exploring nursing as a career option for nonmajors and helped others to better understand the heritage and issues of the profession.

Dolan is especially proud of her involvement (1961–71) with the Committee on Historic Source Materials in Nursing, which was originally formed under the old National League for Nursing Education. This group was organized at a time when the study of nursing history was increasingly perceived as a luxury and was being deleted from nursing curricula in lieu of more scientific content. The invitation to join this prestigious group brought her the opportunity to discuss the problems and issues of promoting and preserving nursing history with such established leaders as Isabel Stewart, Anne Austin, Stella Goostray, and Mary Roberts as well as younger leaders Martha Rogers, Faye Abdellah, and Edith Lewis.

Throughout her career Dolan has been one of nursing's most outspoken advocates for the collection of historical materials and dissemination, teaching, and study of nursing history. During much of this time there was little historical research and writing or support from the profession for such endeavors. Dolan also strongly ascribes to the notion that many current problems have deep roots in the past and are perpetuated by those unfamiliar with nursing history. Her enthusiasm for nursing history has been evident in her teaching, numerous speeches, journal articles, booklets and reviews, keynote addresses, consultancies, and committee memberships. These include chair, board of advisors, History of Nursing Audio/Visual Committee, ANA and NLN (1958–61); member of the National Heritage Committee, Sigma Theta Tau (1979–83); member, board of editorial advisors, *Aesculapius*, the *Journal of the History of Medicine and Allied Sciences*, Medical Heritage Society (1971); contributing author and film consultant for "A History of American Nursing," ANA-NLN Film Service (1961); author and presenter of the widely disseminated videotape series, 'Nursing in Society,' distributed by ANA, Minnesota Video Nursing Council, and Telstar Productions (1965); and chair, Committee on Historical Source Materials, NLN (1965–71).

In addition to Dolan's contributions to nursing history, her career also demonstrates excellence in teaching and scholarship and extensive involvement in service to the profession. She is a member of Pi Lambda Theta (1942) and Sigma Theta Tau (1954). Dolan was the first recipient of the NLN Distinguished Service Award in 1972. In 1980 Dolan's reputation as an excellent teacher was publicly recognized when the Connecticut Nurses' Association established the Josephine A. Dolan Award for Outstanding Contribution to Nursing Education. Mu Chapter of Sigma Theta Tau, which she helped to found, honored her in 1986 by instituting an award for Excellence in Nursing Scholarship in her name. Both of these awards are presented annually to outstanding nurses. In 1983 Dolan was named the Boston University School of Nursing Outstanding Alumna. She holds an honorary doctor of pedagogy from Rhode Island College (1974) and an honorary doctor of nursing science from Boston College (1987).

Throughout her career at the University of Connecticut she was an active member of the university community and served on a variety of university committees. Dolan has an enviable record of professional service at the local, state, and national level, having served on, and chaired, many prestigious committees. She was an active member of the Connecticut State Board of Examiners for Nursing (1951–56); the Connecticut League for Nursing, its board of directors (1964–67, 1977–79) and president (1967–69); the Connecticut Nurses' Association and its board of directors (1960–62); the National League for Nursing, its board of directors (1969–71); and Sigma Theta Tau, serving as the national chair, Nominating Committee (1977–80) and president of Mu Chapter (1962–65).

Dolan's unique contributions to the ongoing presentation and preservation of the proud heritage of nursing has continued in her busy retirement. She has been a visiting lecturer in the University of Connecticut School of Nursing (1976–85). She continues as a consultant in the history of nursing and is professor emeritus, University of Connecticut School of Nursing. Dolan travels extensively and is an active member of her profession and her home community of Holliston, Massachusetts.

PUBLICATIONS BY JOSEPHINE ALOYSE DOLAN

BOOKS

Goodnow's History of Nursing, 10th and 11th eds. Philadelphia: Saunders, 1958, 1963.

History of Nursing, 12th ed. Philadelphia: Saunders, 1968.

Nursing in Society—A Historical Perspective, 13th and 14th eds. Philadelphia: Saunders, 1973, 1978. Japanese edition, 1978.

Editor. *Nursing Clinics of North America*, Vol. 1, No. 1. Philadelphia: Saunders, 1966.

With M.L. Fitzpatrick and E.K. Herrmann. *Nursing in Society—A Historical Perspective*, 15th ed. Philadelphia: Saunders, 1983.

BOOKLETS

The Grace of the Great Lady. Chicago: Medical Heritage Society, 1971.

Bicentennial Calendar. Connecticut: Connecticut Nurses' Association, 1976.

With S. Goostray, K. Dreves, and R. Metheney. *Three Score Years and Ten.* New York: National League for Nursing, 1963.

ARTICLES

"Using Postage Stamps in the Teaching of History of N." *Nursing Outlook* 9 (April 1961): 164–65.

"Nursing Leadership—1895." *Nursing Science* 1 (1963): 223–28.

"Three Schools—1873." *American Journal of Nursing* 75 (June 1975).

With D. Rogers. "The Connecticut Nurses' Association—The Sixth Decade." *Connecticut Nursing News* (January 1965).

BIBLIOGRAPHY

Davis, S.K. Taped interview with J. A. Dolan, February 1987.

Dolan, J.A. Taped interview with author, June 1989.

Herrmann, E.K. Interview with author, May and June 1989.

Widmer, C.L. "Heritage of Accomplishment— the History of the University of Connecticut School of Nursing—1942–1981." Storrs: University of Connecticut School of Nursing, 1982.

Roberta M. Orne

Anita Dowling Dorr

1915–1972

Anita Dowling Dorr was a leader in the field of emergency nursing. She is remembered for progress within her profession that led to the development of ongoing educational programs and dissemination of emergency-care information as mechanisms for achieving optimum emergency health care for all. She was the founder of the Emergency Department Nurses Association and the developer of the first "crisis cart," as well as a representative to numerous agencies involved in planning emergency services in the United States.

Dorr was born on April 18, 1915, in Titusville, Pennsylvania, the daughter of Patrick and Mary Agnes Dowling. The third of seven children, she attended St. Titus High School, graduating in 1932.

The Depression was a major part of her younger life, and in an effort to get a job away from the grinding poverty of these times, she chose to attend nursing school. She enrolled in the program at the E.J. Meyer Memorial Hospital School of Nursing in Buffalo, New York. Upon graduation, she held the position of operating-room supervisor there until joining the Army Nurse Corps (during World War II) as a member of the 23rd Buffalo General Unit. In the Army Nurse Corps she attained the rank of captain, serving in major campaigns in Africa, Italy, France, and Germany. On her return to Buffalo in 1945 at the end of the war, she married John Harold Dorr.

Dorr became the supervisor of the Emergency Department of the Meyer Memorial Hospital in 1960. Increasingly concerned about the crisis in emergency health-care services in the late 1960s, she encouraged nurses to work together and make their voices heard to achieve a common goal of optimum emergency care for all. Initial steps toward this goal were focused on increasing educational opportunities for nurses working in emergency medicine. By the late 1960s, under her leadership, nurses in local emergency departments began pushing for more in-service training, better teaching, and special programs that would bring together experts in the field of emergency health care. Believing that nurses working in the emergency rooms required special training, just as those nurses working in intensive-care units, she developed collaborative relationships with universities and colleges, the American College of Surgeons, American Academy of Orthopedic Surgeons, and the major pharmaceutical companies. This network supported and encouraged educational seminars held around the country.

Additional needs and opportunities identified through these associations eventually led Dorr to found the National Emergency Department Nurses Association in 1970 to expand the educational offerings and networking opportunities around the country. Through the initiatives started in this organization, emergency nurses became involved within their communities and professional organizations as speakers and educators on emergency health-care issues. They became recognized for their expertise and were appointed to local, national, and state emergency medical-services committees. Dorr served as the executive director of the organization until her death in 1972. Since that time, the organization has grown to a membership of over 18,000 emergency nurses worldwide and has shortened its name to the Emergency Nurses Association (ENA).

An additional contribution to emergency health care was the development of the crash cart. Seeing that precious time was being wasted when her staff had to chase around the hospital emergency department to collect the medications and supplies necessary for emergency cases, Dorr developed the first "crisis cart." She gathered and measured those items that might be needed in any emergency. With her husband, John, she designed and built the prototype in her home to house all those items. The "crisis cart," now known as the crash cart, is used in every emergency room in order to save precious time in treating emergencies.

Because of her expertise in emergency nursing, Dorr was chosen as a consultant to numerous local, state, and national agencies involved in emergency care, including the New York State Technical Advisory Board of Emergency Services and the National Committee of the U.S. Public Health Bureau of Emergency Services. She also served as a consultant and lecturer to Paramount Pictures for its medical television programs and as a lecturer to various other medical organizations around the country.

Anita Dorr died on October 4, 1972, from lung cancer. One observer aptly described her a few years later when stating that for Dorr "a hallmark of her career was setting new dimensions in her profession."

PUBLICATIONS BY ANITA DOWLING DORR

"I am a Nurse." Reprinted in *Journal of Emergency Nursing* 16 (1990): 20–21A.

BIBLIOGRAPHY

Atkinson, L.J. "Accountability: The Product of Achievement." *Journal of Emergency Nursing* (1976): 40–42.

Given, J. "January Nurses Crisis Cart Speeds Emergency Care." *Buffalo Evening News*, February 6, 1972, 72.

"In Memoriam." *Road Runner* [a newsletter of Emergency Nurses Assn] 1:1 (Dec 1972): 1.

"In Memoriam." *New York State Council Emergency Department Association* 12: 3 (A Booklet, 1972).

Kelleher, J. "When Dreams Come True." *Journal of Emergency Nursing* 16 (1990): 1.

Linda M. Calley

Mary T. Dowling

?–1947

Mary T. Dowling was a leader in the field of industrial nursing. She was executive secretary of the American Association of Industrial Nurses from 1946 until her death and also was president of the New York Industrial Nurses and the New York Catholic Nurses Club.

Dowling was born in Massachusetts and was a graduate of the Medfield, Massachusetts, Training School for Nurses. She specialized in industrial nursing and medical social work and did graduate work at Fordham University and the City College of New York.

She began her career as an industrial nurse, serving with the Bergen Company of New Jersey and the Rosenwasser Company of New York City. From 1923–31 she was with the Press Publishing Company of New York City.

In 1931 Dowling became associated with the Department of Hospitals in New York City, serving at Riverside Hospital in the Bronx and Staten Island Hospital. For 13 years she was a medical social worker at the Kingston Avenue Hospital in Brooklyn. She was active in the alumnae association of the Medfield School, served on many local and national nursing committees, and was a member of the ANA.

Dowling died of a heart ailment on February 2, 1947, at her New York City home. She had returned to work three weeks earlier after recuperating from a heart attack.

BIBLIOGRAPHY

"Mary T. Dowling." *American Journal of Nursing* 47 (April 1947): 268.

"Miss Dowling Dies; Leader in Nursing." *New York Times*, February 14, 1947.

Alice P. Stein

Rosemary Ellis

1919–1986

Rosemary Ellis was a scholar, educator, researcher, and author whose primary concern was the identification, clarification and transmission of the knowledge that would form the basis for nursing practice and research.

She was born in Berkeley, California, on July 22, 1919, the daughter of banker Willard Drake Ellis and Edna Woods Ellis. She had one brother and then, later, a stepbrother and stepsister when her father married Louise Ficklin.

Growing up in Berkeley, she spent summers in the Northern California mountains with her family, and developed a lifelong interest in natural history. Frank W. Ellis, her brother, recalls that an uncle lived with the family during his medical internship in 1931 and was an influence on him and on Rosemary in choosing health-related careers. In 1936 Ellis graduated from Berkeley High School and first earned a B.A. in economics from the University of California at Berkeley later completing work for a B.S. in nursing at the University of California, San Francisco, in 1944.

Between 1944 and 1952 she served as a head nurse, supervisor, and assistant superintendent of nurses at the University of California Hospital, San Francisco, and also served as second lieutenant with the occupation forces in Japan. Ellis earned

an M.A. in nursing education from the University of Chicago in 1953, remaining there as assistant professor of nursing until 1959. In 1963–64, while doing work for a Ph.D. in human development at the University of Chicago, she was a research assistant in the Department of Psychiatry. Ellis joined the faculty at Frances Payne Bolton School of Nursing, Case Western Reserve University, Cleveland, in 1964 as associate professor and was promoted to full professor in 1968. She became professor emerita in July 1986 when illness forced her retirement. In 1971 Ellis visited Japan as consultant in nursing research and was visiting professor at the University of Edmonton, Canada.

Ellis suffered a stroke in 1972 that left her with left hemiplegia. She shared her experience in an article for the *American Journal of Nursing* about aspects of care for stroke patients. Using a leg brace to assist mobility, she continued traveling, teaching, and lecturing for many years.

Among the many professional organizations in which she was a member were the American Nurses' Association Council of Nurse Researchers, American Association for the Advancement of Science, American Public Health Association, and the National Stroke Association Scientific Advisory Board. She was a fellow of the American Academy of Nursing. The University of California, San Francisco, honored her with the Distinguished Alumna Award in 1985. Other acknowledgments were recognition as Distinguished Contributor to Nursing Science by the American Nurses' Association in June 1986 and a citation by Congress for her accomplishments presented at a meeting of the Greater Cleveland Nurses' Association.

Throughout her tenure at Case Western Reserve University, Ellis contributed to knowledge development in nursing by participating in clinical research and in theory development. She believed that nursing knowledge should be acquired in various ways and that research should include both processes of discovery and validation. She identified at least four types of knowledge in the field of nursing inquiry: scientific knowledge, historical knowledge, philosophic knowledge, and nursing technology. She urged nurse scientists and scholars to give attention to the identification of phenomena essential to nursing science as well as to the application of research methods to study them. Human beings and their responses along with "health," "environment," and "nursing" are concepts central to the discipline of nursing that need to be defined, she believed, in order to identify and clarify nursing's body of knowledge. She advocated a community of scholars, doctorally prepared nurses, thinking and communicating together to assume primary responsibility for developing nursing knowledge. She frequently enjoined nurses to become thinkers as well as doers and to avoid premature emphasis on validation when phenomena to be studied were not clearly defined.

Following a five-week hospitalization with heart and kidney involvement, Rosemary Ellis died on October 10, 1986, in Lakeside Hospital, Cleveland.

PUBLICATIONS BY ROSEMARY ELLIS

"Symposium on Theory Development in Nursing. Characteristics of significant theories." *Nursing Research* 17 (May/June 1968): 217-22.

"The Practitioner as Theorist." *American Journal of Nursing* 69 (July 1969): 1434-38.

"The Nurse as Investigator and Member of the Research Team." *Annals of the New York Academy of Science* 169 (1969): 435-41.

"Values and Vicissitudes of the Scientist Nurse." *Nursing Research* 19 (September/October 1970): 440-45.

"Training for Research." *Journal of Nursing Education* 10 (August 1971): 27-36.

"Unusual Sensory and Thought Disturbances After Cardiac Surgery." *American Journal of Nursing* 72 (November 1972): 2021-25.

"After Stroke. Sitting Problems. Part III." *American Journal of Nursing* 73 (November 1973): 1898-99.

"Conceptual Issues in Nursing." *Nursing Outlook* 30 (July/August 1982): 406-10.

Editorial. *Advances in Nursing Science* 4 (1982): x-xi.

"Philosophic Inquiry." *Annual Review of Nursing Research* 1 (1983): 211-28.

With C.W. Jackson, Jr. "Sensory Deprivation as a Field of Study." *Nursing Research* 20 (January/February, 1971): 46-54.

BIBLIOGRAPHY

Ellis, F.W. Personal communication, 1989.

Ellis, R. "Fallibilities, Fragments and Frames: Contemplation on 25 Years of Research in Medical-Surgical Nursing." *Nursing Research* 26 (May/June 1977): 177. Photo.

Memorial Resolution in Honor of Rosemary Ellis. Cleveland: Faculty Senate, Frances Payne Bolton School of Nursing, Case Western Reserve University, October 21, 1986.

Nursing Archives. Mugar Memorial Library, Boston University, Boston.

Pressler, J.L., and J.J. Fitzpatrick. "Contributions of Rosemary Ellis to Knowledge Development for Nursing." *Image: Journal of Nursing Scholarship* 20 (Spring 1988): 28-30.

"Rosemary Ellis." Obituary. *Cleveland Plain Dealer*, October 17, 1986.

"Rosemary Ellis." *Who's Who in American Nursing*. Washington, D.C.: Society of Nursing Professionals, 1984.

"Rosemary Ellis." *Who's Who in Health Care*, 2nd ed. Rockville, Md.: Aspen, 1981.

Marianne Brook

Bertha Erdmann

1869-1922

Bertha Erdmann was the first superintendent of nurses for what was to become the University of Minnesota School of Nursing. Although illness limited her tenure in this position to one year, her early efforts laid a foundation for later developments in collegiate nursing education at the University of Minnesota and elsewhere. She directed the first "course for nurses," as it was titled, at the University of North Dakota. She is also credited as one of the founders and the first president of the North Dakota (State) Nurses' Association and was very influential in the passage of the first Nurse Practice Act in North Dakota.

Erdmann was born on September 6, 1869, in Milwaukee, Wisconsin, to Andreas and Elisabeth Fuchs Erdmann. She was their fifth child, born after Karl, Elise, Oscar, and Emma. Her father is listed as a sailor on her birth record; probably he served on one of the ships in the Great Lakes.

Her early education was conducted in German. She did enroll for her later schooling in the Milwaukee public-school system. An eye problem precluded her completing high school, but she received private instruction so that she could enter nursing school.

Erdmann graduated from the St. Barnabas Hospital Training School for Nurses, Minneapolis, on August 26, 1899. That same year she was appointed superintendent of Hunter Hospital, Faribault, Minnesota, where she served until 1901, when she became superintendent of nurses at Luther Hospital in St. Paul. She remained there only a short time before being appointed superintendent of nurses at Minneapolis City Hospital, where she served from 1901 to 1903 and from 1905 to 1908, interrupted with a year of teaching first at Luther Hospital and then at Northwestern Hospital, both in Minneapolis. At the City Hospital she introduced the concept, then relatively new, of a preliminary course for probationary students.

About that time other new ideas about nursing education were incubating in Minneapolis. The announcement about the proposed University of Minnesota School for Nurses, as it was originally titled, was made by Dr. Richard Olding Beard before a joint meeting of the American Society of Superintendents of Training Schools for Nurses (forerunner of the present National League for Nursing) and the Associated Alumnae of the United States and Canada (predecessor of the American Nurses' Association). The meeting was held in Minneapolis on June 9, 1909.

Although the University of Minnesota Hospital was yet to be built, Erdmann was appointed its superintendent of nurses in 1908. She then went to Teachers College, Columbia University, for a year's study in the course in Hospital Economics. Here she met a fellow student, Louise Powell, who would later succeed her at the University of Minnesota.

The University of Minnesota School for Nurses officially opened March 1, 1909, as a three-year undergraduate program with four students enrolled. Except for Erdmann, who taught nursing arts along with her administrative responsibilities, the school's faculty were members of the faculty of the medical school. Clinical practice for students was in an old house that served as a temporary university hospital; it accommodated 25 patients.

The program Erdmann inaugurated was similar to one designed by Adelaide Nutting and adopted by the more advanced schools of the time. But it was unique in its setting: the association with the medical school faculty, the prestige of being connected to the university, the carefully selected students who had to meet the university's entrance requirements.

Ill health forced Erdmann's resignation after a year, and the rest of her life was a constant battle against the tuberculosis that eventually led to her death. After extended periods of rest or hospitalization, she would return to employment until illness once again forced her resignation.

In 1910 she was appointed director of the new "course for nurses" at the University of North Dakota, instigated by the university's new president Frank McVey. He came to Grand Forks from the University of Minnesota, bringing with him many ideas that originated there. This unique program appealed to Erdmann, an ardent supporter of collegiate education for nurses. The two-semester nursing program was designed for students who then entered affiliated hospital schools of nursing for the last two years of clinical practice.

She established affiliation arrangements with a number of schools of nursing, not only the Deaconess Hospital in Grand Forks, but also in distant areas such as Augustana Hospital, Chicago; Mercy Hospital, Kansas City; Trinity Hospital, Milwaukee; St. Luke's Hospital, St. Paul; and Bellevue Hospital, New York. The number of students enrolled in this nursing program was never very large, and it was discontinued in 1916.

Erdmann taught many of the courses herself. She also arranged for summer courses, such as dietetics, bacteriology, chemistry, psychology, and sociology, offered to graduate nurses. She firmly believed that good nursing required a sound knowledge base.

Throughout her career, Erdmann was very active in nursing organizations. When the Hennepin County Graduate Nurses' Association was organized in Minneapolis in 1901, she was selected to fill the vacancy created by the illness of the first president, and the next year she was elected to this position. The establishment of the Minnesota State Graduate Nurses' Association was one of the early activities of the fledgling organization, along with its Ramsey County (St. Paul area) counterpart. At the organizational meeting Erdmann was elected temporary chairman of the group. After it was founded, she was among the members of the association who campaigned for a state nurse practice act, which was passed and signed by the governor in 1907.

After she moved to North Dakota, once again Erdmann was involved in organizational activities. She chaired the Committee of the Grand Forks County Graduate Nurses' Association to investigate the possiblity of a state organization. And when the North Dakota State Nurses' Association was founded in 1912, Erdmann was elected its first president. She was re-elected twice, although illness forced her absence from the annual meeting in 1914, where her presidential address was read by a colleague. In 1913 she had been granted a year's leave of absence from the university but resigned the next year.

As was usually true with other state nurses' associations, the early efforts of the North Dakota State Nurses' Association were directed toward the passage of the Nurse Practice Act. Even during her illness and while a patient in the Bismarck Hospital, Erdmann devised means to ensure passage of the proposed legislation. The bill was signed by the Governor on March 9, 1915. A news note in the June issue of the *American Journal of Nursing* that year indicated that the members of the association felt deeply indebted to her for efforts on behalf of the organization.

Erdmann left North Dakota in 1915 to enter Agnes Memorial Sanitarium in Denver. She was very ill at the time but again recovered sufficiently to hold positions of responsibility, including employment at Glockner Sanitarium in Colorado Springs.

In her final illness, she returned to the University of Minnesota Hospital in Minneapolis, where she died on November 5, 1922, at 52 years of age.

Erdmann has been described as a courageous nursing pioneer. A dedicated nurse leader, she was committed to the professionalization of nursing through efforts to secure passage of nurse practice acts as well as promoting sound educational preparation of nurses. Although handicapped by severe illness during much of her career, she made remarkable contributions to the profession that she served so well.

PUBLICATIONS BY BERTHA ERDMANN

"Rest Periods for Nurses." *American Journal of Nursing* 9 (December 1908): 188–89.

BIBLIOGRAPHY

"Bertha Erdmann." Obituary. *American Journal of Nursing* 23 (December 1922): 261–62.

"Bertha Erdmann, R.N. Superintendent of Nurses, 1909–1910." In *Remembering Things Past: A Heritage of Excellence. University of Minnesota School of Nursing Diamond Jubilee, 1909–1984.* B.H. Canedy, ed. Minneapolis: University of Minnesota, 1983. P. 169.

Danielsen, A.O. *North Dakota State Nurses' Association, 1912–1934.* Bismarck: North Dakota State Nurses' Association, 1934.

Gray, J. *Education for Nursing: A History of the University of Minnesota School.* Minneapolis: University of Minnesota Press, 1960. Pp. 19–21.

Heyse, M. Letter to author, November 29, 1971.

Heyse-Cory, M. *Nurse: A Changing Word in a Changing World—the History of the University of North Dakota College of Nursing, 1909–1982.* Grand Forks: University Press, 1983.

Merrill, B.E. *The Trek from Yesterday. A History of Organized Nursing in Minneapolis, 1883–1936.* Privately printed, 1944.

Nursing News and Announcements. Various issues. *American Journal of Nursing* (1912–15).

Powell, M.L. "The History of the Development of Nursing Education at the University of Minnesota." In *Remembering Things Past: A*

Heritage of Excellence. University of Minnesota School of Nursing Diamond Jubilee, 1909–1984. B.H. Canedy, ed. Minneapolis: University of Minnesota, 1983. P. 1.

Sharpless, B.A.T., M.H. Coe, and F.E. Marks. "School of Nursing." In *Masters of Medicine.* J.A. Myers, ed. St. Louis: Warren and Green, 1968.

Shea, M. Letter to author, June 19, 1989.

Wisconsin Department of Health and Social Services. Section on Vital Statistics. Bertha Erdmann Birth Record, September 6, 1869.

Signe S. Cooper

Sara Maiter Errickson

b. 1905

Sara M. Errickson has been called the "matriarch of New Jersey nurses." Her strong presence as executive director of the New Jersey State Nurses' Association moved professional nursing forward in that state.

Sarah Cecelia Maiter Errickson was born in Long Branch, New Jersey, January 12, 1905, the eighth child of Louise (Alberti) Maiter and Frances Xavier Maiter. Both parents were born in Italy and immigrated to the United States at early ages. Her birth occurred three months after the death of her father who had been a grounds superintendent at the McCall estate in Long Branch. Her mother worked as a seamstress to support the family.

Errickson chose nursing because in grade school she had a friend whose mother was bedridden with advanced tuberculosis. She and her friend would provide comfort to the ailing woman. Even as a young child, Errickson was said to carry around bandages at all times. Her career choice was reinforced when she fractured her leg in high school and was hospitalized for several weeks.

Errickson entered Monmouth Memorial Hospital School of Nursing (Long Branch, New Jersey) in 1922 at the age of 17 and graduated in 1925. She joined the American Nurses' Association in 1926; she often relates that she was more concerned with being accepted as an ANA member than with passing state boards. After graduation she did three years of general duty and institutional private-duty nursing at Monmouth Memorial Hospital. During the summers she worked as a camp nurse at Camp Najecko for underprivileged boys from a Philadelphia Episcopal diocese.

In 1928 she began her 22-year public-health nursing career with a position at the Long Branch Public Health Nursing Organization. "My entire career included direct nursing service, organization, supervision and teaching on the local, state, county level in the capacity of staff nurse, assistant supervisor, supervisor, consultant and assistant executive director and executive director."

In 1937 she was employed by the Health Department in Long Branch under the Social Security Act of 1935. She then worked for Monmouth County, developing health programs for schools.

In 1940 at the age of 35 she married Raymond Clifford Errickson, the Public Health Director of Long Branch. A longtime family friend, he was a widower with two grown sons: Raymond Jr. and Louis. Raymond Errickson died only 18 months after their marriage.

Feeling a need for more education, Errickson returned to school receiving a certificate in public-health nursing from University of Pennsylvania in 1942, and a B.S.N. from Seton Hall University in 1946.

Between 1942 through 1944 she worked for the Monmouth County Organization for Social Service (MCOSS) as a supervisor with responsibility for the tuberculosis program. She then obtained a position as a nurse consultant with the New Jersey State Department of Health, where she assisted in the creation of a Bureau of Nursing. She was instrumental in developing a cancer-control program. Errickson also developed a statewide tuberculosis program that included collecting data on the incidence of tuberculosis throughout New Jersey. She qualified as an administrative secretary, a civil service post in which she dealt with tuberculosis control. However, her title remained "nurse consultant."

In 1950 she ended her public-health nursing career by accepting a position as superintendent of a nursing home in Long Island. After two years she returned to New Jersey to care for her ailing mother.

Errickson's eminent work with the New Jersey State Nurses' Association began in 1953 when she was appointed the associate executive director with primary responsibility for implementing ANA functions, standards, and qualification program and editing the *New Jersey Nurse*. By 1955 she was appointed the executive director of NJSNA, a position she held until her retirement in 1972. She was appointed interim director of the organization in 1980. Errickson described the director's position as being a "great challenge in implementing the programs for the association in maintaining high standards of nursing practice and to promulgate good bills to become good laws for health and welfare of the people in New Jersey and certainly to protect the economic and general welfare of the nurses."

Among her accomplishments while executive director were getting civil-service positions integrated with nursing standards, functions, and qualifications; starting refresher courses at Rutgers University; lobbying for a state department of higher education; and participating in a study of nursing needs within New Jersey. She is best known for implementing the Economic and General Welfare Program of the American Nurses Association, after employing agencies did not accept the New Jersey State Nurses' Association plan to negotiate for nurses.

In addition to her membership in the ANA and NJSNA, she was a fellow with the American Public Health Association, affiliated with both the national and New Jersey Organization of Public Health Nurses, a member of the New Jersey League for Nursing Education and a member of Sigma Theta Tau. During her career she also held memberships in the New Jersey Sanitary Association and the American Association for Science.

Errickson has remained an outspoken advocate for one, unified nursing organization: "Unless we unify, unless the nurses come together, unless we have unification of nurses in this country, we are not going anywhere." Although she says, "I never felt that I was doing anything great," Sara Errickson remains a much beloved figure in New Jersey. She was a recipient of the Florence Nightingale Award in 1971 and received the Dean Haley Award from Seton Hall in 1975 for outstanding leadership in nursing. In 1985 Seton Hall University inaugurated the Sara Errickson Medal for Outstanding Achievement in the Promotion of the Profession of Nursing to be awarded annually to a graduate nursing student. A long-time resident of Newark, New Jersey (1955–90), she is presently living in Bethesda, Maryland.

PUBLICATIONS BY
SARA MAITER ERRICKSON

Editor's Column. *New Jersey Nurse* (1953–72). New Jersey State Nurses' Association, Trenton.

BIBLIOGRAPHY

Garrigan, M.A. Oral History, 1975. Boston Archives, Mugar Library, Boston University, Boston, Massachusetts.

Janet L. Fickeissen

Maude Frances Essig
1884–1981

Two periods in Maude Frances Essig's life are of special significance to nursing. The first is her service as a Red Cross nurse with the American Expeditionary Forces in France during World War I, of which she left a detailed account. The second is her tenure at Brokaw Hospital in Normal, Illinois, during which she cultivated the "connection" whose legacy is the School of Nursing of Illinois Wesleyan University.

Maude Frances Essig was born on November 29, 1884, on a farm west of Elkhart, Indiana. The daughter of Lewis and Mary Eliza Leininger Essig, she had two older sisters, Elva and Alice, and a younger brother Frank.

Essig attended public schools in Elkhart and received her nursing education at Passavant Memorial Hospital School of Nursing and the Illinois Training School for Nurses in affiliation with Cook County Hospital in Chicago. Graduating in 1907, she worked for the Chicago Visiting Nurse Association as a school nurse, infant-welfare nurse, tuberculosis nurse, and industrial nurse.

In 1915 she returned to Elkhart to become superintendent of Elkhart General Hospital and Nursing School. During her administration she established an affiliation with Cook County School of Nursing for experience in children's diseases and saw that a modern nurses' home was built separate from the hospital, an innovation for that time.

From September 1917 until May 1920 Essig was on leave from the Elkhart Hospital to serve with the American Expeditionary Forces in France as a member of Base Hospital #32 out of Indianapolis. During these years she documented her experiences in notes and letters to friends and family. Upon her return in the summer of 1919, she assembled these into a handwritten 68-page paper that she entitled "My Trip Abroad with Uncle Sam—1917–1919." The paper was found among her possessions by her nephew after her death in 1981. There is no evidence that she ever attempted to publish or circulate it.

The paper, in the form of a diary, begins with a brief entry dated August 15, 1915, documenting the transfer of Essig's Red Cross membership from Chicago to the Indianapolis chapter, as background for her affiliation with Base Hospital #32. The journal ends on March 22, 1919, with her return to Elkhart. Although the paper was not meant to be a commentary on nursing, nursing duties are described as they directly influence the narrative, and from them it is possible to glean a picture of nursing's role in this crucial segment of government operations during World War I, the base army hospitals.

Essig returned to her position as superintendent at Elkhart, where she served from 1920–22. In 1924 she became director of nurses and of the Training School for Nurses at Brokaw Hospital in Normal, Illinois, and also served as administrator of the hospital from 1938–1940.

When Essig came to Brokaw in 1924, an arrangement was already in place whereby students could receive a bachelor of science degree from Illinois Wesleyan University in the adjoining city of Bloomington, as well as the title of graduate nurse from Brokaw, after a four- or five-year course of study with about half time at each institution. No students had, however, availed themselves of this opportunity.

Essig during her tenure at Brokaw fostered and extended the Wesleyan "connection." In 1925 entrance requirements for the Training School were raised from one year of high school to 15 credits to correspond with those of Illinois Wesleyan. The registrar of Wesleyan was a member of the Training School Committee, and he evaluated the credentials of all applicants.

All students took chemistry and bacteriology at Wesleyan, as well as dietetics at the college in Normal. Classrooms, teaching models, slides, and a microscope were procured, and a library begun. A demonstration room with beds and equipment was set up, and a graduate nurse was hired to teach basic nursing skills.

Essig relieved nurses of many housekeeping tasks and hired maids for that work. Students assumed more responsibility for their expenses, including textbooks, and their monthly allowance was reduced to compensate for the cost of their college courses.

During the next decade Essig continued to improve standards. Incoming students paid an admission fee of $10, and the allowance to first-year students was eliminated. The dietetics course and all sciences were taken at Wesleyan, and the hospital began to employ more graduate nurses to share the responsibility of service to patients. Efforts were made to bring the school up to the standards set by the National Committee on the Grading of Nursing Schools. Affiliations were arranged with Cook County Hospital for experience in pediatric nursing and with the Bloomington Health Department for public-health nursing. In 1930 the first graduate received a bachelor of science from Wesleyan as well as a diploma from Brokaw.

Essig encouraged all who showed interest and ability to consider the degree course of study. Her efforts to improve nursing education at Brokaw resulted in the school receiving a certificate of approval from the National League of Nursing Education in its first attempt to accredit schools of nursing and eliminate those whose only function was to provide labor for hospitals. The Brokaw Hospital School of Nursing became the School of Nursing of Illinois Wesleyan University, with only the baccalaureate course of study, in 1959.

Former students recall Essig as a model of professionalism of the times. She was a stern perfectionist who demanded the best from everyone and gave no less herself. She believed in respect and responsibility, scrupulous honesty, and care of the patient as primary. She made rounds twice a day in the hospital and spoke to each patient and nurse. She remembered and corresponded with her students for many years and followed their lives and activities with interest and concern.

Essig encouraged graduates to join the Red Cross and to become active in professional associations. She set an example by her own activities: in 1933 she was a delegate from 6th District to the 37th Annual Convention of the Illinois Nurses' Association, at which she was elected first vice-president. She attended national and state conventions and meetings and kept the Training School Committee and her students informed of developments in the national nursing arena.

In 1940, during World War II, Essig returned to Passavant Memorial Hospital in Chicago as assistant director of nursing. She retired in 1948, and in 1952 she went to live at the Veterans Center in Dayton, Ohio, a retirement home for persons with military service. She remained there until her death in 1981 and was buried in the National Military Cemetery adjoining the center as she had requested.

PUBLICATIONS BY MAUDE FRANCES ESSIG

"My Trip Abroad With Uncle Sam—1917–1919." Unpublished paper.

"History of Brokaw Hospital." Unpublished paper, 1938.

BIBLIOGRAPHY

Hitz, B.D., ed. *The History of Base Hospital 32.* Indianapolis: n.p., 1922.

Minutes of the Board of Trustees, 1922–1930. Archives, Illinois Wesleyan University, Bloomington, Illinois.

Wooley, A.S. "A Hoosier Nurse in France: the World War I Diary of Maude Essig." *Indiana Magazine of History,* 82 (March 1986): 1.

Alma S. Wooley

Mary Evans
1730–1792

Mary Evans practiced nursing and midwifery in eighteenth-century St. Augustine, Florida. Although documentary evidence of her life and practice is limited, what is known of Evans depicts the role women like her played in colonial America. Her unique status and training enabled her to assist the residents in rustic St. Augustine with childbirth and illness needs.

She was born and raised in South Carolina, the daughter of Susan and Richard Evans. The documentary evidence of her life as a midwife begins in 1763 when she arrived in St. Augustine, with her husband. Widowed soon after moving to Florida, she married Joseph Peavett, a Catholic British military paymaster. Mary practiced as a midwife from the time of her arrival in St. Augustine until shortly before her death. She also worked with her husband running an inn and food store located below their home. In this era, midwives attended normal births and cared for ill women who miscarried or experienced stillbirths. A midwife also helped in the event of child-bed fever. Evans's home in the center of St. Augustine was well located to assist most residents in the town. She remained childless throughout her life, which enabled her to be available to women needing her services day or night.

She and her husband grew quite

wealthy during the years of British rule from 1764–83, as the result of hard work and successful business ventures. In 1783 St. Augustine again came under the Spanish crown, and many of the Protestant British residents moved to other areas of Florida. Those who remained were wealthy landowners and British Catholics like Joseph Peavett. Mary was able to continue practicing as a midwife due to her reputation and marriage to Joseph. Mary was widowed in 1786 and remained in the St. Augustine community to manage her considerable assets.

Within a year after her husband's death, Evans converted to Catholicism and married again. She continued to practice midwifery to some extent but was limited in her activities due to major problems in her third marriage. John Hudson, 28 years her junior, is described in official documents as a profligate wastrel who destroyed her wealth and turned the last six years of her life into a series of financial crises and public ruin. Evans was forced to leave St. Augustine and settle on rural plantation lands not attached to Hudson's debt. She died in 1792, alone at New Waterford Plantation, located outside St. Augustine.

Contemporary writings and depositions filed in St. Augustine attest to Mary Evans's skill, reputation, and the community respect received for her practice as a midwife and caregiver, especially during the twenty years of British rule. Evans represents a fine example of a middle-aged wise woman, trained in birthing arts who served as a nurse in the colonial society. It is fortunate that her wealth and prominence led to the preservation of the fragmentary evidence, documentation, and verbal depositions about her contribution to the health of her community.

BIBLIOGRAPHY

Camper, J. "The History of the Oldest House." In *Evolution of the Oldest House: Notes in Anthropology*, Vol. 7. Tallahassee: Florida State University, 1962.

Griffin, P. *Mary Evans: Woman of Substance*. St. Augustine Historical Society. St. Augustine, Fla.: El Escrubano, 1977.

Mowat, C. *East Florida as a British Province,* *1763–1784*. Facsimile of 1943 edition. Gainesville: University of Florida Press, 1964.

Tanner, H. Vicente Manuel de Zespedes and the Restoration of Spanish Rule in East Florida, 1784–1790. Doctoral Dissertation, University of Michigan, 1961, pp. 58–82.

All documentary evidence of Mary Evans's life, possessions, and practice as a midwife are on file at the St. Augustine Historical Society, St. Augustine, Florida.

Linda Sabin

Margene Olive Faddis
1900–1983

Margene Olive Faddis served for 35 years on the faculty of the Frances Payne Bolton School of Nursing, Case Western Reserve University, Cleveland, Ohio. A highly respected nurse educator, she wrote several nursing textbooks, one of which was translated into Japanese, and two histories of the Frances Payne Bolton School of Nursing.

Faddis was born on August 15, 1900, in Mt. Vernon, Ohio, the daughter of George Albert and Elsie Wright Faddis. Both parents were born in this country, her mother in Ohio and her father in Illinois. The fourth of five children, Faddis had two older sisters, Grace and Helen, an older brother, Elton, who died in the influenza epidemic in France in World War I, and a younger brother, Merrill, who died of a ruptured appendix at age 14.

Faddis grew up in modest circumstances in Mt. Vernon. Her father held various positions, as secretary and cashier of the Mt. Vernon Waterworks Department, as an assistant cashier in a bank, as deputy in the county treasurer's office, after which he was elected to the office of Knox County treasurer. Her mother was a seamstress, noted for her beautiful quilts and other fine needlework.

After graduation from the Mt. Vernon High School, Faddis entered the Lakeside

Hospital School of Nursing in Cleveland. Her niece believes the deaths of her two brothers may have influenced her decision to become a nurse, but also thinks her choice may have been influenced by her compassionate, loving nature and her scientific bent.

The Lakeside Hospital School of Nursing, from which Faddis was graduated in 1923, was the forerunner of the Frances Payne Bolton School of Nursing, Case Western Reserve University. She earned her baccalaureate degree in 1929 and an M.A. in sociology in 1936, both from Western Reserve University.

Faddis began her nursing career as a head nurse at Lakeside Hospital, and in 1925 left Cleveland to serve as supervisor of medical and surgical nursing at the Pasadena (California) General Hospital. Two years later she returned to Cleveland to complete requirements for her B.S. degree.

In 1929 Faddis was appointed to the faculty of the Frances Payne Bolton School of Nursing. She taught medical nursing and pharmacology and achieved the rank of full professor in 1947.

At a time when there were few schools of nursing in university settings, Faddis believed that collegiate nursing education was essential for professional stature. During World War II she was concerned that educational standards that had been carefully established and gradually attained would be eroded to meet the exigencies of the war. After the Cadet Nurse Corps was established, her concerns deepened as students were assigned to clinical practice before they were adequately prepared for it and, with ever increasing shortages of nurses, were often given clinical assignments to meet nursing-service demands rather than their own educational needs.

An advocate for a strong clinical component in nursing education, Faddis was one of the earliest nurses to identify the significant role of the nurse in the care of the chronically ill and the aging. She also recognized the need for geriatric nursing in curricula of schools of nursing and was influential in getting its inclusion in the curriculum of the Frances Payne Bolton School of Nursing.

Faddis was a member of the American Nurses' Association, the National League for Nursing, and the American Association of University Professors, as well as a fellow in the American Gerontological Society. She served as a member of the board of directors of the American Journal of Nursing Company for 12 years and was president of the company from 1953 to 1958. During her tenure on the board, the journals *Nursing Outlook* and *Nursing Research* were established; she chaired the board committee that worked out the arrangements for publication of the latter.

She also chaired the company's first Mary M. Roberts Fellowship Committee. The fellowships, named for a past editor of the *American Journal of Nursing*, were designed to help nurses acquire and develop their writing skills. Initially, the fellowships provided funds for an academic year of study at a recognized college or university; later, winners were awarded funds to attend the summer Bread Loaf Writers' Conference at Middlebury (Vermont) College.

Her contributions to the professional literature, including textbooks and articles in nursing journals, were scholarly, significant, and extensive. Faddis wrote primarily in the areas of pharmacology and medical nursing, with an occasional article on nursing education. Her history of the Frances Payne Bolton School of Nursing is a record of achievement of one of the leading schools in this country.

For several years while she was still working, she cared for her aging parents in her home in Cleveland Heights. Both required help with health problems; her mother had pernicious anemia and her father was diabetic. But they were a help to her, too, in caring for the house and garden.

She retired in 1964 and was named professor emeritus by the university. But retirement did not mean inactivity. She wrote her second history of the Frances Payne Bolton School. She served as chairman of the Chagrin Falls FISH program, a 24-hour a day telephone service for the chronically ill and elderly. Faddis was a well-rounded individual. Her favorite hobbies were photography and weaving, which she had learned at age 50, but she also enjoyed needlework, gardening, cooking, and music and collected Gilbert and Sullivan recordings.

Faddis was presented the first distinguished Alumnus Award from the school of nursing in 1968. In 1973 she was awarded an honorary doctor of humanities degree from Case Western Reserve University. The next year she received an ANA award recognizing her exceptional contributions to the "spirit and advancement of the nursing profession."

Faddis experienced ill health at intervals following her retirement, but the last six months of her life saw her health decline rapidly. She died January 24, 1983, at the nursing care center at Judson Park, the retirement center in Cleveland, where she lived the last eight years of her life.

She is remembered as a devoted aunt to her three nieces (and later to their families), giving them much love and attention after their mother died. She was dedicated to her profession and to her students. She loved teaching and the associations she made in her profession. Her niece notes that she was a very special human being, always concerned with the plight of those in need. She had many friends, loved to travel, was a serious, scholarly person with a good sense of humor.

Colleagues have described Faddis as a visionary in her profession. She was a gifted teacher with high intellectual standards, a forward-thinking educator, a scholar, and a person with warmth and humanity. She had a keen interest in social and political issues. She was an inspiration to her students, who remember her with deep respect and great affection.

PUBLICATIONS BY
MARGENE OLIVE FADDIS

BOOKS

The History of the Frances Payne Bolton School of Nursing. Cleveland: Gilman, 1948.

A School of Nursing Comes of Age: A History of the Frances Payne Bolton School of Nursing. Oberlin, Ohio: Oberlin Printing, 1973.

With J.M. Hayman, Jr. *Pharmacology for Nurses.* Philadelphia: Lippincott, 1940; 2nd ed, 1943; 3rd ed, 1949; 4th ed, 1953; 5th ed, 1959.

With H.E. Grime. *The Mathematics of Solutions and Dosage.* Philadelphia: Lippincott, 1942; 2nd ed, 1944; 3rd ed, 1948.

With J.M. Hayman, Jr. *Care of the Medical Patient.* New York: McGraw-Hill, 1952; 2nd ed, 1954.

ARTICLES

"Nursing Care of Hyperthyroidism." *American Journal of Nursing* 27 (May 1927): 341–42.

"The Use of Pre-Testing in the Nursing School Curriculum." *Annual Report of the National League of Nursing Education,* 1930. Pp. 138–45.

"Two Alluring Aspects of Pharmacology." *American Journal of Nursing* 31 (November 1931): 1269–73 and 32 (February 1932): 138–42.

"What Could You Do in a Home?" *American Journal of Nursing* 34 (January 1934): 31–32.

"Thermometer for Sterile Solutions." *American Journal of Nursing* 34 (April 1934): 339–340.

"Consumer Protection in Cosmetics and Drugs." *Public Health Nursing* 27 (November 1935): 576–80; 28 (January 1936): 28–32.

"Understanding the Laboratory Report." *American Journal of Nursing* 37 (February 1937): 117–22.

"Digitalis." *American Journal of Nursing* 38 (December 1938): 1931–37.

"Clinical Teaching in Medical Nursing." *American Journal of Nursing* 39 (July 1939): 781–84.

"Eliminating Errors in Medications." *American Journal of Nursing* 39 (November 1939): 1217–23.

"Penicillin." *American Journal of Nursing* 47 (January 1947): 31–34.

"Pearl McIver to Become Executive Director of the Journal Company." *American Journal of Nursing* 57 (March 1957): 310.

"Jeanette V. White 1908–1957." *American Journal of Nursing* 57 (April 1957): 461.

"How Rational Drug Therapy Affects Nursing Duties." *Modern Hospital* XCII (July 1959): 93–96.

"On Clinical Teaching." *American Journal of Nursing* 60 (October 1960): 1461–64.

"Drugs, Drugs, and More Drugs." *American Journal of Nursing* 62 (July 1962): 64–66.

"What Is Different About Geriatric Nursing?" *Journal of Nursing Education* 2 (May–June 1963): 13–15.

"This I Believe . . . About Education's Responsibility for Patient Care." *Nursing Outlook* 13 (December 1965): 26–28.

BIBLIOGRAPHY

"ANA Makes Awards to Nurses and Congressmen." *American Journal of Nursing* 74 (August 1974): 1506, 1508.

Faddis, M.O. Curriculum Vita and File. Archives. Case Western Reserve University, Cleveland, Ohio.

Faddis, M.O. In *Who's Who of American Women* (1961–1962), Vol. II, p. 311. Chicago: Marquis, 1962.

Falls, M. Letter to author, July 11, 1989.

"Margene Faddis Retires as Professor of Nursing W.R." *American Journal of Nursing* 64 (December 1964): 46.

"Margene O. Faddis." Obituary. *American Journal of Nursing* 83 (April 1983): 610.

"Margene O. Faddis, Professor at WRU's School of Nursing." Obituary. *Cleveland Plain Dealer*, January 25, 1983.

Merrill, I. Letter to author, June 15, 1989.

Rodabaugh, J.H., and M.J. Rodabaugh. *Nursing in Ohio: A History.* Columbus: The Ohio State Nurses' Association, 1951.

Towns, M. "Margene Faddis says: 'Retirement can be the best time of your life.'" *Chagrin Valley Herald Sun* (Chagrin Falls, Ohio), June 7, 1973.

Signe S. Cooper

Katharine Ellen Faville

1894–1985

Katharine Ellen Faville was a pioneer in both public-health nursing and collegiate nursing education. She encouraged involvement in international aspects of nursing and was nationally recognized for opening doors of educational opportunity for minority nursing students.

Faville was born on December 25, 1894, in Sauk Center, Minnesota, to Henry Wheaton Faville and Rose Mary Apfel Faville. The family moved to a farm near Lake Mills, Wisconsin, when she was quite young. She had a younger sister, Laura Elizabeth, and two brothers, Harry Wheaton and Cassius John.

She majored in chemistry at the University of Wisconsin in Madison and was awarded a B.S. degree in 1915 and an M.S.

the next year. Her record at the university was a distinguished one, and she was elected to Phi Beta Kappa in her junior year. Her first employment was as a chemist in the laboratories of Sears Roebuck and Company in Chicago.

The summer of 1918 she attended the 15-week course of the Vassar Training Camp, an intensive preliminary nursing course offered on the campus of Vassar College, Poughkeepsie, New York. The course was planned so that enrollees could then complete nursing programs in two years, but the school Faville selected, Massachusetts General Hospital School of Nursing, elected not to reduce the length of its program, so she received her diploma in 1921. Shortly afterward, she enrolled in the public-health nursing program at Simmons College in Boston.

Faville began her nursing career in 1922 as a rural public-health nurse in Alcona County, Michigan. She next was appointed director of the Visiting Nurse Service in Wheeling, West Virginia. She then became a nursing field representative for the American Red Cross, serving in Kentucky and Indiana.

From 1927 to 1931 she was an instructor in public-health nursing at Teachers College, Columbia University, New York City. This was a half-time appointment; she also served as educational director for the Association for Improving the Conditions of the Poor.

Faville went to Detroit in 1931 to organize a public-health nursing program at Wayne (now Wayne State) University. She left in 1934 to serve three years as associate dean of the Western Reserve University School of Nursing in Cleveland.

From 1937 to 1943 Faville was director of the Henry Street Visiting Nurse Service (now New York Visiting Nurse Service) in New York City. During World War II she was appointed to the National Nursing Council for War Service, an organization responsible for recruitment of students for the nation's schools of nursing. She also served as a consultant on student recruitment to the subcommittee on nursing of the Health and Medical Committee in the U.S. Office of Defense Health and Welfare Services. In addition, she assisted with the relocation of Japanese-American nurses.

In 1944 she returned to Wayne State University to serve as the first dean of its College of Nursing, a position she held until her retirement in 1963. Here she worked hard to retain the independent status of the College of Nursing in the university. She participated actively in fund-raising campaigns for the school, raising money for nursing scholarships from local and national organizations. Nationally recognized as a leader in collegiate nursing education, Faville established the graduate program in nursing at Wayne State University.

Faville's interest in university education went far beyond the demands of the nursing program. She directed efforts to improve housing on campus, especially for older women students. Her campus involvement included planning housing for physically handicapped students.

One of her former students, Gloria Smith, dean at Wayne State University College of Nursing, believes that Faville influenced everybody with whom she came in contact. She instilled in students a sense of obligation to work in the profession in return for the community's investment in their educations.

Faville went abroad as a nurse consultant to the U.S. delegation to the second assembly of the World Health Organization in Rome, Italy, in 1948. She also received a Rockefeller grant to study nursing in Europe and to help select nurses for scholarships for study in the United States. For several years, prominent European and other foreign nurses received travel grants for study at Wayne State University. Because she, herself, found travel abroad so helpful, she encouraged each department head in the College of Nursing to have similar opportunities and to become consultants in their clinical areas. She considered it important to develop leaders in nursing aware of the world's needs and to encourage graduates of Wayne State University to accept responsible positions abroad.

The College of Nursing admitted students on the basis of qualifications, so black students were admitted. Additionally, Faville was influential in getting them admitted to hospital schools in Detroit. Through affiliation agreements with hospitals, the college demanded that all students be given opportunities for clinical experience. Hospitals that previously refused to accept black students in their schools of nursing were forced to reconsider their restrictive policies. For her effort in securing equal opportunities for minority students, Faville was presented the Mary Mahoney Award at the convention of the American Nurses' Association in 1966.

The Greater Detroit District, Michigan Nurses Association, selected her as "Nurse of the Year" in 1960. She was honored by the professional association for the many services she had rendered to nursing and nurses. She was also honored as an outstanding graduate of the Massachusetts General Hospital School of Nursing for pioneering in public-health nursing, for her dynamic leadership in nursing education, and for the high standards she brought to the nursing profession.

Faville was active in a number of professional and health-related organizations. She was a fellow in the American Public Health Association. She served on the board of directors, National Organization for Public Health Nursing (1932–40), on the ANA Committee on Nursing in International Affairs; as president (1954–56) and on the board of directors of the Michigan League for Nursing; and on the Board of the Michigan Society for Mental Health. She was a consultant to the U.S. Veterans Administration and was a member of the Advisory Committee to the U.S. Children's Bureau.

She wrote extensively, and, more than most nurses, she published in other than nursing publications. In part, this was related to her recruitment activities during World War II. Writing for these publications demonstrated her recognition that effective recruitment required nursing to tell its story more broadly.

Faville retired as dean at Wayne State in 1963 and lived in Faville Hall on campus in a residential apartment named in her honor. The Katharine E. Faville Lectureship was established in 1975.

She died June 23, 1985, at the Henry Ford Hospital in Detroit.

Faville has been described as a forceful and dynamic person with a critical intellect, vision, and the courage of her convictions. She was an early advocate for nursing education in institutions of higher learning and for the admission of minority students in schools of nursing. She had a significant influence on the advancement of collegiate nursing education and the promotion of social justice in nursing education.

PUBLICATIONS BY KATHARINE ELLEN FAVILLE

"The Nurse as Counselor in Troubled Homes." *Red Cross Courier* 4 (August 15, 1925): 14–15.

"Fifth Annual Conference of State Directors of Maternity and Infancy Work." *Public Health Nurse* 20 (June 1928): 308–09.

"RN: Rural Nurse and Real Neighbor." *American Journal of Nursing* 28 (June 1928): 567–70.

"Nurses from Other Lands." *Public Health Nurse* 21 (May 1929): 234–35.

"The Philosophy of Education Applied to Staff Education for Public Health Nurses." *Public Health Nurse* 21 (October 1929): 512–13.

"Another Course in Public Health Nursing." *Trained Nurse and Hospital Review* 87 (August 1931): 192.

"Postgraduate Preparation for Industrial Nursing." *Public Health Nursing* 24 (February 1932): 79–83.

"Channels for Improvement (in Schools of Nursing and Postgraduate Courses)." *Public Health Nursing* 26 (June 1934): 329–35.

"New Deals for Nurses, II. Professional Education." *Survey* 71 (May 1935): 137–38.

"Private Agency in the Defense Program." *Public Health Nursing* 34 (January 1942): 4–10.

"New Opportunities for Nurses." *Occupations* 20 (February 1942): 327–32.

"Nursing Needs Challenge Junior College." *Junior College Journal* 13 (October 1942): 76–79.

"The Nursing Profession and the War Effort." *School and College Placement* 3 (October 1943): 7–13.

"Developments in Nursing School Programs." *American Journal of Nursing* 45 (September 1945): 757.

"Organizing the Community for Public Health Nursing." *Public Health Nursing* 39 (February 1947): 101–03.

"Michigan Plans for Nursing Service and Nursing Education." *Fifty-fifth Annual Report*, National League of Nursing Education, 1949. Pp. 232–40.

"The Second World Health Assembly." *American Journal of Nursing* 49 (December 1949): 766.

"College of Nursing Moves into the Community." *Nursing World* 124 (October 1950): 456–58, 474, 479.

With D. L. Frackelton. "Opportunities in Nursing for Disadvantaged Youth." *Nursing Outlook* 14 (April 1966): 26–28.

BIBLIOGRAPHY

Clappison, G.B. *Vassar's Rainbow Division, 1918*. Lake Mills, Iowa: Graphic Publishing, 1964. Pp. 206–207.

"Courage of Their Convictions." *Nursing Science* 2 (August 1964): 322–23.

Faville, K. Curriculum Vita and File. Wayne State University College of Nursing, Detroit, Michigan.

Faville, K. In *Who's Who of American Women, 1966–1967*, Vol. 4, p. 366. Chicago: Marquis, 1967.

Faville, K. Letter to author, July 4, 1973.

"Henry Street Director Resigns." *Trained Nurse and Hospital Review* 110 (September 1943): 205.

Miller, H.S. *Mary Elizabeth Mahoney, 1845–1926, America's First Black Professional Nurse*. Atlanta: Wright, 1986. Pp. 64–66.

"Miss Faville Commended." *Trained Nurse and Hospital Review* 116 (June 1946): 450.

"New Era for Wayne State." *Nursing Outlook* 13 (August 1965): 11.

Perkins, S. *A Centennial Review*. Massachusetts General Hospital School of Nursing, 1873–1973. Boston: Massachusetts General Hospital Nurses Alumnae Association, 1975.

Schorr, T. and A. Zimmerman. "Gloria R. Smith." In *Making Choices, Taking Chances: Nurse Leaders Tell Their Story*. St. Louis: Mosby, 1988. Pp. 322–26.

Smith, G. Letter to author, October 11, 1988.

White, E. Letter to author, December 6, 1988.

Signe S. Cooper

Gertrude LaBrake Fife

1902–1980

In 1931, with the founding of what would come to be called the American Association of Nurse Anesthetists, Agatha C. Hodgins fulfilled a long-cherished dream. Less than two years later, however, she suffered a serious heart attack, and her role in the organizations' further development was restricted. The burden of carrying through the work fell to her assistant at Lakeside Hospital (Cleveland), Gertrude LaBrake Fife. Fife proved to be a capable successor to Hodgins. She not only implemented the goals Hodgins had set, but also extended them. As second president of the association, as treasurer, and as founder and editor of its journal (all the while continuing as a full-time educator and notable clinical practitioner), she worked with dedication and energy. Of particular importance was her guiding the association to a program of certification of nurse anesthetists through a national qualifying examination and of accreditation for nurse anesthesia schools.

Fife was born Gertrude LaBrake in 1902 in Rutland, Vermont. She graduated from the Fanny Allen Hospital School of Nursing, Winooski, Vermont, in 1923. It was there that as a student nurse she gave her first anesthetic. At the time there were no formally trained nurse anesthetists in the state, but the example of the sisters at Fanny Allen in administering anesthesia encouraged Fife to become an anesthetist. She later wrote of them, "Of all the nurses with whom I have been associated in my many years in hospital work, they remain to me outstanding examples of women with unvarying devotion to their calling."

She was trained in anesthesia at the Lakeside Hospital (University Hospitals) School of Anesthesia, Cleveland, Ohio, under its founder, Agatha C. Hodgins. After graduation in 1924, she quickly became the first assistant and began an impressive clinical career. She was anesthetist for some of the most outstanding surgeons of the day, including Drs. George W. Crile and Elliot Cutler. She had a long and special association with pioneering heart surgeon, Dr. Claude S. Beck, with whom she perfected the anesthesia technic for pericardectomy. She also worked with Dr. Frederick R. Mautz in the development and use of the respirator, and, with Beck, pioneered the use of the automatic respirator in open-chest surgery.

Sometime before 1931 she was married to Matthew Fife, but the date is unknown.

On June 17, 1931, Fife was present at the organizational meeting of what was initially the International Association of Nurse Anesthetists (in 1932 it became the National Association of Nurse Anesthetists and in 1939 the American Association of Nurse Anesthetists). It was Fife who made the formal motion that the association be formed and she was one of the signers of the articles of incorporation and a member of the first board of directors. When Hodgins, founder and administrative leader of the association fell ill on January 1, 1933, Fife not only assumed her role as director of the University Hospitals School of Anesthesia, but also took up the task of continuing the development of the young professional association of nurse anesthetists.

In later reminiscences Fife made clear that she did so at the urging of John R. Mannix, then assistant director of University Hospitals and administrator in charge of the Anesthesia Department. She recalled that he "was an organizer. He was interested in the development of the hospital, and, incidentally, he was the one that started the Blue Cross plan." Mannix insisted that Fife continue the association work and put her in touch with the American Hospital Association, a linkage that provided crucial support for the young nursing group. The first annual meeting of the National Association of Nurse Anesthetists was thus held concurrently with that of the AHA, on September 13–15, 1933, in Milwaukee, Wisconsin. The program (which had been planned by Fife and colleague Helen Lamb) was a great success. It was attended by 120 people representing 27 states.

In her address at this meeting, Fife focused on the most pressing, practical issue facing nurse anesthetists: standardization of education. She outlined the necessary course of action, one in which nurse anesthetists would take control over their own accelerating professionalization. Fife called for a committee to investigate all schools of nurse anesthesia with the object of creating a list of "accredited" schools because the national association "should at all times be able to furnish information to hospitals or surgeons desirous of employing anesthetists regarding the standing of schools and the qualifications of members of the National Association desirous of obtaining positions." It was also necessary, she said, to establish "national board examinations for nurse anesthetists" that "would place in the surgeon's hands an official record showing that her knowledge of the subject has met with the approval of an examining board—a board chosen and functioning to safeguard the surgeon's interest, the interest of the hospitals, and the interest of the public."

But gaining acceptance for the plan of a national certifying examination was not easy, chiefly because Hodgins (retired but keeping a watchful eye on matters) favored another approach to establishing the position of the professional nurse anesthetist: state registration. Her reasons for doing so may have been the result of her conviction that the work fell under neither the category of medicine nor that of nursing and that nurse anesthetists needed the protection of a separate legal status. Hodgins may also have been affected by years of listening to the charge leveled by physician-anesthetists hostile to the existence of nurses in the field, that they were "unlicensed" practitioners.

To this concern Fife responded (and was correct in her prediction) that "in a few years the superintendents and surgeons generally would require their anesthetists to be recognized by the National Association. After all, the superintendents and surgeons are not interested in whether the examining board has obtained legislative sanction—they are interested in making certain that their anesthetists are equipped to give anesthetics."

Fife's plan was embraced at the 1936 national meeting, in part because it was realized that a state-by-state registration effort presented a prohibitive financial burden as well as strategic legal risks. The plan was also accepted because, the association's Educational Committee reported that year, there was now a "definite trend in the direction of National Boards of

Examinations by various professional groups, as noted by the recently created American Board of Surgery [for national examination and certification of general surgeons], and also the Council on Dental Education, organized only two months ago 'for the examination and listing of [dental] specialists.' A carefully worked out plan looking forward to eventual national examination and certification for nurse anesthetists would therefore seem to be *peculiarly* in keeping with the current trend of professional thought in our fields" (emphasis added). What Fife knew—and told in an unpublished 1974 memoir—was that Dr. Carl H. Lenhart of University Hospitals, Cleveland, and Dr. Howard Karsner of Western Reserve University, both active in developing physician national boards of examination and both supportive of nurse anesthetists, had discretely counseled her, thereby helping to direct the professionalization of the nurse specialty group.

Fife had been elected the association's second president at the Milwaukee meeting, a position she held for two terms (1933–35). After that meeting, she established the *Bulletin of the National Association of Nurse Anesthetists* and continued as its editor for 12 years. She was association treasurer, 1935–50, and over the years served on various national committees. She also remained as director of University Hospitals School of Anesthesia until 1946 and continued her own distinguished clinical work. In 1956, on the occasion of the twenty-fifth anniversary of the American Association of Nurse Anesthetists, Fife reflected on the achievement of the profession. Her words also capture the significance of her own lifework:

> We are justly proud of our accomplishments and particularly so when we realize that the work was done by our members. We did not seek grants or solicit large contributions. We started out with only a few dollars in the treasury. Women holding full-time, responsible jobs in anesthesia traveled miles over week ends to meet with other members to map out programs. We were fortunate in that we had farseeing men in the hospital and

surgical groups interested in our work and our progress. They gave us moral support, advice, and the stimulus to go forward. We are grateful to them.

Little has been said or written about the actual work of the nurse anesthetist. When lung surgery, heart surgery, and brain surgery were in their infancy, the nurse anesthetist was at the head of the table. When I left University Hospitals in 1946, we had performed so many heart operations that the anesthesia was a relatively simple procedure. At least we were past the pioneer stage. We, as nurse anesthetists, had been given a job to do, and we did it.

In recognition of her contributions to the development of the profession, Fife was honored several times by the American Association of Nurse Anesthetists. She was made an honorary member in 1946 and received its Award of Appreciation in 1950. In 1978 she was presented with the Agatha Hodgins Award for Outstanding Accomplishment.

Fife died of a heart attack in Cleveland, in 1980. Her husband Matthew had died in 1975.

BIBLIOGRAPHY

Bankert, M. *Watchful Care, A History of America's Nurse Anesthetists*. New York: Continuum, 1989.

"Gertrude L. Fife, One of AANA Founding Members, Dies," *AANA News Bulletin* (November 1980).

Gertrude L. Fife Biographical Materials, folder. Archives. American Association of Nurse Anesthetists, Park Ridge, Illinois.

Marianne Bankert

Alice Fisher

1839–1888

Alice Fisher was an expert organizer, educator, and reformer in nursing. An Englishwoman, Fisher spent the last four years of her 13-year nursing career in the United States. She significantly reorganized the Philadelphia Hospital in Pennsylvania and transformed scandalous conditions through the provision of proper nursing care. She established the Training School for Nurses at the Philadelphia Hospital and served as chief nurse until her death at age 49.

Born into a prominent family on June 14, 1839, at Queen's House, Greenwich, England, Alice Fisher was the oldest of two daughters. Her father, the Reverend George Fisher, fellow of the Royal Society, was an instructor in mathematics at the Royal Navy School. He served as headmaster of the Greenwich Hospital School. Her grandfather had been headmaster of Eton College at Windsor. Her mother died when Fisher was 11 years of age. Her father suffered a long illness, and Fisher cared for him until his death in 1873. Until she entered nursing two years later, Fisher, fond of painting and books, pursued a literary career. She had moderate success with two fiction novels. Her first, *Too Bright to Last*, was published the same year as her father's death. That was followed by a three-volume work, *His Queen*, published in 1875. In her mid-30s Fisher enrolled in the Nightingale Training School at St. Thomas's Hospital in London, England. While there, the tall and thin Fisher experienced her first bout of inflammatory rheumatism. She suffered valvular heart damage. She would experience episodic cardiac symptoms for the rest of her life and eventually die from this condition.

After graduation from the training school in 1876, Fisher became assistant superintendent at the Royal Infirmary at Edinburgh. Six months later, hearing that the Fever Hospital, Newcastle on Tyne, had difficulty filling the position of superintendent, Fisher applied and was accepted. She arrived in June 1876 and found many cases of typhus. Although she stayed less than one year, Fisher successfully ameliorated the reputation of the hospital as pest house through her training of nurses, eradication of filthy conditions, and reformation of the hospital. While there, Fisher collaborated with Rachel Williams to produce a handbook for nurses titled *Hints for Hospital Nurses*, published in 1877. She later brought this early nursing text with her to the United States.

Fisher's notable administrative skills led her to her next position as superintendent of Addenbroke's Hospital, Cambridge, England, on May 14, 1877. Her reputation growing, she was chosen out of 21 candidates. While there, she significantly uplifted the low standard of nursing that prevailed upon her arrival and established a small training school for nurses. Her stay of five years would be the longest of her nursing career at any one hospital.

In April 1882 Fisher accepted the position of matron at the Radcliffe Infirmary, Oxford, England. Before resigning to take a new position six months later, Fisher once again demonstrated her superb organizational abilities by smoothly initiating a nursing system during that short period.

Fisher began her next position as superintendent at the General Hospital, Birmingham, England, on November 1, 1882. She was chosen this time out of 44 candidates. Eighteen months into her position, in May 1884, the influential Fisher proposed the founding of a nursing school. Although her health deteriorated at one point, exacerbated by overwork, Fisher successfully established a three-year training program. This underway, she left on October 10, 1884, feeling well enough to tackle a new challenge in the United States. Sorely needed and uniquely qualified for what lay ahead, she came to Pennsylvania.

Early in 1884 a movement was begun by the board of guardians at the Philadelphia Hospital, Pennsylvania, to address the abominable conditions resulting from years of gross mismanagement, corrupt inefficiency, and errant political involvement. Begun as an almshouse in 1730, the hospital, known popularly as "Old Blockley" or "Blockley," was sadly in need of reform. A recent publicized scandal starkly illuminated the truly wretched conditions of this hospital and almshouse, which together housed approximately 3,000 patients—a combination of the ill, mentally ill, and infirm. The board,

while still possessing a few irresponsible and unaccountable individuals, nonetheless, had several admirable members interested in serious reform. A proposal was set forth to establish a training school for nurses as part of a necessary solution. Considerable difficulty was experienced in finding a suitable candidate for this daunting position. A lengthy nationwide search proved fruitless. The president of the board, George Childs, owner of a daily newspaper in Philadelphia, appealed to Florence Nightingale for advice. The position was offered to Fisher upon learning of her impressive accomplishments and encompassing knowledge in the intricacies of institutional management. She accepted and arrived in Philadelphia in November 1884.

Considerable controversy reigned over Fisher's selection. Objections were voiced over her "importation" and several board members refused to agree to pay her requested salary of $1000. Childs, along with another influential board member, Anthony J. Drexel, paid personally for her transportation, expenses, and part of her salary as well as those of the assistant who accompanied her. Edith A. Hornor was Fisher's co-worker at Cambridge and Oxford and recipient of the Victoria Cross for her services during the Zulu War of 1879. Many on the board were completely unappreciative of the function of an assistant and questioned her value, despite the magnitude of the task ahead. Fisher successfully weathered initial resistance and even several disconcerting displays of hostility. "The English Nurse" had rotten eggs thrown onto her windows, received threatening letters, and once was the intended recipient of an explosive sent through the mail, which fortunately was halted at the post office. Despite these dismaying incidents, Fisher exhibited the force of her unique character and proceeded to revolutionize nursing at Blockley.

Before sailing from England, Fisher had written the board requesting that all nurses of good quality and integrity be retained. This small group of nurses formed the nucleus of the new training school that formally opened January 1,

1885. Upon Fisher's arrival, the majority of the nursing care was provided by other inmates of the almshouse, most totally unfit for the work. Fisher held classes for the nurses, while Hornor provided bedside instruction. She arranged for the attending staff to provide lectures twice weekly. The main hospital building was remodeled and repaired to provide living quarters for the nurses. Through skillful management and direction, drawing upon her wealth of experience, Fisher effected profound changes in the hospital within six months. Despite her considerable work load, she was able to leave for two months in the late spring of 1885 to lend her expertise and organize a hospital training service during the typhoid epidemic at Plymouth, Pennsylvania.

The first commencement of the Training School for Nurses of the Philadelphia Hospital was held January 16, 1886. There were 15 graduates. Because several simultaneous classes graduated at different times of the year, the first year totaled 45 graduates. By 1889 the enrollment had increased to 87 students. Two types of nursing courses were offered. The one-year program prepared nurses for private duty, while the two-year program qualified nurses for institutional work. The quality of nursing care and conditions improved dramatically under Fisher with a subsequent reduction in the mortality rate. Skilled at interpersonal relations, Fisher fostered and maintained excellent rapport with staff and physicians, winning their support and cooperation. For four years as chief nurse, Fisher worked unstintingly to attract a better class of women to nursing and to upgrade them through education.

Fisher died of valvular heart disease on June 3, 1888, eleven days shy of her fiftieth birthday. For the year prior to her death her health had progressively worsened, but she still performed an enormous amount of work, even making rounds by wheelchair. Her private physician and friend, Dr. J. William White, expressed the view that given her physical condition, her long-standing intensity of effort had assisted in shortening her life. Fisher was buried at Woodlands Cemetery on June 5, 1888, within sight of Blockley,

a site she had personally chosen. Over her casket, per her request, was draped the British ensign of the Royal Navy. Dr. (later Sir) William Osler, then professor of clinical medicine at the University of Pennsylvania, served as pallbearer. A brief tribute to Fisher in the *Philadelphia Medical News* lamenting her death has been attributed to him. Also a pallbearer was United States Senator Joseph R. Hawley, who had married her assistant Edith Hornor in November 1887.

After her death, early alumnae meetings were held at the Alice Fisher Club, at a location close to the Philadelphia Hospital Training School. Five years later the Alice Fisher Alumnae Association was formally established. Marion E. Smith, Fisher's successor and a graduate of the school in 1886, was elected president, and Fisher's former pupil Roberta M. West was elected secretary. On the first anniversary of her death, a brass tablet bearing her inscription and a portrait of Fisher wearing the school uniform was presented to the school. Osler sent a telegram regretting his inability to attend. As late as 1929 the custom of visiting Fisher's grave on each Easter Sunday afternoon after a memorial service was still observed by the nurses, staff, and alumnae of the school.

PUBLICATIONS BY ALICE FISHER

With Rachel Williams. *Hints for Hospital Nurses.* Edinburgh, Scot.: Maclachlan and Stewart, 1877.

FICTION

Too Bright to Last. N.p., 1873.

His Queen. London: King, 1875.

BIBLIOGRAPHY

"Alice Fisher." In *Early Leaders of American Nursing.* New York: National League of Nursing Education, 1922.

Alice Fisher: Chief Nurse of the Training School for Nurses, Philadelphia Hospital. Philadelphia: Sower, 1890. Microfiche.

Clayton, S.L. "School of Nursing." In *History of Blockley: A History of the Philadelphia General Hospital from Its Inception, 1731–1928.* J.W. Croskey, compiler. Philadelphia: Davis, 1929.

Cope, Z. "Alice Fisher—Matron and Reformer." *Nursing Mirror* 107 (June 27, 1958): i, 968.

Cope, Z. *Six Disciples of Florence Nightingale.* London: Pitman Medical, 1961.

"A Devoted Nurse: Death of Miss Alice Fisher of Philadelphia." Obituary. *New York Times*, June 6, 1888. (From the *Philadelphia Ledger*, June 4, 1888.)

Hawley, E.A. "Some Eminent Nurses-II: Alice Fisher." In *How to Become a Trained Nurse.* J. Hodson, ed. New York: Abbatt, 1898.

Institutional Records of the Philadelphia General Hospital and School of Nursing, 1885-1977. Historical Collection, Center for the Study of the History of Nursing, University of Pennsylvania, School of Nursing, Philadelphia.

Lawrence, C. *History of the Philadelphia Alms-houses and Hospitals.* Philadelphia: The author, 1905; repr., New York: Arno Press, 1976.

Medical News 52 (June 9, 1888): 642.

"Nightingale Letter to Alice Fisher in Philadelphia." *American Nurse* 8 (January 31, 1976): 2.

O'Brien, P. "'All a Woman's Life Can Bring': The Domestic Roots of Nursing in Philadelphia, 1830-1885." *Nursing Research* 36 (January-February 1987): 12-17.

Rives, R.E. "The Passing of Old Blockley." *American Journal of Nursing* 27 (September 1927): 747-49.

Smith, M.E. "The Pioneer Work of Alice Fisher in Philadelphia." Address. Nurses' Associated Alumnae of the United States, May 14, 1904. *American Journal of Nursing* 4 (July 1904): 803-08.

West, R M. *History of Nursing in Pennsylvania.* Philadelphia: Pennsylvania State Nurses' Association, 1927.

Sharon Murphy

Julia Otteson Flikke

1879-1965

Julia Otteson Flikke was the sixth superintendent of the Army Nurse Corps, holding this position from 1937 to 1943. She had served in the corps since May 1918, when Augustana Hospital, Chicago, where she was then assistant superintendent of nurses, sent an affiliated medical unit overseas after the United States entered World War I.

Flikke was born on March 16, 1879 in Viroqua, Wisconsin, the daughter of Solfest and Kristi (Severson) Otteson. She graduated from Viroqua High School in 1899 and married Arne T. Flikke, who died on October 15, 1911. In 1912 she entered nursing school at Augustana Hospital Training School, Chicago, and graduated in 1915. Building on some previous teaching experience in Wisconsin, she studied administration and nursing education at Teachers College, Columbia University in 1915 and 1916, returning to Augustana Hospital in 1916 as assistant superintendent of nurses until the mobilization in 1918.

Flikke served overseas from 1918 to 1920, first as chief nurse, Base Hospital No. 11, France, then in 1919, as head nurse, Nantes Evacuation Unit No. 28 and Hospital Train No. 55. Returning to the United States in 1920, she remained in the Army Nurse Corps serving at the Army and Navy General Hospital, Hot Springs, Arkansas. Overseas tours of duty took her to Ft. McKinley, the Philippines, and Tientsin, China. In 1922 she was assigned to Walter Reed General Hospital, serving there as principal chief nurse until 1934. For her service there she received citations for "outstanding service and proficiency." During this time, in 1925, she studied further at Teachers College, Columbia. In 1934 she was assigned to Ft. Sam Houston, Texas. From 1927 to 1937 her (relative) rank was captain and she was assistant superintendent of the Army Nurse Corps (ANC). In 1937 she was appointed chief of the ANC and assigned the rank of major.

Flikke assumed the post of Chief when the corps was still operating under peacetime conditions. In 1938, at the ANA convention, the corps announced that it would increase its strength from 600 to 675 nurses; by July 1941 the Corps was striving to reach 4000 nurses; by D-Day, 1943, there were 10,000 U.S. Army nurses in Great Britain alone.

The pressing problem of recruitment was the one Flikke addressed in her public statements and writings. *Nurses in Action*, published in 1943 was written to inform nurses and potential nurses of the history of the Army Nurse Corps and to encourage them to enlist as army nurses.

Rapidly changing conditions for military nurses after the onset of the war required changes in regulations concerning uniforms, marital status of army nurses, and the status of the ANC in the army itself.

In 1942 Flikke was promoted to colonel (relative rank), the first woman to hold this rank in the U.S. Army. She retired in June 1943 for reasons of health. In June 1944 she was awarded an honorary doctor of science degree from Wittenberg University, Springfield, Ohio.

Julia Flikke was a lifelong member of the Lutheran Church. She was also a member of the 20th Century Club of Washington, D.C., and of the American Legion.

She entered the National Lutheran Home for the Aged in June 1958 and died there at the age of 86 on February 23, 1965.

PUBLICATIONS BY JULIA OTTESON FLIKKE

BOOKS

Nurses in Action. Philadelphia: Lippincott, 1943.

ARTICLES

"Invitation to Service." *Journal of the Medical Society of Cape May County, New Jersey* 4 (June 1942): 6-7.

BIBLIOGRAPHY

Aynes, E.A. *From Nightingale to Eagle.* Englewood Cliffs, NJ: Prentice-Hall, 1973.

Bullough, V.L., and B. Bullough. *The Emergence of Modern Nursing.* Toronto: Macmillan, 1969.

"Julia O. Flikke." Obituary. *American Journal of Nursing* 65 (April 1965): 155-56.

Letters and Unpublished Papers. Wittenberg University Library Special Collections, Springfield, Ohio.

Pennock, M.R. *Makers of Nursing History.* New York: Lakeside, 1940.

Roberts, M.M. *American Nursing: History and Interpretation.* New York: Macmillan, 1954.

Roberts, M.M. *The Army Nurse Corps: Yesterday and Today.* Washington, D.C.: U.S. Army, 1958.

Robinson, C. "Colonel Julia O. Flikke, Chief of the Army Nurse Corps." *Journal of the Medical Society of Cape May County, New Jersey* 4 (June 1942): 3-6.

"They Directed the Army Nurse Corps." *American Journal of Nursing* 55 (November 1955): 1350-51.

Marianne Brook

Beulah Sanford France

1891-1971

Beulah Sanford France was a prolific writer and syndicated columnist on child health from 1930-60. Her work appeared in such popular magazines as *Life and Health* and *American Baby.* She also did extensive broadcasting on health subjects in the New York City area.

France was born in Redding, Connecticut, on October 18, 1891, the daughter of George Turney and Florence May (Hill) Sanford. She graduated from Centenary Hill Collegiate Institute in 1907. She took her nurses' training at St. Luke's Hospital School of Nursing and Sloane Hospital for Women in New York City, graduating in 1920. She did graduate work at Columbia University from 1921-23, George Peabody College (Nashville, Tenn.) from 1925-26, and Pratt Institute (New York City) in 1927. She was awarded an honorary Litt.D. by Hartwick College (Oneonta, N.Y.) in 1961.

France began her career as a public-health nurse in 1920 in Larchmont, New York, staying there for one year. From 1921-26 she was supervisor of public-health nurses for the Metropolitan Life Insurance Company in New York City.

She married Harry C. France, who gained fame as a syndicated financial columnist and author, on March 26, 1927, and they had one daughter.

She returned to work in 1930, writing and broadcasting health programs for the New York City Department of Health. From 1932-44 she did health-education work for the pharmaceutical firm E.R. Squibb and Sons and from 1934-60 did free-lance writing, radio and television broadcasting, and lecturing on health. From 1932-42 she conducted courses in child care at the Brides' School of Scientific Housekeeping in New York City.

France was child-care editor of *Country Gentleman* (later called *Better Farming*). She was editorial director of *American Baby Magazine* from 1940–63 and then editor emeritus until her death. Her syndicated daily column, "Child Care," appeared throughout the country for four years, and she contributed to health magazines in the United States, Canada, England, and Latin America.

A fellow of the American Public Health Association and a member of the Royal Society of Health of London, France also was a member of the Public Health Association of New York City, the Maternity Center Association of New York City, the American Nurses' Association, the International Council of Nurses, as well as many other organizations. She was business manager of the bulletin of St. Luke's Hospital Alumnae Association from 1930–54 and child-welfare chairman of the League of Women Voters from 1930–32. From 1932–46 she served as RN trustee of Centenary College (Hackettstown, N.J.).

France died on December 28, 1971, in New York City, two weeks before the death of her husband.

BIBLIOGRAPHY

"Beulah Sanford France." *American Journal of Nursing* 72 (February 1972): 352.

"France, Beulah." Deaths. *New York Times* December 31, 1971.

"France, Beulah Sanford." In *Who's Who in America*, 1970-1971. Vol. 36, p. 758. Chicago: Marquis, 1971.

Alice P. Stein

Sister Charles Marie Frank

b. 1906

In Sister Charles Marie Frank's own words, she considers herself to be a "nurse educator ... a teacher of nursing across the board." During her career that role assumed many forms including those of teacher, professor, dean, consultant in nursing, and author. It also made her an internationalist in nursing education taking her expertise to Peru, Columbia, Venezuela, Brazil, and Puerto Rico. In the Catholic University of America's (CUA) *The Olivian*, the author of an article about Sr. Charles Marie called her "one of the giants in nursing and in the history of CUA."

Born Mary Carolyn Frank on December 7, 1906, in St. Louis, Missouri, she was the daughter of Caroline Catherine Popp and John William Frank. She was the older of two children having a brother two and a half years her junior born June 27, 1909. Her mother died when Mary Carolyn was 8 years old, leaving a big void in her life.

Both her primary and two years of secondary education were obtained at various schools in St. Louis. At the time, two to four years of secondary education were recommended but not mandatory for nursing-school applicants. The entrance of the United States into World War I greatly influenced Mary Carolyn's choice of nursing as a career. She was caught up in the patriotic fervor that abounded, making speeches about patriotism in her own and other classrooms. A popular song of the era "My Little Red Cross Nurse" made a lasting impression on her and was one stimulus for her entry into nursing.

At the age of 17 she enrolled at the St. Louis Mullanphy Hospital School of Nursing against her father's wishes but with the welcome blessings of her paternal grandmother and a great aunt. Both of the older women had desperately wanted to be nurses for the Confederacy during the American Civil War but were prohibited from doing so because of parental disapproval. They said words to the effect that "someone in this family must do what she wants to do" and persuaded Mary Carolyn's father to allow her to pursue a nursing career notwithstanding parental objection. An uncle also gave his support for her choice.

The St. Louis Mullanphy Hospital School of Nursing was affiliated with the St. Louis University School of Medicine and provided a well-balanced education for nurses. The professors from the medical school instructed the nurses and took a special interest in their career development. Student nurses lived in an apartment house, and social skills as well as nursing skills were emphasized. The rules for students were quite liberal for the times.

In 1926, three months prior to graduation, Mary Carolyn left nursing school to enter the convent in Normandy, Missouri, affiliated with the Sisters of Charity of the Incarnate Word. She spent her two-year novitiate period in the convent, 1926–28, where her name was changed to Sister Charles Marie. After completion of the novitiate she was sent to St. Joseph's Hospital School of Nursing in Paris, Texas, to complete her training as a nurse. However, in order to qualify for completing her nursing work in two years at St. Joseph's, a transcript of her work at St. Louis Mullanphy had to be submitted to, and approved by, the Texas State Board of Nurse Examiners. That body enforced a rule requiring that a transfer student to a nursing school in Texas spend two years at the school from which the diploma was to be awarded and also submit a transcript of previous work for approval. At the time of her matriculation at Mullanphy, record keeping in schools of nursing was poor at best, and at this particular school records of students who left the nursing school before graduation were not retained. The director of nurses at Mullanphy was new and did not remember Mary Carolyn Frank. However, a transcript for Mary Carolyn Frank, now Sister Charles Marie Frank, was able to be reconstructed from those of her classmates. Fortunately, Mullanphy did have a standard curriculum in place at the time.

Sister Charles Marie remembers the situation at St. Joseph's to be less than ideal with "16 students and about the same number of patients." However, while in a student capacity at St. Joseph's, she instructed students in nursing skills and functioned in various leadership roles. Thus, she spent considerably more time in "training" than did her contemporaries: 33 months in Missouri and 24 in Texas. She finally became a registered nurse in 1930.

For the years that immediately followed her graduation from nursing school, Sister Charles Marie worked in numerous and varied capacities. She functioned as supervisor and instructor in various hospitals and schools of nursing conducted by the Sisters of Charity of the Incarnate Word of San Antonio, Texas. Between 1931 and 1942, she held positions as x-ray technician and instructor of nursing at Santa Rosa Hospital, San Antonio; St. John's Hospital, San Angelo; and director of nurses at St. Anthony Hospital, Amarillo—all in Texas.

In 1932 Sister Charles Marie began part-time studies at Incarnate Word College in San Antonio. Without a high-school diploma she had to demonstrate a knowledge base equivalent to that of students who had received a diploma. To do so, she took a battery of tests over a period of a week, passing all of them.

She returned to Incarnate Word College in 1937 and graduated magna cum laude in 1939 with a bachelor of science in nursing education. After working three years as the director of the School of Nursing at St. Anthony Hospital in Amarillo, Texas, she enrolled at the Catholic University of America (CUA), where she received the master of science degree in nursing education in 1943.

Immediately after graduation, Sister Charles Marie returned to Incarnate Word College in San Antonio as chairman of the Department of Nursing and reached the rank of professor. She remained in this position until 1954, during which time she was able to enroll in some postmasters courses in psychiatric nursing during the second semester and summer of 1947 at CUA. In 1953, while still in the leadership role at Incarnate Word College, she started phasing into the role of supervisor of health services and consultor general, Sisters of Charity of the Incarnate Word, a role that she assumed on a full-time basis until 1957. At that time she returned to CUA as dean of the School of Nursing and earned the rank of professor. She remained at CUA as dean until 1964, when she left for missionary work in Chembote, Peru.

During the years between 1950 and 1965, Sister Charles Marie served as consultant to numerous agencies both in the United States and abroad. Her work as a consultant included functioning as special consultant to the United States Public Health Service, National Institute of Mental Health; nursing consultant to the U.S. Fourth Army; and nursing consultant to the U.S. Veterans Administration, Department of Medicine and Surgery in Washington, D.C.; Pittsburgh, Pennsylvania; Tuskegee, Alabama; and Puerto Rico.

While serving as dean of the School of Nursing at Catholic University, 1957–64, Sister Charles Marie did much to advance the prestige of the school. She supervised a tremendous growth in the numbers of students enrolled in the master's program, an increase of 362 percent in just two years. She also witnessed the change in the school's name from the School of Nursing Education to the School of Nursing. She initiated action to start a doctoral program in nursing. A new nursing-school building was erected during her tenure at CUA. Sister's skill at negotiating proved to be very valuable during this time. She bartered, for example, to get architectural features, such as an auditorium, added because they would better accommodate the needs of the nursing school.

While functioning as dean at CUA, Sister Charles Marie was called upon to assist several South American countries with various aspects of nursing education. In 1958 she went to Bogota, Colombia, as a consultant to the Ministry of Health and five university schools of nursing. In this role she was instrumental in the redesign of the nursing curricula for the entire country of Colombia. In 1960 she was in Rio de Janeiro for three months serving as a consultant to the Brazilian Nurses' Association for a survey of nursing needs for that country. She spent another month consulting with various groups and agencies in Santiago, Chile; Lima, Peru; and Bogota and further directed an extended nursing project for the Colombian schools from 1962–64.

Prior to her five-year residency in Peru, Sister Charles Marie spent the summer of 1964 at the Ponce Institute for Intercultural Communication at the Catholic Uni-

versity of Puerto Rico pursuing course work in anthropology, Spanish culture, and language. While in Peru, she served as the superior of the new mission and public-health nurse at the Incarnate Word Mission in Centro Santa Clara at Chimbote. This was followed by a three-year period, 1966–69, spent at the University of Trujillo establishing a basic degree nursing program under the auspices of Project HOPE, the People-to-People Health Foundation. Her tenure at the University of Trujillo was not a peaceful one because a national revolution and prolonged student strikes created difficulties for the American nurse educators who were involved with this project.

From 1969–72 Sister Charles Marie served in various capacities to Project HOPE. She worked as a consultant on a short-term basis in Laredo, Texas, and spent three months as a consultant and instructor at the Universidad de Cartegena in Colombia and later at the Universidad de Zulia in Maracaibo, Venezuela.

Sister Charles Marie's membership in a religious order did not preclude affiliations with the military. During World War II she was a member (1944–45) of the National Committee on Recruitment for the National Nursing Council for War Service. From 1953–57 she served as nursing consultant to the U.S. Fourth Army, and from 1955–59 and again in 1969, she was a lecturer at the Medical Field Service School for the Army Nurse Corps at Fort Sam Houston, Texas. In addition to these activities, from 1972–1973 and again in 1974, she was a member of the Defense Advisory Committee for Women in the Armed Services, U.S. Department of Defense, 1972–73 and 1974.

In 1971 she assumed the role of coordinator of rehabilitation services of the Villa Rosa Psychiatric Service at Santa Rosa Medical Center in San Antonio. From 1972–78 she served in pastoral ministry at the same medical center, and from 1978–85 was the health nurse for senior members at the Incarnate Word Convent.

Throughout her career Sister Charles Marie has been active in nursing professional organizations. At various times she served as a board member and third vice-president of the National League for Nursing. She also was second vice-president of the Texas Nurses' Association and its president from 1952–54. She also has been an American Red Cross Nurse since 1942.

The word "retirement" is one that is rarely used in religious orders. At the age of 83 Sister Charles Marie is writing the histories of the congregation's four Peruvian missions.

Sister Charles Marie's contributions to nursing and health care have not gone unnoticed. In 1960 she received a Certificate of Merit from the Brazilian Nurses' Association. In 1961 she received the coveted Florence Nightingale medal. This award, granted by the International Committee of the Red Cross, is one of the highest honors that can be bestowed upon a nurse. In 1964 Catholic University of America awarded Sister Charles Marie its Alumnae Award. She received the Silver Medal and Diploma of Honor and Merit from Trujillo, La Libertad, Peru, in 1969. The Texas Nurses' Association gave her its Service Award in 1976, and, in that same year, Incarnate Word College initiated a lecture series in her honor. In 1987 the National University of Trujillo granted Sister Charles Marie "the title of Honorary Professor, in order to acknowledge the many important services she has rendered to this institution, as well as having fulfilled all the requirements established by law." In addition she is a member of Sigma Theta Tau International Honor Society and Pi Gamma Mu.

Sister Charles Marie resides at the Incarnate Word Mother House and Retirement Center in San Antonio, Texas.

PUBLICATIONS BY SISTER CHARLES MARIE FRANK

BOOKS

The Historical Development of Nursing. Philadelphia: Saunders, 1952.

Foundations of Nursing, 2nd ed. rev. Philadelphia: Saunders, 1959.

The History of the School of Nursing of the Faculty of Medical Sciences of La Universidad de Trujillo. Lima, Peru: People-to-People Health Foundation, 1971.

One Collegiate School of Nursing. The History of The Division of Nursing of Incarnate Word College. San Antonio: Incarnate Word College, 1977.

With L. Heidgerken, eds. *Perspectives in Nursing Education: Educational Patterns, Their Evolution and Characteristics.* Washington, D.C.: Catholic University of America, 1963.

With S.T. Elizando, *Desarrollo de la Enfermería.* (Adaptation of *The Historical Development of Nursing* by Sor Teresa Elizondo.) Mexico: La Prensa Mexicana, 1961.

ARTICLES

"Where Does Nursing Education End and Nursing Service Begin?" *Hospital Progress* 30 (June 1949): 169–72.

"Hospital Nursing and its Problems." *Texas Hospitals* 9 (March 1954): 7, 13–15, 18.

"The Heart of the Matter." *Nursing Outlook* 3 (November 1955): 596–97.

"Leadership in Nursing Education—Nursing Service." Texas League for Nursing. *TLN Newsletter* 2 (December 1958): 1–2.

"The Utilization of Nursing Personnel." *Nursing Outlook* 8 (April 1960): 202–03.

"On Continuing Growth." *American Journal of Nursing* 60 (October 1960): 1488–90.

"The Way Ahead." *Hospital Progress* 41 (October 1960): 84, 88, 90, 92.

"Truth Seekers." Guest Editorial. *American Journal of Nursing* 61 (May 1961): 43.

"Nursing Education for Whom, Where and When." *American Journal of Nursing* 62 (April 1962): 50–55.

"Satisfaction in Nursing Practice." *Nursing Outlook* 10 (May 1962): 302–04.

"Consultation in Retrospect." *Nursing Outlook* 10 (November 1962): 750–52.

"Viewing the Patient from the Stratosphere." *Nursing Outlook* 11 (January 1963): 62–65.

"Tomorrow's Reality." *Nursing Science* 1 (December 1963): 332–40.

BIBLIOGRAPHY

Anonymous. "The Second Dean." *The Olivian* 11 (Fall 1988): 2–3. (Although the article is unsigned, Sister Charles Marie stated that it was written by Barbara Conway, who had been administrative assistant to CUA's deans for 45 years prior to retirement.)

Frank, C.M. Interview with author, February 27, 1989.

Harriman, E.R. Notes for American Red Cross Florence Nightingale Awards, May 8, 1961.

Memorandum from Carlos Chirinos Villanueva, Rector, National University of Trujillo to Reverend Mother [No Name] regarding Sister Charles Marie Frank, August 7, 1987.

Young, G.F. "Nun Makes a Habit of Helping."
    Sunday Express-News (San Antonio) May
    8, 1983.

Eleanor L.M. Crowder

Stella Louisa Fuller

1878–1966

Stella Fuller was the first of five nurses designated a Jane Delano nurse and in this role was an early public-health nurse in Alaska. She also served as a Red Cross nurse in France in World War I, and after the war lectured on the Chautauqua circuit.

Fuller was born on April 26, 1878, in Lawrence (Brown County), Wisconsin. Her parents were Loyal M. and Alice Clark Fuller. Both parents were born in this country, her father in New York and her mother in Wisconsin. The second of two children, Fuller had a brother Rolie.

She grew up on a farm and attended "common" school for 10 years, graduating in April 1894. She did not attend high school, nor was it required when she entered a school of nursing, but in 1931 she received a high-school diploma after successfully passing a written examination. From 1895 to 1903 she taught in rural schools in Brown County.

Fuller graduated from the Milwaukee County Hospital Training School, Wauwatosa, in 1907. For the next three years she practiced as a private-duty nurse, often caring for patients in their own homes.

She then left Wisconsin for a brief time and served as night supervisor at Minnequa Hospital, Pueblo, Colorado. When she returned to Milwaukee, she joined the staff of the Visiting Nurse Association (VNA), where she was employed for five years (1911–16). During this time the Milwaukee VNA gave her services to the Children's Free Hospital (now the Children's Hospital of Wisconsin) as a social worker. She is credited with being the first hospital social worker in the state. For a short time she was an industrial nurse at the United

States Glue Factory at Carrollville (now Oak Creek, a Milwaukee suburb).

In 1916 Fuller was appointed superintendent of Maple Crest, the Manitowoc County (Wisconsin) tuberculosis sanitarium, at Whitelaw. The following year she joined the staff of the Wisconsin Anti-Tuberculosis Association (WATA—now the American Lung Association of Wisconsin) as a demonstration nurse. To encourage the employment of public-health nurses, the WATA rewarded counties having the largest Christmas-seal sales with the services of a public-health nurse for a month; in this time the demonstration nurse was supposed to convince county boards of supervisors of their value so they would then hire a nurse.

After several months as demonstration nurse, Fuller became director of the WATA's public-health nursing course, a program initiated in 1916. Most of Wisconsin's early country nurses were graduates of this program; there were no collegiate schools of nursing in the state at the time. Since tuberculosis was then a leading cause of death, the WATA sponsorship of the course was appropriate. Fuller was active in nursing organizations, serving as president of the Alumni Association of the Milwaukee County Hospital Training School. She edited the Department of Nursing section of the *Wisconsin Medical Journal*, a periodical available to nurses before the Wisconsin (State) Nurses' Association had its own publication.

She left the WATA in April 1918 and served for a year as a Red Cross nurse in France. Following military service, Fuller was selected as one of 31 Red Cross nurses as a lecturer on the Chautauqua circuit the summer of 1919. Chautauqua provided education, entertainment, and culture to rural communities throughout the United States; participants traveled from one community to another. For their part of the program, the nurses described their experiences overseas during World War I and incorporated a health message in their talks.

Fuller then returned to Wisconsin in 1919 as field director for the Red Cross but left the state to serve a short time on the staff of the National Organization of

Public Health Nursing. After that she joined the staff of the southern division of the American Red Cross in Atlanta. While there, she was invited to become a Jane Delano public-health nurse. Under the terms of Jane Delano's will, funds were provided to support nurses in communities unable to afford the services that nurses provided.

According to a letter in her file in the Red Cross archives, Fuller was the first to be selected as a Delano nurse, and she was sent to Alaska the fall of 1922. Her headquarters were in Seward, but her patients were as far away as Onalaska at the end of the Aleutian Peninsula, a two-week, 1,250-mile boat trip.

Typhoid fever, trachoma, and tuberculosis were common among her patients. In addition to administering to their needs, she attended women in labor and cared for their infants. She endured incredible hardships in her attempts to provide care; even securing transportation was a challenge. She had to adapt her work to the schedule of the boat that took her to many of her patients. Eventually, a sense of futility overcame her, as doctors, dentists, hospitals, and medical supplies were lacking; singlehandedly, Fuller was unable to accomplish much. Originally, it was planned that she would serve three years in Alaska, but the Delano Committee withdrew the service in 1924.

This experience was followed in 1925 by another return to Wisconsin, this time to Kenosha. Here she was employed as a public-health nurse by the Kenosha Health Department, and for a short time she was director of nursing of the Kenosha Hospital.

In 1937 Fuller became a writer for the New York Life Insurance Company with headquarters in Green Bay; how long she served in this capacity is not known. She spent her retirement years in Green Bay, where she was very active in church work at the St. Paul Methodist Church. She maintained her own apartment, until a stroke forced her to enter a nursing home.

Fuller died on August 14, 1966, at St. Mary's Hospital in Green Bay.

A niece remembers her as a very friendly, outgoing person and a serious, studious person with a good mind.

Fuller had a colorful and checkered career. She was a restless person who sought—and found—adventure and challenge. She served as pioneer industrial nurse, a public-health nurse, a teacher of nurses, an army nurse, and other roles. Many of her numerous and significant contributions to the profession were pioneering in nature.

PUBLICATIONS BY STELLA LOUISA FULLER

"Training the Surgical Nurse." *Trained Nurses* 46 (March 1911): 159–60.

"Visiting Nurse in Milwaukee." *Trained Nurse* 48 (April 1912): 219–20.

"The Atlanta Convention." *American Journal of Nursing* 20 (June 1920): 720–22.

"Hints on Writing." *Public Health Nurse* 12 (December 1920): 1019–20.

"Surgery in the Aleutian Islands." *Public Health Nurse* 15 (December 1923): 625–27.

"When It's Boat Day in Alaska" *Milwaukee Journal*, November 28, 1936.

BIBLIOGRAPHY

"American Red Cross Nursing Services in Alaska: A Capsule Summary." Mimeographed, n.d. Archives, University of Alaska, Fairbanks.

"Carrying on for Jane A. Delano." *American Journal of Nursing* 37 (July 1937): 737.

"The Delano Red Cross Nurses." *American Journal of Nursing* 23 (October 1922): 35–37.

"The First Delano Red Cross Nurses." *Public Health Nurse* 15 (October 1922): 546.

Kernodle, P. *The Red Cross Nurse in Action, 1882–1948.* New York: Harper, 1949. Pp. 287–89.

Mayer, M.J. Letter to author, January 16, 1989.

"Miss Stella Fuller." Obituary. *Green Bay Press Gazette*, August 15, 1966.

Noyes, C.D. "The Delano Red Cross Nurses." *American Journal of Nursing* (November 1924): 1113–21.

Rice, Mrs. R. Letter to author, June 26, 1989.

Stella Fuller File. Archives, American Red Cross, Washington, D.C.

U.S. Census Records. Brown County, Wisconsin, 1880.

Wisconsin Department of Health and Social Services. Section on Vital Statistics. Stella Fuller. Birth Record, November 7, 1878. Death Certificate, August 14, 1966.

Signe S. Cooper

Harriet Fulmer

ca. 1877–1952

Harriet Fulmer was a leader in the development of visiting nursing and in the professionalization of nursing. Through her work at the Visiting Nurse Association of Chicago (VNA), she created and implemented many innovative programs of nursing practice. She founded the Graduate Nurses' Association of the State of Illinois (later the Illinois Nurses' Association) and was its first president. She was a leader in the fight for the registration of nurses. Fulmer was a fairly prolific writer and founded her own journal, the *Visiting Nurse Quarterly*, as well as participating in the formation of the *American Journal of Nursing*.

Harriet Fulmer was born about 1877 in Fulmerville, Pennsylvania, the daughter of John Roericke Fulmer and Emma Jane (Beardsley) Fulmer. After graduation from a Nebraska high school, she attended St. Lukes Hospital Training School for Nurses in Chicago.

She began her career by doing private-duty nursing for one year. In 1897 she began a long tenure, first as a staff nurse, then head nurse/superintendent at the Visiting Nurse Association of Chicago. She was appointed head nurse in 1898 at the age of 21 years. The title was changed to superintendent several years later. It was while in this position that she made her greatest contributions to nursing.

Harriet Fulmer brought a new dimension of professionalism to the VNA. She used a scientific approach and was very practical as well. Under her leadership, the VNA started programs of industrial nursing, home visiting for insurance-policy holders, and baby-welfare work, among others. One of her major accomplishments was related to the identification and treatment of tuberculosis.

In 1902 Fulmer approached the VNA board and requested that they take the lead in developing a "broad" approach to the Great White Plague, as tuberculosis was then characterized. This led to the development of an effective multidisciplinary and multiagency approach to combat this contagious and highly prevalent disease. This collaborative approach to the delivery of health-care service was characteristic of much of her subsequent work as well. Some of the activities in which Fulmer took the lead included the establishment of neighborhood clinics, the development of a comprehensive tracking system, public education, and tent colonies for the isolation and treatment of persons with tuberculosis.

Fulmer had a particular interest in children, and under her leadership the VNA established a number of child-health programs. A school nursing program was established. Credit for this is often given to the social reformer, Jane Addams, but it was Harriet Fulmer who had established pilot projects in the schools some years earlier and was responsible for the implementation of a comprehensive program beginning about 1903.

Another concern of hers related to the medical treatment of sick babies. Under her leadership a system of baby tents for the care of ill infants was established. These tents were erected during summer months in high-risk neighborhoods. Mothers, who were often afraid to take their babies to hospitals, brought them to the tents each morning. The infants spent the day in a clean, quiet environment and received both medical and nursing care. Fulmer established a mechanism by which visiting nurses made home visits to these families in order to teach them prevention measures and illness care.

Prevention was a recurrent theme in her work. One rather appealing, and effective, scheme was the creation of the Chicago Clean City League. This was a club for children that promoted personal hygiene, preventive health practices, and environmental safety and beautification. Fulmer wrote a letter to public-school children offering 15 suggestions for "How to be Healthy this Summer." Activities of the league included the distribution of soap, towels, and toothbrushes as well as flower seeds and window boxes for "any boy or girl who will care for them." Contests were held to judge the results of these gardening efforts. The nurses distributed buttons that signified League membership, and children were instructed that, in times of trouble, they could go to the nurse for help.

Harriet Fulmer was instrumental in the development of a number of other innovative VNA programs. She organized and implemented a large program of industrial nursing, negotiating contracts with major companies to provide nursing services. The VNA began to respond to disasters during her tenure with the organization. She was cited for heroic action during rescue attempts at the site of Chicago's Iroquois Theater, which had been struck by a major fire during a performance.

Fulmer was very committed to the education of pupil nurses as well as her own staff. She established affiliations and a program of education with several schools of nursing. She also started a system of orientation and in-service education for the staff nurses. She hired the first African American nurse, Tallahassee Smith, in 1905.

Fulmer attended and spoke at many conferences including as a delegate to the International Congress of Women (1901, in Berlin) and the International Congress of Nurses (1906 in Paris) and a speaker at the Jubilee Congress of District Nursing, the 40th anniversary of district nursing celebration (1907 in Liverpool, England). She gave a brief speech about visiting-nurse qualifications at the jubilee. Interestingly, she was introduced as being of English birth and having received nurses' training in an English school, neither of which facts were true.

As the first president of the Graduate Nurses' Association of the State of Illinois, Fulmer led the fight for state registration of nurses. She had long been supportive of registration for nurses as she believed that this was a measure of quality. In her role as VNA superintendent, she sought graduates of the "best" schools of nursing, and, as registration became available to nurses, she hired only registered nurses. The VNA had established a group of "emergency nurses" (the approximate equivalent of today's home health aides) in 1892. These were neighborhood women who were trained to provide home care. Fulmer, supportive of registration, expressed regret that these women would lose their jobs because of the registration requirement.

Recognizing a need for more information for nurses practicing her specialty, she started her own journal, the *Visiting Nurse Quarterly*, which she published in 1905 and 1906. This journal covered a variety of topics of interest to visiting nurses, including meeting announcements and reports, editorial commentary, and "how to" articles of such diversity as school nursing and tuberculosis care. Letters of support from leaders such as Lillian Wald encouraged Fulmer to continue this work. Subscriptions were received from other countries as well as the United States. Despite the value of this publication, there was insufficient financial support from either subscriptions or the VNA board, and the publication ceased. The concept and related materials were given to the Cleveland VNA, who later started publication using the name *Public Health Quarterly*. In 1912 the journal was given to the National Organization of Public Health Nurses and became the *Public Health Nurse* and, finally, *Public Health Nursing*.

Fulmer was a member of the Committee on Periodicals of the Associated Alumnae of the United States and Canada (later the American Nurses' Association). This committee planned the formation of the *American Journal of Nursing*, and Fulmer served as the editor for public-health nursing reports in this journal beginning in 1908. In addition to the columns in the *American Journal of Nursing* and the *Visiting Nurse Quarterly*, she published four articles during her tenure as superintendent, one on the history of visiting-nurse work.

The VNA board was aware of the professional activities of their head nurse, but its members seemed to have a benevolent, but limited, interest in them. This did not stop Harriet Fulmer, who repeatedly credited her successes to them. The board noted her "spontaneity and new and effective methods of promoting the work of the organization."

In 1911 she was given eight months' paid vacation. Soon after that (1912), she terminated her position with the VNA. The reasons for the leave and termination are not recorded, but it is likely that it was because of illness or family circumstances as she worked only for one year after she left the VNA (1913–14 as secretary of the Illinois State Association for the Prevention of Tuberculosis), and she did not work again until 1917, when she became the supervisor of rural nursing services in Cook County, Illinois, which position she held until 1940.

Harriet Fulmer was a very dedicated nurse who used her many skills and innovations to promote the profession of nursing and visiting nursing in particular. She was recognized for her contributions. She herself was very self-effacing and often gave credit to others for her ideas. She was recognized for her kindness and humanity as well as her philosophy of nursing. She wrote, "The sooner we eliminate commercialism from the medical and nursing profession, the more rapidly will we accomplish our real service to mankind."

Fulmer died November 27, 1952, in Chicago at 65 years of age. She was characterized as inspiring her nurses to "love for the people and enthusiasm for their daily task."

PUBLICATIONS BY HARRIET FULMER

ARTICLES

"History of Visiting Nurse Work in America." *American Journal of Nursing* 2 (March 1902): 411–25.

"Address to Graduates of the Michael Reese [Chicago] Training School, 1905." Quoted in "Editor's Miscellany." *American Journal of Nursing* 6 (April 1906): 261–62.

"Visiting Nurse Tent Colony for Tubercular Poor, Glencoe, Illinois." *Visiting Nurse Quarterly* 2 (July 1906): 100–02.

"The Theory and Practice of Visiting Nursing and the Attitude of the Profession Towards It." *American Journal of Nursing* 6 (October 1906): 821–23.

OTHER PUBLICATIONS

Editor and publisher of the *Visiting Nurse Quarterly* in 1905 and 1906.

BIBLIOGRAPHY

Brainard, A.M. *The Evolution of Public Health Nursing.* Philadelphia: Saunders, 1922.

"Chicago Clean City League." *Visiting Nurse Quarterly* (July 1906): 90–91.

Minutes, Board of Directors, Visiting Nurse Association of Chicago, June 5, 1902.

Minutes, Board of Directors, Visiting Nurse Association of Chicago, November 6, 1902.

Minutes, Board of Directors, Visiting Nurse Association of Chicago, November 5, 1903.

Minutes, Board of Directors, Visiting Nurse Association of Chicago, January 7, 1904.

"A New Effort for Care of Sick Babies." *Visiting Nurse Quarterly* (July 1906): 84.

"Report of Proceedings." Jubilee Congress of District Nursing (Liverpool, England), May 12–14, 1909.

"Report on Tuberculosis Work." Visiting Nurse Association of Chicago, Chicago, 1902.

Wendy Kent Burgess

Bertha J. Gardner

1861–1917

Bertha J. Gardner was a founder of the New Jersey State Nurses' Association and was pivotal to that state's early nursing legislation. Later she served as the assistant business manager of the *American Journal of Nursing.*

Born August 3, 1861, in Newark, New Jersey, she was one of three children of Ira and Sara (Smith) Gardner. Nothing is known of her family or her childhood. At the age of 16 she graduated from the Orange Memorial Hospital Training School in 1877 and practiced as a private-duty nurse for several years in Orange. She worked as a graduate nurse in Massachusetts and California before she returned to New Jersey in 1894 because of her mother's illness and subsequent death. Gardner briefly worked as the night superintendent at Orange Memorial Hospital before resuming private-duty nursing. Within New Jersey she was regarded as a tower of strength in private-duty nursing.

When the graduates of Orange Training School formed their alumnae association in 1895, Gardner was elected second vice-president. She eventually served two terms as the alumni president and was chosen as delegate to the Congress of Nurses in Buffalo held in September 1901.

Nursing organizations continued to be her focus, and in December 1901 she chaired the first meeting of the New Jersey State Nurses' Association (NJSNA). Bertha Gardner is considered the founder of NJSNA and served two nonconsecutive terms as president (1903–05, 1909–11). During her second term she was the prime mover of the bill to create New Jersey's first Board of Nurse Examiners. Many of her nursing colleagues wanted physicians to serve on the Board of Nurse Examiners, but Gardner was a strong advocate for an autonomous nurse board. During an association debate on the composition of the proposed board, Gardner is quoted in the meeting's minutes as saying with "some indignation that nurses were capable of conducting their own affairs, the doctors had done nothing to advance the cause of nurses."

While networking to gain support for the bill, Gardner met with Sophia Palmer, editor of the *American Journal of Nursing.* From Palmer she gained not only insights into lobbying for the bill, but also started a friendship that would last until her death. Gardner also met with the speaker of the New Jersey Assembly and with Governor Woodrow Wilson, lobbying for their support. At a public hearing Gardner testified for an autonomous nurse board. Finally, in 1912 the bill was passed creating New Jersey's Board of Nurse Examiners composed of five registered nurses.

Gardner's untiring efforts lobbying for the bill were not forgotten; she was honored posthumously when NJSNA issued a commemorative stamp featuring her bust on the association's twenty-fifth anniversary.

A recognized leader within the American Nurses' Association, Gardner presented two papers at the Sixteenth Annual Convention of the ANA in 1913. She spoke to the Private-Duty Section on "Private-Duty Emergencies," a tribute to the resourceful private-duty nurses. In her second paper to the convention on educa-tional standards, in addition to the requisite high-school education, fair health, and knowledge of simple domestic duties, she advocated "assertion" for private-duty nurses who often lived for prolonged spells in a patient's home.

Leaving the strenuous field of private-duty nursing, Gardner once again applied her organizational skills for the benefit of the nursing profession. From 1914 until her death in 1917 she served as the assistant business manager of the *American Journal of Nursing* and was credited with reorganizing its business management and subscription service.

Bertha J. Gardner, stricken with endocarditis, died at the age of 55.

PUBLICATIONS BY BERTHA J. GARDNER

"Minimum Education Standards." *American Journal of Nursing* 13 (September 1913): 964–66.

"Private Duty Emergencies." *American Journal of Nursing* 13 (September 1913): 1005–07.

BIBLIOGRAPHY

"Bertha J. Gardner." Obituary. *American Journal of Nursing* 17 (July 1917): 1027.

New Jersey State Nurses' Association, Minutes of proceedings, Trenton, December 14, 1911.

"Nursing in New Jersey 1902–1952." Trenton: New Jersey State Nurses' Association, 1952.

Palmer, S. "Editorial Comment." *American Journal of Nursing* 14 (December 1913): 162–63.

Palmer, S. "Editorial Comment." *American Journal of Nursing* 17 (August 1917): 1041.

"Some Account of the Orange Training School." Orange, NJ, 1899.

Janet L. Fickeissen

Mildred Garrett (Primer)

b. 1905

Mildred Garrett Primer left her mark in nursing in the field of public-health nursing. She began her career in public health as a county nurse in Potter County, Texas, and retired as the program director, public-health nursing, in the Texas Department of Public Health. Over the intervening 42 years she spent slightly over a year in college and several years as a city-county nurse. Moving to the state Department of Health in 1936 she served there as nurse advisor, director of nurse education, state supervising nurse, director of the Division of Public Health Nursing, and the director of departmental nursing. Concomitantly, she was very active in public-health and nursing organizations.

Born on July 13, 1905, to Nellie Eliza Lay and Harrison Potilla Garrett, Mildred Garrett was the oldest of seven children. Her siblings and the years of their birth are Harrison Jr., 1906; Lurline Imogene (Owen), 1911; James Archie, 1913; Reginald Emmett, 1916; Dot, 1919; and Nell (Carson), 1923. Garrett was born at home outside of Hempstead, Texas, in rural Waller County. Her father was a Baptist minister.

Garrett's first eight years of formal education were at Pine Island School in rural Waller County, Texas. The family moved to Grady, New Mexico, in 1920, where she attended Grady High School for one and a half years. In 1922 the family moved again, this time to a rural area near Clovis, New Mexico. She finished her last year and a half of high school at Clovis High School, graduating in 1923. The moves were made because her father was called to pastor churches in different locations.

Garrett contends that "I don't remember a time when I didn't want to be a nurse." She believes that she was probably influenced by her family's physician, who was a neighbor. She started her career as a nurse aide at the Baptist Hospital in Clovis. After three weeks of service she was put on night duty with another nurse, who soon began leaving Mildred alone with the 14 patients entrusted to their care. The job lasted a total of nine months with one interruption. She left to enter nursing school.

Garrett's first choice of a nursing education program was Baylor Hospital School of Nursing in Dallas, Texas. However her parents feared her going to a big city to school. Consequently, in 1924 she enrolled in Northwest Texas Hospital

School of Nursing in Amarillo. The 75-bed hospital had opened in March 1924. The hospital superintendent, the director of the nursing school, and the supervisors of each of the patient services were graduate nurses.

Students worked on the nursing units eight hours per day. Classes were held during "time off" and/or in the evening. Students were constantly admonished to give good care to the patients and "make a good impression on the community" so the "new" hospital could continue to operate. Student nurses had some experience there at the "T.B. Cottage" through relieving the staff nurse during her four hours off each day from taking care of tubercular patients.

Garrett's course of training also included a three-and-a-half-month rotation at John Sealy Hospital in Galveston for experience in obstetrics and gynecology, pediatrics, and orthopedics.

Immediately after graduation Garrett went to her parent's home in San Jon, New Mexico, to make white graduate uniforms. She returned to Amarillo after a month and did private-duty nursing. In the fall of 1928 she entered Montezuma Baptist College in New Mexico, where she enrolled in the usual freshman courses. She also did some private-duty nursing. In 1929 she was invited to be the college nurse for the summer term. Her remuneration was to be free room and board as well as tuition and fees. Unfortunately, she became ill and had to give up classes but did remain to the end of the session as the college nurse. She then returned to Amarillo where she did private-duty nursing. One case in particular in this period was responsible for her career in public health in Texas.

Garrett was called to the Kritser Ranch outside of Amarillo to care for Mr. Kritser. He died, and she was asked to stay on to care for an ill child. Later the original patient's sister-in-law asked her to stay with her children while she traveled, which Garrett did.

Several weeks after she returned to Amarillo to private nursing, she was again called to the sister-in-law's home to care for a young Kritser brother who had sustained a fractured leg and was bedridden until it healed. After approximately three weeks her employer, a Mrs. Weymouth, asked Garrett to come into the living room for a talk. Garrett thought the talk would be about the family's ability to take over the care of the boy. Instead, Garrett was reminded of recent articles in the local newspaper concerning Potter County's intention of hiring a nurse to work in a proposed children's clinic. Garrett was offered the job. She protested, saying that she had no experience in public-health nursing. It seems the county commissioners had authorized the Junior Welfare League, a forerunner of the Junior League, to secure a nurse. Mrs. Weymouth was a member of that organization and had visited the State Department of Health to get ideas about the necessary credentials. She was told that they needed a nurse who "could get along with all the doctors and was good with children." She believed that Garrett "fit the bill."

After consultation with the Northwest Texas Hospital superintendent, her private physician, and her father, Garrett decided to accept the challenge. The arrangement was unusual in that the county was responsible for hiring her, but her salary was supplemented by the Junior Welfare League, which operated the children's clinics.

Garrett began her career in public health on April 1, 1930, in a self-fashioned uniform carrying a bag with supplies bought at Walgreen's Drug Store. Her office, which also served as a well- and ill-baby clinic, was a portion of the basement of the public library. Garrett's responsibilities included operating the children's clinics, making needed home visits, and supervising health-related services for the nine schools in the county.

By November 1930 the Health Department reorganized, and a Health Unit was established for the city of Amarillo and Potter County. Garrett's position evolved to that of a city-county nurse for those jurisdictions.

During the summer of 1931 Garrett attended Vanderbilt University for a six-week course in public-health nursing. The course opened new vistas for her. Soon

after returning to Texas from summer school, she reorganized the office and obtained a Works Progress Administration (WPA) project. The project furnished a nurse for the office, freeing Garrett to do more home visiting.

In 1935 Shirley Titus offered Garrett a "working scholarship" at Vanderbilt University. The working part involved being the evening hostess in the nurses' dormitory from 6:30 P.M. until 11 P.M. Her tuition of $250, as well as room and board, were covered by the scholarship. Garrett raised spending money by renting her car to a friend in Amarillo for $10 per month. Her initial goal in attending Vanderbilt was to earn a certificate in public-health nursing. However, summoning Garrett to her office, Dean Titus explained to her that she could obtain a bachelor of science degree in nursing (B.S.N.), with a major in public-health nursing, if she stayed at Vanderbilt and fulfilled a two-month-field-experience requirement in public health. Garrett did so, graduating in June 1936 with a B.S.N.

Shortly before graduation, Garrett had been offered a position as "state advisory nurse" for the state Department of Health in Austin, and on September 1, 1936, she became the state advisory nurse. The position was funded with Social Security Administration monies and paid $150 per month plus an expense account. The allowances were 35 cents for breakfast, 75 cents for lunch, $1 for dinner, and $2 per night for a hotel room. The job required considerable travel and frequently taxed Garrett's ingenuity. In 1938 Garrett became the director of nurse education for the state Department of Public Health. Over the ensuing 34 years she progressed up the Texas Department of Public Health hierarchy into roles of ever increasing responsibility. She retired in 1972 from the position of program director, public-health nursing, Texas Department of Public Health.

During Garrett's tenure at the State Health Department she was able to accomplish much. Soon after the Division of Public Health Nursing was established in 1943, discrimination, in both pay scales and educational stipends, for black nurses was abolished. In-service training courses were initiated on a casual basis at first and later were conducted on an annual basis for directors, consultants, supervisors, and teachers of public-health nursing.

During the Depression federal monies were available for the education of registered nurses in public health. Prior to the establishment of the Division of Public Health Nursing Garett designed and implemented an orientation course for nurse trainees who had Social Security scholarships to study public-health nursing. The nurses received the orientation prior to enrolling in out-of-state schools for the study of public health.

During the years of World War II public-health nurse manpower was substantially reduced because of nurses entering the military services. Postwar, Garrett was involved in activities of the Public Health Department in establishing and implementing nursing protocols to be used in time of national disaster in the state disaster control center. Although they were part of national activities, as a result of the cold war they were also designed to be used in case of civil disasters. In 1954, during the Rio Grande River flood, she was the first State Department of Health employee to serve in the state disaster control center.

Beginning in 1962, Garrett was active in formulating the plans to provide nursing services for migrant farm workers working in Texas. The Migrant Health Project met health-care needs of migrant workers in areas where no local health department existed. In areas where such departments did exist, nurses employed by the project worked with the migrants through those departments.

Throughout her career Garrett was a member of many professional organizations, including the American Nurses' Association and the National League for Nursing and their state constituents, the American and Texas Public Health associations, the United States-Mexico Border Public Health Association, and the American Red Cross Nursing Service. The extent of her activities is demonstrated in the number of offices that she held in those

organizations over the course of her professional career. Representative offices held were president of TGNA 1946–50, vice-president of the Texas Organization for Public Health Nurses, 1935–39; first vice-chairman of the ANA Public Health Nurses' Section, and Chairman of the Council of State Directors of Public Health Nursing, 1941.

Four years after her retirement Mildred Garrett married Dr. Benjamin M. Primer, Sr., a physician with whom she had worked in the Amarillo-Potter County Health Unit. She makes her home in Austin, Texas.

PUBLICATIONS BY
MILDRED GARRETT (PRIMER)

"Balancing the Program of a City-County Nurse." *Public Health Nursing* 24 (March 1932): 147–49.

"Improvised Equipment for Small Fry." *Trained Nurse and Hospital Review* 109 (July 1942): 25.

"Nursing Contributions to Health Programs for School Children." *Journal of the Texas Public Health Association* 2 (December 1950): 223–25.

"What the Records Show." *Texas Health Bulletin* 5 (June 1952): 10–14.

"A Survey of Nursing Resources." *Texas Health Bulletin* 8 (November 1955): 16–18.

"The Ladies in Civil Defense." *Texas Health Bulletin* 9 (September/October 1956): 9–11, 16.

"The United States-Mexico Border Public Health Association." *Nursing Outlook* 7 (1959): 295–97. Spanish translation printed in *Boletin de la Oficina Sanitaria Panamericana* 46 (1959): 370–72.

"Facing up to it." *TPHA Journal* 20 (November/December 1968): 224–25.

"Community Health Nursing in Texas: Yesterday, Today and Tomorrow." *TPHA Journal* 24 (May/June 1972): 1244–28.

BIBLIOGRAPHY

Garrett, M. Interview with the author, May 16, 1980.

Garrett, M. Letter to Lillian Taubert, January 5, 1972.

Marett, A. "Mildred Garrett, Public-Health Nurse Retires after 42 Years." *Austin American-Statesman*, July 30, 1972, F10.

Eleanor L.M. Crowder

Mary Ann Garrigan

b. 1914

Nurse educator and administrator, Mary Ann Garrigan founded the nursing archives in the Department of Special Collections, Mugar Memorial Library at Boston University, in order to improve the teaching of nursing history, to foster historical research, and to provide and preserve resource material in nursing history.

Mary Ann Leonarda Garrigan, was born on January 24, 1914, in New York City, one of five children of Thomas Edward and Wilhelmina (Fredericks) Garrigan. Her parents were of German/Hungarian and Irish descent. She attended school in Westchester County and graduated from Westchester School of Nursing in Valhalla, New York, in 1935. The following year she received a certificate in maternity nursing from the Women's Hospital of New York. During the next four years she studied and worked. She taught nursing at her alma mater, and in 1941 she received a bachelor of science degree from Teachers College, Columbia University. Before joining the U.S. Army Nurse Corps in 1943, Garrigan worked as a staff nurse and advisor at the Henry Street Visiting Nurse Service and also served as director of Precinct #43 New York-Disaster Relief. While stationed as a member of the Army Nurses Corps Halloran Hospital on Staten Island, she was assigned the management and training of all nurse cadets in the eastern area.

Garrigan received a master's degree in education from Boston University in 1947 and was invited to become an instructor at the school. She was promoted to assistant professor in 1951, associate professor the following year, and full professor in 1956. Her primary responsibility was directing the newly instituted four-year baccalaureate nursing education program, which continued under her leadership for the next ten years.

Her interest in nursing history led her to initiate the establishment of the Nursing Archives at Boston University in March 1966, and in 1971 it was named the official depository for the American Journal of Nursing Company and the American Nurses' Association. She was also instrumental in founding the *Journal of Nursing History* in 1985.

Garrigan's many honors include honorary doctorate of humane letters degrees from the University of San Diego and from Boston University in 1979 and the Edith Moore Copeland Founders Award of Sigma Theta Tau. Upon her retirement she was named curator emerita of the Nursing Archives.

She currently resides in Marblehead, Massachusetts, and continues to serve as a mentor for researchers in nursing history.

PUBLICATIONS BY MARY ANN GARRIGAN

"Guidance in the School of Nursing: A Suggested In-service Program for Faculty" Master of Science Thesis, Boston University, 1947.

"Woolsey Sisters of New York. A family's involvement in Civil War and a new profession (1860–1900)." *Nursing Research* 21 (1972); 170–71. (Book review.)

"In the Spirit of '76." *American Journal of Nursing* 76 (July 1976): 1101.

BIBLIOGRAPHY

"A Tribute to Mary Ann Garrigan." *Journal of Nursing History* 2 (November 1986): 3–15.

Lilli Sentz

Lucy Doman Germain

1903–1988

Lucy D. Germain had an outstanding career as a nurse educator and nursing-service administrator. From 1959–64 she was executive director of the American Journal of Nursing Company and actively participated in the planning and development of the *International Nursing Index*.

Germain was born on November 28, 1903, in Petrolia, Ontario, Canada. Her father, Robert A. Germain, of French descent, was a harnessmaker by trade and a successful small-town businessman. Her mother, Caroline Parker Germain, a first-generation Canadian, had English ancestors. Her mother died in her late thirties, and her father remarried a woman who was very supportive of Germain and her only brother, G.C. Ronald Germain. He died in 1982.

Germain attended grammar school in Alvinston, Ontario, and was graduated from the Petrolia, Ontario, High School. Her mother's illness influenced her decision to become a nurse. The care given by the registered nurse who attended her mother deeply impressed Germain.

In 1924 she enrolled in the Farrand Training School for Nurses (later known as the Harper Hospital School of Nursing) in Detroit and graduated three years later. The program included an affiliation in contagious-disease nursing at the Herman Kiefer Hospital in Detroit.

Germain completed requirements for the bachelor of science degree in nursing from Teachers College, Columbia University, New York City, in 1931. She was awarded a master's degree in education from the University of Michigan, Ann Arbor, in 1940.

Her first employment was as a private-duty nurse, and then she was appointed instructor at the School of Nursing, Port Huron Hospital, Port Huron, Michigan, where she served for two years. Returning to Harper Hospital in 1930, she held a variety of positions, including instructor of nursing arts, head nurse on an orthopedic unit, supervisor of surgical nursing, assistant director of nursing service and assistant director of the School of Nursing (1937–40).

In 1940 Germain was appointed a field representative for the *American Journal of Nursing*. In this position, she traveled all over the United States, helping local committees encourage nurses to subscribe to and read the *Journal* and speaking to groups of nurses on ways to use the publication more effectively. During World War II she was on loan to the National Nursing Council for War Service.

In 1946, Germain returned to the Harper Hospital as director of nursing ser-

vice and nursing education and assistant administrator of the hospital. In this position she was committed to promoting equal opportunities for all racial and ethnic groups. This was demonstrated in 1948 by her appointment of Mary Marshall as head nurse, the first known black woman to hold such a position in the state of Michigan. Germain supported the practice of hiring private-duty nurses of color, but as head nurse Marshall had to ask the patients if they would accept the nurses. In 1954 Marshall became the first black instructor in any nursing school in Michigan when she was appointed to the Harper Hospital School of Nursing faculty. Under Germain's direction, the Harper Hospital School of Nursing accepted its first black students in the early 1950s.

Germain encouraged and supported the staff in many ways. She invited them for high tea every Friday, especially when influential nursing leaders were visiting Detroit. She urged them to meet leaders when attending nursing conferences or conventions.

Returning to New York in 1959, Germain was appointed executive director of the American Journal of Nursing Company. During her five-year tenure in this position, she actively promoted the development of the *International Nursing Index* and chaired its Advisory Committee after it became a reality.

In 1964 Germain left New York for Philadelphia, where she served as vice-president for nursing at the Pennsylvania Hospital. Here she was responsible for reorganizing the nursing program, facilitated a merger of two separate schools of nursing (one for men, another for women), helped establish nursing service at the neighborhood health center operated by the hospital, developed a home-care program, and initiated a comprehensive in-service education program.

Germain retired from her position at the Pennsylvania Hospital in 1970 but soon accepted another as a part-time faculty member at the University of Oklahoma College of Nursing as director of its continuing-education program. For several months she was on loan to the University of Oklahoma Hospital as its director of nursing. She retired in 1976.

But retirement did not mean inactivity. Germain was one of the founders of the El Reno, Oklahoma, Mobile Meals services and was on its board of directors. She helped establish a Canadian County (Oklahoma) Health Department and for six years served on the Oklahoma State Health Advisory Committee for home care.

Throughout her professional career, she was very active in local, state, national, and international nursing associations. Germain was truly an organizational woman, serving on many boards and committees. She was third vice-president and treasurer of the American Nurses' Association (ANA) and chaired its finance committee. In 1958 she was nominated for the presidency of the ANA but lost the election. She represented the ANA as an advisor to the National Student Nurses' Association and served on the board of directors of the American Nurses' Foundation. She also served as a member of the board of directors of the National League for Nursing and chaired its Committee on Perspectives.

A person with many international interests, she chaired the ANA's first Committee on Nursing in International Affairs. She was actively involved in the International Council of Nurses, serving as an ANA delegate to several of its congresses and chairing its Ways and Means and Public Relations committees. She was instrumental in bringing many exchange nurses from foreign countries to Harper Hospital.

Germain wrote extensively for professional nursing and hospital journals, including articles in foreign nursing journals. She was frequently sought as a speaker and conducted workshops in various parts of the country.

She received many honors throughout her professional career. A fellowship from the American-Scandanavian Foundation permitted her a four-month educational tour of Denmark, Norway, Sweden, and Finland. In 1952 she was named one of Detroit's Women of Achievement, and six years later she was among the city's Top Ten Women Who Work and selected the Michigan Nurse of the Year. She was awarded honorary membership in the Alumni Association of the Harper Hospital School of Nursing, and in 1959 the association established the Lucy D. Germain Scholarship Fund. After her retirement, the University of Oklahoma College of Nursing honored her by naming its continuing-education program the Lucy D. Germain Continuing Education Program.

Germain was a member of Pi Lambda Theta, an education honorary society; Sigma Theta Tau, the nursing honorary society; the American Hospital Association; the American Public Health Association. She also was an active participant in women's organizations such as Soroptimist International and the Women's City Club of Detroit. A deeply religious person, she was an active member of the Methodist Church.

She was a cheerful, friendly person, with a marked sense of humor. She had boundless energy, a love of life, and enthusiasm in all that she did. Her deep professional commitment was demonstrated not only in her work, but also in her extensive participation in nursing organizations. As a nursing administrator, she is remembered for her interest in her staff, her willingness to teach and encourage them to greater achievement. Sometimes the staff felt she was building castles in the air but, nonetheless, accepted the challenges she offered. She was a farsighted visionary, with the courage of her convictions in support of patients, individuals, and social causes.

Germain died on April, 3 1988, at the Harper-Grace Hospital in Detroit.

PUBLICATIONS BY LUCY DOMAN GERMAIN

"Orthopaedic Nursing." *Irish Nursing and Hospital World* (October 1936): 10–11.

"Pharmacy-Nursing Teamwork Improves Care of Patient." *Hospital Management* 69 (June 1950): 78–82.

"How Hospital Nurses Helped with the Harper Hospital Study." *American Journal of Nursing* 53 (October 1953): 1197–99.

"How Close Are We to a Nursing Index?" *American Journal of Nursing* 64 (May 1964): 106.

"Impact: How Federal Health Legislation Will

Affect Nursing Service." *Hospital Progress* 47 (October 1966): 86–98.

"A New Position Was Created." *International Journal of Nursing Studies* 4 (December 1967): 295–300.

"Needed: Changes in Hospitals to Utilize the New Practitioners in Nursing." *Journal of Nursing Education* 8 (August 1969): 25–29.

"Who Should the Director of Nursing Be?" *Nursing Clinics of North America* 5 (June 1970): 289–96.

"Symposium on Nursing Leaders Look at Clinical Nursing." *Nursing Clinics of North America* 6 (June 1971): 215–16.

BIBLIOGRAPHY

Addams, R. "Lucy Germain Becomes Executive Director of Journal Company." *American Journal of Nursing* 59 (August 1959): 1113.

Germain, L.D. Papers. Archives, Harper Hospital, Detroit, Michigan.

Germain, L.D. Professional resume, 1984.

Germain, L.D. Resume. American Journal of Nursing Company, 1958.

Haynes, I. Letter to author, February 19, 1990.

Hill, C.E. Letter to author, March 15, 1990.

"Lucy D. Germain: An Appreciation." *Nursing Clinics of North America* 6 (June 1971): 267–69.

"Lucy Germian Dies at 84." *American Journal of Nursing* 88 (May 1988): 750.

Marshall, M. Letter to the author, April 3, 1990.

Myers, E.J. Letter to the author, March 3, 1990.

Rado, M., and B. Strohl. "Nursing to Maintain a Tradition." *Nursing at the Detroit Medical Center* 2 (Winter 1987): 12–13.

Signe S. Cooper

Sister Agnes Mary Gonzaga Grace

(1812–1897)

Director of the St. Joseph's Orphan Asylum and in charge of the Satterlee Hospital in west Philadelphia during the Civil War, Sister Gonzaga was an outstanding administrator and nurse who devoted her life to helping the poor and the orphaned.

Anne Grace was born in Baltimore, Maryland, on February 22, 1812, of Protestant parentage. Her father, a seaman, died two years after her birth, and her mother died in 1816 of yellow fever. Shortly before her death, Mrs. Grace became a Roman Catholic, and Anne was raised in the Catholic faith by Elizabeth Michel, a young woman of 17 who cared for Anne's mother during the final stages of her illness. After her baptism Anne became known as Agnes Mary Grace. She entered St. Joseph's Academy, Emmitsburg (Maryland), in December 1822, where she spent the next four years. On March 11, 1827, she joined the community of the Sisters of Charity of St. Vincent De Paul, the order founded by Mother Elizabeth Seton, and three years later she made her final vows as Sister Gonzaga.

Prior to taking her vows, Sister Gonzaga had opened a school in Harrisburg, Pennsylvania, with two older sisters. In 1830 she was assigned to St. Joseph's Orphan Asylum, located next to Holy Trinity Church in Philadelphia. When the sister in charge of the orphanage died in 1843, Sister Gonzaga assumed the administrative responsibilities. One year later she was sent as assistant to the Novitiate of the Sisters of Charity in Donaldsonville, Louisiana, and to New Orleans, but in 1851 she returned to St. Joseph's Orphanage. In 1855 she left, this time for the Mother House in Paris. She returned for a brief assignment to St. Joseph's, Emmitsburg, as procuratrix and then went to Philadelphia again to St. Joseph's Orphanage.

The Civil War was to mark the most eventful epoch in the career of Sister Gonzaga and developed her extraordinary gifts and qualities of administration. When Satterlee Hospital, the army hospital, was established in Philadelphia at the beginning of the war, the physicians requested that it be staffed with Catholic sisters, stating that the sisters had two qualities that the so called Dix Nurses, i.e., the army nurses under the direction of Dorothea Dix, lacked: silence and obedience. On June 9, 1862, Sister Gonzaga and 40 sisters began service at the hospital. They were not paid, but the orders to which they belonged received reimbursement for their services.

During the war Sister Gonzaga and her assistants kept a journal of hospital life, and she recalled vividly the battles of Bull Run and Gettysburg. When the hospital closed in 1865, more than 60,000 soldiers had been treated, and a total of 91 nuns had been on duty during that time. While working at Satterlee Hospital, Sister Gonzaga continued to be in charge of St. Joseph's Orphanage.

Sister Gonzaga returned full time to the orphanage after the war. In 1877 she celebrated her golden jubilee in the sisterhood and received the blessing of Pope Pius IX. Ten years later she was recalled to the Mother House to take it easy, but the people of Philadelphia signed petitions for her return, and the request was granted.

During the last years of her life she suffered from increasing infirmities and died at the orphanage on October 8, 1897 at the age of 85. After her death the Gonzaga Memorial Asylum was built in Germantown, Philadelphia, in her memory.

BIBLIOGRAPHY

Barton, G. *Angels of the Battlefield*, 2nd ed. Philadelphia: Catholic Art Publishing, 1898. (Includes Sister Gonzaga's journal first published in the *Records of the American Catholic Historical Society*, ed. by S.T. Smith, December 1897.)

Donnelly, E.C. *Life of Sister Mary Gonzaga Grace of the Daughters of Charity of St. Vincent de Paul 1812–1897*. Philadelphia, 1900.

Jolly, E. R. *Nuns of the Battlefield*. Providence, R.I.: Providence Visitor Press, 1927.

Matthews, I. Interview with the author.

Taylor, F.H. *Philadelphia in the Civil War*. Philadelphia: Rudolph Blankenburg for the City, 1913.

Lilli Sentz

Amelia Howe Grant

1887–1967

As an outstanding administrator, educator, and writer in the field of public-health nursing, Amelia Howe Grant enriched the lives of not only the patients needing public-health nursing care, but also the nurses and students working in the field. She made major contributions to the development of the philosophical and conceptual base in public-health nursing for both practice and education through her example as the head of the New York City Health Department, her 10 years as a faculty member at Columbia Teachers College and the Yale School of Nursing, and through her numerous publications. She was truly a leader of her field.

Born in Utica, New York, on September 23, 1887, to George A. and Allie Stowell Grant, Grant spent her early childhood on a farm in central New York with her three siblings. She was first educated in a one-room school house and subsequently attended and graduated from Afton (N.Y.) High School.

Grant obtained her initial nursing education at Faxton Hospital School of Nursing in Utica, New York, graduating in 1910. In 1919 she completed a one-year course in public-health nursing at Simmons College, Boston. In 1922 she completed a baccalaureate and, in 1923, a master's degree at Teachers College, Columbia University.

Her first position upon completing basic nursing education was as a private-duty nurse, which she practiced from 1910 until 1917. Her experiences in this area gave her a good foundation in nursing and also led her to choose the new field of public-health nursing for her further professional development.

After completing the one-year program in public-health nursing at Simmons College, she became a supervising nurse at the Henry Street Visiting Nurse Service in New York City. The director of the service at that time was Annie Warburton Goodrich, who was developing a student affiliation with Teachers College at Columbia University. Working with the early students in that program, Grant furthered her interest in education and also began to develop her philosophy about public-health nursing. These early educational and professional experiences prepared her for further development in her career.

Grant began her teaching career in 1920 when she left the Henry Street Visiting Nurse Service to become an assistant instructor in the Department of Nursing Education at Teachers College. From 1923 on, she was involved in developing educational programs in public-health nursing, first as an assistant professor in nursing education at Yale University School of Nursing, 1923–26, and, subsequently, as a lecturer at Teachers College, Columbia. She was one of five people Goodrich took to New Haven to create the Yale University School of Nursing. Its program was one of the first to address both the curative and preventive aspects of nursing.

It was Grant's responsibility as an assistant professor and supervisor of the New Haven Dispensary to develop the public-health curriculum for the undergraduate program. Grant is credited during this time with the development of the conceptual and philosophical theories that identified the place of the outpatient department as a connecting link between the hospital and the family. She continued her work in education as a lecturer at Teachers College in the area of public-health supervision and administration and through her numerous publications.

Grant authored numerous articles for *Public Health Nursing*, the journal of the National Organization of Public Health Nurses. She wrote on the importance of social hygiene to the cause and prevention of disease and the need for public-health nurses to teach these principles to the families and parents with whom they worked. She emphasized the important role of the nurse as a teacher both within the home and within the school setting. In her writing she also encouraged the inclusion of public-health nursing principles in the undergraduate curriculum, stressing the importance of educating nurses in normal growth and development.

In 1926 Grant embarked on a career as an administrator. She first served as an assistant director of Bellevue Yorkville Health Demonstration funded by the Milbank Memorial Foundation for research in community health in New York City. In that position she demonstrated that a nursing department could function more effectively on a generalized rather than a specialized basis. She also had the opportunity to demonstrate her skills as an administrator.

With this background and her demonstrated ability as a public-health administrator, Grant was chosen director of the newly organized New York City Department of Health Bureau of Nursing. Prior to this time there were few positions in official public agencies that required or allowed nursing leadership. As the director of the Bureau of Nursing, Grant demonstrated the contribution nursing could make in all areas of public health.

At that time the New York Department of Health was the largest official agency of its kind in the country. A major challenge for Grant was moving the nursing staff to the new bureau. This required reorganization of almost all departments in the Department of Health since until that time the 700 nurses in the department had been working in various bureaus without nursing leadership.

Under Grant's professional nursing leadership supervisors were brought together in a generalized program where their experience and knowledge could be utilized to plan and develop the essential nursing components of the public-health program. They also identified the needs of nurses for professional development in public health, which led to the recognition of the need to develop continuing-education programs and to secure funding for further specialized education for select nurses.

Grant's contributions and leadership, particularly in the area of planning, extended to many national and local organizations. In the area of administration she made major contributions at the national level as the president of the National Organization for Public Health Nursing. Here she used her knowledge of planning and financial management to guide the organization through a change in mission during a time of financial uncertainty in the country. In her role she demonstrated the need for and the methodology of both incremental and long-term strategic planning. At the local level she served on many community organizations and is credited with promoting the plan for district health centers in New York City.

In the area of education she served in many capacities—most notably, as the chair of the National League of Nursing Education and as the chair of the Joint Committee of the American Social Hygiene Association and the National League for Nursing. In these positions she contributed to studies regarding the role of the outpatient department in the education of a nurse, the curricular issues in social hygiene for nurses, and the social content of the curriculum.

Amelia Howe Grant died August 8, 1967, in Amsterdam, New York. Throughout her career she received numerous honors for her professional work. Her many professional and personal interests combined to "make her a real person as well as an able leader in an important field for human betterment" (Wales, 1940).

PUBLICATIONS BY AMELIA HOWE GRANT

BOOKS

Nursing: A Community Health Service. Philadelphia: Saunders, 1942.

ARTICLES

"The Principles of Public Health Nursing in the Undergraduate Course." *National League of Nursing Education: Annual Report.* New York: National League for Nursing, 1925.

"The Public Health Nurse as a Health Teacher." *American Journal of Nursing* 25 (February 1925): 106–07.

"The Nurse in School Health Services." *Journal of School Health* 7 (December 1937): 243–45.

BIBLIOGRAPHY

"Amelia H. Grant Dies: Headed New York Health Department." *Nursing Outlook* 16 (October 1967): 13.

"Amelia H. Grant, 79: A Leader in Nursing." *New York Times*, August 15, 1967, 1, 39.

Howes, D., editor. *American Women 1933–1940: A Composite Biographical Dictionary.* Vol. 1, p. 387. Detroit: Gale Research, 1981.

Wales, M. "Amelia Grant." *National League for Nursing Biographical Sketches.* New York: National League for Nursing, 1940.

Linda M. Calley

Carolyn E. Gray
1873–1938

A nursing educator and author, Carolyn Elizabeth Gray was one of the first educators to be involved in collegiate schools of nursing. She coauthored the second edition of Kimber's *Anatomy and Physiology for Nurses*, which became a classic textbook for nursing students. Diana E. Clifford Kimber, who had written the first nurse-authored anatomy and physiology text in 1894, had been an instructor at City Hospital School of Nursing (New York City) when Gray was a student.

Gray was born in New York City, the eldest of four daughters. Her mother died when she was a young girl, and so, at an early age, Gray was enrolled at St. Mary's Academy in Newburgh, New York. Gillett (n.d.) described her as attractive (having very curly auburn hair), keen of mind, articulate, and ready to stand up for her beliefs. Gray's first employment, at age 16, was that of rural schoolteacher in Croton Falls, New York.

Gray's nursing career began in 1891 when she entered City Hospital School of Nursing on Welfare Island, New York City. She graduated in 1893.

Her first position as a graduate nurse was superintendent of nurses at Governeur Hospital (1893–95). She was 20 years old and the only graduate nurse on the staff of this hospital located near the waterfront on New York's Lower East Side. The hospital was surrounded by tenements and factories. At that time the hospital itself consisted of an abandoned police building and two tenements to house patients and staff. Gray's responsibilities included not only taking charge of the hospital, but also teaching the student nurses sent from City Hospital for additional experience. The hospital served 3,000 patients yearly.

From 1895 to 1907 she held a similar position at Fordham Hospital, located in the Bronx, New York City. Gray was again the only graduate nurse on the staff. She taught not only nursing students who came to Fordham for additional experience, but also the postgraduate nursing courses that were offered.

After 12 years at Fordham, Gray accepted a position as science instructor at City Hospital, teaching from 1907 until 1911. "We frequently hear nurses who were students in the school at that time speak of the good instruction they received in her classes" (Gillett, n.d.). During this time she was selected by Kimber to revise her anatomy and physiology textbook. The text later underwent numerous revisions by Gray and Kimber and, later, by Gray and Carolyn E. Stackpole.

Gray was superintendent of nurses at Pittsburgh Homeopathic Hospital from 1911 until 1913. Her efforts to reorganize the School of Nursing resulted in higher admission standards, separation of students in sequential classes, dietetics as a component of the curriculum, and increased instructional time.

Gray returned to New York City to City Hospital School of Nursing as principal in 1914. She made various improvements there: increasing the length of time of study, increasing course content by expanding affiliations, and improving the theoretical knowledge of students by both increased hours of classroom work and additional content. Gray also established a government mechanism for students and was one of the first to initiate the eight-hour day for students. She also encouraged City Hospital to raise funds to establish a scholarship for graduates to continue their education at Teachers College, Columbia University. The scholarship was known as the Darche-Kimber Scholarship. Louise Darche had been the superintendent of nurses at City Hospital while Gray had been a student. Gray left her position at City Hospital in 1919, but she remained the chair of the scholarship committee until her death.

During her tenure at City Hospital, Gray was enrolled at Teachers College, where she earned her B.S. degree in 1917 and her M.A. in 1920. Also during this period she worked for *Modern Hospital* magazine. In 1918 Gray and Annie Warburton Goodrich were joint associate editors of a nursing column. In 1919 Gray became the sole editor for the column, "Nursing and the Hospital." She continued her association with *Modern Hospital* until 1925.

Gray publicized nursing as a career. While at Pittsburgh Homeopathic, she had produced a circular that described the school's course of study. At City Hospital, she worked with a physician who was interested in photography. He made lantern slides of the students' daily life at City Hospital School of Nursing. Gray would take the slides and a portable stereopticon and present the program to groups of young women.

Gray was secretary to the State Board of Nurse Examiners from 1919 to 1920. She also served during that time as chair of the Committee on Classification of the National League of Nursing Education. This committee's work led to the formation of the Committee on the Grading of Nursing Schools.

From 1920 to 1921 she was assistant secretary of the Committee of the Rockefeller Foundation for the Study of Nursing Education. The "Goldmark Report," *Nursing and Nursing Education in the United States*, was published by that committee. Gray was involved with some of the field work studying the schools of nursing.

Gray was appointed the first Dean of Western Reserve University School of Nursing (Cleveland) in 1923. Prior to that, she had been employed as associate professor of nursing education in the College for Women at Western Reserve in preparation for the establishment of the School of Nursing.

After leaving Western Reserve, she served as a consultant and gave lectures and courses on nursing education throughout the country. One course, offered at Teachers College, Columbia University, was specifically oriented to collegiate schools of nursing. She also taught at the College of St. Teresa in Winona, Minnesota, and the University of California, Berkeley. In addition to teaching and consulting work, other activities, such as chairing the National League of Nursing Education Committee for the Study of Nursing Education in Colleges and Universities, filled most of her time until her retirement in 1933.

Gray had always been active in the National and New York State Leagues of Nursing Education. She had been president of the New York City and New York State leagues and a vice-president at the national level.

Gray's last full-time position involved her return to City Hospital in 1931. She was principal of the school and was charged with closing the program from which she had graduated. At this time she was in poor health, and when arrangements had been made to close the school, Gray retired.

Gray had moved to Florida in hopes of improving her health. She died in Miami on December 29, 1938.

In a 1922 interview in the *Cleveland Press*, Gray provided some personal data. She spoke of the demand for nurses, her desire for collegiate nursing programs, and the attraction of nursing in terms of dramatic interest and opportunities for great service. Her heroines were Florence Nightingale, Edith Cavell, and M. Adelaide Nutting, and her reading preferences were books on social and economic problems.

Gray's contributions to nursing were primarily those of an educator. She taught, was an innovative educational administrator, served professional organizations seeking to upgrade educational standards, and authored a classic textbook and many articles on nursing education.

Gray was, along with other noted nurses such as Annie Warburton Goodrich, Lillian D. Wald, and M. Adelaide Nutting, a member of the Committee of the Rockefeller Foundation for the Study of Nursing Education. The report of that group stimulated increased interest in university education for nurses. In Cleveland the "Goldmark Report," along with the success of the Vassar Training Camp for nurses during World War I, strengthened the commitment of Western Reserve University to develop a nursing program. With the financial backing of Frances Payne Bolton, the nursing program at Western Reserve was established with Gray as the first dean. Her work with curriculum development for the Vassar Training Camp, as well as previous work in nursing education, had prepared her well for this role. That program, now the Frances Payne Bolton School of Nursing at Case Western Reserve University, is still an acknowledged leader in the field of nursing education.

Gray was particularly concerned that nursing education not exploit students and that it be of high quality. She fought for an eight-hour day for students that included both the clinical and classroom requirements; many "eight-hour days" of the period were eight hours of clinical experience with additional time required for classroom participation. Her concern was not only with the student's health, but also the patient; she felt that overworked nurses were unable to provide quality care. In one of her articles ("Health, Hours, and Assignments," 1935) she suggested that "silent" roller skates or some form of motorized transportation be developed to eliminate fatigue in nurses.

Gray's coauthorship of Kimber's anatomy and physiology text made her name known to generations of nursing students. The text was considered a classic and had consistently good reviews through its many editions. Gray and her coauthors were careful to update the text with each edition, reflecting her belief that students need current scientific knowledge. Gray also had many articles pertaining to nursing education published. Topics included the aims of nursing education (1921), recruitment of students (1921), ideals of the profession and education (1922), the use of anatomical models (1922), the desirable mix of student and professional staff on maternity units (1928), comprehensive and honest school catalogues (1929), teaching anatomy and physiology (1933), and hours of student work and their impact on health (1935).

As one of the early and excellent pioneers in nursing education, Gray developed innovations and set standards for the education of professional nurses. Her active involvement in the profession helped to bring the education of nurses out of the apprenticeship orientation and into the educational mainstream.

PUBLICATIONS BY
CAROLYN E. GRAY

BOOKS

With Diana E. Clifford Kimber. *Anatomy and Physiology for Nurses.* New York: Macmillan, 1910, 3rd edition, Kimber revised through 1934, 8th edition.

With Diana E. Clifford Kimber and Carolyn E. Stackpole. *Textbook of Anatomy and Physiology.* New York: Macmillan, 1934, 9th edition, through 1938, 10th edition.

ARTICLES (SELECTED)

"A Campaign for Recruiting Nurses." *American Journal of Nursing* 21 (January 1921): 251–56.

"What Are the Aims of Nursing Education." *American Journal of Nursing* 21 (February 1921): 308–13.

"Gummed Paper Models." *American Journal of Nursing* 23 (October 1922): 20.

"The Ideals of the Nursing Profession for Schools of Nursing." *American Journal of Nursing* 23 (November 1922): 87–91.

"As Seen by an Observer." *American Journal of Nursing* 23 (March 1923): 238–39.

"Personnel for a Maternity Unit." *American Journal of Nursing* 28 (November 1928): 1103–04.

"School of Nursing Catalogues." *American Journal of Nursing* 29 (January 1929): 47–53.

"Teaching Anatomy and Physiology Effectively." *American Journal of Nursing* 33 (September 1933): 1075–83.

"Health, Hours, and Assignments." *American Journal of Nursing* 35 (June 1935): 529–37.

"A Nursing Service for Nurses." *American Journal of Nursing* 35 (November 1935): 1017–21.

BIBLIOGRAPHY

"Carolyn E. Gray." News article. Case Western Reserve University Archives. 1922. Photocopy.

"Carolyn E. Gray." Obituary. *American Journal of Nursing* 39 (February 1939): 217–18.

"Carolyn E. Gray." Obituary. Case Western Reserve University Archives. 1938. Photocopy.

Friedman, A.H. "Gray, Carolyn Elizabeth." In *Dictionary of American Nursing Biography.* M. Kauffman, ed., Westport, Conn.: Greenwood, 1988. Pp. 167–68.

Gillett, H. *Carolyn E. Gray.* Biographical sketch. Copyright National League for Nursing Education. Special Collection, Milbank Memorial Library, Teacher's College, Columbia University, New York. Photocopy.

Goodnow, M. *Nursing History,* 9th ed. Philadelphia: Saunders, 1953. Pp. 215–16.

Roberts, M. *American Nursing and Interpretation.* New York: Macmillan, 1959. Pp. 215–18.

"Who's Who in the Nursing World." *American Journal of Nursing* 23 (September 1923): 1022.

Leslie M. Thom

Katharine Greenough
1920–1975

An active organizational woman, Katharine Greenough served in an administrative capacity in two state nurses' associations and as president of the American Nurses' Foundation. At the time of her death she was director of the American Journal of Nursing Company's Educational Services Division.

The oldest of three children and the only girl. Greenough was born in New York City, January 16, 1920, to James and Frances Hartwell Greenough. Her father was a distinguished surgeon whose family was from Boston. Her brothers were James, who became a chemist, and Robert, an engineer.

When Greenough was a small child, the family moved to Cooperstown, New York, after her father accepted a position as chief of staff of the Mary Imogene Hospital. The family lived on a 23-acre farm on the outskirts of town. She was about 13 years old when she was sent to Boston to live with her Grandmother Greenough to attend high school.

Greenough enrolled in Radcliffe College, majoring in political science, and was graduated in 1941. She wanted to enroll in medical school, but at that time it was difficult for women to get into medical school, and her father discouraged her. A long-time friend, Jane Roe, believes that he may have felt that she would be taking the place of a man, a frequently stated argument of the time. She enrolled in the Columbia Presbyterian School of Nursing in New York City, where she was an excellent, competent, and innovative nurse, not very studious, but very serious about the patients.

Upon completion of the nursing program in 1944, she was appointed a head nurse at the Presbyterian Hospital in New York. After two years she left for six months in Minneapolis as a polio nurse, then from 1947–49 was an operating-room nurse at St. Luke's Hospital in Bethlehem, Pennsylvania. It was here that she met Barbara Schutt, who recruited her for the position of assistant executive secretary of the Pennsylvania Nurses' Association.

Schutt and Greenough worked very closely over the next several years, traveling throughout the state, helping organize local units for collective bargaining. She claimed that she and Schutt invented the structure of the local units to facilitate collective bargaining by nurses. During this time, she developed her understanding of and expertise in the economic and general welfare program of the American Nurses' Association (ANA). She considered her involvement in these early years of nurses' activity in labor relations as exciting ones. But she and Schutt were subjected to abuse and derogation; they were called "Reds" and "Commies" by their own colleagues and were not always welcome in many communities.

Much of what she learned in Pennsylvania she used when she served as executive secretary of the Texas (Graduate) Nurses' Association from 1957–63. These were difficult years for her, largely because of opposition by hospital administrators and by nurses to the economic and general welfare program.

Greenough left Texas to enroll in the graduate program at the University of California, San Francisco, completing her master's degree in 1965. Following graduation, she continued study as a postmaster's student and then was admitted as one of the first five students in the new doctor of nursing science program at the University of California, San Francisco.

While enrolled in the doctoral program, Greenough supported herself by working in a number of short-term nursing posi-

tions. During the summer of 1966 she was employed by the California Nurses' Association during a series of strikes by nurses in the state. She worked primarily with the nurses at San Francisco General Hospital; she also worked with the 3,300 nurses in the Bay area united in action for better working conditions.

She later served as a lecturer at the University of California at San Francisco School of Nursing, as a nurse specialist in coronary care at the Veterans Administration Hospital, Fort Miley, California, as a research coordinator for Planned Parenthood of California, and as research coordinator, San Francisco Pre-Hospital Coronary Care Project, San Francisco Heart Association.

The Coronary Care Project matched her clinical interest in patients who had suffered myocardial infarction. At this time innovations in the treatment of these patients, including the creation of coronary care units and more emphasis on rehabilitation, increased the number of recoveries. The Pre-Hospital Coronary Care Project investigated the efficiency of the response of ambulance services to calls of patients with myocardial infarction, to establish a corollary between rapidity of response and positive outcome. The study resulted in improved ambulance service and eventual installation of a 911 system, then just being explored in various parts of the country. Greenough had planned to use the data collected as a basis for her doctoral dissertation, which she was working on at the time of her death.

In 1971 she was invited to serve as a consultant to a special committee of the International Council of Nurses (ICN) to develop a proposal for a change in structure of the organization. She spent several months in Geneva on this project. The next year she served as staff to the committee, chaired by Hildegarde Peplau, when its report was presented at the ICN Congress in Mexico City.

Greenough was reluctant to leave San Francisco, where she shared a house with her good friend Maura Carroll, but she felt that the next opportunity afforded her was too good to turn down. She was appointed director of the Educational Services Division of the American Journal of Nursing Company in 1973. Her responsibilities included the development of new educational materials, particularly those designed for the continuing education of practicing nurses.

During much of her career the time and energy that Greenough devoted to the ANA were exemplary. She served on its board of directors from 1962–70 and on various committees, including the Nominating Committee. As a member of the Finance Committee, she agonized over the desperate financial crisis of the organization in 1969. She served on the committee that designed and named the Congress on Nursing Practice and was instrumental in its establishment. She fought for the creation of the American Academy of Nursing and served on the committee to draft criteria for membership in the academy. She served as president of the American Nurses' Foundation (1970–72) and on its board of trustees, assignments she relished because of the foundation's tie to research.

Greenough became ill in December 1974, with vague symptoms; by March she was severely ill and was then diagnosed as having acute leukemia. She was treated with chemotherapy and had a short period of remission. She died at St. Luke's Hospital in New York, September 5, 1975.

Greenough is remembered as a very serious person when promoting her ideas. An intelligent person who relished a good argument, she could make fun of herself when she realized the argument had gone on too long.

Her special interest and skill was in organizational management, but during her years of study this was not considered a particularly respectable area for nurses to pursue, so she specialized in clinical nursing research. In her organizational work Greenough has been described as someone who avoided the limelight but acted in the background to make things happen. Thus, her contributions to nursing may not be as well known as those of others. Nevertheless, her contributions were significant, and her untimely death was a serious loss to the profession.

PUBLICATIONS BY KATHARINE GREENOUGH

"Public Relations Program in Two States." *American Journal of Nursing* 51 (July 1951): 428.

"Membership Institute." *American Journal of Nursing* 52 (November 1952): 1339.

"Why Do They Join?" *American Journal of Nursing* 54 (July 1954): 816–18.

"Iatrogenic Cardiac Invalidism: Can the Coronary Care Unit Be Responsible?" *Journal of Rehabilitation* 34 (June 1968): 16–17.

"Determining Standards for Nursing Care." *American Journal of Nursing* 68 (October 1968): 2153–57.

BIBLIOGRAPHY

Carroll, M.C. Letter to the author, with biographical data on Katharine Greenough, February 28, 1990.

Greenough, K. "Curriculum Vita." New York: American Journal of Nursing Company, 1973.

"Katharine Greenough." In *Who's Who of American Women, 1961–1962*, 2nd ed. Chicago: Marquis, 1962.

"Kay Greenough Dies, Headed AJN Company Educational Services, Was Former TNA Executive Director." *American Journal of Nursing* 75 (October 1975): 1872.

Quinn, S. *ICN, Past and Present.* Harrow, Eng. Scutari, 1989. P. 191.

Roe, J.S.J. Letter to the author, June 6, 1990.

Zimmerman, A. Letter to the author, May 22, 1990.

Signe S. Cooper

Cordelia Adelaide Perrine Harvey

(1824–1895)

Although not directly educated as a nurse, Cordelia Adelaide Perrine Harvey performed as such in her role as a volunteer sanitary agent during the Civil War. Her generous acts led to her being called the "Wisconsin Angel" and the "Florence Nightingale of Wisconsin."

Born to John and Mary Hibbard Perrine on December 27, 1824, she first became a public figure when she married the honorable Louis Harvey of Madison, Wisconsin, on November 2, 1847. In 1862 Louis Harvey became the governor of Wisconsin and was an advocate of the Wisconsin military involved in the Civil War. Within 100 days of taking office, the governor went to visit the Wisconsin troops but never returned to his home state because on April 19, 1862, he drowned on his return trip.

Cordelia Harvey was extremely shaken by her husband's death. However, encouraged by a letter from him written two days prior to his death informing her of the good he accomplished by going to the camps, she channeled her energy into continuing the work her husband had started.

She contacted the Western Sanitary Commission and was appointed as a sanitary agent. Sanitary agents served as the governor's personal representative, visited and inspected hospitals and camps, reported the number of sick and wounded and arranged for transport home of disabled soldiers, distributed gifts and medical supplies and made available extra surgeons and nurses for the wounded.

Harvey's first assignment was in St. Louis, which was the site of active military operations. The job she undertook not only provided comfort to soldiers, but also took her mind away from her own sorrow. She inspected hospitals and camps, comforted the sick, and offered fruit and wine to Wisconsin soldiers. Following her assignment in St. Louis, Harvey moved to Cape Girardeau (Missouri), where she was appalled at the conditions for convalescing soldiers. She worked to procure furloughs for the wounded and discharges for the permanently disabled to get them away from "a place of death." During the spring of 1863 she moved to Vicksburg (Mississippi) and became very ill with miasma.

She returned to Wisconsin for convalescence, convincing her further of the need for northern convalescent hospitals. Her crusade for such facilities, however, was met with resistance from officials. Her belief was so strong that she arranged a meeting with President Lincoln to discuss the matter. Distant convalescent hospitals were not looked upon favorably by the federal government because it was believed that a hospital away from combat and close to home would further encourage desertion. In a personal account of her five appointments with President Lincoln and one with Secretary of War Edwin M. Stanton, Harvey described the various emotions and behaviors displayed by the President. In the end her perseverance and art of persuasion were successful. The President authorized the secretary of war to approve a convalescent hospital away from the front line named after Harvey's late husband.

Thus, came the establishment of the Harvey U.S. Army General Hospital, which was the former Farwell house, a three-story octagonal building on the edge of Lake Monona in Madison (Wisconsin). The establishment of this hospital led to the opening of two more army hospitals in Milwaukee and Prairie du Chien in 1864. After obtaining permission for the establishment of the Harvey U.S. Army General Hospital, Harvey returned to Memphis and arranged for over 100 men at Fort Pickering to move to the Harvey Hospital. As proof of her firm belief that northern convalescent hospitals were beneficial, of the original number of soldiers transferred, only seven died and five were discharged. The rest of the soldiers returned to active duty following convalescence.

Following the war, Harvey turned her energies to war-orphaned children. She again traveled to Washington to obtain the federal government's approval to convert Harvey Hospital to an orphan's home. Again her mission was successful, and she became its first superintendent. The home operated from 1866 to 1874, when most of the orphans reached their teens. The Soldiers Orphan's Home housed 200–300 children at a time.

The rest of Harvey's life is not as well documented as her activities during the Civil War. She married the Reverend Albert T. Chester of Buffalo, New York, on November 27, 1876. Cordelia Adelaide Perrine Harvey Chester died February 27, 1895, leaving many warm memories of her warm, sincere efforts toward ill soldiers during the Civil War.

PUBLICATIONS BY CORDELIA ADELAIDE PERRINE HARVEY

"A Wisconsin Woman's Picture of President Lincoln." *Wisconsin Magazine of History* 1: (March 1918): 233–55.

BIBLIOGRAPHY

Cooper, S.S. *Wisconsin's Nursing Pioneers.* Madison: Regents of the University of Wisconsin-Madison, 1968.

Current, R.N. *The History of Wisconsin II: The Civil War Era 1848–1873.* Madison: State Historical Society of Wisconsin, 1976.

Hurn, E.A. *Wisconsin Woman in the War Between the States.* Madison: Wisconsin History Commission, 1911. Pp. 118–33.

Quiner, E.B. *The Military History of Wisconsin: A Record of the Civil and Military Patriotism of the State in the War for the Union.* Chicago: Clark, 1866. P. 102.

Rogge, M.M. Nursing and Politics: A Forgotten Legacy. *Nursing Research* 36 (1987): 26–30.

Stimson, J., and E. Thompson. "Women Nurses with the Union Forces in the Civil War." *Military Surgeon* 62, (1928): 215.

Michaelene P. Mirr

Lulu K. Wolf Hassenplug

b. 1903

Educator and founder and dean of the School of Nursing at the University of California at Los Angeles, Hassenplug was an innovator in nursing education and influenced the advance of the nursing profession throughout the country.

Lulu K. Wolf Hassenplug was born in Milton, Pennsylvania, on October 3, 1903, the daughter of Fred Wilhelm and Hettie D. Armand (Wetzel) Wolf. She entered the Army School of Nursing, Washington, D.C., in 1921 against the wishes of her father, who thought her too talented for a career in nursing. She was paid a monthly salary of $30, enabling her to become financially independent of her family. An added benefit of the school was its location in Washington with its rich cultural life, especially the theater. Hassenplug had

wanted to become an actress, but her father opposed her aspirations. After receiving her diploma in 1924, Hassenplug taught nursing at the Piedmont Hospital in Atlanta and earned a B.S. from Teachers College, Columbia University in 1927. She had entered the field of nursing to discover if she liked it as a life career. Finding it challenging, she embarked on a life-long mission to revolutionize nursing education and to reform deficiencies in the profession.

Before becoming the first dean of the School of Nursing at the University of California at Los Angeles in 1948, Hassenplug served as the educational director at the Jewish Hospital in Philadelphia, an associate professor at the Medical College of Virginia in Richmond, and professor of nursing at Vanderbilt University in Nashville. She spent a year as a fellow with the Florence Nightingale International Foundation at the University of London and later as a Rockefeller fellow at Johns Hopkins University, where she received a master of public-health degree in 1947.

Hassenplug was persuaded to go to Los Angeles to design the UCLA school of nursing. When she arrived, the Department of Nursing was located in a basement next to the women's restroom. Her first goal was to establish a solid baccalaureate program within the university, and in 1954 UCLA presented its first baccalaureate graduating class in nursing. The program met the standards of other baccalaureate degrees of the university with an upper-division major in nursing, and the students were free to marry and live where they chose. A second goal was to institute a graduate program, and in 1952 the master of science degree was awarded to two nurses. In 1954 the school moved into a newly built Center for Health Sciences with eight faculty members.

Hassenplug was also active in state and regional organizations. She helped found the Western Council for Higher Education of Nurses and chaired a committee that instituted a program enabling nurses from 13 western states to share the latest developments in nursing practice. Through her work in national organizations, she was able to influence nursing education and working conditions for practicing nurses throughout the country.

In 1958 Hassenplug was chosen by the *Los Angeles Times* as Woman of the Year in Education. Other honors include the Mary Adelaide Nutting Award from the National League for Nursing and the Crystal Star from the National League for Nursing Board of Directors. She was the first to receive the Jessie M. Scott Award, the highest honor of the American Nurses' Association. She also received an award for distinguished service to the university at the UCLA Golden Anniversary, and a scholarship was established in her name at the School of Nursing. In 1979 the California Nurses' Association also established an award in her honor. She received two honorary doctor of science degrees from the University of New Mexico in 1964 and from Bucknell University in 1965.

A prolific author, Hassenplug published more than 60 articles on nursing and nursing education, and wrote two textbooks and coauthored another. She served as consultant to a number of universities in the United States and Canada, to the University of Cali in Columbia, South America, and to several governmental committees.

After 20 years as dean of the School of Nursing at UCLA, Hassenplug retired in 1968. She and her husband Harry, whom she had married in 1953, moved to Palm Desert, two hours outside Los Angeles. Since her husband's death in 1983, she spends much of her time swimming, traveling, keeping up on current affairs, and trying to stay out of the mainstream of nursing. In the fall of 1988 the UCLA School of Nursing started a two-year campaign to establish the Lulu Wolf Hassenplug Endowed Chair in honor of its founding dean.

PUBLICATIONS BY LULU K. WOLF HASSENPLUG

BOOKS

The Principles of Nursing Care. Philadelphia: Lippincott, 1937.

Nursing. New York: Appleton-Century, 1947.

With M.R. Smith et al. *A Study Guide Testbook in the Principles and Practices of Nursing.* New York: Macmillan, 1930.

ARTICLES (SELECTED)

"Time and Intelligence Study." *American Journal of Nursing* 28 (November 1928): 1105–07.

"A Laboratory in Clinical Experience." *American Journal of Nursing* 49 (December 1949): 799–800.

"The Expanding Role of the Nurse." *Oklahoma Nurse* 44 (November 1969): 1–5.

"This I Believe—About University Nursing Education." *Nursing Outlook* 18 (May 1970): 38–40.

"Discussion of 'Dimensions of Role Commitment: Career Patterns of Deans in Nursing.'" *Communicating Nursing Research* 4 (July 1971): 103–06.

"Discussion of 'Professional-Bureaucratic Conflict and Integrative Role Behavior.'" *Communicating Nursing Research* 4 (July 1971): 77–81.

"Nursing Can Move from Here to There." *Nursing Outlook* 25 (July 1977): 432–38.

"Unified Action—Nursing's Ticket to Viability and Visibility in the 1980s." *Journal of the New York State Nurses Association* 8 (December 1977): 7–14.

"Resocializating the Nursing Role Commitment." NLN Publication 52-1675 (1977): 1–5.

"2001 is Here!" NLN Publication 52-1724 (1978): 1–5.

With M.O. Wolaning, V. Stone et al. "Personal Perspectives on Aging and Nursing." *Journal of Gerontologic Nursing* 8 (January 1982): 23–29.

BIBLIOGRAPHY

Alperin, S.H. "What They're Saying." *Nursing World* 133 (1959): 10, 32.

Barnum, B.J. "Reminiscences by Lulu Wolf Hassenplug." *Nursing and Health Care* 11 (March 1990): 150–52.

Chaisson, G.M. "70+ and Going Strong. Roleless in Retirement—Not Lulu." *Geriatric Nursing* 3 (January/February 1982): 61–62.

Goss, T.C. "From Unpaid Workers to Respected Scholars: Reminiscences of Lulu Wolf Hassenplug." *Nursing Outlook* 38 (May/June 1990): 125–28.

Gregory, L. "Lulu Wolf Hassenplug." *UCLA Nursing* 5 (1988): 4–7.

Hassenplug, L.W. Correspondence. Nutting Collection, Columbia University, New York.

Hassenplug, L.W. Papers. Nursing Archives, Mugar Memorial Library, Boston University.

Kalisch, P., and B. Kalisch. *The Advance of American Nursing.* Boston: Little, Brown, 1978.

Safier, G. *Contemporary American Leaders in Nursing. An Oral History.* New York: McGraw-Hill, 1977.

Who's Who of American Women. Chicago: Marquis, 1970–1971, 1974–1975.

Women in Public Office. Center for the American Woman and Politics. New York: Bowker, 1976.

Lilli Sentz

Wilma Scott Heide

1921–1985

Thinking the thinkable was a philosophy strongly held by Wilma Scott Heide as she approached a multiple professional life—a life as a nurse, sociologist, writer, and lecturer. She was a self-described feminist, a recognized humanist, a political activist, and a scholar. She served two terms as president of the National Organization for Women (NOW) and encouraged the American Nurses' Association (ANA) to become politically involved, resulting in the formation of Nurses Now.

Heide was born on February 26, 1921, in Ferndale, Pennsylvania. She was the third child of four born to Ada and William Scott. At the time of her birth her father was a brakeman for the Baltimore and Ohio Railroad and her mother was a homemaker. In 1932 the family moved to Connellsville, Pennsylvania, where Heide lived until graduating from high school with honors in 1938. The family had been unable to send the two older children to college, and, in spite of a partial scholarship, the family felt it unfair to allow Wilma to attend college. The result was a job as a sales person in a department store, and during this period she played semiprofessional basketball. In 1940 she became an attendant at the state mental hospital in Torrence, which led to her entering nursing school in 1942 at the Brooklyn State Hospital in Brooklyn, New

York, where she was accepted as a cadet nurse, graduating with a diploma in 1945.

Heide received a bachelors degree in sociology in 1950 from University of Pittsburgh and, while continuing with graduate work, met and married Eugene Heide in 1951. Her husband was involved in higher education administration. The Heides had two daughters: Terry Lynn born in 1956 and Tamara Lee born in 1959. In 1955 Heide received a master's degree in sociology and nursing from the University of Pittsburgh. She was accepted for doctoral studies in 1970; however, the demands of her involvement in NOW postponed studies until 1975, when she entered the Union Graduate School and received a Ph.D. in psychology with the writing of the thesis "Feminism for the Health of It: A Covenant with Truth."

Heide held many positions in nursing, education, and the women's movement during her life. She lectured throughout the United States and wrote prolifically for newspapers, magazines, and journals in the United States and England. Following the completion of nursing school, she returned to work at Torrence State Hospital as a staff nurse for three years, and at this time her awareness of socioeconomic ills became heightened. She continued her education and chose sociology as the field that would assist her to the understandings for impacting change.

During the years 1947–49 Heide held a variety of positions in nursing; employed as a nurse at Pennsylvania College for Women, taught health education in Oswego, New York, became a school nurse, and was the educational director at the School of Nursing of the Orangeburg Regional Hospital in South Carolina. During this period she became a wife and mother, received bachelor and master degrees, and was active in community activities, such as YWCA, Girl Scouting, PTA, the civil rights movement, and the federal antipoverty program. Heide's journalistic career also began in the 1960s as a direct result of her involvement with the civil rights movement. She wrote a series of articles in 1964 for two Pennsylvania newspapers concerning the effects of civil rights on the lives of black people and in 1965 wrote a 12-part series called "Poverty is Expensive." During her involvement in civil rights and poverty issues she became aware of the injustices of women under the patriarchal system. Her fervent interest in the women's movement culminated in her becoming the national president of NOW. She was appointed to the Pennsylvania State Human Relations Commission and, as the only woman on the commission, spent a great deal of energy and time educating the commission on issues of sexism. Heide also served on the American Civil Liberties Union and on the editorial board of *Social Policy Magazine*.

A *New York Post* article on Heide, dated September 30, 1971, stated that Eugene Heide introduced his wife to NOW in 1967: "He was reading the paper one day and came across an article about NOW. In what has to be the gross understatement of the year, he said, 'Wilma, I think you might find this interesting.'" Heide immediately became involved by organizing a local chapter of NOW, becoming the Pennsylvania coordinator, and serving on the national board of NOW. In February 1968 she became the national membership coordinator, and in 1970 she was elected to chair NOW's national board. During this time she continued her involvement with civil rights and the Human Relations Commission. The amount of time and energy centered on the women's movement, NOW, and political activity placed a strain on her family life, and in 1972 she and Eugene Heide were divorced.

In 1971 Heide had become president of NOW, a position she held for two terms until the spring of 1974. During her presidency NOW made tremendous growth. It became the largest feminist organization in the world with a membership in 1974 of 50,000 and a budget of over $750,000. Heide was involved in every facet of women's discrimination, taking on multinational corporations, such as AT&T, major national newspapers, and broadcast media. Issues that she directed her attention to were passage of the Equal Rights Amendment (ERA), segregation of job advertisements in newspapers, sexist language, equal pay for women in all fields, sexism and religion, health care for women, child care, poverty, illiteracy, racism, and the strengthening of the international women's movements.

The ANA did not support the ERA when Heide became president of NOW. The objection was based in part on the issue of giving up "protective legislation" for women. Heide was able to assist the ANA to change its position and support the ERA in 1971. She also worked with the ANA to encourage the organization to assume active political stands on the issue of sexism in nursing and health care. She believed a direct result of her discussions led the ANA in May 1974 to form the political arm, Nurses' Coalition for Action in Politics (N-CAP). She carried the same persuasive activities to other organizations, such as the American Federation of Labor-Congress of Industrial Organizations (AFL-CIO), the Leadership Conference on Civil Rights, and other national organizations.

In her tenure as president of NOW, Heide was enormously successful in persuading national organizations to support the ERA and in impressing legislators and large companies that sexism held a negative impact on the daily life of all citizens in the United States. She traveled extensively, gave innumerable speeches, and presented testimony before legislators. Her approach included negotiating, direct action, fact finding, court action, and education. Heide's commitment to feminism, however, went beyond passage of the ERA and the passage of legislation to a moral and ethical stand that can be elicited in her later writings and teaching.

During the years between 1974 and 1980 Heide explored other ways to carry out her goals for women. Her connections with NOW decreased, but not her activities for the passage of the ERA and other women's issues. Her new activities included involvement with peace-making, and to this end she attended and spoke at conferences throughout the world. Her focus in the early 1980s was so directed. She saw that both the issues of peace and feminism were congruent and that the patriarchal political structure was much in need of the visions and values of feminism to maintain world peace. During this period she continued her teaching career.

In spite of the multitude of interests that took Heide from nursing to feminism and to the blending of feminism and peace activities, she really never left nursing. "Like nursing, feminism deals with human development and nurturing." Throughout her life Heide envisioned profound societal and universal changes as a consequence of feminism. She advocated a feminist synthesis of feminine strength and masculine values, resulting in "the power of love in the sense of caring about ourselves and others [can] begin and continue to exceed the love of power over others."

Heide died on May 8, 1985. She was driving home from a visit with her daughters and friends in Boston and Connecticut, and while on the Pennsylvania Turnpike, she experienced chest pain. She was taken to a hospital, where she died. Her body was cremated, and a commemoration and celebration was held for her in the Chapel of Reconciliation at the University of Pennsylvania in Philadelphia.

PUBLICATIONS BY WILMA SCOTT HEIDE

BOOKS

Feminism for the Health of It. Buffalo: Margaretdaughers, 1985.

CHAPTERS IN BOOKS

"Feminism, RX for Health Nursing." In *American Nurses' Association Clinical Sessions.* New York: Appleton-Century-Crofts, 1975.

"Introduction." In *Hospitals, Paternalism and the Role of the Nurse.* J.A. Ashley. New York: Teachers College Press, 1976.

"Feminism: Making a Difference in Our Health. In *The Woman Patient.* Vol. I. M. Notman and C. Nadelson, eds. New York: Plenum, 1979.

"The Quest for Our Humanity via Higher Education." In *Learning Tomorrows, Commentaries on the Future of Education.* Peter H. Wagschal, ed. New York: Praeger, 1979.

"Feminist Activism in Nursing and Health Care." In *Socialization, Sexism and Stereotyping.* J. Muff, ed. St. Louis: Mosby, 1981.

ARTICLES

"Poverty is Expensive." 12-part series. *Valley Daily News, New Kensington Daily Dispatch,* and other area newspapers, April 1965.

"Women's Liberation Means Putting Nurses and Nursing in Its Place." *Imprint* 18 (May/June 1971): 4–5, 16.

"The New Feminism and the Health Profession." *Sociological Abstracts* (August 1972).

"Nursing and Women's Liberation—A Parallel." *American Journal of Nursing* 73 (May 1973): 824–26.

"Feminism and the 'Fallen Woman.'" *Criminal Justice and Behavior* 1 (December 1974): 369–73.

"Why Don't We? A Womanifesto for Change." *MS.* (June 1976): 88–89.

"Scholarship/Action in the Human Interest." *Signs* 5 (Autumn 1979).

BIBLIOGRAPHY

Archives. Collection #83-M133, Box 1, Files 10–11. Schlensinger Library, Cambridge, Mass.

Haney, E.H. *A Feminist Legacy: The Ethics of Wilma Scott Heide and Company.* Buffalo: Margaretdaughters, 1985.

Jean Marie Symonds

Virginia Henderson

b. 1897

Virginia Henderson has been called "the first lady of nursing" and "the first truly international nurse." She has been compared to Clara Barton, Florence Nightingale, and Annie Goodrich. Her nursing career has spanned almost 70 years, during which she nursed in hospitals, homes, and clinics; she has taught clinical nursing and nursing research and performed laboratory and field-based studies. Her published work on nursing principles have been translated into 25 languages, and she oversaw the creation of the first and only annotated index of nursing research for English-language speakers.

Henderson was born on November 30, 1897, in Kansas City, Missouri, the fifth of eight children of Lucy Minor Abbot and Daniel Brosius Henderson, an attorney whose practice was focused on the rights of Native Americans. Henderson's paternal grandfather, Charles Henderson, was an industrialist in Hancock, Maryland.

Her maternal grandfather, William Richardson Abbot, a classics scholar, was principal of Bellevue (Va.) High School from 1870 until the school closed in 1910. Before her fourth birthday, Henderson and her family returned to Bedford County, in northern Virginia, the state for which young Virginia had been named. She resided there until adulthood in two homes—first in Bellevue and later in Trivium.

Henderson's education centered in the home. She studied with her aunts and later with her older sister Jane, a Sweet Briar College graduate. As a teenager, Henderson attended classes taught by her uncle, Charles Abbot, at a school that he ran for neighborhood boys.

In a desire to assist the World War I effort, Henderson applied to Annie Warburton Goodrich for acceptance in the Army School of Nursing, Washington, D.C., where she began three years of study in the autumn of 1918. Nursing courses were taught by distinguished nurse educators attracted to the Army School by Goodrich. Related medical and some biological science courses were taught by physicians. Theory of public health was taught at Teachers College, Columbia University, in New York City.

Following a four-month preliminary course of classroom work, Henderson had a schedule of student rotations at various hospitals, including Columbia Hospital (Washington, D.C.), Boston Floating Hospital for Children, Bloomingdale psychiatric hospital (White Plains, N.Y.), and in the Hell's Kitchen neighborhood of New York City, through an affiliation with the Henry Street Visiting Nurse Association (HSVNA). In these settings she developed a keen interest and skill in treating communicable diseases.

Henderson passed the New York State Board examination by waiver and was licensed to practice nursing in the spring of 1921. Following licensure, she joined the HSVNA to nurse the poor in the Bronx borough of New York City. At Goodrich's request, she left HSVNA after six months to direct a summer camp for 30 underprivileged city children. Upon completion of this task and recuperation from ex-

haustion, Henderson took the Virginia State Nursing Board examination, which she passed with high scores. Her next position was with the Visiting Nurse Association of Washington, D.C.

The love of teaching that characterized her family for generations soon became apparent in Henderson. In 1924 she accepted a position at Norfolk Protestant Hospital School as the first full-time nursing instructor in Virginia. In order to implement the 1917 standard curriculum developed by the National League of Nursing Education (now the National League for Nursing—NLN), Henderson restricted entry to the school to twice a year in contrast to the rolling admission policy in place at that time.

During her five years at the school she replaced a number of physician instructors and taught anatomy, physiology, and pharmacology herself. She gradually enlisted teaching assistance from nursing supervisors in obstetrics/gynecology and surgery and from nonnurse experts in bacteriology and chemistry from both the hospital and the community. Henderson initiated an on-site nursing library (stocked largely with donated materials from publishers and with government documents) and a nursing laboratory (with donations from manufacturers). Concerned for the quality of life of her students, she designed recreation programs for them, including the building of a hospital tennis court.

During this period Henderson's involvement with the Virginia State Nursing Association included chairing the Education Section and exposing practicing nurses to much of the same educational material that she used in the classroom. Her own continuing education occurred during the summers when she studied at Teachers College.

Thinking that she needed a stronger science background, Henderson left Norfolk Protestant Hospital School in 1929 and entered Teachers College. She carried the maximum load of 32 "units," which included chemistry, physics, anatomy, physiology, and bacteriology, as well as English literature, history, and statistics. She was deeply influenced by the educational theory and methods of Edward Thorndike and the nursing leadership of Isabel Stewart. Although she worked part time as a live-in private-duty nurse, financial limitations forced her back into full-time practice after one year of advanced schooling.

In 1930 Strong Memorial Hospital (Rochester, N.Y.) employed Henderson as the teaching supervisor of its Outpatient Department. In this capacity she attended interdisciplinary community health meetings. At these meetings she met representatives from all the health-related disciplines in the area. These meetings became for her a model for the promotion of community health care, which she continues to advocate strongly after more than 60 years of practice and teaching.

In 1931 the Rockefeller Foundation awarded Henderson a fellowship to complete her post-basic program at Teachers College. To supplement these funds, she also undertook an instructorship at the college, working with several faculty members. She took courses at Columbia University Medical School and Postgraduate Hospital and completed a B.S. in 1932 and an M.A. in 1934—both degrees in nursing education. Henderson's master's thesis on medical and surgical asepsis involved (1) an animal experiment to determine whether steam under pressure was more efficacious than boiling in eliminating pathogens from surgical instruments and (2) a review of state sanitary codes.

After graduation, Henderson remained on the college's faculty as instructor and associate professor of nursing education from 1934–48. She taught research and medical-surgical nursing. She initiated nursing clinics during which patients would critique the nursing care that they had been given. During this period she also undertook her first revision of the late Bertha Harmer's *Textbook of the Principles and Practice of Nursing*.

Henderson left Teachers College in 1948. She spent the following five years in New York City working on the fifth edition of the Harmer text, in the process making it "my text." It was published in 1955 as *Principles and Practice of Nursing*. Culling and condensing the central principles

of this text, she—with the International Council of Nurses—published *Basic Principles of Nursing* in 1960, which is now translated into 25 languages.

During this intensive writing period, Henderson was approached by Leo Simmons, a sociologist from Yale University, to assist with a survey and assessment of nursing research. Upon completion of her own text, Henderson in 1953 moved to New Haven as research associate to the new project, first funded at the Yale School of Nursing (YSN) under Dean Elizabeth T. Bixler by the Nursing Division of the U.S. Public Health Service (USPHS). Impetus for the project came from a study after World War II by the Nursing Service Committee, chaired by Marion Sheahan and composed of nurses and others. The committee confirmed the absence not only of an index of nursing literature, but also the absence of nursing literature from most libraries.

A USPHS grant funded the project, which permitted Henderson to embark on extended fieldwork throughout the United States. She visited the deans of nursing and medical schools, practicing nurses, nursing students, and others regarding (1) research that they had undertaken as nurses or (2) that they knew about, as well as (3) what research they might undertake if adequate resources were available. The survey documented that most research examined the nurse as a worker or how such workers should be educated rather than outcomes of nursing care. Clinically focused research was rare.

Henderson also read available nursing-related holdings of libraries on the East Coast of the United States. She abstracted all doctoral dissertations written by nurses from the 1930s to the end of the 1950s. These numbered fewer than 200 and primarily involved education-related and social-research questions.

With the assistance of Dean Florence Wald at YSN, Henderson was funded as the director of the Nursing Studies Index Project from 1959–71. She set up an advisory board of publishers, librarians, scholars, and clinicians, who substantiated the inadequacy of existing library resources for nursing; established regional bodies for information gathering; and recommended a national or international nursing index. Building on her extensive file of annotations, the publishing company J.B. Lippincott (with the backing of the American Nursing Foundation) published in 1963 the *Nursing Studies Index, 1957–1959*, an annotated guide to reported studies, research in progress, research methods, and historical materials related to nursing in periodicals, books, and pamphlets published in English. Retrospective indices to 1900 were subsequently published. (The advisory committee that Henderson originally established for the project survives today as the Inter-Agency Council on Library Resources for Nursing, with interdisciplinary representation from 20 agencies.)

Following the completion of the project, Henderson was named Research Associate Emeritus of YSN and embarked—at 75 years of age—on an international schedule of speaking and teaching in North America, Scandinavia, the British Isles, Europe, the Middle East, the Orient, and Australia. She continued to advocate comprehensive, universal, tax-supported health care for all United States citizens and ardently defended the consumer movement. She has spoken widely on the need to interest men in nursing careers, the obligation of the health-care system to open the health record to the patient, and the inherent overlap of medical and nursing care and tasks.

Henderson has received honorary degrees from the University of Western Ontario (doctor of laws, 1970), the University of Rochester (doctor of science, 1972), Rush University (doctor of science, 1975), Pace University (doctor of humane letters, 1979), Catholic University (doctor of science, 1980), Yale University (doctor of science, 1982), Old Dominion University and Boston College (doctor of science, 1983), Thomas Jefferson University (doctor of letters, 1985), Emory University (doctor of science, 1985), St. Joseph's College (doctor of science, 1986), the University of North Carolina (doctor of science, 1988), and the l'Escola d'Infermeria de la Universtat de Barcelona (1988).

She holds honorary memberships or fellowships in the YSN Nursing Alumnae Association (1973), the Registered Nurse Association of Ontario (1975), the American Academy of Nursing (1977), the Association of Integrated and Degree Courses in Nursing and the Irish Nurses' Organization (1977), the Royal College of Nursing (London, 1978), Sigma Theta Tau, Vanderbilt University (1979), the Japanese Nursing Association (1985), and the Norwegian Nurses Association (1987). She was also named Vice–President for Life of the Royal College of Nursing, London (1987).

Prizes awarded to Henderson include the award for "distinguished and exemplary service, nursing leadership and social consciousness in furthering the worthy cause of nursing and health care" (American Nurses' Association, 1974), the Presidential Bicentennial Award (Boston College School of Nursing, 1976), the Mary Adelaide Nutting Award (National League for Nursing, 1977), the Annie W. Goodrich Teaching Award (YSN student body, 1981), the Christianne Reimann Prize (International Council of Nurses, 1985), the Merit Award (National Association of Nurses of Columbia, South America, 1985), and the Excellence in Education Award (now the Virginia Henderson Award, National Association for Home Care, 1985).

PUBLICATION BY VIRGINIA HENDERSON

BOOKS AND PAMPHLETS

Textbook of the Principles and Practice of Nursing, 4th ed. New York: Macmillan, 1945.

Principles and Practice of Nursing. New York: Macmillan, 5th ed., 1955; 6th ed., 1978.

International Council of Nursing (ICN) Basic Principles of Nursing Care. Geneva: ICN, 1960; rev., 1969.

Nursing Studies Index. Philadelphia: Lippincott, Vol. IV, (1957–59), 1963; Vol. III (1950–56), 1966; Vol. II (1930–49), 1970; Vol. I (1900–29), 1972.

Nursing Research: A Survey and Assessment. New York: Appleton-Century-Crofts, 1964.

The Nature of Nursing. New York: Macmillan, 1966.

Being Informed: Nursing Resources for the Information Age. No. 15–1974. New York: National League for Nursing, 1985.

ARTICLES (SELECTED)

"Oxygen Therapy: A Study of Some Aspects of the Operation of an Oxygen Tent." *American Journal of Nursing* 38 (1938): 1203–16.

"Medical and Surgical Asepsis: The Development of Asepsis and a Study of Current Practice with Recommendations in Relation to Certain Aseptic Nursing Methods in Hospitals." *Nursing Education Bulletin* (June 1939).

"Annie Warburton Goodrich." *American Journal of Nursing* 55 (1955): 1488–92.

"Research in Nursing—When?" *Nursing Research* 4 (February 1956): 99.

"A Survey and Assessment of Research in Nursing." In *The Yearbook of Modern Nursing—1956.* New York: Putnam, 1957.

"The Nature of Nursing." *American Journal of Nursing* 64 (August 1964): 62.

"Some Comments for Nurses Today." *Alumnae Magazine of Columbia University-Presbyterian Hospital School of Nursing* 63 (Spring 1968): 5–15.

"Library Resources in Nursing—Their Development and Use." *International Nursing Review* 15 (1968): 164, 236, 348.

"Library Activities in Regional Medical Programs." *Bulletin of the Medical Library Association* 59 (January 1971): 53–64.

"Health Is Everybody's Business." *Canadian Nurse* 67 (March 1971): 31–34.

"On Nursing Care Plans and Their History." *Nursing Outlook* 21 (June 1973): 378–89.

"Annie Warburton Goodrich." *Dictionary of American Biography, Suppl 5, 1951–55.* New York: Scribner, 1977.

"Awareness of Library Resources: A Characteristic of Professional Workers." In *Reference Resources for Research and Continuing Education.* Kansas City, Mo.: American Nurses' Association, 1977.

"The Concept of Nursing." *Journal of Advanced Nursing* 3 (March 1978): 113–30.

"Professional Writing." *Nursing Mirror* 146 (May 1978): 15–18.

"Preserving the Essence of Nursing in a Technological Age." *Nursing Times* 75 (November 1979): 2012–23, 2056–68.

"Nursing—Yesterday and Tomorrow." *Nursing Times* 76 (May 1980): 905–07.

"The Nursing Process—Is the Title Right?" *Journal of Advanced Nursing* 7 (March 1982): 103–09.

"Ma conception des sions infirmiers—Un modele ouvert pour le developpement d'une judgment clinique." *Sions* 440 (October 1984): 9–16.

"Ma conception des sions infirmiers—Une conception variable selon les cultures." *Sions* 440 (October 1984): 35–40.

"The Essence of Nursing in High Technology." *Nursing Administration Quarterly* 9, No. 4 (1985): 1–9.

"Some Observations on Health Care by Health Services or Health Industries." Editorial. *Journal of Advanced Nursing* 11 (January 1986): 1–2.

"The Nursing Process—A Critique." *Holistic Nursing Practice* 1 (May 1987): 7–18.

BIBLIOGRAPHY

Halamandaris, V.J. "A Tribute to Virginia Henderson: The First Lady of Nursing." *Caring* 7 (1988): 56–65.

Henderson, V. Interviews with the author, July 22 and September 6, 1990.

Shamansky, S.L. "Community Health Nursing Revisited: A Conversation with Virginia Henderson." *Public Health Nursing* 1 (1985): 193–201.

Smith, J.P. *Virginia Henderson, The First Ninety Years.* Middlesex, U.K.: Scutari Press, 1989.

Judith C. Hays

Lenah Sutcliffe Higbee

1874–1941

The second superintendent of the U.S. Navy Nurse Corps, Lenah Higbee was the first woman to receive the Navy Cross while still living, and in 1944 the destroyer U.S.S. Higbee was named for her.

Lenah Agnes Wiseman Sutcliffe Higbee was born in Chatham, New Brunswick, Canada on May 18, 1874, the daughter of the Reverend Ingraham and Anna A. (Brent) Sutcliffe. She was educated at Mount Alison Seminary, Sackville, New Brunswick, and was an alumna of Hamilton College, Ontario where she received a degree of master of liberal arts, a two-year program. She also attended a special course in English literature and science at the University of Toronto. She graduated from the New York Post-Graduate Hospital School of Nursing in 1899 and shortly thereafter married Lieutenant Colonel

John Henley Higbee, United States Marine Corps.

After her husband's death in 1908, Higbee did postgraduate work at Fordham Hospital in New York City and was among the first twenty nurses, the "sacred twenty," to be selected for appointment to the Navy Nurse Corps in 1908. Following her appointment on October 1, 1908, she reported to the Naval Medical School Hospital in Washington, D.C., for four to six months of indoctrination and training. She served as chief nurse of the naval Hospital at Norfolk, Virginia, from 1909 until she was appointed superintendent of the Nurse Corps on January 20, 1911. She guided the development of the Nurse Corps throughout World War I, and on November 11, 1920, President Woodrow Wilson presented the Navy Cross to Higbee in recognition of her distinguished service in the line of her profession and devotion to duty. She was the first woman to receive the Navy Cross in her lifetime.

Higbee retired from the Nurse Corps on November 30, 1922, and moved to Winter Park, Florida, where she resided with her lifelong friends, Miss Isabel Strong and Dr. Lawrence W. Strong. She died suddenly on January 10, 1941, in the Orange General Hospital at the age of 66. Higbee is buried beside her husband at Arlington National Cemetery.

On November 13, 1944, the destroyer U.S.S. *Higbee* was launched by the Bath Iron Works in Maine. It was commissioned on January 27, 1945, and earned one battle star for service in World War II and seven battle stars for service in the Korean War.

PUBLICATIONS BY
LENAH SUTCLIFFE HIGBEE

"Nursing as It Related to War—the Navy". *American Journal of Nursing* 18 (August 1918): 1061–64.

"Work of the Navy Nurse Corps." In *Annual Report, 1919,* National League of Nursing Education, and *Proceedings of the 25th Convention.* Baltimore: Williams & Wilkins, 1919.

"Navy Nurse Corps." *Trained Nurse* 66 (March 1921): 221–24.

"Nursing in Government Services. Second Paper." *American Journal of Nursing* 22 (April 1922): 524–46.

"Nurse and Dietitian: A Team." *Hospital Management* 13 (May 1922): 65.

BIBLIOGRAPHY

Dunn, L.K. "A Special Race of Women: The Navy Nurse Corps, 1908–1935." Unpublished manuscript.

"Mrs. Higbee's Resignation." *American Journal of Nursing* 23 (January 1923): 293.

"The Navy Nurse Corps." *Pacific Coast Journal of Nursing* 19 (January 1923): 11–12.

"Navy Nurse Corps Honored." *Nursing Outlook* 2 (May 1954): 258.

"The New Navy Nurse Corps Superintendent." *American Journal of Nursing* 11 (May 1911): 474.

Obituary. *New York Times,* January 12, 1941, 46.

Roberts, M. M. *American Nursing: History and Interpretation.* New York: Macmillan, 1954.

Woman's Who's Who of America: A Biographical Dictionary of Contemporary Women of the United States and Canada, 1914–1915. New York: American Commonwealth, 1914.

Lilli Sentz

Jane Elizabeth Hitchcock
1863–1939

Jane Elizabeth Hitchcock pioneered in the field of public-health nursing practice and education. For over 20 years, she served at the Henry Street Settlement in New York City. She also taught public-health nursing and began special programs in public-health nursing. She became a leader and spokesperson for this area of specialization during its emerging period. Her long and varied career provides a valuable image of the opportunities open to nurses in her era.

She was born to Dr. Edward and Mary Lewis (Judson) Hitchcock. Her family traced its ancestry back to the early settlers of Massachusetts. She was educated in Massachusetts at Mt. Holyoke College and in New York at Cornell University as a special student (1885–88). She graduated in 1891 from the New York Hospital Training School for Nurses. She returned to Massachusetts and practiced as a head nurse in the Newton Hospital.

From 1896 to 1922 Hitchcock practiced and lived at the Henry Street Settlement in New York. She began as one of the first four practicing public-health nurses and was later promoted to the position of supervisor. During this period she began teaching public-health nursing at the Lincoln Hospital School of Nursing in New York. She also initiated the nursing service offered to policyholders of the Metropolitan Life Insurance Company.

Hitchcock served with the American Red Cross during a crucial period following World War I. She worked with the Placement Bureau, helping returning military nurses readjust to civilian life and assisting them in finding employment. She only left Henry Street once during her long tenure. For several weeks shortly after the turn of the century she served as a supervisor of visiting nurses during a severe outbreak of typhoid fever in Ithaca, New York.

As a leader during the early years of the Henry Street Settlement, Hitchcock delivered major speeches and wrote numerous articles in nursing periodicals about public-health nursing. Her primary effort throughout her career was devoted to the development and standardization of public-health nursing within education and practice. She worked very hard to encourage the inclusion of public-health nursing in all basic nursing curricula. She educated nursing students in this field throughout most of her career.

In addition, Hitchcock actively participated in the developments within the young nursing profession in New York. She served on the Board of Nurse Examiners from its beginning in 1903 to 1919 as secretary. She helped to write public-health nursing questions for the board's licensing exams. She also served as officer and active participant in the National Organization of Public Health Nursing and the New York Hospital Alumnae Organization.

At age 65 she retired from active nursing to Amherst, Massachusetts, and lived quietly until her death from pneumonia in North Hampton, Massachusetts, in 1939 at the age of 76.

PUBLICATIONS BY JANE ELIZABETH HITCHCOCK

"Standardizations of Public Health Nursing." *Visiting Nurse Quarterly* (April 1912): 8–13. This article was reprinted in *Public Health Nursing* 29 (February 1937): 35.

"How to Celebrate the Children's Year." *Bulletin of the National Organization for Public Health Nursing* No. 3 (May 1918): 12–13.

"Five Hundred Cases of Pneumonia." *American Journal of Nursing* 21 (December 1921): 894–95.

"How Many Public Health Nurses?" *Public Health Nursing* 33 (January 1941): 21.

BIBLIOGRAPHY

Brainard, A. *The Evolution of Public Health Nursing.* Philadelphia: Saunders, 1922.

Fitzpatrick, M. *The National Organization for Public Health Nursing, 1912–1952: Development of a Practice Field.* New York: National League for Nursing, 1975.

Obituary. *American Journal of Nursing* 39 (May 1939): 371.

Roberts, M. *American Nursing: History and Interpretation.* New York: Macmillan, 1954.

Linda Sabin

Myn M. Hoffman

1883–1951

Lieutenant Commander Myn M. Hoffman was the fourth superintendent of the U.S. Navy Nurse Corps, serving from 1935–38.

Hoffman was born in Bradford, Illinois, on May 12, 1883, and was graduated from the Illinois State Normal School. After teaching in Illinois public schools, she entered the St. Joseph's Hospital School of Nursing in Denver, Colorado, graduating March 4, 1915.

She practiced nursing for two years in Colorado and Illinois and then entered the Navy Nurse Corps in 1917 at Norfolk, Virginia. Promoted to the rank of chief nurse two years later, she served at various naval hospitals and at a hospital on St. Croix, Virgin Islands.

She became chief nurse of a Washington naval hospital in 1925. She was named assistant superintendent of the Nurse Corps in 1934 and in December of that year was promoted to superintendent. Disability forced her to retire in 1938.

She died at her retirement home in Bronxville, New York, on January 4, 1951, and was buried in the nurses' section of Arlington National Cemetery with full military honors.

BIBLIOGRAPHY

"Comdr. Hoffman Dies: Was Chief Navy Nurse." *Washington Star*, January 8, 1951.

"Comdr. Myn M. Hoffman." Obituary. *Times-Herald* (Washington) January 9, 1951.

"Miss Hoffman Retires." *Trained Nurse and Hospital Review* (November 1938): 437.

Pennock, M.R. ed. *Makers of Nursing History*. New York: Lakeside, 1940.

Alice P. Stein

Aileen I. Hogan

1899–1981

Aileen I. Hogan was a pioneer in nurse-midwifery and childbirth education in both the United States and Canada. She was the first executive secretary of the American College of Nurse-Midwives and developed its archives. For 15 years, she traveled throughout North America doing childbirth education for the Maternity Center Association.

Hogan was born in Ottawa, Ontario, on November 10, 1899, to James M. and Christina McMaster Hogan. Her parents were Catholics of Scottish and Irish descent, and she had two older brothers and one younger brother and sister. The clan had been in Canada for four or five generations, and Hogan's father was a farmer in the tradition of his family.

After graduating from high school at age 16, Hogan took a secretarial course and worked in the Canadian Federal War Department during World War I. During the influenza epidemic of 1917–18 both parents died. In 1920 Hogan and three other family members immigrated to New York City, where she found work as a medical secretary and attained U.S. citizenship.

In her late 30s Hogan decided to become a nurse and took the three-year program at Columbia Presbyterian Hospital School of Nursing in New York. During her training she rotated as a staff nurse in the various departments of the Sloane Hospital at the Presbyterian Medical Center. In 1942, after two years in this rotation, she was named head nurse in the labor and delivery service.

With the nation at war, she joined the Presbyterian Hospital Unit that sailed for Ireland in July 1942. The group served in Oxford, England, in 1943 and early 1944, went to France in July 1944, and returned to the United States the following year. In addition to her duties with the wounded and sick, Hogan gave informal guidance in parenting to soldier fathers.

After the war Hogan studied nursing at Teachers College, Columbia University, under the G.I. Bill, earning a B.S. in 1947 and an M.A. in 1948. Although she had planned to continue her education for her Ph.D. she accepted a position to chair the Maternity Nursing Department at Case Western Reserve University in Cleveland. In Ohio she also served on the Educational Advisory Committee of the state Department of Health.

She resigned in 1950 and in 1951 became a consultant with the Maternity Center Association (MCA) in New York. For the next 15 years, she set up parent-education programs in cooperation with nurses throughout North America. The programs covered the principles of midwifery and stressed the importance of family health, continuity of care, and a cooperative, team approach. In Canada the work was federally sponsored, and each province planned a program of one to three two-week workshops. In the United States each state arranged its own programs.

At the time she began working for the

MCA, nurse-midwives had been organized within the structure of the National Organization of Public Health Nursing. When this group dissolved, the nurse-midwives aligned themselves with the new National League for Nursing. At its first convention Hogan was elected chair of its Maternal Child Health (MCH) Interdivisional Council. However, the nurse-midwives soon decided to become independent. With the cooperation of the American Nurses' Association and the National League for Nursing, an organization committee established the American College of Nurse-Midwives (ACNM). Hogan held several offices in the college.

After retiring from the MCA in 1965, she moved to Santa Fe, New Mexico, to take part in ACNM work at the Catholic Maternity Institute there. The altitude proved unhealthful for her, and she returned to New York to become executive secretary of the college. In 1970 the ACNM archives were set up, and Hogan chaired the committee that administered them. In 1971 she assisted in organizing the worldwide convention of the International Congress of Midwives in Washington, D.C.

Hogan retired in 1974. She died of a cardiopulmonary disorder on January 7, 1981, at a home she shared with her surviving sister, Mrs. Frederick Peters, in Whiting, New Jersey.

PUBLICATIONS BY AILEEN I. HOGAN

"Bomb-Born Babies." *Public Health Nurse* 43 (July 1951): 383–85.

"The Premature Baby." *American Journal of Nursing* 54 (May 1954): 575–77.

"A Tribute to the Pioneers." *Journal of Nurse-Midwifery* (Summer 1975): 6–11.

BIBLIOGRAPHY

Tom, S.A. "Spokeswoman for Midwifery: Aileen Hogan." *Journal of Nurse-Midwifery* 26 (May/June 1981): 7–11.

Alice P. Stein

Lydia Holman
1868–1960

Lydia Holman was a pioneer of rural public-health nursing. She served the people of Mitchell County, North Carolina, for nearly 40 years, working with isolated families in mountainous, rugged country where she was the only health-care practitioner for over 20 years. Holman often found it was necessary to perform the duties of physician and dentist along with nursing. She was especially dedicated to improving the quality of maternal and child health and decreasing infant mortality. She began her work in northwestern North Carolina at Ledger. In 1911 she moved to Altapass, where she established a small hospital.

Holman, the daughter of Robert and Elizabeth Ann Holman, was born in Philadelphia, Pennsylvania, on January 5, 1868. She began her nursing career in 1894 as the charge nurse at a hospital for typhoid patients at Mt. Carbon, Pennsylvania. The following year she graduated from the Philadelphia General Hospital School of Nursing.

Holman worked for two years as a private-duty nurse in Pottsville, Pennsylvania, and is reported as having been the head nurse at the County Alms Hospital at Schulykill Haven, Pennsylvania, in 1897. Holman then moved to Lexington, Kentucky, where she was a nurse at the John Blair Hospital. During the Spanish-American War she worked in Macon, Georgia.

She then accepted a private-duty assignment to nurse a typhoid patient at Ledger, North Carolina. The patient, who was living at her summer home, was an educated woman of considerable means. Holman stayed and nursed her until May 1901.

The recovery of a typhoid patient Holman cared for privately so impressed the residents of Ledger that they began bringing their sick and injured to her for care. To those in this region typhoid usually resulted in death. News of the "healing" nurse spread quickly, and more cases showed up at her doorstep. Holman felt it was her duty to help care for those living in this rough and remote country. Holman found herself enjoying the rural life and was increasingly drawn to the lifestyle, traditions, and beliefs of the mountain people. Many of their health problems were related to the life of those in the region. Large families were often crowded into small cabins with little ventilation, as windows were sealed and chinks in cabin construction were tightly closed. The diet was inadequate, consisting mainly of "pork and pone." Conditions were often unclean; bathing was considered unhealthy. Holman described life in the North Carolina region as one of "terrible isolation, almost changeless lives, from birth to death." There was a high incidence of tuberculosis, typhoid, and pellagra. Infant mortality was high. Holman was especially concerned about the lack of obstetric care.

After completing her nursing assignment at Ledger in the spring of 1901, Holman returned to Philadelphia to better prepare herself to serve the people in rural North Carolina. In order to do so, she spent the next two years gaining additional experience in maternal and child nursing. During this time she worked among Philadelphia's poor and in New York City's Henry Street Settlement with Lillian Wald.

In July 1902 Lydia Holman returned to Ledger on salary to nurse her former typhoid patient. Holman's arrangement with her patient allowed her to care for residents who came to her needing nursing services. Soon she was devoting all of her time caring for those who sought her help.

Holman established the Mountain Visiting Nurse service at Ledger in 1902. Records indicate that she was the only nurse on staff. She accepted medical, surgical, obstetrical, contagious, and tuberculosis cases. There was no regular salary, and hours were described as irregular, "calls answered whenever received." Compensation for her services was determined on an individual basis. If patients were unable to afford standard charges, Holman asked people to pay what they could. Fees for obstetric cases ranged from $2 to $10. Some paid in crops or livestock, and others could not afford any payment for her nursing services. It was only with this small compensation that Holman supported herself and maintained a three-room cabin.

Mitchell County, where Holman worked, was a mountainous and remote area. Roads were poor, and during the winter months often impassable. Holman found that horseback was the best method of travel. Patient visits sometimes required her to ride up to 30 miles a day through difficult country. Holman answered calls whenever they came, day and night, good weather and bad. She would often return home from a full day of patient visits only to find someone at the cabin needing her to travel immediately to another case.

Long distances between visits made it necessary for Holman to include considerable health education for patients and their families. She often gave instruction in hygiene, dietetics, and treatment regimens. The family was then responsible for carrying out her orders between nursing visits. She made as many as 42 visits a month and handled a variety of problems from tooth extractions and skin conditions to surgical procedures, traumatic injuries, and obstetric cases.

Still, her primary concern for her district was obstetric cases. She was a trained midwife and attended several hundred deliveries during her career and handled many difficult births. She carefully tended new mothers after childbirth. Before Holman's arrival, area women frequently did not fully recover after childbirth. All too often birth resulted in death for the mother. It was generally believed that if a woman remained in bed for more than three days after giving birth, she would not survive.

Though Homan was a public-health nurse by training, she described herself as a "combination country doctor and visiting nurse." She attended acute illnesses and trauma cases brought to her. When confronted with difficult problems, she had only her own collection of medical books to consult. Though she felt her nursing education did not adequately prepare her for her work, she believed it was her duty to do what she could to help the mountain people.

Holman's life at Ledger was difficult. During her 10 years there, she lived alone, tending to her own housework along with caring for her horse. She traveled out of the area only for supplies. Holman solicited donations of clothes and supplies from friends in the Philadelphia area.

The work at Ledger grew to be overwhelming for one person. Holman made a trip to Baltimore to secure support from influential friends. She received assistance from organizations in Boston and Baltimore as well as from the alumnae of the Johns Hopkins' School of Nursing. Her successful pleas resulted in the creation of the Holman Association in 1911. An early report of the association described it as "an organization for the promotion of rural nursing, hygiene and social service." The Holman Association was incorporated in the state of Maryland with a nine-member board of directors, including Dr. William Welch. A large part of the association's support came from the Johns Hopkins University Medical School. Medical students spent time working with Lydia Holman, and the school also provided her with supplies.

The Carolina Clinchfield and Ohio Railroad gave the Holman Association land at Altapass, North Carolina, where Holman established a small infirmary—initially a one-room hut.

Although the Holman Association existed for only two years, it allowed Lydia Holman to expand her work and improve conditions in the region. After the association was dissolved, she continued to receive financial assistance, support, staff, and supplies from Baltimore and Boston, and by 1920 Lydia Holman had raised enough money to build a small hospital. The "Holman Committee" in Boston reported that the hospital recorded 1,800 visits during its first year of operation. By 1924, at age 56, Holman was working with another nurse and had the assistance of a housekeeper. Holman continued her work among the people of Mitchell County at Altapass until her retirement.

At Altapass Holman was involved in both nursing and social work. She held classes in housework, cooking, and sew-ing, conducted a kindergarten, and held parties for neighbors. She tended a garden, where she grew fresh vegetables to give to those who came by.

Holman received recognition from her colleagues for her accomplishments as a rural public-health nurse in Mitchell County. She was elected to the first board of directors of the National Organization of Public Health Nurses in 1912. At the English-Speaking Conference for Maternal-Infant Welfare held in London in 1924, Carolyn Conant Von Blarcom, an authority on obstetrical nursing, cited Lydia Holman as a special example of a public-health nurse who worked to improve the conditions surrounding motherhood. Von Blarcom credits Holman with "alleviating distress and averting disaster in Altapass, North Carolina."

Holman was elected to the Mitchell County Board of Health in 1936. She continued her nursing work until her retirement in the 1950s. Her efforts in the North Carolina mountains have been continued by state and federal agencies as well as the Red Cross.

She died on February 25, 1960, in the Veterans Administration Hospital at Oteen, North Carolina, after suffering a long illness.

PUBLICATIONS BY LYDIA HOLMAN

"Visiting Nursing in the Mountains of Western North Carolina." *American Journal of Nursing* 7 (August 1907): 831–37.

Reports of the Holman Association. Unpublished, 1911.

BIBLIOGRAPHY

Brainard, A.M. *The Evolution of Public Health Nursing.* New York: Garland, 1985.

Dock, L. *History of American Red Cross Nursing.* New York: Macmillan, 1922.

Fitzpatrick, M.L. *The National Organization for Public Health Nursing, 1912–1952: Development of a Practice Field.* New York: National League for Nursing, 1975.

"Lydia Holman." Obituary. *American Journal of Nursing* 60 (May 1960): 634.

Kaufman, M., ed. *Dictionary of American Nursing Biography.* Westport, Conn.: Greenwood, 1988.

Kernodle, P.B. *The Red Cross Nurse in Action 1882–1948.* New York: Harper, 1949.

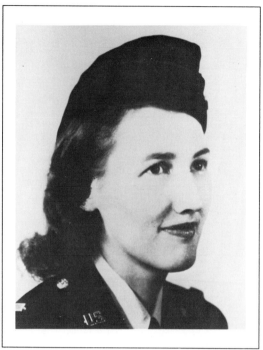

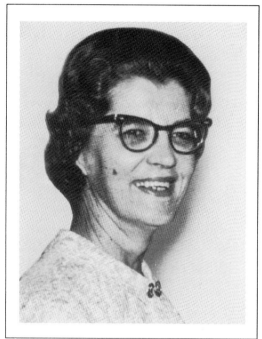

Ellen Gertrude Ainsworth   Marian Alford

Lydia E. Anderson   Edith Augusta Ariss

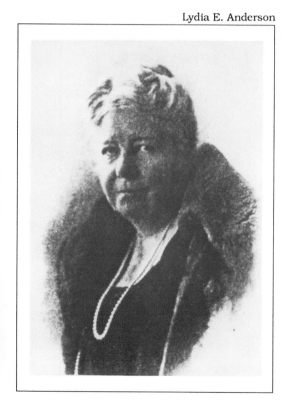

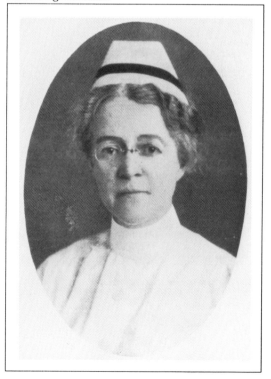

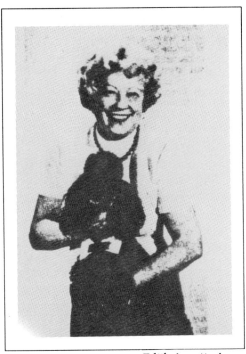

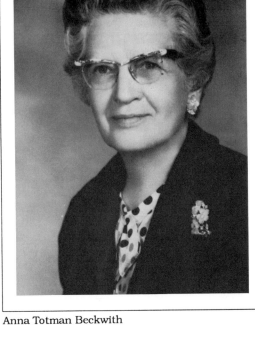

Edith Annette Ayres   Anna Totman Beckwith

Edna Behrens   Ella Best

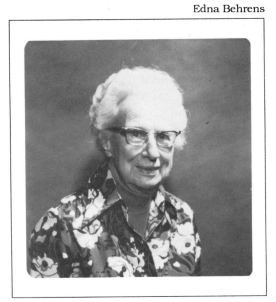

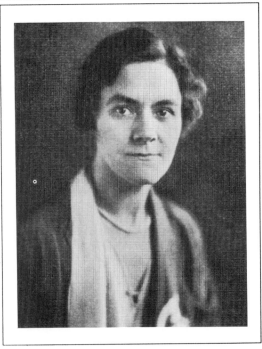

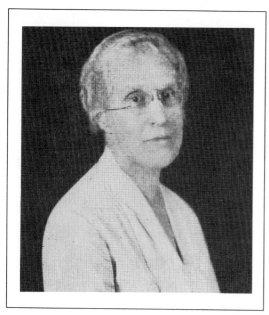

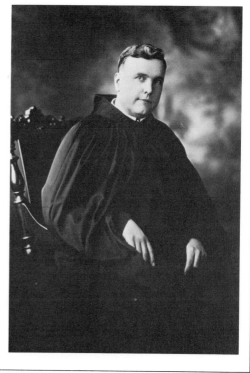

Annie M. Brainard

Brother Sebastian Brogan

Amy Frances Brown

Martha Marie Montgomery Brown

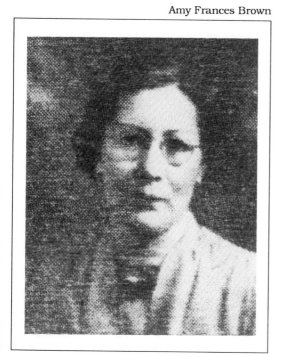

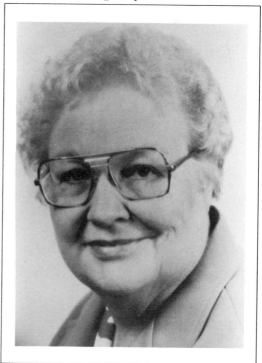

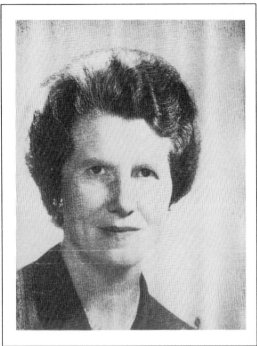

Helen Edith Browne

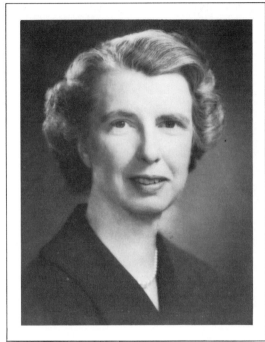

Helen Lathrop Bunge

Charlotte Burgess

St. Francis Xavier (Mother) Cabrini

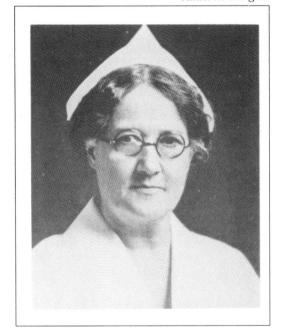

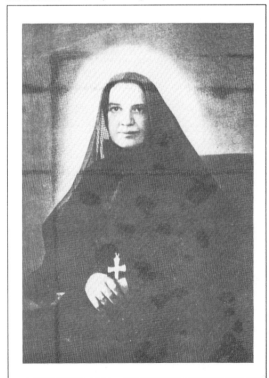

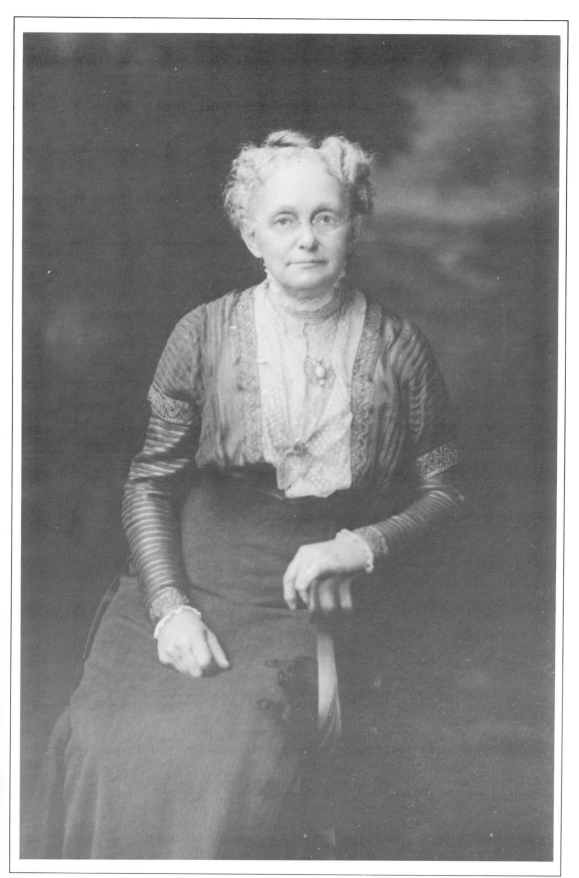

Martha Jenks Wheaton Chase

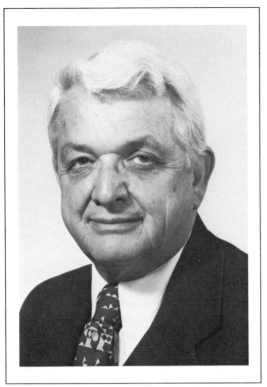

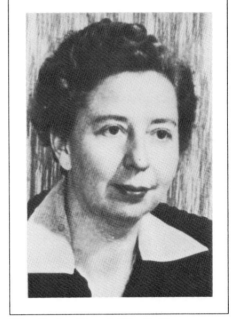

Luther P. Christman   Ellen Evalyn Church (Marshall)

Anna Laura Cole   Charity E. Collins

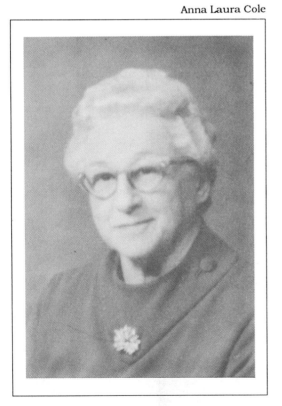

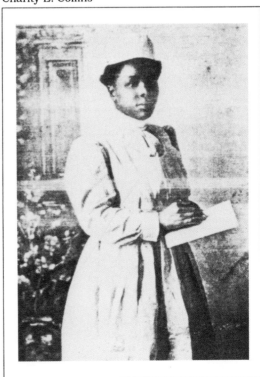

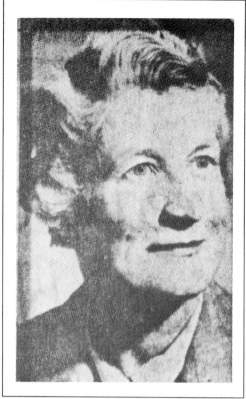

Pearl Parvin Coulter

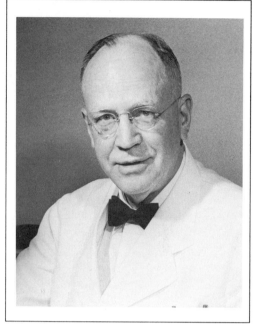

LeRoy N. Craig

Namahyoke Gertrude (Sockum) Curtis

Louise M. Darche

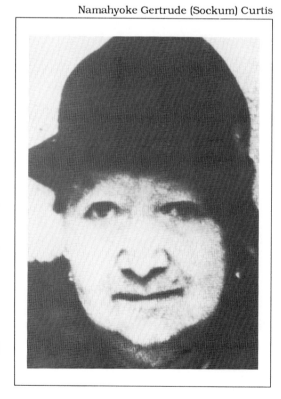

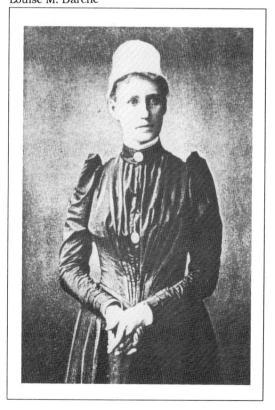

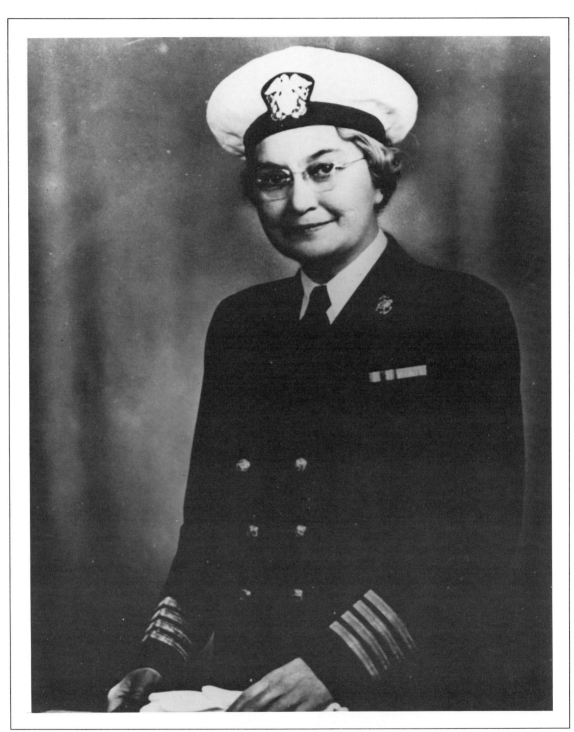

Sue Sophia Dauser

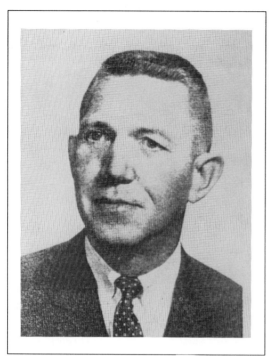

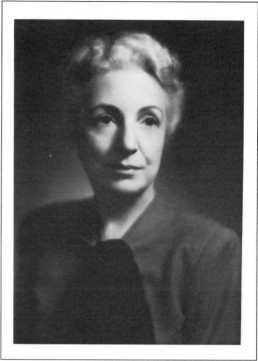

Philip Edson Day   Clare Dennison

Kezia Payne de Pelchin

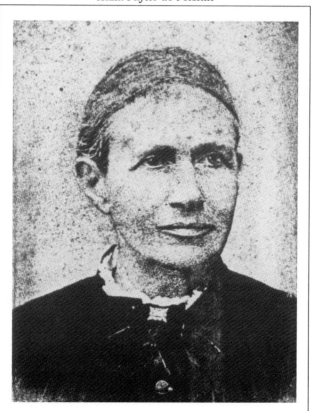

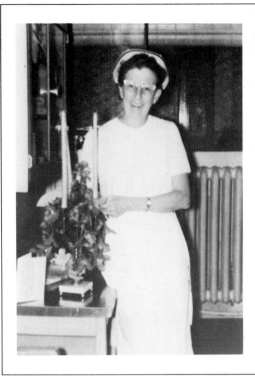

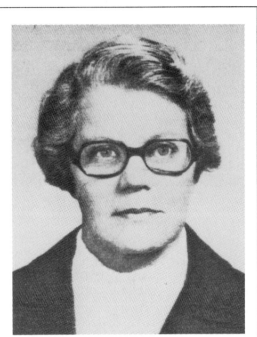

Anita Dowling Dorr   Rosemary Ellis

Bertha Erdmann   Sara Maiter Errickson

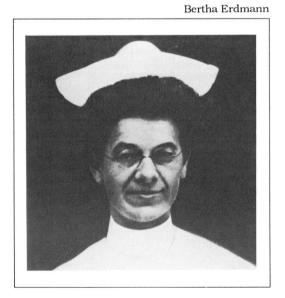

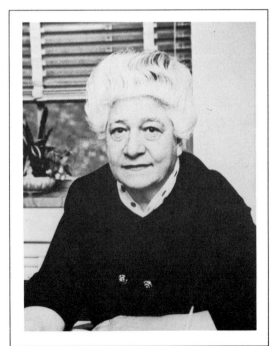

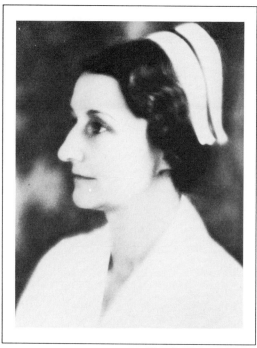

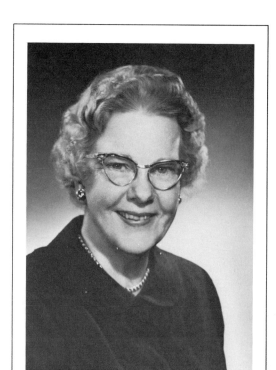

Maude Frances Essig   Margene Olive Faddis

Katherine Ellen Faville   Gertrude Labrake Fife

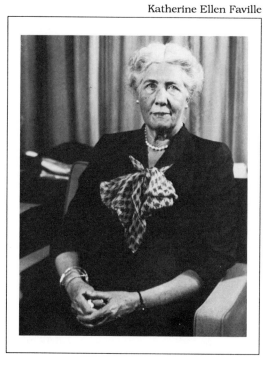

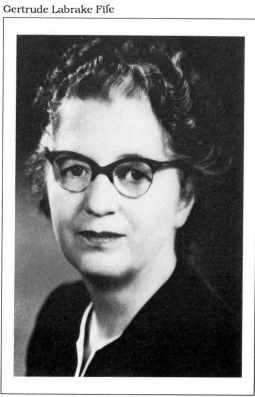

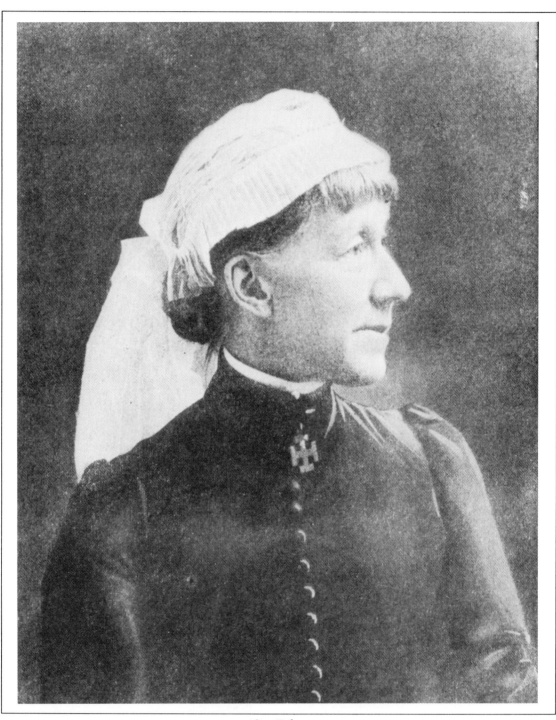

Alice Fisher

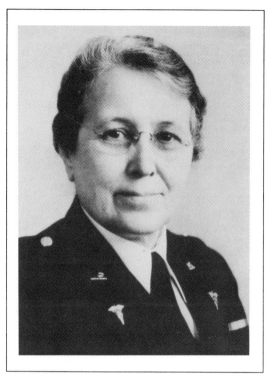

Julia Otteson Flikke

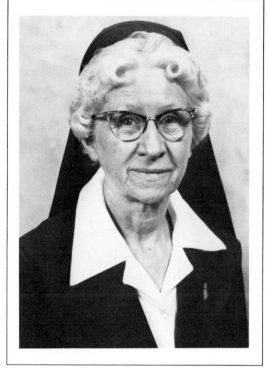

Sister Charles Marie Frank

Stella Louisa Fuller

Harriet Fulmer

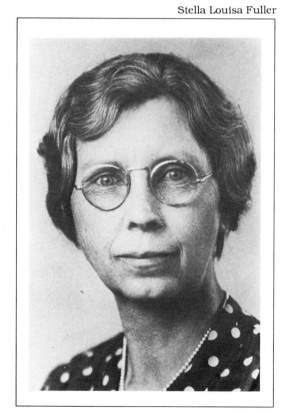

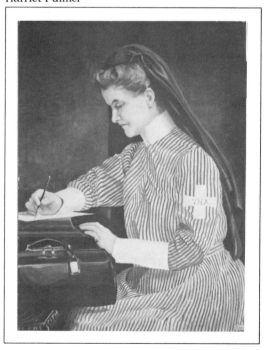

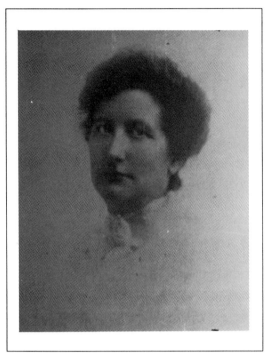

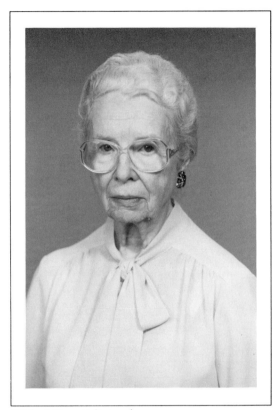

Bertha J. Gardner   Mildred Garrett (Primer)

Lucy Doman Germain

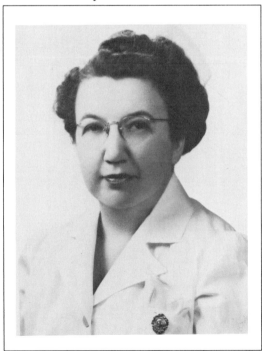

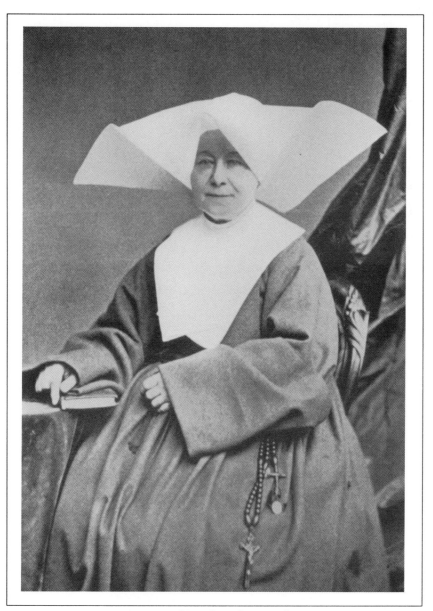

Sister Agnes Mary Gray Conzaga Grace

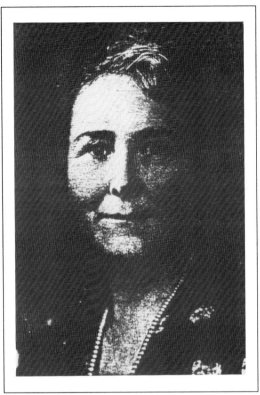

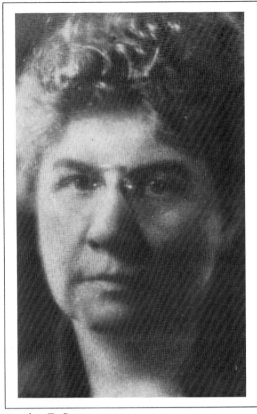

Amelia Howe Grant   Carolyn E. Gray

Katherine Greenough   Cordelia Adelaide Harvey

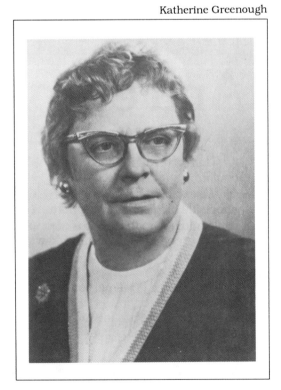

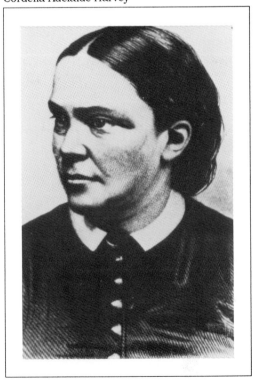

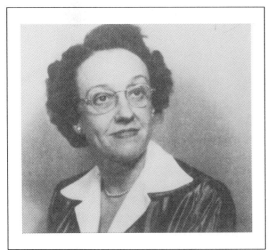

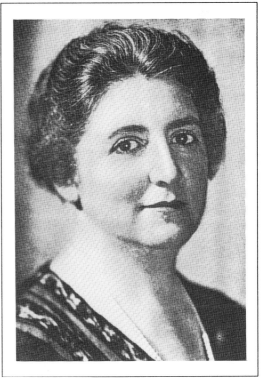

Lulu Wolf Hassenplug   Marion Gertrude Howell

Virginia Henderson

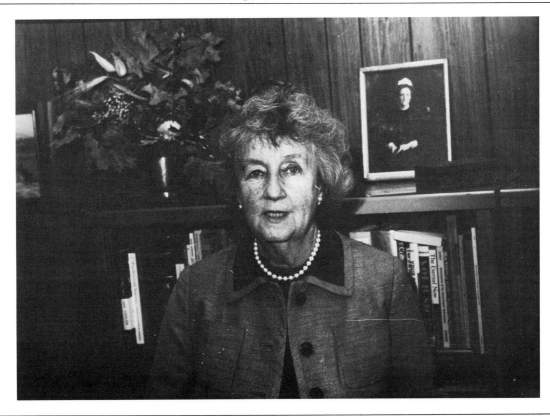

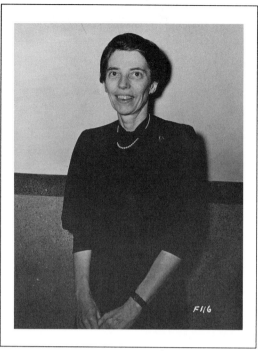

Ruth Weaver Hubbard

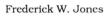

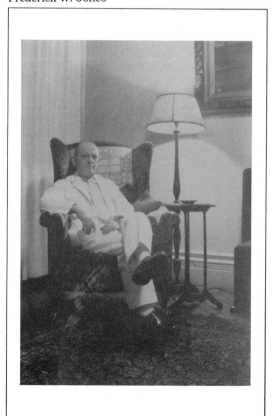

Ethel (Mary Incledon) Johns

Freddie Louise Powell Johnson

Frederick W. Jones

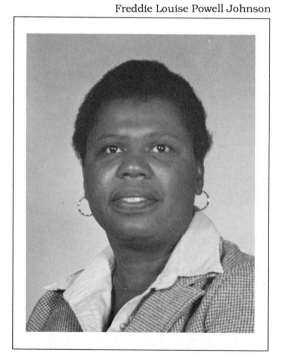

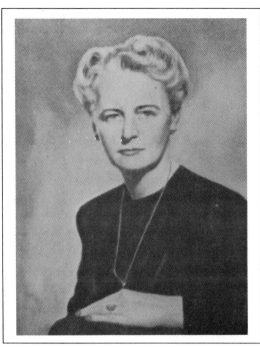

Catherine M. Kain

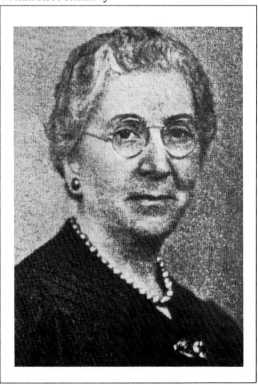

Manelva Wylie Keller

Elizabeth L. Kemble

Cecilia Rose Kennedy

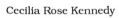

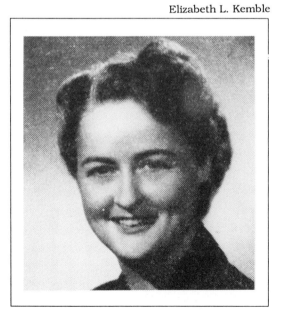

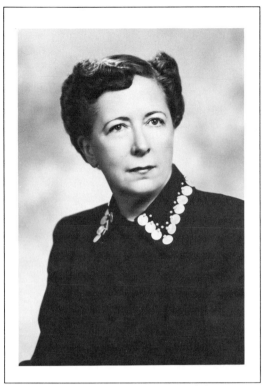

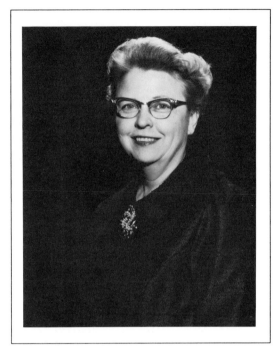

Gladys Kiniery   Ruth Perkins Kuehn

Lucille Petry Leone   Edith Patton Lewis

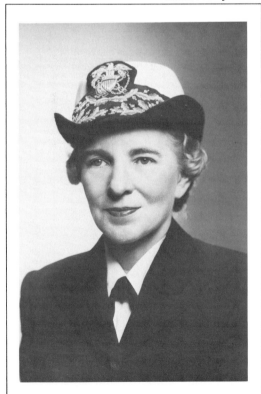

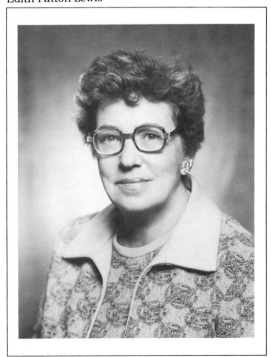

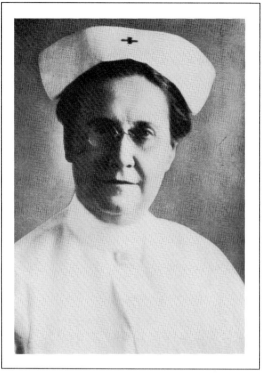

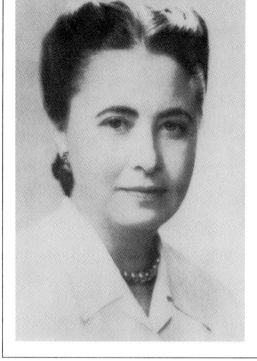

Emily Lemoine Loveridge   Theresa I. Lynch

Helen Grace McClelland   Annabella McCrae

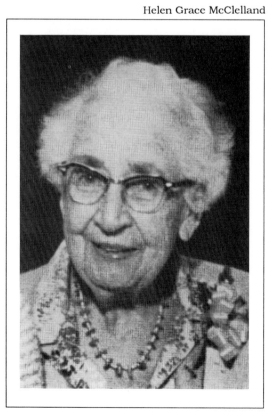

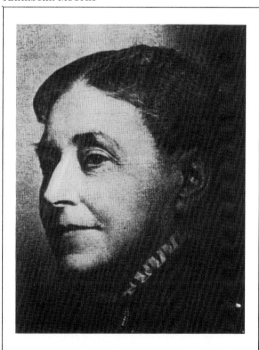

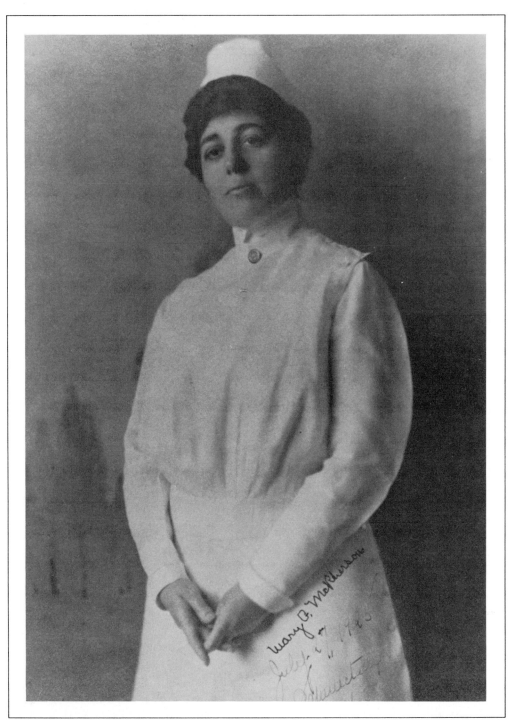

Mary G. McPherson

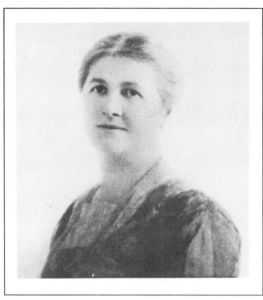

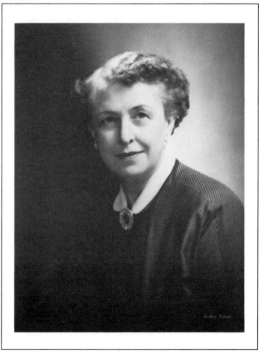

Clara Barton McMillen   Florence McQuillen

Ann Kathryn Magnussen   Mary Ann Maher

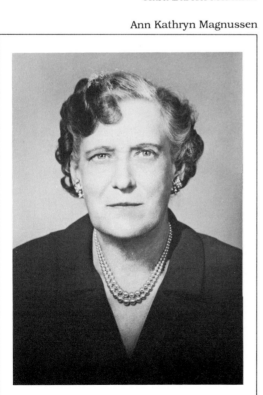

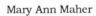

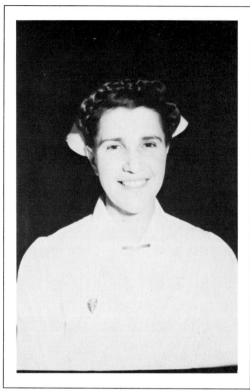

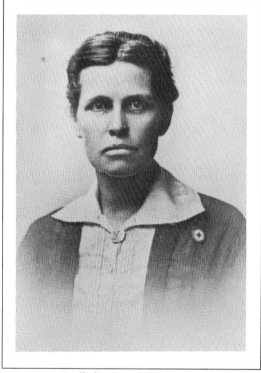

Marguerite Lucy Manfreda

Julia St. Lo Mellichamp

Lucy Jane Rider Meyer

Marya Annice Miller

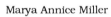

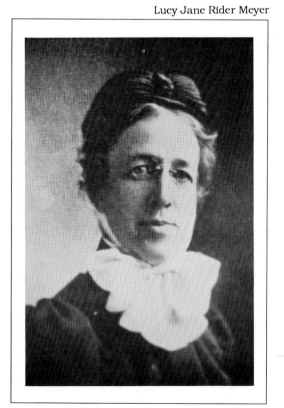

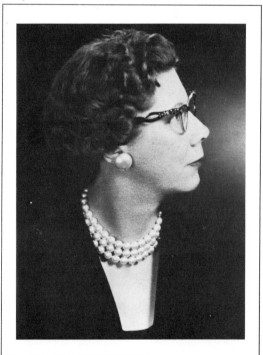

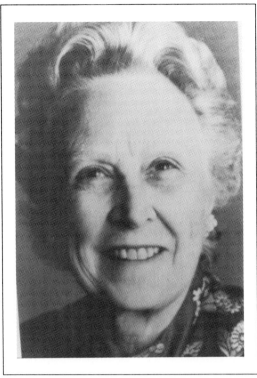

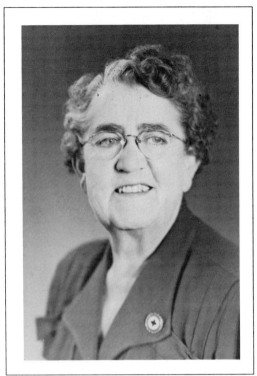

Mildred Montag   Elba Lila Morse

Mary Kelly Mollane   Tressie Virginia Myers

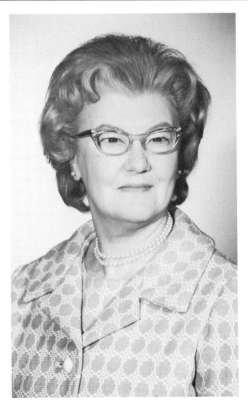

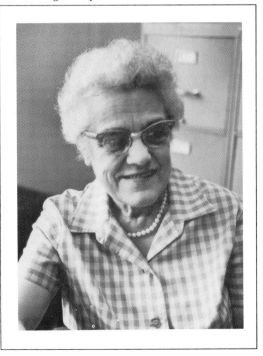

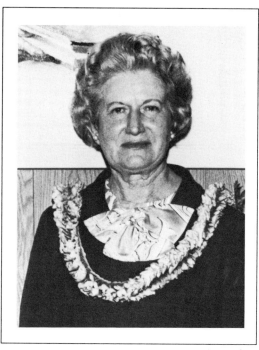

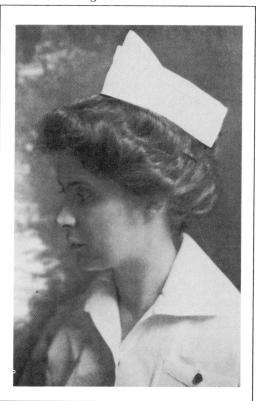

Helen Nahm Lalu Nathoy

Lucille E. Notter Ethel Janette Odegard

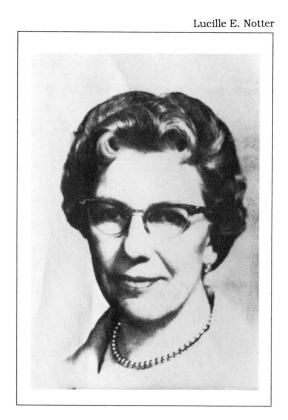

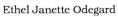

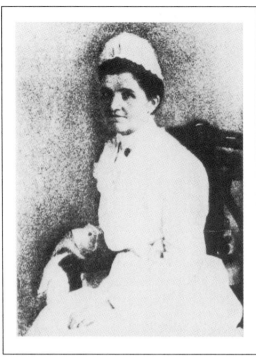

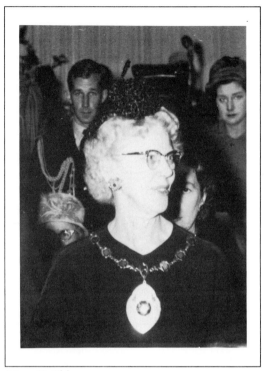

Mary Agnes O'Donnell   Agnes K. Ohlson

Virginia Ohlson   Hildegard Peplau

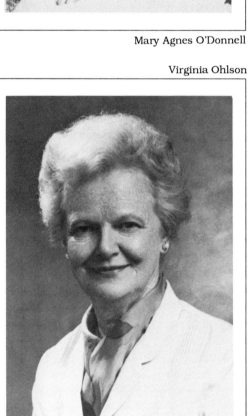

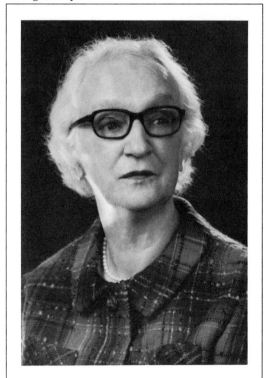

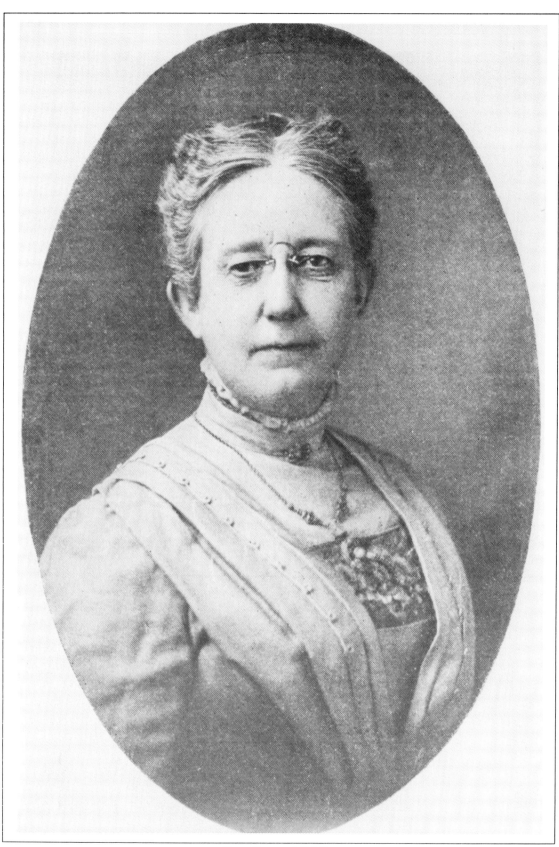

Mary Margaret Riddle

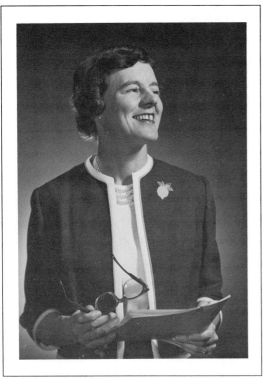

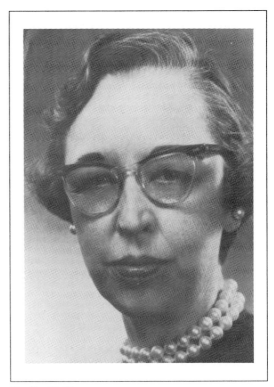

Alice M. Robinson   Martha E. Rogers

Marjorie E. Sanderson   Frances Schervier

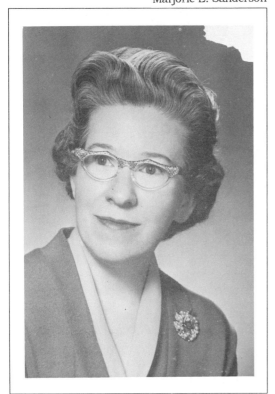

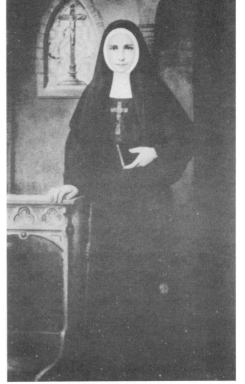

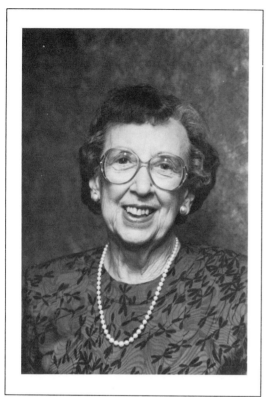

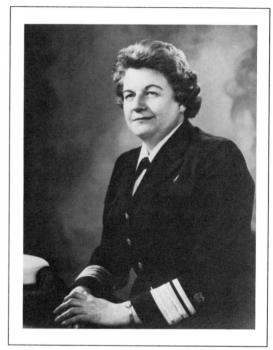

Rozella May Schlotfeldt   Jessie M. Scott

Barbara Gordon Schutt

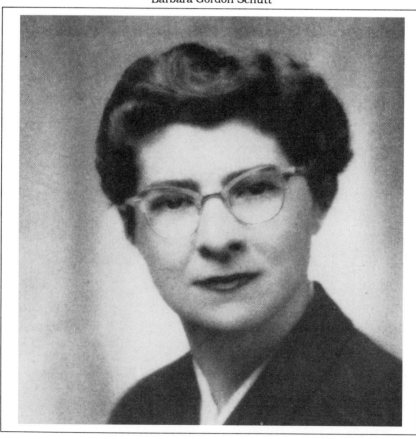

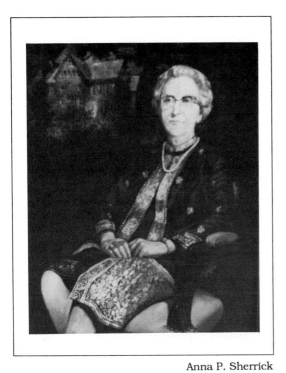

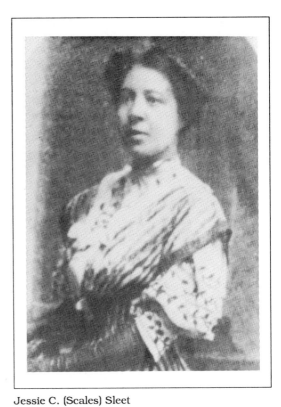

Anna P. Sherrick

Jessie C. (Scales) Sleet

Brother Camillus Snyder

Eugenia Kennedy Spalding

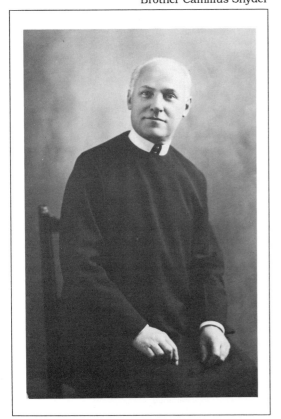

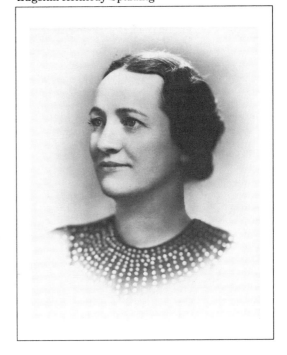

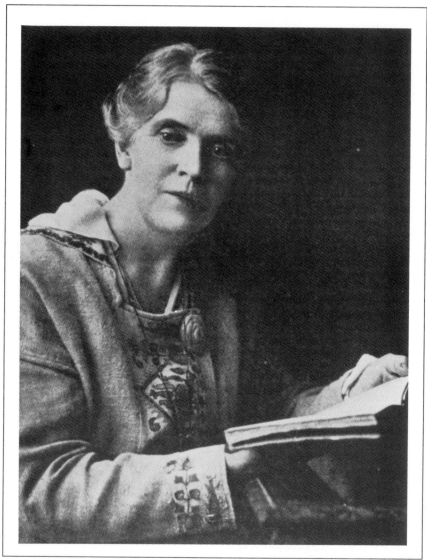

Margaret Elliott Frances Sirch

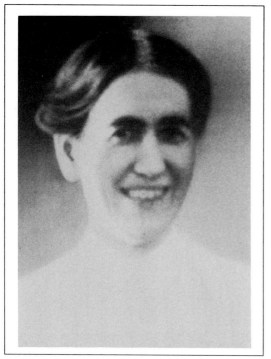
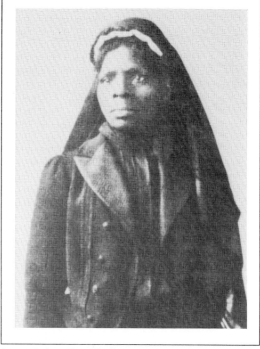

Marietta B. Squire   Susie Baker King Taylor

Julie Chamberlain Tebo
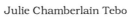

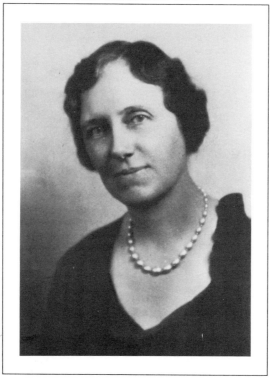

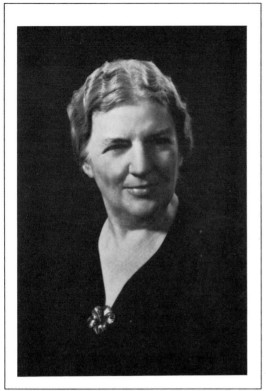
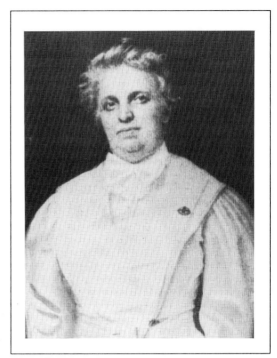

Margaret Anthony Tracy   Susan Tracy

Joyce E. Travelbee

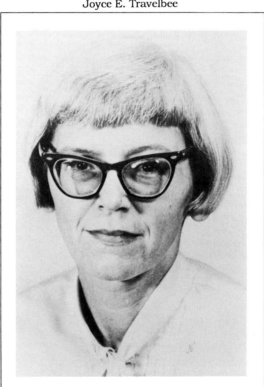

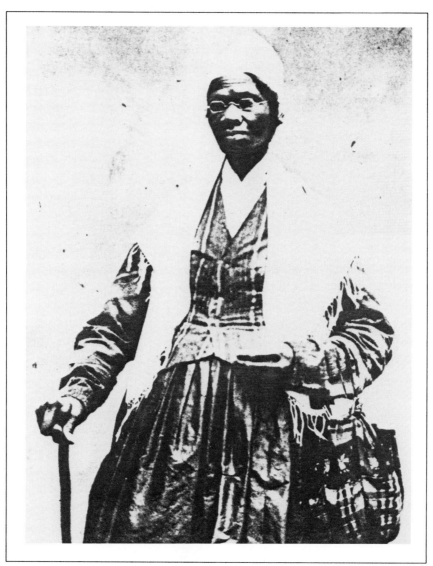

Sojourner Truth

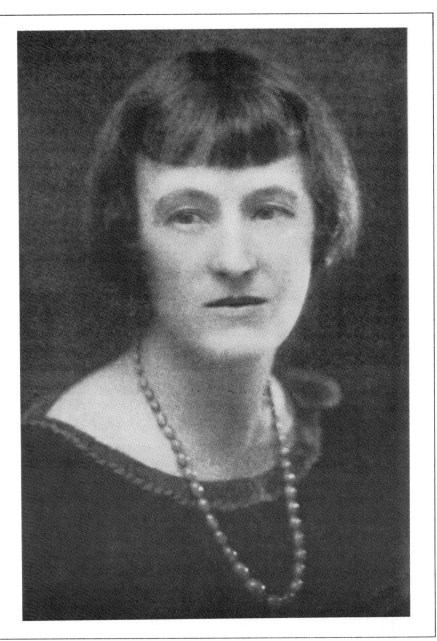

Stella Booth Vail

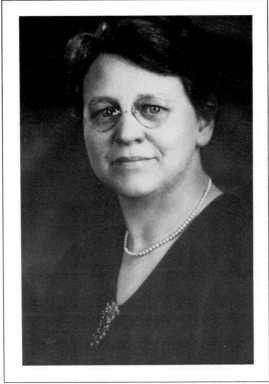

Jane Van de Vrede

Phyllis Jean Verhonek   Mrytle Viola Werth

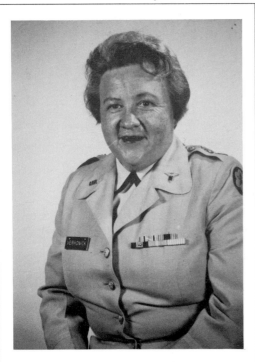

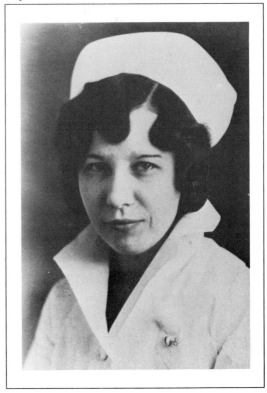

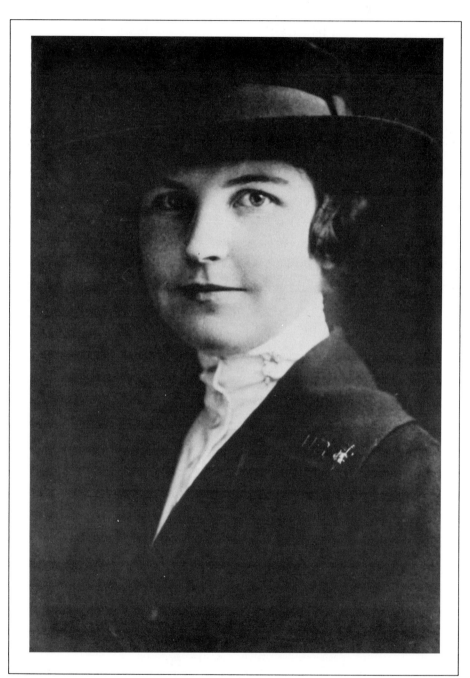

Sophie Gran Jeune Winton

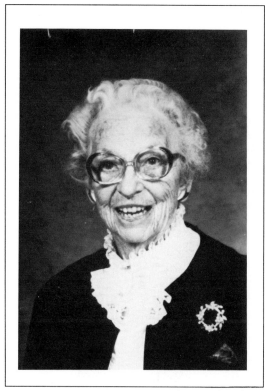

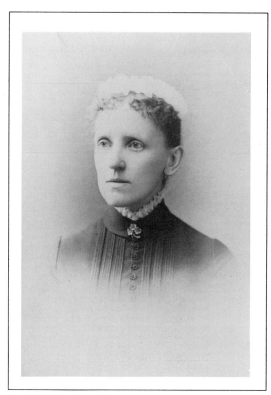

Carolyn Ladd Widmer Lucie E. Woodward

Ann Zimmerman

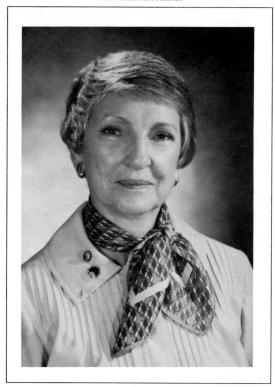

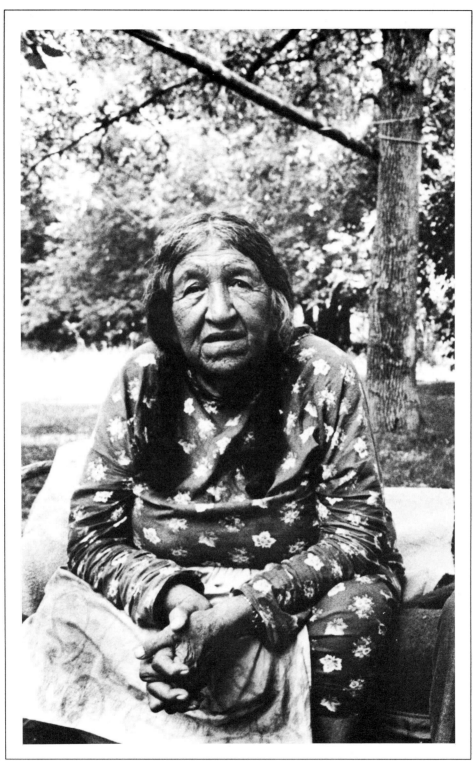

Susie Yellow Tail

North Carolina State Archives, Board of Nurse Registration and Nursing Education, Raleigh.

"Sixteenth Annual Report." *Johns Hopkins Nurses Alumnae Magazine.* 7(August 1908): 166–68.

Von Blarcom, C.C. *Obstetrical Nursing.* New York: Macmillan, 1932.

Waters, Y. *Visiting Nursing in the United States.* New York: Macmillan, 1909.

William Henry Welch Papers. Alan Mason Chesney Medical Archives of the Johns Hopkins Medical Institutions, Baltimore, Maryland.

Wyche, M.L. *The History of Nursing in North Carolina.* Chapel Hill: University of North Carolina Press, 1938.

Susan N. Craft

Marion Gertrude Howell

1887–1975

Marion Gertrude Howell was dean of the Frances Payne Bolton School of Nursing of Western Reserve University in Cleveland. She saw the school through the tumult of both the Great Depression and World War II. She had a special interest in public-health nursing.

Howell was born on September 26, 1887, in Freeport, Ohio, to John G. and Mary Jane Knox Howell. Her father was a physician and inspired her to pursue a nursing career.

In 1912 she received a Ph.B. degree from the College of Wooster, Ohio, and began teaching English at Minerva (Ohio) High School. She remained there until 1918. After attending the Vassar Training Camp during World War I, she studied nursing at the Lakeside Hospital School of Nursing (Ohio), spending two months of her senior year in training at University Public Health Nursing District. She received her R.N. in 1920. The following year she received an M.S. and a certificate in public-health nursing from the School of Applied Social Sciences at Western Reserve University. While there, she held an Edward Fitch Cushing scholarship and was a member of Delta Delta Delta. She later received an honorary doctorate from Western Reserve.

From 1921–22 Howell worked as a school nurse in the Fairmont, West Virginia, public schools. During the following academic year she was an instructor in public-health nursing in the University Nursing District in Cleveland.

She began her career at Western Reserve University in 1923, when she was named assistant professor of public-health nursing in the School of Applied Social Sciences. She became an associate professor in 1924 and a full professor in 1927.

She was acting director of the university's Public-Health Nursing Department, 1923–24, and director, 1924–32. One of the projects during that time was preschool clinics for area children.

In 1932 the School of Nursing and the Nursing Service of the three university hospitals underwent a period of reorganization. Howell was named to the dual posts of dean of the School of Nursing and director of the Nursing Service of the university hospitals. Associate administrators in each sector shared the administrative details.

Early in her tenure, the work hours of graduate nurses were reduced from 52 to 48 hours per week, and both students and graduates were given one full day off per week. Volunteer ward clerks relieved some of the pressure of the assigned nurses by answering the phone and otherwise assisting at the nurses' station. The first class of college graduates to enroll in the School of Nursing was admitted in 1934, with 23 students representing 19 colleges. Beginning in 1933, the school helped to organize and became active in the Association of Collegiate Schools of Nursing. The school's name was changed to Frances Payne Bolton School of Nursing in 1935, honoring a benefactor. An undergraduate program was added in 1941.

During World War II Howell was chairman of the government subcommittee of the National Nursing Council. She was a president and first vice-president of the National Organization for Public Health Nurses and a vice-president of the Association of Collegiate Schools of Nursing.

Howell was very active in organizations concerning her profession. She was a member of the American Nurses' Association, the National League of Nursing Education, the American Association of Social Workers, the American Public Health Association, the American Congress of Obstetrics and Gynecology, the Cleveland Hospital Council, the Cleveland Child Health Association, the American Red Cross, and the Maternal Health Association.

On the community level, she was a member of the Cleveland Museum of Art, the Musical Arts Association in Cleveland, the Consumers League of Ohio, the Guild of St. Barnabas for Nurses, the League of Women Voters, the Women's City Club of Cleveland, and the Women's Faculty Club of Western Reserve University. Her hobbies included music, theater, and reading.

Because of ill health, Howell took a leave of absence in January 1946 and then retired in June. She moved to Beaver Falls, Pennsylvania, and died there August 16, 1975, after a brief illness.

PUBLICATIONS BY MARION GERTRUDE HOWELL

With L.W. Ware. "At the ICN." *Public Health Nursing* 29 (October 1937): 576–77.

BIBLIOGRAPHY

Bower, I.M. *Public Health Nursing in Cleveland.* Cleveland: School of Social Science, Western Reserve University, 1930.

Faddis, M.O. *A School of Nursing Comes of Age.* Cleveland: Alumni Association of the Frances Payne Bolton School of Nursing, 1973.

Faddis, M.O. *The History of the Frances Payne Bolton School of Nursing.* Cleveland: Western Reserve University Press, 1948.

Farnham, E. *Pioneering in Public Health Nursing Education.* Cleveland: Western Reserve University Press, 1964.

Goodrich, A.W. "Marion Gertrude Howell." Unidentified manuscript, undated. Frances Payne Bolton School of Nursing, Case Western Reserve University, Cleveland.

Howes, D. ed. *American Women 1935–1940: A Composite Biographical Dictionary.* Detroit: Gale, 1981.

"Marion G. Howell." *American Journal of Nursing* 75 (October 1975): 1887.

Alice P. Stein

Ruth Weaver Hubbard
1897–1955

Ruth Weaver Hubbard was one of the major leaders in public-health nursing in the United States in the decade following World War II. She was the general director of the Visiting Nurse Society of Philadelphia for 26 years and the president of the National Organization for Public Health Nursing (NOPHN) for the period 1946–50. Her wide participation in health and nursing activities, her knowledge of public-health nursing practice and education, and her ability to communicate her vision of the public-health nurse through her publications distinguished her nursing career.

Hubbard was born in 1897 in Brooklyn, New York, the daughter of Dr. William S. Hubbard and Mrs. William S. Hubbard, a graduate nurse of about 1893. She had two known siblings, Elizabeth Weaver Hubbard (Seymour) and William Stimpson Hubbard.

Hubbard was a 1921 diploma graduate of the Army School of Nursing, Walter Reed Hospital, Washington, D.C. She received a B.S. in 1925 from Teachers College, Columbia University, New York City. She did additional graduate work at Yale University, New Haven, Connecticut, between 1927 and 1929 and at the University of Pennsylvania, Philadelphia, between 1935 and 1941. As the recipient of a Rockefeller Foundation fellowship, she toured Eastern Europe, Scandinavia, and the British Isles for three months in 1931 to study nursing education and public-health nursing.

Hubbard began her recorded professional experience working as a staff nurse at the Brooklyn Visiting Nurse Association for five months in 1922. After receiving her B.S. degree, she was the head nurse in the Pediatric Clinic at the New Haven, Connecticut, Dispensary, 1925–27. The following two years she served as the education director of the Visiting Nurse Association of New Haven. In June 1929 she was appointed to succeed Katherine Tucker as the general director of the Visiting Nurse Society (VNS) of Philadelphia and continued to lead this prominent agency until her death. Tucker and Hubbard were together credited with transforming the Philadelphia VNS from a multipurpose home-welfare agency into a modern professional nursing organization.

Concurrent with her nursing-practice roles, Hubbard was active as a public-health nursing educator. Between 1925 and 1926 she taught at the Yale School of Nursing, first as an assistant instructor, then as an instructor. For 20 years (1935–55) she was a lecturer on the organization and administration of public-health nursing at the University of Pennsylvania School of Nursing. She was also a visiting lecturer at the University of California at Berkeley during summer school in 1936 and 1942 and at the University of Minnesota in 1948.

Through her publications, Hubbard supported the integration of public-health nursing concepts into all facets of nursing education, emphasizing the use of appropriately trained instructors. She encouraged wide acceptance of the "health approach" to nursing, the understanding of the patient as an individual whose own characteristics determine needed care. While acknowledging that not every public-health nursing agency could accommodate students due to size and standards, she challenged the suggestion that a student program would be costly for an agency by underscoring the interdependence of educational institutions and service agencies.

Hubbard was a member of the Education Committee of the NOPHN from 1930 until at least 1946 and was its chair, 1940–42. At the Philadelphia VNS she also developed a new public-health nursing affiliation for senior cadet nurses in 1944. In the late 1940s she was part of the professional advisory committee for Esther Lucille Brown's national study of nursing education.

Hubbard advocated the adoption of the many successful programs of the Philadelphia VNS during her presentations at many nursing and public-health meetings and her frequent publications. And she called on organizations to experiment with public health programs. She championed hourly nursing, the extension of public-health nursing to the paying patient, and assurance to all members of the community of access to professional nurses at a reasonable cost. In the field of industrial nursing, Philadelphia in 1933, extended public health concepts to industry through the use of VNS staff nurses for part-time work in plant dispensaries in their district. Hubbard promoted the use of generalized nurses in the implementation of all specialized services and that existing resources be used to provide such service if possible.

Hubbard assured the survival of the VNS through the Depression of the 1930s, at one point demanding to take a greater cut in salary than anyone else on the staff. Rather than submitting to crisis, she continued to plan for the future of the VNS. Hubbard utilized the opportunity of funding through the Federal Emergency Relief Act Ruling No. 7 beginning in 1933 to extend service to new populations in Philadelphia, to acquaint additional physicians with VNS work, and to promote closer working relationships with other community service organizations.

One of the most innovative programs developed by Hubbard at the Philadelphia VNS was the Intensive Home-Care Plan in 1949, later the Philadelphia Home-Care Plan (PHCP). The objective of the PHCP was to achieve better coordination and intensification of long-term home services to promote maximal patient recovery. Though modeled on the hospital-centered, physician-controlled home-care program of Montefiore Hospital, New York City, the Philadelphia VNS adaptation of home-care programs emphasized agency-control, nurse-coordination, and served as a model itself to other nursing organizations.

Hubbard was concerned in other ways with assuring the funding of public-health nursing for home health and sickness care. A member of the Nursing Advisory Committee of the Metropolitan Life Insurance (MLI) Company Nursing Service, Hubbard coordinated a joint NOPHN-MLI pilot study to estimate the probable effects of the withdrawal of MLI sponsorship of VNAs in the early 1950s and to develop strategies to adjust. She worked locally to attempt to expand the extension of nursing service under voluntary pre-payment health plans.

The combination of the VNS and the Philadelphia Department of Health Nursing in 1959 into Community Nursing Services was the legacy of Hubbard's leadership in local public-health affairs since 1945. As a member of many committees and survey groups, she advocated family orientation of care that would be assured with the use of the generalist nurse. She developed a pilot combination program with the Starr Center Association in the late 1940s that demonstrated its feasibility.

Hubbard's two terms as president of the NOPHN occurred at a time of crisis in the organization over shrinking membership and inadequate funding. A member of the Committee on Structure of National Nursing Organizations, Hubbard called for reorganization as the best means to develop and assure nursing-service standards, to advance the various branches of nursing, and to secure adequate salaries. After her presidency ended in 1950, she continued on the Executive Committee until the NOPHN merged to form the National League for Nursing on January 1, 1953.

Because of her natural leadership ability and her substantive contributions to meetings and conferences, Hubbard was appointed to numerous professional committees. She served on the Commission on Chronic Illness and its Technical Advisory Committee. She represented the NLN on the Council of Federal Nursing Services and was the rotating chair of the Interassociation Committee on Health. She was also a member of the editorial board of the *American Journal of Public Health.* Her international work continued throughout her life, and she served on the International Council of Nurses, Committee on Nursing Service.

Hubbard received recognition for her achievements in nursing, including the 1949 Bronze Medal for Distinguished Service to Nursing from the Pennsylvania Nurses' Association, the Philadelphia Friendship Fete Award for outstanding

service to humanity in 1955, and the Distinguished Daughter Award in 1955 from the Commonwealth of Pennsylvania.

After a long illness during which she kept up many aspects of her work, Ruth Weaver Hubbard died on December 6, 1955, in the Rush, New York, home of her sister. Her friends and community leaders in Philadelphia established the Ruth Weaver Hubbard Foundation to perpetuate her work by providing scholarships to nurses for advanced education and special studies.

PUBLICATIONS BY RUTH WEAVER HUBBARD (SELECTED)

"Bag Technic and the Hourly Nurse." *American Journal of Nursing* 28 (June 1928): 557–59.

"Hourly Nursing from the Visiting Nurse Association Viewpoint." *Public Health Nursing* 22 (July 1930): 391–93.

"Nursing Care for Relief Board Clients." *Public Health Nursing* 27 (February 1935): 63–67.

"How Shall We Secure Adequate Experience in Public Health Nursing?" *American Journal of Nursing* 35 (August 1935): 772–78.

"Use of Existing Visiting Nurse Services for Industrial Work in Small Plants." *American Journal of Public Health* 31 (January 1941): 27–33.

"Philadelphia Visiting Nurse Society Program for Senior Cadets." *Public Health Nursing* 36 (March 1944): 132–34.

"Nursing for Health in Tomorrow's Family." *Public Health Nursing* 40 (June 1948): 293–98.

"Public Health Nursing: 1900–1950." *American Journal of Nursing* 50 (October 1950): 608–11.

"Working Together for Public Health." *The Canadian Nurse* 48 (February 1952): 111–14.

"Field Instruction: Costs and Benefits." *Public Health Nursing* 44 (October 1952): 531–35.

"The Continuity." *Public Health Nursing* 44 (December 1952): 657–58.

With M. Scheuer. "Referral Plans: Organization of Referral Programs." *Nursing Outlook* 4 (January 1956): 18–19.

BIBLIOGRAPHY

American Journal of Nursing Company. Records. Nursing Archive, Special Collections, Mugar Memorial Library, Boston University. Boston.

"Death of Ruth Hubbard, 12/6/1955." *NLN News* 3 (December 1955): 4.

Fitzpatrick, M.L. *The National Organization for Public Health Nursing: Development of a Practice Field.* New York: National League for Nursing, 1975. Pp. 166–201.

Hirsch, L.V., M.S. Klein, and G.W. Marlowe. *Combining Public Health Nursing Agencies: A Case Study in Philadelphia.* New York: National League for Nursing, 1967. Pp. 1–26.

Philadelphia Evening Bulletin. Clipping files "Ruth W. Hubbard" and "Visiting Nurse Society." Urban Archives, Temple University, Philadelphia.

Visiting Nurse Service of Philadelphia. Records. Box 14, Folders 19–22; Box 33, Folders 130–131. Center for the Study of the History of Nursing, School of Nursing, University of Pennsylvania, Philadelphia.

Janna L. Dieckmann and Susan N. Craft

Helen Hartley Jenkins

1860–1934

Helen Hartley Jenkins was a philanthropist who was the first to make a major endowment to a nursing-education program in the United States. Her gift as a trustee of Teachers College, Columbia University, enabled the college to establish its department of nursing and health, under the directorship of Mary Adelaide Nutting. Jenkins also was a principal donor of the New York Polytechnic Hospital. She devoted much of her adult life to organizations whose goal was to raise the standards of nursing education.

Jenkins was born on August 16, 1860, into a family long known for its philanthropic enterprises. Her father, Marcellus Hartley, headed a company that made firearms and munitions and founded Hartley House, a settlement house in New York City. Her mother was Frances Chester (White) Hartley, and she had two sisters who lived to adulthood including a twin, Grace. Educated in private schools, she was married in 1894 and later separated from a lawyer and businessman, George Walker Jenkins. Their children were Helen, who died in 1920, and Grace.

When Marcellus Hartley died in 1902, daughter Helen embarked on a full-time career in philanthropy and became president of the Hartley Corporation, of Hartford, Connecticut, which she organized to administer the work.

She was a trustee of Teachers College from 1907–34, and in 1909 endowed its nursing program. This was the first major endowment of a nursing-education program in the United States. Jenkins was instrumental in attracting Nutting to be the first head of the Department of Nursing and Health there, and she endowed professorships for the department in 1910 and 1923.

She supported the School of Nursing, Memorial Hospital, Morristown, New Jersey, which was later named for her. Beside making a substantial donation to the New York Polytechnic Hospital, she personally oversaw its housekeeping department for several years. In 1910 and 1921 she endowed the Marcellus Hartley Chair of Materia Medica at the New York University Medical School. In 1922 she donated Grace Hospital to Banner Elk, North Carolina, and it was named for her twin. She was on the boards of directors of numerous other hospitals and was a trustee of Yenching University, Peiping (Beijing) China.

Jenkins also was active in social-welfare causes, especially improved housing for low-income families. She assisted several immigrant organizations and was decorated by the governments of Montenegro and Serbia. She worked for bipartisan government in New York and for prison reform. Her home was often the scene of meetings of charitable, educational and social committees.

Jenkins was awarded the gold medal of the National Institute for Social Sciences in 1916 and was its president in 1923. New York University awarded her an honorary doctorate of humane letters in 1922 and Trinity College, Hartford, Connecticut, a master's degree in 1924.

Jenkins died at her home in Morristown, New Jersey, April 24, 1934, after four years of myocarditis, exacerbated in 1930 by a disastrous fire that she was in. After her death her work was continued by the Hartley Corporation of Hartford.

BIBLIOGRAPHY

Fridlington, R.J. "Jenkins, Helen Hartley." In *Notable American Women, 1607–1950.* E.T. James et al., eds. Cambridge: Belknap Press of Harvard University Press, 1971.

"Jenkins, Helen Hartley." In *Makers of Nursing History.* M.R. Pennock, ed. New York: Lakeside, 1940.

"Mrs. G.W. Jenkins Dies at Age of 73." Obituary *New York Times*, April 25, 1934.

Alice P. Stein

Ethel Mary Incledon Johns

1879–1968

Ethel Mary Incledon Johns was a nursing pioneer whose innovative leadership shaped and reformed Canadian nursing during the first half of the century and though her influence on American nursing was not quite as great was a significant figure in the United States as well. Johns held numerous prestigious positions in nursing. She worked as a private-duty nurse, head nurse, superintendent/director of nursing services, and consultant for national and international studies. As a consultant Johns provided data for national studies that revealed the status of American nursing and directions for future research. She emphasized the importance of nursing history, realizing that she participated in history in the making, and took pride in her role as a leader creating reform for the future. She believed that writing history provided the necessary guidance for those who would follow. As editor, author, and public advocate, Johns championed nurses' registration and gave a strong voice as to what the future education and service of nursing should be.

Johns was born on May 13, 1879, in the village of Meanstoke, Southampton, England, to Henry Incledon Johns and Amy Robinson Johnson, a year after the marriage of her parents. Her father, a member of a prominent family in church and public service, was curate of the local church in Meanstoke. Her mother came from the Islands of Anglesey off the coast of Wales. Ethel had two younger brothers, Owen and Alexander.

In 1888 Johns father took an assignment as a missionary on the Wabigon Indian Reserve in northwestern Ontario, leaving his wife and two children behind in Denbigh, North Wales, where they had been staying with her mother's father. After the death of her grandfather in 1888 the children were placed in boarding schools in Denbigh, and her mother migrated to Canada to join her husband. It was not until 1892 that the children were able to join their parents in Canada and meet their new younger brother.

The family lived in a log cabin on the reservation and the Johns children who attended school on the reservation quickly became fluent in the language of the Indians on the reservation. In 1895, their father died, and Amy Johns, faced with supporting her three children, applied for the position as reservation teacher, and Ethel (then 16) agreed to become her assistant.

In 1896 a visiting free-lance journalist, Cora Hind, visited the reservation, and spent the night with the Johns family. She became a lifelong friend of Ethel, and clearly acted as mentor to the young woman. In June 1899, following the advice of Cora Hind, Johns entered the Winnipeg (Manitoba) Hospital Training School for Nurses. Though Winnipeg was the closest major city to the reservation, it was also the home of Cora Hind.

The school of nursing was in its twelfth year when Johns entered with 18 other students, the largest group yet to be admitted. Among her classmates was Isabel Maitland Stewart who became her lifetime friend. After Johns graduated in June 1902, she held a variety of positions starting as a private-duty nurse, then head nurse in the operating room, superintendent of nursing, and, night supervisor at Winnipeg General. In between her various appointments in Winnipeg she also worked at other places, including a year-long stint at St. Lukes Hospital in St. Paul, Minnesota. In 1905 Johns and her friend Stewart became involved in two newly established organizations, the Alumnae

Associations of the Graduate Nurses of the Winnipeg General Hospital and the Manitoba Association of Graduate Nurses. Johns edited the *Alumnae Journal* of Winnipeg General Hospital while Stewart served as business manager. Johns also began to write about issues in nursing for the *Canadian Nurse* which had begun publication in 1905.

In April 1911 Johns was elected president of the Manitoba Association of Graduate Nurses, and soon after this left Winnipeg to become lady superintendent at the McKeller General Hospital in Fort William as well as director of the School of Nursing there. It was in this position that she came to believe she needed additional education.

Following through on this, she enrolled at Teachers College, Columbia University in New York City for the academic year 1914–1915, and again in the summer of 1924. Her teachers were Adelaide Nutting, Annie Goodrich, and Lavina Dock. Returning to Manitoba in 1915, she became superintendent and principal of the nurse-training school at the Winnipeg General Children's Hospital. She also became active in the Manitoba Association of Registered Nurses and the Canadian Society of Superintendents of Training Schools. The latter group appointed her to a committee to study nursing education and the report she made on this in 1917 proved to be critical of the lack of regulations governing nursing education. She was soon able to do something about nursing in Manitoba through her appointment as one of the nine Commissioners of Public Welfare in Manitoba. She became a spokesperson for organized nursing urging improvements in nursing registration and nursing education.

In 1919, she resigned her position at Children's Hospital because of differences of opinion with the hospital administration and in September of that year took a position as director of nursing at Vancouver General Hospital and dean of the Department of Nursing at the University of British Columbia in Vancouver. She developed a two-track program for students, one training students in the hospital where they received a diploma, and the second, a combined program at the university and hospital where the students received both a degree and a diploma. In 1921 she resigned as director of nursing but retained her role as director of the education program in the training school and became a full-time member of the faculty at the University.

A 1924 visit to the University by a representative of the Rockefeller Foundation studying nursing education, led to an invitation for her to become a "Special Member of the Field Staff in Nursing Education" set up by the Foundation to establish nursing schools in Europe. Before departing for Europe, however, the Foundation requested she do a study on the status of "Negro Women in Nursing," a task which entailed field trips to 16 cities and 23 hospital schools. The study marked the entry of the Rockefeller Foundation into the support of Black nursing schools.

Early in 1926 she sailed for Paris, where she worked in Romania, Bulgaria, Turkey, France, Belgium, and Hungary. She participated in selecting fellows for training in American nursing schools, advised them, and provided advice and assistance when they returned to their positions. She also reorganized the School of Nursing at Debrecen, Hungary.

In 1929 Johns returned to New York City to become director of studies for the Committee on Nursing Organization of the New York Hospital-Cornell Medical College Association. As part of the project she analyzed costs for nursing service, and set up an independent budget for nursing education, thus separating service from education. When this project was completed in November 1931, Johns joined the staff of the Committee on the Grading of Nursing Schools, a joint effort of various nursing organizations and foundations, including the Rockefeller Foundation. The director of the project was May Ayres Burgess while Johns was nurse associate.

In 1933 she returned to Canada as editor and business manager of the *Canadian Nurse*, the official organ of the Canadian Nurses' Association. Under her leadership the journal was upgraded and expanded, and she continued in this position until her retirement at age 65. She continued to write professionally after her retirement, including her histories of the Johns Hopkins School of Nursing and the Winnipeg General Hospital School of Nursing. She also began her autobiography but completed only three chapters.

In 1949 she moved to Vancouver, where she continued to be active in nursing organizations until the last few years of her life. She received numerous awards, including the Mary Agnes Snively award, the Edith Cavel-Marie Depage medallion, a medal from the Counsel of General Hospital Administration of Lyons (France) and an honorary degree of Doctor of Laws from Mt. Allison University in 1948. She died on September 2, 1968, at the age of 89. Her ashes were interred at the Mount Royal Cemetery in Montreal in a gravesite shared with her mother and brother.

PUBLICATIONS BY ETHEL MARY INCLEDON JOHNS

ARTICLES (SELECTED)

"The Training of Superintendents in Small Hospitals," *Modern Hospital* (Oct. 1915). 241–42.

"Nursing Education in Western Canada," *Canadian Nurse* 15 (June 1919). 1772–85.

"The University in Relation to Nursing Education," *Modern Hospital* 15 (August 1920): 105–09.

"It Took Thirty-Three Years," *Canadian Nurse*, 39 (August 1943): 509–11.

The ICN Responsibility for International Education of Nurses," *International Nursing Bulletin* 7 (Winter 1950): 20–23.

Numerous editorials and brief articles.

BOOKS

With Blanche Pfefferkorn. *An Activity Analysis of Nursing.* New York: Committee on the Grading of Nursing Schools, 1934.

With Blanche Pfefferkorn. *The Johns Hopkins Hospital School of Nursing 1889–1929.* Baltimore: The Johns Hopkins Press, 1954.

The Winnipeg General Hospital School of Nursing, 1887–1953. Winnipeg: Alumnae Association, 1957.

UNPUBLISHED REPORT

The Status of the Negro Woman in Nursing in the U.S. Rockefeller Archive Center Collections, Pocantico Hills, NY.

BIBLIOGRAPHY

Street, Margaret M. *Watch Fires on the Mountain: The Life and Writings of Ethel Johns.* Toronto: University of Toronto Press, 1973.

Various items in the Adelaide Nutting College, Teachers College, Columbia University, including application of Ethel Johns to Teachers College, and various letters and references.

Althea T. Davis

Freddie Louise Powell Johnson
1931–1982

Freddie Louise Powell Johnson was a major trailblazer for minorities in nursing in the Midwest. She was the first black graduate of the University of Nebraska School of Nursing and the first person to earn a doctorate through the American Nurses' Association Fellowship Award for Ethnic Minorities. Johnson was an active researcher in gerontological nursing and had a particular interest in minority elderly. She served as a research mentor to numerous students and other faculty. Balancing roles of wife, mother, nurse, teacher, researcher, community leader, and advocate for racial minorities and the elderly, Johnson spent all but three years of her nursing career at the University of Nebraska Medical Center in Omaha.

Johnson was born on March 6, 1931, in Vicksburg, Mississippi, the second daughter of the Reverend R.H. and Vera Powell. She attended high school in St. Joseph, Missouri, where her father served a Methodist congregation. Reverend Powell's transfer to Lincoln, Nebraska, brought Johnson to the University of Nebraska School of Nursing in Omaha, where she received her bachelor of science degree in nursing in 1952. Her interest in obstetrical nursing led her to the Margaret Hague Maternity Hospital in Jersey City, New Jersey, where she received a postgraduate certificate in 1953.

After completing her postgraduate

study, Johnson returned to Omaha and from 1953–58 held positions as staff nurse, assistant head nurse, and head nurse in obstetrics at the University of Nebraska Hospital. It was during this time that she met a young serviceman from Philadelphia who was stationed at Offutt Air Force Base near Omaha. She and Van L. Johnson were married on August 6, 1955, in Colorado Springs, Colorado, with her father performing the wedding ceremony. Van Johnson joined the staff of the Nebraska Psychiatric Institute on the University campus in 1957 as an electronics technician. (In 1990 he completed 33 years of service to the university.) The couple's first child, Vanetta Louise, was born on March 7, 1958, and a second daughter, Valerie Lynn, was born on September 17, 1962. Johnson's husband and daughters provided support and encouragement throughout her career.

The only break in Johnson's tenure at the university came in 1958 when she resigned to accept a nursing supervisor position at the Salvation Army's Booth Memorial Hospital. When she returned to the university in 1961, she joined the faculty of the School of Nursing and spent the remainder of her professional life as a nurse educator and researcher. She taught initially in the baccalaureate nursing program in the areas of medical-surgical nursing, nursing leadership, quality assurance, and gerontology. Her clinical interests became focused on nursing administration and the care of the elderly.

Johnson continued her formal education, and in 1963 she received a master of arts degree in nursing education from the University of Omaha (now the University of Nebraska at Omaha). In 1976 she was awarded the doctor of philosophy degree in adult and continuing education from the University of Nebraska–Lincoln. Funding for her doctoral work came from an American Nurses' Association Fellowship Award for Ethnic Minorities. Her dissertation focused on the territorial rights of institutionalized elderly clients, reflecting her interest in the needs of the elderly population. She also held a clinical associate position with the Visiting Nurse As-

sociation and served as a volunteer primary nurse in a health-maintenance clinic for the elderly.

Soon after receiving her Ph.D., Johnson was promoted to the rank of associate professor and was asked to join the graduate faculty to teach gerontological nursing and advanced research methods in nursing. She also served as research advisor to many graduate nursing students. An outstanding teacher and mentor, Johnson encouraged her students to explore, to take risks, to question current practices, and to dream for the future. She was honored with an Outstanding Teacher Award in 1982. Other honors included recognition by the College of Nursing Alumni Association in 1977 and membership in Sigma Theta Tau in 1978. She was listed in *Who's Who in Nebraska* in 1977 and in *Who's Who Among Notable Americans* in 1979.

Johnson's administrative duties included serving as assistant to the director of the Nursing Care Research Center in the College of Nursing and as acting director of the center in 1981. She also served on many college and university committees throughout her career. Her work relating to recruitment, retention, and advisement of minority students was of great significance to the health-education programs at the Medical Center.

Johnson's involvement in professional organizations began early and continued throughout her career. She was a member of the American Nurses' Association, the National League for Nursing, the Adult Education Association, the American Heart Association, the American Gerontological Association, Delta Sigma Theta Sorority, and the National Black Nurses' Association. She was a president of the Omaha Black Nurses' Association. She served as an accreditation visitor for the National League for Nursing and was a member of the review board and a site visitor for the National Institutes of Mental Health (NIMH) from 1979–82. She also served as an elected member of the governing board of the Midwest Nursing Research Society (MNRS) from 1980–82.

Despite a rigorous schedule as an educator, researcher, and related professional activities, Johnson was also very involved in school, church, and community activities. She and her husband served as Girl Scout and Boy Scout leaders and were active in the Parent Teacher Association (PTA). Johnson served as president of the PTA at North High School and was an honorary life member of the Nebraska PTA. She was a Sunday school teacher at Trinity United Methodist Church.

Johnson's commitment to the black community was shown through her efforts to establish a health-care clinic and other social services in northeast Omaha, the heart of the black population in the 1960s. She served as vice-president of Northeast Omaha Health Services, Inc., and later as a member of the executive board of Community Plaza for Human Resources. These organizations and their leaders were responsible for bringing needed services to the people of the community. Much of the work was done by Johnson and other nurses who donated their time for health screening, health teaching, and referral to other professionals.

Johnson's research on territoriality in the institutionalized elderly and the life satisfaction of rural and urban elderly persons was beginning to attract national attention in the early 1980s. It seemed certain that she would make significant contributions to the care of the increasing number of older people in our population, when her life and career were cut short by her death on November 3, 1982, at age 51, after a yearlong battle with pancreatic cancer. She was survived by her husband, Van; daughters, Vanetta and Valerie; mother, Vera Powell; and sister, Robbie Bean. Her body was donated to medical science, and memorial services were held on November 14, 1982, at Trinity United Methodist Church. Hundreds of relatives and friends attended the service to show their love and respect for a remarkable woman who had touched so many lives in such special ways. Memorial funds received after her death were used to establish the Freddie Powell Johnson and Class of 1952 Nursing Scholarship through the University of Nebraska Foundation.

PUBLICATIONS BY FREDDIE LOUISE POWELL JOHNSON

"Territorial Behavior of Nursing Home Residents." *Issues in Mental Health Nursing* 1 (Spring 1978): 43–52.

"Responses to Territorial Intrusion By Nursing Home Residents." *Advances in Nursing Science* 1 (July 1979): 21–34.

With Hatcher, W. "The Patient With Sickle Cell Anemia." *Nursing Forum* 13 (1974): 259–88.

With Foxall, M.J., E. Cook, E. Kelleher, E. Kentopp, and E.A. Mannlein, "Life Satisfaction of the Elderly American Indian." *White Cloud Journal* 3 (1984): 3–13.

With Foxall, M.H., M. Kidwell-Udin, G. Miller, and M.E. Stolzer. "Life Satisfaction in the Minority Elderly." *Issues in Mental Health Nursing* 6 (1984): 189–207.

With Cook, E., M.J. Foxall, E. Kelleher, E. Kentopp, and E.A. Mannlein. "Life Satisfaction of the Elderly American Indian." *International Journal of Nursing Studies* 23 (1986): 265–73.

With Foxall, M.H., E. Kelleher, E. Kentopp, E.A. Mannlein, and E. Cook. "Comparison of Mental Health and Life Satisfaction of Five Elderly Ethnic Groups." *Western Journal of Nursing Research* 10 (October 1988): 613–18.

BIBLIOGRAPHY

"Dr. Johnson Dies of Cancer." Obituary. *Omaha World-Herald*, November 5, 1982.

"Memorial Services for Dr. Johnson Saturday." *Omaha Star*, November 11, 1982.

Schneckloth, N.W. *University of Nebraska College of Nursing: 1917–1987* Omaha: University of Nebraska Medical Center, 1987.

Yeaworth, R.C. Memorial Tribute. Annual Business Meeting of the Midwest Nursing Research Society (April 12, 1983), Iowa City, Iowa.

Nancy Warren Schneckloth

Sally May Johnson
1880–1957

An innovator in both nursing and nursing education, Sally May Johnson introduced new courses of study and new categories of nursing workers to meet the demands of an expanding profession. She was superintendent of nurses and director of the School of Nursing at Massachusetts General Hospital from 1920–46 and received the Florence Nightingale Medal.

A native of New England, Johnson was born in East Morris, Connecticut, on May 10, 1880, to Francis and Statira Judson Johnson. Her parents were of English descent, and her father was a farmer. Her one brother was 11 years older.

After obtaining her elementary education at a one-room district school, Johnson attended high school in nearby Litchfield. She commuted by horse and buggy with a cousin, who later entered medicine and who influenced her thinking about her career.

After graduating from the New Britain Normal School in 1898, Johnson spent nine years teaching Grade 5 in the Winsted, Connecticut, public schools, near her birthplace.

In August 1907 she entered the Massachusetts General Hospital Training School for Nurses. She spent a month as a relief supervisor in the school's office before graduating in 1910 and later took a six-month postgraduate course in psychiatry at McLean Hospital. Waverley, Massachusetts. In 1932 she received a B.S. degree from Teachers College, Columbia University.

After leaving McLean, Johnson spent a year as an instructor in practical nursing at St. Luke's Hospital, New Bedford, Massachusetts. She then became an instructor and, in 1913, assistant superintendent of nurses at Peter Bent Brigham Hospital School of Nursing in Boston. There it was her style to seize every possible opportunity for teaching on the wards. In later years the hospital presented her with a pin and honorary diploma in recognition of her work.

Beginning in January 1917, she served as superintendent of nurses and principal of the School of Nursing at Albany (New York) Hospital. Under her influence, the duty time of special nurses was reduced from 24 to 12 hours. With the onset of World War I, she organized the nursing service of the hospital's American Red Cross Base Hospital, which she placed under the direction of her assistant when it was sent overseas.

On leave from Albany, she directed the Army School of Nursing at Walter Reed Hospital in Washington, D.C., and taught courses in nursing there from July 1, 1918, until the November signing of the Armistice.

She began 26 years of service as superintendent of nurses and principal of the Massachusetts General Hospital School of Nursing on October 1, 1920; before her, none had held the position longer than a decade.

Immediately, Johnson set out to improve student programs. She was instrumental in establishing a coordinated program with Radcliffe College under which students graduated with both a diploma and a baccalaureate degree in nursing. She used regular inventories to standardize ward equipment and enhanced the curriculum and the correlation of theory and practice. During her tenure the school doubled and then trebled in enrollment, and nearly 2,000 nurses graduated from the program.

In the hospital she introduced several new specialized categories of workers, including ward helper, ward secretary, staff nurse, and assistant nurse. She was a leader in securing an eight-hour day for private-duty nurses and payment of salaries wholly in cash.

In 1923 she began serving also as superintendent of nurses at the Massachusetts Eye and Ear Infirmary and, beginning in 1930, directed the nursing service at Baker Memorial Hospital. She was an associate in nursing at Simons College.

During the period immediately following World War I, Johnson was active on the legislative committee of the New York State Nurses' Association.

She was a director of the National League of Nursing Education, the American Journal of Nursing Company, and the American Nurses' Association and was president of the New England Division of the ANA, the Massachusetts League, and the Suffolk County Directory for Nurses.

On October 16, 1939, the Massachusetts General Hospital Nurses' Alumnae Association presented the hospital with a portrait of Johnson painted by Emil Pollak-Ottendorf. In the portrait she wears the pins of Massachusetts General and Peter Bent Brigham hospitals. She received the Florence Nightingale Medal of the International Red Cross in 1937.

Johnson died at Phillips House of Massachusetts General Hospital on March 24, 1937, of an infarction of the cerebellum and cerebro-vascular disease.

PUBLICATIONS BY SALLY MAY JOHNSON

"Intake, Output and Treatment Charts." *American Journal of Nursing* 24 (October 1924): 1035–37.

"A Trial of the Eight-Hour Day for Special Nurses." *Bulletin of the American Hospital Association* 9 (January 1935): 123–30.

"How One Nurse Superintendent Surmounts Wartime Obstacles." *Hospital Management* 58 (September 1944): 66, 68, 70, 72.

"A Nursing Council Plans for Field Experience." *Public Health Nursing* 40 (March 1948): 133–35, 150.

With others. "Practical Objectives in Nursing Education." *National League of Nursing Education Annual Report, 1924,* and *Proceedings of the 30th Convention.* Baltimore: Williams & Wilkins, 1925. Pp. 174–80.

BIBLIOGRAPHY

"Alumnae Association Affairs: Alumnae Present Miss Johnson's Portrait." *American Journal of Nursing* 39 (December 1939): 1387–88.

Hall, C.M. "Sally Johnson." National League of Nursing Education (n.d.).

"Miss Sally M. Johnson." *New York Times,* March 25, 1957, 25.

"Obituaries: Sally M. Johnson." *American Journal of Nursing* 57 (May 1957): 650–51.

Alice P. Stein

Elizabeth Rinker Kratz Jones

1868–1937

Elizabeth Rinker Kratz Jones was one of the pioneers in military nursing during the Spanish American War.

Jones was born in Hilltown, Bucks County, Pennsylvania, on September 18, 1868, the daughter of Dr. and Mrs. Harvey Kratz. She had at least one brother and one sister. The family in 1890 moved to New Britain, Pennsylvania.

On May 12, 1893, Kratz entered into nurses training at the Blockley Hospital (later to become known as the Philadelphia General Hospital School of Nursing). After completing her training in 1895, she remained at the hospital for another year, and from 1896–97 she was a nurse at Dr. E. E. Montgomer's Private Hospital in Philadelphia. For a brief period she also nursed the elderly in Ohio.

When the Spanish American War broke out, she volunteered as an army contract nurse. From August 2, 1898, to September 3, 1899, she was stationed at a 200-bed hospital in Fort Meyer, Virginia. On January 17, 1899, she embarked on the U.S. Army transport *Manitoba,* bound for Cuba, where she served at Velado for seven months and later in Havana. It was not until 1901 that a letter appointing her to the Army Nurse Corps, which had been mailed two years earlier, finally caught up with her. She attended the first annual Spanish-American War Nurses' Convention in 1901 in Washington, D.C., and attended the reception for the nurses held by President and Mrs. Theodore Roosevelt.

On her return to the United States she first became head nurse of Delaware Hospital, Wilmington, and then held a similar position at Meadville Hospital in Pennsylvania. On December 15, 1901, she returned to Philadelphia to care for smallpox patients at the Municipal Hospital and worked there until March 1904. At that time she joined a group of nurses who had been recruited by Dr. Anita Newcomb McGee for work in Japan to care for the Japanese wounded during the Russo-Japanese War. The group worked without pay, but they did demonstrate to the Japanese the importance of good nursing. Jones was made a life member of the Japanese Red Cross for her help in educating Japanese women about nursing skills.

From 1905–08 she worked as head nurse of the Men's Medical Department of the Episcopal Hospital in Philadelphia. In 1908 she was invited to be a head nurse at the California State Hospital in Patton but turned that down in order to go to Panama, where she nursed ill workers constructing the Panama Canal. On her return she went to Boise, Idaho, where she had family, and then she started a nursing home in Washington State with another nurse. She later served as head nurse at Wenatchee Hospital in that state. It was here that she met her husband, Theodore Everett Jones. The two were married on February 21, 1911. They made their home in Sequin, Washington. As was customary at the time, Jones retired from nursing after her marriage, and she and her husband operated a fishing boat until his death in 1929. However, Jones continued to keep in touch with her former colleagues and attended the reunion of the 35th Encampment of the Spanish-American War Veterans in 1933.

She spent the last years of her life in Burbank, California, where she died in November 1937.

BIBLIOGRAPHY

Archives. Pennsylvania Hospital, Philadelphia.

Matthew, I. Telephone interview by Lilli Sentz, 1990.

West, R.M. *History of Nursing in Pennsylvania.* Philadelphia: Pennsylvania State Nurses' Association, 1926.

Francine Wallace and Lilli Sentz

Frederick W. Jones

ca. 1890–ca. 1948

Frederick W. Jones was closely associated with the development and restructuring of the curricula of two distinguished men's nursing schools in the United States. Jones first served as the director of the reorganized Mills School of the Bellevue and Allied Hospitals Training School for Nurses, in New York City, from 1921–29. He was subsequently recruited to organize and develop the St. Vincent's Hospital School of Nursing for Men Nurses, in New York City. He remained as the director of St. Vincent's Men's School from 1930 until the school's closure in 1938. During the years that he provided decisive educational leadership in these institutions, he was responsible for instituting improvements in the curriculum that resulted in the advancement of quality professional education for men in nursing.

When Jones was admitted to the Mills School of the Bellevue and Allied Hospitals Training School for Nurses on February 11, 1909, he listed an address in Manchester, New Hampshire, as his home. He resided in New York City during his years in nursing school and remained in the New York City area throughout his lengthy career in nursing education.

Jones completed all course requirements at the Mills School on January 18, 1911. His class was the last to graduate from what was later called "the old Mills Training School at Bellevue Hospital." Shortly after the 1911 class graduated, the Mills Training School altered its curriculum from one in which men were provided with the education to become registered nurses to one in which men were only prepared as male orderlies.

After graduation in 1911, Jones worked for a short time as an assistant at the Mills School during the period when its mission was to train male orderlies. He resigned in January 1912 but returned in July 1912 to take charge of the dispensary. He was rapidly promoted to the position of head nurse and in January 1913 was made supervising nurse at Bellevue Hospital.

His career at the Mills School was interrupted during World War I. During the early days of the war Jones volunteered for service and went abroad to serve in the Chanticleer Ambulance Service, where he remained until the Armistice was signed. He was wounded during the war and was later decorated by the French government for his meritorious service in the Ambulance Corps.

Former students relate that Jones was very reticent about his personal life but proudly displayed his medals in his office at the St. Vincent's school. He never married and seldom disclosed any information about his background or personal life to his colleagues or to his students. He had a sister living in Brooklyn, whom he visited on the rare occasions he allowed himself a respite away from his professional duties.

In 1920 the Mills School was fortunately once again reorganized to meet its original professional mission of educating men to be qualified to take the New York State Board examination to become registered nurses. The orderly training program was discontinued, and the nursing program was reinstituted and restructured under Jones's initiative. Jones was appointed as the first director of the reorganized Mills School in 1920. By 1925 he had the additional title of superintendent of nurses, along with the related responsibilities. Jones provided vigorous leadership in these positions until he left the school in 1929.

Written testimonials including the "Fifty-Second Report of the Bellevue Training School for Nurses," attest to his accomplishments during the eight important years when the school rebuilt its reputation as an excellent educational institution that prepared men for careers as registered nurses. An expanded nursing curriculum, which included such innovations as a more lengthy three-year course of study, and extensive theoretical instruction in addition to practical experience, was offered under his direction.

Several student publications, official reports, and school handbooks, published during those years recognized Jones for his excellent abilities as a teacher. He was also cited for his understanding and fair treatment of his students.

Jones's recruitment as the founding director at St. Vincent's School for Men Nurses was considered a key factor necessary to the establishment of this new school of nursing for men in New York City. He was successfully recruited from his position at the Mills School, and in 1929 he began the difficult steps that were necessary to organize and operate the School for Men Nurses at the St. Vincent's Hospital School of Nursing.

Under his leadership the school was opened in February 1930. Fourteen male students were admitted during the first year of operation. A nursing school for women at St. Vincent's had been in place for a number of years. The two schools, however, remained completely separate in curriculum and instruction.

In addition to serving as the founding director of the men's school at St. Vincent's, Jones also instructed some nursing classes. The school offered a three-year course of instruction, which included courses in the basic sciences, materia medica, urological nursing, psychology, massage, nutrition, professional ethics, and professional problems, as well as many additional courses related to specialty areas of nursing practice. Applicants had to be in the upper one-third of their senior high-school class, indicating that acceptance standards were rigorous.

The School for Men Nurses grew rapidly in size and reputation until unfortunate financial difficulties related to the St. Vincent's School of Nursing for Women's affiliation with the College of Mount St. Vincent made the separate existence of the school for men no longer viable. Thus the St. Vincent's School for Men Nurses closed in 1938.

Additional information about Jones's professional career and personal life, after the school's closing, is fragmentary. A letter that Jones wrote to a former student in June 1947 notes that he remained at St. Vincent's Hospital as personnel manager until September 1946. He subsequently accepted a position at the Hospital of the Holy Family in Brooklyn, beginning in November 1946. The date of his death is uncertain, but on the basis of historical materials available, it is believed to be during 1948.

Throughout his nursing career, Frederick W. Jones maintained a commitment to the promotion of high standards of educational preparation for men nurses. Under his professional direction, during the years he served as the director of the Mills School and at St. Vincent's, he achieved his goal through the quality instruction based on innovative curricula that he insisted upon in the programs under his direction.

PUBLICATIONS BY FREDERICK W. JONES

"Men Nurses in the United States." *International Nursing Review* 6 (March 1931): 142–44.

"Vocational Opportunities for Men Nurses." *American Journal of Nursing* 34 (February 1934): 131–33.

BIBLIOGRAPHY

Byrne, Sr. M.L. "A History of St. Vincent's Hospital School of Nursing." Ph.D. dissertation, Catholic University of America, 1941.

"Class History." In Mills Training School *Annual*, 1931. P. 32.

Correspondence with Carol Clarke, associate executive director, Nursing/Patient Care Services Administration, Bellevue Hospital Center, New York City.

Correspondence with graduates of St. Vincent's School of Nursing for Men: Cyril Speicher, Joseph E. Lorenz, Charles F. Sipos.

Correspondence with Lorinda Klein, assistant director, Bellevue History Project, Bellevue Hospital Center, New York City.

Dolan, J.A. *Goodnow's History of Nursing*, 10th ed. Philadelphia: Saunders, 1958. P. 272.

Downey, J.F. "The Future of Men in Nursing." *Trained Nurse and Hospital Review* 75 (September 1925): 258–61.

"Fifty-Second Report of the Bellevue Training School for Nurses," 1925. P. 33.

"History of Mills School." Student Handbook. Mills School of Nursing for Men, New York City, n.d.

Minutes of the meeting of the Executive Committee of the Board of Managers of the Bellevue and Mills Schools of Nursing, November 1, 1921.

"My Oath." Fiftieth-anniversary publication of the Mills School of Nursing. New York: Bellevue Hospital, 1937.

Nash, H.H. "Men Nurses in New York State: Historical Sketch with Notes on Present Problems." *Trained Nurse and Hospital Review* 97 (August 1936): 123–29.

Prospectus. New York: St. Vincent's Hospital School of Nursing for Men, 1935.

Speicher, C. "St. Vincent's Men's School of Nursing." *Alumnae Newsletter* 28 (Spring 1986).

Walsh, Sr. M. de L. *With A Great Heart: The Story of St. Vincent's Hospital and Medical Center of New York, 1849–1964*. New York: St. Vincent's Hospital and Medical Center of New York, 1965.

Karen L. Buchinger

Catherine M. Kain
1909–1963

As chief nursing advisor to the Agency for International Development (AID), Catherine M. Kain was responsible for sending American nurses and American nursing skills throughout the world. From 1947 until her death she recruited the majority of professional nurses serving AID in 19 countries. She directed her actions toward improving all facets of health care and made a major effort to convince foreign governments to spend more money on health services and education as a basis of social consciousness and economic development.

Kain, born January 11, 1909 in Milwaukee, Wisconsin, was the youngest child of James S. Kain and Isabelle McHugh Kain. Her sister, Mary Isabelle, was the oldest in the family with her brother, James Simon, next in age. Their parents died within six months of each other when Kain was 10 or 12 years old, and her aunt was appointed the children's guardian. Kain attended Immaculate Conception Catholic Grade School and St. John's Cathederal Catholic High School in Milwaukee. Perhaps because her mother had been a nurse and because she based all her actions on a strong Christian philosophy, the 16-year-old Kain entered St. Mary's Hospital School of Nursing in her hometown on August 29, 1925.

Her 96 classmates soon became aware of her as a dedicated and conscientious student. She missed only one day of training—on March 26, 1927, when she went home because of a death in the family. She graduated from nursing school on July 31, 1928. Her interest in and awareness of other people made everyone feel as if they were her or his best friend, and throughout her life she kept up a large correspondence with people she met during her varied career.

After graduation, while working at St. Mary's Hospital, Kain attended Marquette University, where she earned her B.S. degree in 1931. She continued graduate school at Marquette and at the University of Washington in Seattle before World War II. The war interrupted her formal education, but she returned to school in the early 1950s, obtaining her M.S. from Catholic University of America, Washington, D.C., in 1953.

As part of her career, Kain felt it important to be active in local and national nursing organizations. She was assistant registrar of the Milwaukee District Nurses' Association and a member of the board of directors of the Wisconsin League for Nurses from 1932–33. She also served on the International Affairs Committee for the American Nurses' Association. Though away from the state for many years, she always retained her membership in the Wisconsin Nurses' Association. For a time she was secretary for the National Committee of the American Nurses' Association. As her interests widened, she joined the American Public Health Association and the Association for Military Surgeons.

From 1933 until 1940 Kain was educational director of St. Mary's School of Nursing. Then, moving to the state of Washington, she became an instructor at the Seattle College of Nursing, 1940–42. One of her former students remembers her as an exacting but supportive teacher who set high standards for herself and her pupils.

When World War II began, she joined the U.S. Navy as a lieutenant commander in the Navy Nurse Corps. Her assignments included director of the Navy Cadet Nurses, U.S. Naval Hospital, Portsmouth, Virginia, and chief nurse of the U.S. Naval Operating Base Dispensary, Rio de Janeiro, Brazil. In South America she spent 16 months supervising the care of navy men hospitalized in the American wing of the Brazilian Air Force Hospital. In 1946 she received a commendation for her work in Brazil from the commander-in-chief of the U.S. Atlantic Fleet.

After the war Kain returned to Brazil as a consultant nurse in the field party of the Health and Sanitation Division of the Institute of Inter-American Affairs. The role played by American nursing advisors serving in the United States foreign-aid programs began with a project in Brazil in 1943, proceeded through the development of a format of operation under the Point IV Program introduced by President Harry Truman after World War II, and later continued under the Agency for International Development.

Truman's fourth major point in the foreign-policy part of his January 20, 1949, inaugural address proposed that since more than half the world's population were living in conditions approaching misery, victims of disease and starvation, the United States should embark on a bold new program for making the benefits of scientific advances and industrial progress available for the improvement and growth of underdeveloped areas. Kain agreed completely and felt that although health was only one part of the AID program for developing areas of the world, no other technical activity of foreign aid better fostered close personal communication between the American advisor and the people of the assigned country. After her assignment in Brazil, Kain continued her work, becoming the regional nursing advisor in Latin America. She served as a consultant nurse in Santiago, where she received an honorary degree from the University of Chile.

In 1958 she accepted the post of chief nursing advisor of AID. Her position required extensive travel in Asia, the Middle East, Africa, and Latin America along with a speaking knowledge of the languages and customs of the countries involved with the agency. She believed that the role played by American nursing advisors serving in the United States foreign-aid programs was as important to the security of the United States as it was to the social and economic growth of the countries in which these programs were in operation.

Kain educated the AID nursing personnel to meet emergency needs, to improve health services and educational facilities, and to train national nursing professionals. She also wanted AID nurses to set up long-range programs to continue after the AID people were withdrawn. Under her guidance, whatever the health related activity was in an individual country, all AID nursing projects were designed to upgrade nursing practices and develop or improve educational institutions. However, she realized that in each country the advisor confronted a different level of development and different cultural traditions. The nurse's success depended upon her ability to cope with these differences while keeping in mind the social and economic development of the country, as well as the U.S. relations with it.

Kain insisted that all projects reflect the correct stage of development of the country where the advisory nurse was assigned. Where modern health concepts were just beginning to emerge, she stressed the most basic public-health standards and training. Under more advanced circumstances, the nursing advisor helped with the standardization of school curriculum, the translation of texts, and the establishment of a nursing code and licensing procedures. Particular emphasis was placed on preparation of local leaders to continue the programs. Kain had trained many foreign nurses herself while on assignment in other countries, so she had the practical experience necessary to help the Americans establish health programs for native professionals.

In order to further educate these professionals, Kain encouraged AID to make contracts with American universities, not only to accept foreign students, but also to provide the university personnel and technical assistance for nursing education abroad. After Kain's death her colleagues at the Catholic University of America (CUA) set up a memorial fund in her name to be used to assist foreign students enrolled in the CUA School of Nursing who had to support themselves.

Kain also considered it important to coordinate the nursing advisor's projects with the programs of other international organizations. AID joined with the World Health Organization and the United Nations Children's Fund in the battle to control disease. It also cooperated closely with other U.S. government organizations, such as the National Institutes of Health, the Peace Corps, the Defense Department and the U.S. Public Health Service. Collaborating private organizations included the Association of American Medical Schools, the Rockefeller and Kellogg foundations, and the National League for Nursing.

Kain felt that it was a part of her mission to try to free all peoples from their basic problems of illness and poverty. She knew that good health was an important part of a country's strength, both in self-help toward social and economic achievement and in defense of its own independence. She wanted to help all countries gain full and self-sustaining membership in a world dedicated to peace and progress. At the time of her death, 71 nursing advisors assisted with health projects in 42 countries. Of these, 44 were direct employees of AID. When Kain received a letter of commendation from the U.S. surgeon general for her work, the assistant administrator of AID declared that it was an understatement to just label Kain as their chief nursing advisor since her influence went far beyond what the title would imply.

Though she had spent many years away from her birthplace, when her health began to fail, she returned to Whitefish Bay near Milwaukee to be with her brother and sister and to spend some time with friends in Suring, Wisconsin. While there, her condition deteriorated, so she returned to Milwaukee and immediately entered St. Mary's Hospital. Critically ill with cancer, Kain is reported to have said, "I am home now." Thus her illustrious nursing career ended where it began, and she died the next day, October 30, 1963.

In 1965 the St. Mary's School of Nursing Alumnae Association donated a portrait of Kain to the school library, and the library was dedicated as the Catherine Kain Memorial Library. A plaque in her memory was placed on the door.

PUBLICATIONS BY CATHERINE M. KAIN

"Nursing and the Agency for International Development." *Nursing Outlook* 11 (December 1963): 902–04.

BIBLIOGRAPHY

"AID Nursing Chief Died." *Nursing Outlook* 11 (December 1963): 860.

"Catherine Kain, Nursing Expert." *Washington Post,* November 1, 1963, C6.

"Five Wisconsin Nurses." *Wisconsin Nurses Association Bulletin* 33 (January–February 1964): 8.

Kain M. (Mrs. James S. Kain). Telephone conversation with the author, May 27, 1989.

"News." *American Journal of Nursing* 47 (June 1947): 224.

"News of War Nurses–New Chief Nurse." *Trained Nurse and Hospital Review* 114 (June 1945): 429.

Oberbreckling, C.M., ed. *St. Mary's School of Nursing 1894–1969.* Milwaukee: Alumnae Association, St. Mary's School of Nursing, 1969. Pp. 37–38.

"Obituaries." *American Journal of Nursing* 64 (January 1964): 52, 54.

St. Mary's Hospital School of Nursing Roll Call—September 1924–August 1934. Madison: Wisconsin State Historical Society Archives, 1934.

"Students' Loans Memorialize State Department Nurse." *American Journal of Nursing* 64 (July 1964): 148.

Mary Van Hulle Jones

Mildred Keaton

1898–1980

She feared the white fury of neither storm nor polar bear. Carried her medicines in her mukluks so they wouldn't freeze. Smoked a pipe as she drove her dog sled "to keep my nose warm." She was Mildred Keaton, traveling nurse for the Bureau of Indian Affairs in Alaska. In her 45 years of service, thousands of grateful Indians and rural settlers came to revere her as "the angel in furs" and "the most beloved woman in Alaska." A popular saying of the time was: "When it's too rough outdoors for man or beast, call the traveling nurse."

Of Irish lineage, Keaton was born to J.P. and Ella Jane (Huffman) Keaton in Carter County, Kentucky, in 1898. Her 10 brothers called her "Buster" and instilled in her the rugged stamina and love of adventure that characterized her maverick style of nursing.

The family moved to Alabama, then Wyoming, and finally to Snohomish, Washington. She attended a girls' school in Alabama and finished her elementary and secondary schooling in Snohomish.

Keaton attended the University of Washington at Seattle and considered careers in both medicine and music. She began her nurse's training at Providence Hospital, Everett, Washington, and completed it at St. Peter's Hospital in Olympia, Washington.

Her early nursing was done in and near Snohomish. She was a nurse for the Three Lakes Lumber Company from 1917–21, a surgical assistant at Snohomish Hospital, and private-duty nurse at Providence Hospital from 1921–23.

According to one account, a toss of a coin led her to her true calling. It is said that two public-health positions were advertised, one in Alaska and the other in Hawaii. She and another interested nurse tossed for them, and Keaton drew Alaska. For the next 22 years, she worked in a succession of nursing positions that took her all over Alaska. She began as a village nurse in Kake from 1924–27 and spent the next year in Juneau as a surgical nurse at St. Anne's Hospital and superintendent of the Juneau American Legion Baby Clinic. For the following three years, she was a surgical nurse at Juneau's Alaska Native Service Hospital.

She was a field nurse in the Alaska Native Service from 1932–36. Training her own dogs, she traveled by sled, Coast Guard cutter, and Eskimo boat to bring nursing service to Indians on the Kotzebue and Seward peninsulas.

She helped victims of the Nome fire of 1934 and the influenza epidemic that struck Point Barrow, Point Lay, and Wainwright in 1935. She worked among nomadic Eskimos on the Arctic Slope from 1936–41, making 1,800-mile annual trips from Point Barrow to Demarcation Point by dog sled. During this time she gathered data on the Eskimos for the government. When World War II struck, she helped to evacuate natives from the Aleutian Islands and worked aboard the Coast Guard cutter *North Star.* For eight months in 1941 she was in sole charge of the Barrow Hospital, at which time it was without a physician.

Her knack for making friends and her wilderness survival skills won her wide acceptance and respect in the sparsely populated area that she served. She performed medical procedures not ordinarily assigned to a nurse such as appendectomies and dental extractions. She was often called upon to serve as judge, marshal, commissioner, and interpreter as well as nurse. News of her daring exploits spread throughout the continent, and in 1937 she was featured in an article in *Collier's Magazine.*

In Nome, from 1943–46, she served as a field nurse. She left the Indian Service in 1947 and returned to Washington but was back in Nome in 1951 for a two-year assignment as a welfare agent for the Lower Kuskokwim and Yukon River valleys. She worked as head of the White Pass Hospital at Skagway and spent about a decade as a nurse for the White Pass and Yukon Railroad in southeastern Alaska. From 1964–72 she was a volunteer nurse in the Cooper River Boarding School at Glenallen.

Retiring in 1972, she returned to Snohomish to live with a brother, Robert, who had made his career with the Alaska Juneau gold mine. She died in a Snohomish nursing home May 15, 1980, and within 90 minutes, her brother, too, was dead.

Keaton was a member of the National Red Cross Nursing Service and the National Organization for Public Health Nursing.

BIBLIOGRAPHY

"Biographical Sketches: Women's History Month #19." Typescript. Anchorage: Alaska Women's Commission. Undated.

"Keaton, Mildred Huffman." *Tewksbury's Who's Who in Alaska.* Juneau, n.p. 1947. P. 43.

Courtney, W.B. "Angel in Furs." *Collier's Magazine* 100 (November 20, 1937): 67.

"Mildred H. Keaton." *Anchorage Times,* June 6, 1980.

"Mildred H. Keaton." *Alaska Magazine* (August 1980).

Alice P. Stein

Manelva Wylie Keller
?–1965

Manelva Wylie Keller was a nurse, photographer, and author whose photographic work facilitated identification of pathological conditions. She was instrumental in establishing the photographic service offered by St. Luke's Hospital in New York City and operated it from 1921–50. She originated and edited *St. Luke's Hospital Bulletin,* and was coauthor of the *Textbook of Surgical Nursing,* which became a standard textbook in many schools of nursing. She also wrote and edited the *History of the St. Luke's Hospital Training School for Nurses,* published in 1938.

Keller was born in Sulphur Springs, Ohio, of Dutch and Scottish descent. After attending primary and secondary schools in Sulphur Springs, she transferred to Heidelberg Preparatory School in Tiffin, Ohio. She received a B.S. degree in 1906 from Heidelberg College, where her uncle was on the faculty. She was the first female editor of *The Kilikilik,* Heidelberg's student newspaper.

At the time, about the only career open to a female with a college degree was teaching, and Keller determined to do what was expected of her. She really wanted to be a newspaper reporter, but that was socially unacceptable. She began as a substitute teacher and, in the course of the next few years, taught every primary and secondary grade. However, she disliked teaching's disciplinary aspects and sought the advice of the dean of women at Heidelberg on an alternative career. The dean suggested nursing, and Keller, still without enthusiasm, entered St. Luke's Hospital Training School for Nurses in 1907. She was one of the few college graduates in the school.

After graduation in 1910, Keller served successively as graduate assistant night supervisor, operating-room assistant, and chief operating-room nurse. In 1912 she became the hospital's first nurse anesthetist. On October 3, 1914, she began a tour of duty at Hospital B of the American ambulance unit in Neuilly and then Paris, France. She returned to the United States to teach home nursing for the Red Cross.

Then in 1917, with the United States at war, she served with the Presbyterian Hospital Unit, Base Hospital No. 2. Later, she transferred to Mobile Hospital No. 2 and remained with it until the signing of the Armistice. With the Army of Occupation, she served with the Mobile Unit at Trier, Germany.

Together with Dr. Ralph Colp, she wrote *Textbook of Surgical Nursing*. She did subsequent editions with other co-authors, and the book was reissued under her name alone in 1936.

Combining her interest in photography with her sensitivities as a nurse, she began taking pictures to document the work of a New York City physician, a Dr. Lyle. Together, they established the St. Luke's Hospital Photographic Service, which eventually included 7,000 plates. Until 1950 she held the position of clinical photographer at the hospital. From then until her retirement in 1952, she did special photographic assignments.

She was editor of the quarterly *St. Luke's Hospital Bulletin* from its inception in 1939 and illustrated it with her photographs. She wrote the hospital history at the request of Lincoln Cromwell, president of the board of managers, but her name does not appear on the title page.

After her retirement, Keller continued to work on the hospital alumnae roster. She died at the Long Island Home, South Oaks, Amityville, New York, on February 23, 1965.

PUBLICATIONS BY MANELVA WYLIE KELLER

BOOKS

Textbook of Surgical Nursing. New York: Macmillan, 1936.

History of St. Luke's Hospital Training School for Nurses. New York: St. Luke's Hospital, 1938.

BIBLIOGRAPHY

"Four Outstanding Graduates Die, . . . Manelva W. Keller." *St. Luke's Alumnae Bulletin* (Spring 1965): 16.

Hughes, A. "Miss Keller Retires." *St. Luke's Alumnae Bulletin* (Fall 1952): 4–5.

"Keller, Manelva Wylie '10." In *History of The St. Luke's Hospital Training School for Nurses*. New York: St. Luke's Hospital, 1938.

MacFee, William F. "Manelva W. Keller." *St. Luke's Hospital Bulletin* (October 1952): 3–5.

Makers of Nursing History. M.R. Pennock, ed. New York: Lakeside, 1940.

"Manelva Keller, '10, Receives Recognition of her Alma Mater." *St. Luke's Alumnae Bulletin* (December 1938): 11.

"Manelva Wylie Keller, B.S., R.N." *Trained Nurse and Hospital Review* 84 (February 1930): 210, 217.

Alice P. Stein

Dorothy Kelly
b. 1911

Dorothy Kelly has been a public-health nurse, writer, and editor of nursing publications. She was an early advocate of unity among nurses and of collective bargaining through the professional organizations. She is the sister of Mary Kelly Mullane, whose biography is included in this volume.

Kelly was born in New York City on March 6, 1911, the daughter of Thomas J. and Ann Nilan Kelly. She completed high school at the Academy of the Holy Cross in 1928. After graduating from Holy Name Hospital School of Nursing, Teaneck, New Jersey, in 1931, the same year as her older sister, Kelly entered the field of public-health nursing and worked in the Detroit Department of Public Health and the Montclair New Jersey Bureau of Public Health Nursing. She continued her education, earning a B.S. in nursing from Wayne State University, Detroit, in 1946 and a master's degree in public health from Harvard University in 1953.

For three and a half years during World War II Kelly was a member of the U.S. Army Nurse Corps, serving at a field hospital in India. From 1946 to 1953 she was assistant director of the Detroit Visiting Nurse Association, practicing with Emilie Sargent. During this time she began to write about nursing organizations for the *Michigan Nurse*, published by the Michigan Nurses' Association, and about administrative topics in the public-health field for other publications. Kelly became editor of the *Catholic Nurse* in 1954, continuing in this position until publication of that journal ceased in 1969. Concurrently, she served as executive director of the Council of Catholic Nurses until it was disbanded in 1970. She then became editor of *Supervisor Nurse*, retiring from that position in 1978.

Editorials written by Kelly during her tenure as editor of *Supervisor Nurse* were insightful and outspoken and addressed the variety of current concerns of the profession and of the working nurse. Kelly supported accountability of nursing service to the patient; she believed that direct accountability was a hallmark of a profession. A strong supporter of the American Nurses' Association (ANA), Kelly frequently called in her editorials for the right and responsibility of all nurses to belong to the ANA and to dialogue with that organization over perceived differences between the needs of the working nurse and the position of the ANA. She saw the ANA as the collective-bargaining body for all nurses. From 1964–68 she served on the ANA Committee on Economic and General Welfare and from 1968–72 on the ANA Commission on Economic and General Welfare.

In addition to her writing, Kelly was known as a speaker on behalf of nursing. She addressed many state nurses' associations as keynote speaker and also spoke for nursing at national conferences of nonnursing groups. Dorothy Kelly's distinguished service and contributions to the nursing profession were recognized in 1978 when she was presented the ANA Honorary Recognition Award at the association's biennial meeting.

Kelly's retirement years have been spent living with her sister, Mary Kelly Mullane, in Washington, D.C., and Florida, caring for older family members, traveling, and doing volunteer work.

PUBLICATIONS BY DOROTHY KELLY

"The Michigan Nursing Center Association." *Public Health Nursing* 40 (May 1948): 256.

"Automobile Plan in a Private Agency." *Public Health Nursing* 44 (June 1952): 338–39.

"Practical Nurse Students and the Cancer Patient." *American Journal of Nursing* 55 (April 1955): 454–56.

BIBLIOGRAPHY

"Dorothy Kelly Recipient of Honorary Recognition Award." *American Nurse* 10 (June 15, 1978): 10.

"70+ and Going Strong. Dorothy Kelly and Mary Mullane: Footloose and Fancy Free." *Geriatric Nursing* 3 (May/June 1982): 196–98.

Marianne Brook

Helen Winifred Kelly

1865–1956

Helen Winifred Kelly was an early leader in nursing in Wisconsin. Her fearlessness and determination helped pave the road for registration and organization of nurses in Wisconsin.

She was born on February 9, 1865, on a farm to Bernard and Sarah O'Connell Kelly in Monches, Wisconsin. Kelly graduated from the Illinois Training School for Nurses, also known as the Cook County Hospital School of Nursing, in Chicago in 1895.

Following graduation, she worked three to four years as a private-duty nurse. Her nursing career was varied and included positions such as the assistant superintendent at Illinois Training School, superintendent of nurses at the California Hospital, Los Angeles, principal of Milwaukee County Training School (1909), as well as superintendent at Mercy Hospital in Janesville, Wisconsin (1928). In 1924 Kelly became the registrar of the Wisconsin Nurses' Club and Registry in Milwaukee and was influential in this role in making nursing a powerful force in the Milwaukee area. She was also a supervisor of field nurses for the Chicago Department of Health. Her career also took her to Big Bend Desert, Washington, as a Red Cross public-health worker, and to Baker,

Oregon, where she organized school health work. Kelly also took postgraduate courses at Teachers College, Columbia University (at that time called hospital economics), the Chicago School of Civics and Philanthropy, the School of Sociology of Loyola University, Chicago, and the University of Chicago.

During her employment as superintendent of Milwaukee County Hospital of Nursing, Kelly became involved with Stella Mathews in attempting to organize the nurses in Wisconsin. A temporary organization was begun in 1909. Articles of incorporation of the Wisconsin State Nurses' Association were filed with the state on January 1910. At the time of incorporation the nurses were more regionally oriented than state minded. It was the legislative efforts regarding registration of nurses that united the group as a state organization, and Kelly played an instrumental role, serving as the state organization's first president. The association had decided to concentrate on registration in the 1913 legislative biennium, but a change of plans occurred when a bill was introduced in the 1911 legislative session. Though the association was not able to provide the input that would reflect the legislation that they had hoped for, the bill was enacted and marked the beginning of nurse registration in the state of Wisconsin. One of its provisions called for a survey of schools of nursing in Wisconsin, a project which Kelly carried out.

Kelly maintained high standards for herself as well as others. Her conviction that nurses maintain high standards was evident in her legislative efforts as well as her efforts in her work as a registrar. In 1924, she published an article in the *American Journal of Nurses* on "The Relation of the Private Duty Nurse to the Directory." In the article she alluded to the fact that nurses should only sign with official registries that have high standards and not any group that calls them for work.

Personal correspondence between Kelly and Edith Partridge, the executive secretary of the Wisconsin State Nurses' Association (1924–56) indicates that Kelly was very firm in her beliefs. For example, as editor of *An Historical Sketch*, the early

history of the Wisconsin State Nurses' Association, Kelly did not want to include the name of an individual in the credits because she did not believe the individual contributed enough to the book. She was very blunt and open with Partridge and refused to be swayed on the matter. When Partridge took the matters in her own hands, Kelly was respectful, but honest, in her reply to Partridge's action on the situation.

In addition to serving as the first president of the Wisconsin State Nurses' Association, Kelly served as president of her school of nursing alumnae group and as president of the First District Association of Illinois. Kelly received the first Red Cross Badge (No. 2100) issued through the Wisconsin Red Cross Committee and was a delegate to the International Council of Nurses (ICN) in 1912 in Cologne, Germany. In 1928 she was featured as "Who's Who in the Nursing World" in the *American Journal of Nursing.*

Helen Winifred Kelly lived to the age of 91. She died at Villa St. Ann in Oconomowoc, Wisconsin, on October 16, 1956. The nursing profession in the state of Wisconsin owes much of its history and prestige to this courageous and determined individual.

PUBLICATIONS BY HELEN WINIFRED KELLY

BOOKS

Editor. *An Historical Sketch.* Milwaukee: Wisconsin State Nurses' Association, 1935.

With M. Bradshaw. *A Handbook for School Nurses.* New York: Macmillan, 1918.

ARTICLES

"The Relation of the Private Duty Nurse to the Directory." *American Journal of Nursing* 24 (September 1924): 960–63.

BIBLIOGRAPHY

"Founder of WSNA Dies." *Bulletin of the Wisconsin State Nurses Association,* 25, No. 4 (Winter 1956): 4.

Kelly, H.W. Personal correspondence to Edith Partridge, 1934–35. Wisconsin State Historical Society, Madison, Wisconsin

"Who's Who in the Nursing World" (1928). *American Journal of Nursing* 28 (April 1928): 374.

Michaelene P. Mirr

Elizabeth L. Kemble

1907–1981

Elizabeth Kemble was the first dean of the school of nursing at the University of North Carolina at Chapel Hill. As dean, she established a nursing baccalaureate program and the first nursing master's degree program in the state. Prior to becoming dean at Chapel Hill, Kemble was director of the National League of Nursing Education's Department of Measurement and Guidance. As director, she was responsible for the expansion and coordination of educational testing programs for nursing students, practical nurses, and graduate nurses.

Elizabeth L. Kemble was born in 1907 in Greenville, Ohio. She received a diploma from the University of Cincinnati College of Nursing and Health and a B.S. from New York University. She was awarded an M.A. degree and Ed.D. from Columbia University.

Kemble held positions as assistant director, supervisor, and instructor at nursing schools in Ohio, New Jersey, and New York. She was also an instructor at St. Johns University, Hunter College, and New York University, in New York.

From 1941–45 Kemble was assistant, and later associate, director of the nurse testing division of the Psychological Corporation. In 1946 she became director of the Department of Measurement and Guidance of the National League of Nursing Education (NLNE). Her experience at the Psychological Corporation prepared her for the rapidly expanding NLNE testing department. Under her leadership the department expanded and improved testing tools for pre-admission, advanced placement, achievement tests for nursing students, practical-nurse testing, and graduate-nurse testing coordinated with a state board test pool.

Kemble successfully coordinated state licensing boards across the nation into the NLNE test pool managed by her department. Standard testing and licensing had long been a goal for nursing in the United States. Under Kemble's direction the Department of Measurement and Guidance experienced a dramatic in-crease in activity, including the registration of nurses and aptitude testing for nursing-school applicants.

In the articles that Kemble wrote about the programs and goals of her department she described the psychometric-testing process and outlined the role of her department in coordinating test development, testing, and scoring. The testing programs of the NLNE department were considered a service to the nursing profession and a factor in the increasing enrollment in nursing schools.

In 1950 Kemble was appointed as first dean of the nursing school of the University of North Carolina at Chapel Hill. She established the state's first baccalaureate program the following year, a master's level nursing program in 1955, and in 1963 a continuing-education program for nursing.

As dean, she sat on the board of the University's Division of Health Sciences. She served as chairman of the American Nurses' Association's Technical Committee to the Program of Studies of Nursing Functions, which reviewed research applications and awarded funding to study what nurses were doing and what they should do. Kemble was also a consultant to the surgeon general of the U.S. Air Force in the 1960s.

On November 16, 1963, she was presented with an award for her outstanding contribution to the profession by New York University's Department of Nursing Education. Kemble retired as dean in 1967 but continued to teach at Chapel Hill until 1971.

Elizabeth Kemble died in Raleigh, North Carolina, on November 30, 1982, at the age of 74 after suffering a long illness. Following her death, the American Nurses' Association placed a tribute to her in the association's record.

PUBLICATIONS BY ELIZABETH L. KEMBLE

"Shopping for a School of Nursing." *American Journal of Nursing* 42 (February 1942): 166–67.

"What Applicants Hope and Fear About Schools of Nursing." *American Journal of Nursing* 45 (October 1945): 829–30.

"Shorter and Sharper Testing Tools for the Pre-Nursing and Guidance Test Services." *American Journal of Nursing* 47 (May 1947): 327–30.

"The Value and Method of Administering Tests." *Journal of the American Association of Nurse Anesthetists* 17 (February 1949): 5–12, 74.

"International Aspects of the Testing Program." *American Journal of Nursing* 49 (February 1949): 113.

"This is Your Program of Research in Nursing Functions." *American Journal of Nursing* 51 (February 1951): 92–93.

"The Dean—Born or Made." *Nursing Outlook* 11 (October 1963): 737–40.

With E. Spaney. "Studying Students or Testing Teachers." *American Journal of Nursing* 47 (July 1947): 481–83.

With E. Spaney. "State Board Test Pool Examinations." *American Journal of Nursing* 47 (August 1947): 552–55.

BIBLIOGRAPHY

American Journal of Nursing 50 (August 1950): 28.

"Elizabeth L. Kemble Receives NYU Award." *Nursing Outlook* 12 (January 1964): 8.

"Elizabeth L. Kemble." Obituary. *American Journal of Nursing* 82 (February 1982): 320–21.

Kaufman, M., ed. *Dictionary of American Nursing Biography.* Wesport, Conn.: Greenwood, 1988.

"News from National Headquarters." *American Journal of Nursing* 46 (September 1946): 628; 50 (April 1950): 247.

Roberts, M.M. *American Nursing History and Interpretation.* New York: Macmillan, 1954.

Stewart, I.M. and A.L. Austin. *A History of Nursing.* New York: Putnam, 1962.

Susan N. Craft

CECELIA ROSE KENNEDY

1885–1981

A leader in Red Cross nursing both in the United States and abroad, Cecelia Rose Kennedy received the Distinguished Service Cross for her work during World War II.

Cecelia (also called Cecile) Kennedy was born in July 1885 in Drifton, Luzerne County, Pennsylvania, the eldest of nine children. Her mother was a music teacher and her father a mining engineer. The family moved often, and Kennedy spent part of her childhood in Schuykill County, Pennsylvania, in Oneida, New York, in West Virginia, and in Canada County, Pennsylvania. She attended high school at St. Mary's Academy in Scranton, Pennsylvania, and at the Atlantic High School and later took preparatory courses privately in order to qualify for college.

In 1906 she entered the Philadelphia General Hospital Nursing School at the advice of her aunt, who was a graduate of the school. Kennedy received her diploma in 1909. For several years she did private-duty nursing, traveling abroad with her patients. Between travels she attended night courses in social work at the University of Philadelphia. In 1916 she left for Europe to become a social worker with the Red Cross in England.

Three months before the Armistice of World War I she was transferred to France. When it was discovered that she was trained as a nurse, she worked in that capacity until the end of the war. She remained in Europe appraising the relief needs of war and civilian disasters and eventually became head of the disaster service for the International Red Cross with headquarters in Geneva.

In 1934 Kennedy returned to the United States. She took a position with the American Red Cross in Pennsylvania as a state relations officer, working as a liaison between the American Red Cross and public and private agencies at the state level. Because of her effectiveness, she was sent to many states on disaster-relief duty. She organized Gray Ladies Volunteer Programs in hospitals all over the country and taught the first classes herself in Pittsburgh, Pennsylvania. She also helped establish nationwide Red Cross courses in first aid, life saving, and home nursing.

During World War II Kennedy directed the Red Cross in Pennsylvania, for which she was awarded the Distinguished Service Medal, the first woman to be so honored. She also received citations from the governors of five states where she assisted in disaster relief. For many years she served as a special service representative between various Red Cross chapters in the East, maintaining normal peacetime activities to the community, such as home services, nursing, first aid, blood program, water safety, and accident prevention. She was offered a scholarship to Simmons College in Boston by the American Red Cross but decided instead to take a degree in social services from New York University.

Kennedy retired from the Red Cross in 1959 after 40 years of service. She continued to serve on President Eisenhower's Peace Committee and on the National Safety Council.

Possessing a keen sense of humor, Kennedy was a master of the art of public relations, and her eyes sparkled when she described her work. In her retirement she received honorary degrees from Villanova University and Duquesne University in Pittsburgh.

Kennedy died on January 9, 1981, at St. Francis Country Home, Darby, Pennsylvania.

BIBLIOGRAPHY

American Red Cross Archives, American Red Cross National Headquarters, Washington, D.C.

Matthews, I. Interview with the author. 1990.

Nunan, E. Transcript of oral interview with Kennedy in September 1977 and November 1978.

Philadelphia General Hospital Archives. Philadelphia, Pa.

Rabenstein, M. Transcript of oral interview with Kennedy in 1959.

Red Cross Courier April 1932; May 1939; August 1946; January 1948.

Lilli Sentz

Diana E. Clifford Kimber (Sister Mary Diana)
?–1928

Diana E. Clifford Kimber was the author of the first scientific book ever written by a nurse specifically for nurses. Her *Anatomy and Physiology for Nurses* was issued in repeated editions between 1893 and 1948.

The daughter of a prominent Oxfordshire, England, family, Kimber received a broad education in England and Germany. She came to the United States and entered the Bellevue Hospital Training School in 1884. There, she met several people who greatly influenced her life, including Louise Darche, who was to become her close friend and companion, and Lavinia Dock.

When she completed her training, she spent about six months as night superintendent and head of a surgical ward. She then became assistant superintendent of the Illinois Training School for Nurses, an affiliate of Cook County Hospital, serving under Isabel Hampton.

Late in 1887 Darche was named superintendent of the Training School for Nurses at Old Charity Hospital on Blackwell's Island (later Welfare Island), New York City, and asked Kimber to be her assistant. On January 1, 1888, they began a decade of service together in which the progress of the school was a product of their combined judgment and efforts to promote the school in the face of political conflict. Darche conducted the public dealings, while Kimber planned the curriculum and taught. It was her desire to serve her students better that prompted her to write her textbook.

In 1897 Kimber presented a plea for an equitable schedule and salary scale for nurses at the fourth annual convention of the American Association of Superintendents of Training Schools.

When Darche's deteriorating health forced her to resign in February 1898, Kimber assumed her duties for the remainder of the academic year. She then took Darche back to England and nursed her until Darche died.

After living at home for a time, Kimber

joined an Anglican sisterhood, taking residence in the Convent of the Holy Name in Malvern. The chief work of the sisterhood was public-health nursing among the poor in England's large manufacturing cities. Kimber worked to establish more economical private-duty nursing for people of moderate or modest means, using district nurses and charging on an hourly basis. She also contributed to the welfare of sick nurses.

At the convent Kimber at last found time to indulge her lifelong enthusiasm for gardening and became noted for her roses. In October 1927 her already frail health began to fail, and she died at the convent on January 11, 1928.

PUBLICATIONS BY
DIANA E. CLIFFORD KIMBER

With C.E. Gray. *Anatomy and Physiology for Nurses.* New York: Macmillan, 1893, 1902, (subsequent editions to 1948 with various secondary authors).

BIBLIOGRAPHY

"Diana Clifford Kimber." *American Journal of Nursing* 28 (May 1928): 486–87.

Dolan, J.A. *Nursing in Society.* Philadelphia: Saunders, 1973. PP. 209, 258.

Pennock, M.R. ed. *Makers of Nursing History.* New York: Lakeside, 1928. Pp. 80–81.

Alice P. Stein

Gladys Kiniery

1904–1988

Gladys Kiniery was a pioneer in baccalaureate education in the state of Illinois. As the dean of the Loyola University School of Nursing, the first accredited baccalaureate program in the state, and as a nursing leader in the state, Kiniery was influential in upgrading nursing education throughout Illinois. She later had the important role of the staff person responsible for the evaluation report of the first national Nurse Training Act. She had a sense of purpose in upgrading nursing education and dedication to the concept of quality education as a means to improve patient care.

Kiniery was born on November 14, 1904, in Footville, Wisconsin, the ninth of 10 children born to William and Julia Kiniery. Her father, an Irish immigrant, had come to Wisconsin with the help of his uncle to work in railroad construction. He built a hotel (the Hotel Canary), where he rented rooms and lived with his family. He was involved in construction, livery, and real estate. Gladys' mother not only took care of her children, but cooked for the railroad workers as well.

Kiniery attended high school in Janesville, Wisconsin, and Mercy Hospital School of Nursing there. Following graduation in 1925, she worked for a short time as staff nurse at Mercy Hospital and then worked at the University of Wisconsin Hospital in Madison, before moving to Detroit, where she found life in a large city much more suitable to her tastes. In Detroit she worked as a staff nurse, head nurse, and private-duty nurse at Harper Hospital. Encouraged by her brother, Dr. Paul Kiniery, who had joined the faculty at Loyola University in Chicago, she began taking night courses to complete her bachelor's degree. She was awarded a bachelor in philosophy, cum laude, from Loyola University in 1936. She completed a postgraduate course in communicable disease and pediatric nursing and ward administration at Cook County Hospital in 1931. She returned to school in 1938 and obtained a certificate in public-health nursing in 1939 and a master's degree in public health from the University of Michigan in 1940.

While pursuing her studies in Chicago from 1930–36, Kiniery worked as a head nurse and supervisor in the Children's Hospital of Cook County Hospital. In addition to her responsibility for all aspects of the service (including admissions and outpatient units), she was responsible for clinical instruction of affiliating basic students and postgraduate students. On graduation in 1936, she transferred to the University of Chicago clinics, where she was a supervisor and public-health instructor in the outpatient clinics and home-delivery services conducted by the

Chicago Lying-In Hospital. In the hospital and clinics, she taught and supervised basic and registered nurse students in all aspects of maternity and newborn care. During this time she also was a supervisor of nurseries at Chicago Lying-In Hospital.

Following her graduation from the University of Michigan, she worked as a staff nurse in a rural county health department in Coldwater, Michigan, then as assistant professor and coordinator of the basic nursing programs at Wayne State University from 1943–46 in Detroit. For three years she then worked as a supervisor for the Visiting Nurse Association in Detroit. With almost 20 years experience in nursing and with this varied background in public health, obstetrics, pediatrics, and medical-surgical nursing, and with experience as a practitioner, teacher, and administrator, Kiniery was more than qualified to apply for the deanship at Loyola University. With her brother Paul on the faculty in the History Department and her younger sister Ruth residing in Chicago, this position brought her career advancement as well as proximity to her family.

Kiniery came to Loyola University as dean and professor in 1947. She brought the School of Nursing to prominence as one of the first 24 nationally accredited programs in the country and the first fully accredited college of nursing in Illinois. Achieving these accomplishments was often difficult because at the time hospital diploma nursing programs were strong and numerous in Chicago. Not only did Kiniery have to withstand the resistance of these strong nursing diploma programs, but also the resistance of the male-dominated Jesuit university with its traditional views of women and women's work. Her strong belief in a liberal education coupled with a scientific background, however, was the basis for her mission in establishing a strong, generic baccalaureate program.

For many years, Kiniery was the only woman serving as an administrator in the university. She had to cope not only with being the sole woman administrator, but also with being the dean of the unique female-dominated program of nursing.

For all the time that she was at Loyola, she commanded the respect of the Jesuits with whom she worked. While she was dean, the school expanded its enrollment in the baccalaureate program, and in 1963, under her leadership, Loyola University started its master's program in teaching and administration for associate-nursing degree programs. This graduate program, supported by a grant from the W.K. Kellogg Foundation, was the first in Illinois to prepare faculty for developing junior-college nursing programs. The graduate program also offered a curriculum to prepare clinical specialists in medical-surgical nursing. During Kiniery's tenure as dean, the Loyola Public Health Training Center was established in nearby Evanston to provide experience to Loyola nursing students in caring for the health needs of families. In 1963 Kiniery guided the establishment of the Alpha Beta chapter of Sigma Theta Tau, the national honor society of nursing at Loyola.

While at Loyola, Kiniery fostered efforts to encourage more minorities into nursing and was responsible for the university being one of the 10 baccalaureate schools of nursing to obtain funds from the Sealantic Fund, a project for the disadvantaged in nursing, funded by the Rockefeller Foundation.

Also during her tenure as dean, she also served on advisory boards for St. Elizabeth, St. Francis, and Provident hospitals. She served on the board of directors of the National Conference of Catholic Schools of Nursing and also on the Advisory Council of the Illinois Department of Registration and Education. She chaired the Committee on Baccalaureate and Higher Degree Programs of the Illinois League for Nursing and also the Jesuit Education Association's Conference on Schools and Departments of Nursing. She served as a vice-president of the Chicago Council on Community Nursing.

On her retirement as dean in 1966, Kiniery was recruited to be a special consultant in the Division of Nursing, United States Public Health Service. She served as chief of the Program Review Unit, Nursing Education and Training Branch, responsible as the staff director to the Program Review Committee to evaluate the impact of the Nurse Training Act of 1964 (Public Law 88-581). With the enactment of this law, Congress provided for financial support in the area of expansion and improvement of nursing education. This evaluation, (published in 1967 as the *Program Review Report* under the guidance of Kiniery) was a significant report. It resulted in subsequent nursing legislation and the continuation of federal funding for nursing.

As a staff member of the Nurse Education and Training Branch of the Division of Nursing, Kiniery was one of the group that received a Superior Service Unit Citation in recognition of "diligence and imagination which they brought to the task of the program review of the Nurse Training Act of 1964." On completion of the committee work, Kiniery continued as a nurse consultant in the Division of Nursing, implementing legislation for the Nurse Construction Grant Program.

Loyola University awarded an honorary doctorate in human letters to her during commencement ceremonies in May 1982.

Kiniery retired from the U.S. Public Health Service in 1972 and moved to South Pasadena, Florida, where she lived with her widowed sister, Ruth Palmer. Kiniery took care of her sister Ruth at their home, where Ruth died of cancer. Kiniery also died of cancer on March 4, 1988.

A memorial service was held for her in Chicago on April 12, 1988, at the chapel of the Lake Shore campus of Loyola University.

Kiniery endowed the Marcela Niehoff School of Nursing at Loyola University with funds to provide for research symposia and faculty inservices in memory of her beloved sister, Ruth Palmer.

PUBLICATIONS BY GLADYS KINIERY

"The Registered Nurse Goes to College." *Chart* 54 (November 1957): 4–6.

BIBLIOGRAPHY

Application for Federal Employment. Standard Form 57. Completed by Gladys Kiniery in 1966. Archives of Loyola University, Chicago.

Archives, Gladys Kiniery. Loyola University School of Nursing, Chicago.

Division of Nursing. U.S. Department of Health, Education, and Welfare. *Nurse Training Act of 1964, Program Review Report.* PHS Public. No. 1740. Arlington, Va.: U.S. Public Health Service, 1967.

Golden Jubilee Program, School of Nursing, Loyola University. Archives of Loyola University, Chicago.

Homily by Julia Lane, Dean, School of Nursing. Gladys Kiniery Memorial Services. Loyola University. Archives of Loyola University, Chicago.

Susan Dudas and Mary Ann Krol

Bertha L. Knapp

1880–1965

Bertha L. Knapp is best known as the superintendent of the training school and of the nursing services at Wesley Hospital in Chicago and saw the school become part of Northwestern University. She was a strong advocate of personal patient care and upgrading nursing.

Knapp was born on September 19, 1880, in Dewitt, Michigan. She attended the nursing school at University Hospital, which was affiliated with the University of Michigan in Ann Arbor. After graduation in 1903 she was named a supervisor of the children's and medical departments, and soon after this assistant superintendent of nurses. In 1907 she became a nursing supervisor with the Chicago Visiting Nurse Association, a position she left in 1908 to become superintendent at the Wesley Hospital in Chicago.

At Wesley Hospital she emphasized the importance of personal patient care but also insisted that students have time off from their duties for specialized instruction. Wesley Hospital very early in her administration required four years of high school even though Illinois laws only required one year. Knapp was one of the earliest superintendents to hire a full-time instructor for the school, and by 1912 she not only had the instructor but two assistant superintendents, a night supervisor, one surgical and three floor nurses, a dietitian, and a masseuse. She also made certain that students had clinical experience in psychopathic nursing, pediatric nursing, and community health as well as experience with patients with communicable disease.

Always one of the innovators in nursing education, Knapp gave students two half days off a week and four weeks of annual vacation time. Extracurricular events were an integral part of the training school life. The students had a yearbook, a chorus, and a volunteer Bible study group. In 1925 Knapp hired a social director, who also served as counselor, librarian, and advisor to the yearbook staff.

The financial difficulties of the hospital in the 1930s forced her to cut out the nurse training program in 1935 rather than lower her standards. She continued as superintendent of nurses, however, and managed to maintain a continuing-education program for the staff. The nursing crisis of World War II allowed her to reopen the school again in 1942 and to strengthen the tenuous connection that had existed with Northwestern University. In 1943 the hospital and the university established a five-year combination degree with students receiving a B.S. degree from Northwestern and a diploma from the hospital's training school.

Knapp was the first chairperson of the Illinois Board of Nurse Examiners when it was established in 1917. She was also a director of the Illinois League of Nursing Education, the Illinois State Nurses' Association, and the Central Council for Nursing Education. She retired on September 1, 1943, after 35 years of service to Wesley Hospital, and the Bertha L. Knapp Scholarship Fund was established in her honor by the alumnae association.

On her retirement with the title of superintendent of nurses emeritus, she returned to the family home in Michigan. In 1958 she married Dr. Richard A. Smith, who had first proposed to her while they were students at Michigan, 60 years earlier. They were married at her summer home in Neillsville, Wisconsin. She died there on August 1, 1965.

PUBLICATIONS BY BERTHA L. KNAPP

"The Recruiting, Admission and Graduation of Student Nurses," *American Journal of Nursing* 24 (January 1924): 323–6.

"Discipline in Schools of Nursing is Most Effective When Voluntary," *Hospital Management* 21 (March 1926): 31.

BIBLIOGRAPHY

Hawkins, J.W., "Bertha L. Knapp," *Dictionary of American Biography*, Edited by M. Kaufman, New York: Greenwood Press, 1988. Pp. 220–222.

"News About Nursing: About People You Know: Bertha L. Knapp," *American Journal of Nursing* 43 (July 1943): 687.

"New Schools, New Programs." *American Journal of Nursing* 42 (August 1942): 960–61.

Sacharski, S. unpublished history of the Northwestern Memorial Hospital, Chicago, in the Northwestern Memorial Hospital Archives and Library.

Francine Wallace

Ruth Perkins Kuehn

1900–1986

Ruth Perkins Kuehn was responsible for establishing the University of Pittsburgh School of Nursing, and during her 22 years as the school's dean she provided the leadership in developing a master's program in 1942 and the third nursing doctoral program in the nation in 1957. She devoted more than 35 years to the advancement of nursing nationally and internationally. Her primary goal throughout the years was the improvement of patient care.

Kuehn was born on May 13, 1900, in Sharon, Wisconsin, to Anson and Lura Perkins. She graduated from Sharon High School in 1918. During high school she played the piano for many of the school functions. Following graduation, she studied the pipe organ at Carroll College, Wisconsin.

She completed the nursing program at Children's Memorial Hospital, Chicago, in

1925. This program of study included one year of experience at Evanston General Hospital. Following graduation, Kuehn was first employed as a private-duty nurse in Chicago and then as a night supervisor at her alma mater Children's Memorial Hospital. She then became a supervisor and instructor in pediatric nursing at St. Luke's Hospital School of Nursing. Kuehn moved to Columbus, Ohio, in 1928 and became a supervisor and instructor in pediatric nursing at the Ohio State University School of Nursing. She received her bachelor of science in 1931 and her master of arts (nursing) in 1934 from Ohio State while she continued to work as an instructor and finally as director of nursing education at the School of Nursing. For the next few years she was director of the school. On December 8, 1935, she married Conrad Kuehn, a practicing urologist.

Kuehn's major dissertation advisor at Ohio State University was Dr. W.W. Charter, who was a friend of Dr. Bowman, chancellor at the University of Pittsburgh. At that time Pittsburgh was thinking of developing a collegiate school of nursing. Charter suggested his student, and Bowman asked to meet with Kuehn. He then offered her the position of dean of the proposed school of nursing. She consented on the condition that the school would be an autonomous school of nursing.

Kuehn was formally appointed dean of the University of Pittsburgh School of Nursing in September 1939. The following year she initiated the nation's first continuing-education workshop for nursing faculty. The program included workshops on the new curriculum guide, on preparing instructional material, on planning guidance programs, and how to develop techniques to evaluate teachers. When Kuehn earned the doctor of philosophy degree in 1942 from Ohio State University, she became the first dean of a school of nursing to hold this degree.

Kuehn formulated the graduation ceremony for baccalaureate students at the Pittsburgh School of Nursing and designed the pin for the school, which incorporates symbols of the university, nursing, and Pittsburgh. The former seal of the University of Pittsburgh forms the center of the pin, and the candle represents the light of learning. Below the candle is engraved the date of 1787, reminding us that the School of Nursing is a part of the University of Pittsburgh, which was founded in Pennsylvania that year. The space between the flames of the candle represents the three rivers coming together in Pittsburgh. The branches of laurel on either side of the candle are symbolic of honor and distinction. The Pinning Ceremony [graduation] conducted today is the same as that first performed in 1943. It includes the "Passing of the Light," a ritual that symbolizes graduates' commitment to the ideals of superior nursing practice. The student who has achieved the highest standing in nursing in the class becomes the "Keeper of the Light" and its custodian until it is time to pass it on to the next class.

Kuehn was a pioneer in nursing research. She initiated several research studies in the 1950s. A major program in the field of method improvement in nursing was done in collaboration with the Department of Industrial Engineering at the University of Pittsburgh School of Engineering. Studies were also done on the types of hospital bed design and bedmaking. A major comprehensive study on utilization of personnel and patient care was completed in 1955. The Kellog Foundation funded the School of Nursing to develop management techniques to improve the functioning of operating rooms, recovery rooms, and central supply.

Her student body was always foremost on Kuehn's mind. Her school was the first in Pennsylvania to admit black students, the first to admit married women, and the first to permit students to marry and complete their program. As the student body grew, Kuehn campaigned for a nurses' residence, which was completed in 1953.

During her deanship Kuehn belonged to, and provided leadership for, many organizations. She was president of Sigma Theta Tau and a member of Pi Lambda Theta and Alpha Tau Delta. She served as vice-president of the American Nurses' Association and as delegate to the International Council of Nurses and the Inter-

American Congress of Nurses in Rio de Janeiro (1947–48). Her international interests were not new, for she had recruited international students from the time she became dean.

She was also a member of the National League for Nursing, the American Hospital Association, the Association of Collegiate Schools of Nursing, the National Education Association, and other nursing and nonnursing associations. She served as a member of the board of directors of the Association of Collegiate Schools of Nursing, a member of the Executive Committee, National Committee for the improvement of nursing services, a member of the National Mental Health Advisory Council; the National Advisory Committee of the American Nurses' Foundation Research Project; and a member of other national committees and councils. She served as a consultant to many universities in the United States as well as in Sweden, England, and Ireland.

In 1961 Kuehn retired as dean of the University of Pittsburgh School of Nursing. After an educational leave she became the first full-time director of continuing education in nursing at the University of Pittsburgh. As professor of nursing education, she developed the graduate program in nursing administration.

Kuehn fully retired in 1964 and returned to Sharon, Wisconsin, with her husband. She died November 15, 1986.

PUBLICATIONS BY RUTH PERKINS KUEHN (SELECTED)

BOOKS

Essentials of Pediatric Nursing. Philadelphia: Davis, 1933.

With F. George. *Patterns of Patient Care.* New York: Macmillan, 1955.

ARTICLES

"Who Should Supervise the Mock Laboratory?" *Modern Hospital* 36 (1931): 77–82.

"Making the Most of Case Studies." *American Journal of Nursing* 34 (1934): 1068–69.

"University Relationships Between Schools of Nursing and Hospitals." *Hospitals* 15 (1941): 60–63.

"Nurse Power in Mobilization." *American Journal of Nursing* 51 (1951): 395–98.

"Should the Development of Sound Basic Collegiate Programs be Accelerated?" *American Journal of Nursing* 52 (1952): 1116–17.

"There's Method in These Nursing Studies." *Modern Hospital* 85 (1955): 74.

BIBLIOGRAPHY

Archives. University of Pittsburgh, Pittsburgh, Pennsylvania.

Gilbertson, H. Interview with the author, April 26, 1990, Sharon, Wisconsin.

Kuehn, C. Interview with the author, April 26, 1990, Sharon, Wisconsin.

Malone, A.C. Interview with the author, April 25–26, 1990.

Salisbury, M. Interview with the author, April 26, 1990, Sharon, Wisconsin.

Young, L. "Ruth Perkins Kuehn." University of Pittsburgh School of Nursing Alumni Newsletter (Spring 1964).

Enid Goldberg

Harriet L. Leete

1875?–1927

Harriet Leete was a pioneer in child-health nursing. In 1906 she joined the staff of the Infant's Clinic in Cleveland as the first superintendent of nurses at the newly opened Babies' Dispensary located in Cleveland's Haymarket District. The dispensary took care of sick infants and, under the direction of Leete and others, initiated a program to do well-baby care by encouraging mothers to bring their babies to be weighed and examined even if not ill. The procedures and concepts that she helped establish there were later adopted by infant dispensaries throughout the United States.

Leete's birth date is unknown, as are her parents. She is believed to have been born in Cleveland, probably in 1875. Trained at the Lakeside Training School for Nurses in Cleveland, she graduated on March 23, 1901. After working for brief periods as a private-duty nurse in sanatoria in New York City, Rochester, and elsewhere, she returned to her native city to become supervisor of the men's surgical ward at the Lakeside Hospital. In 1906 she joined the nursing staff of Infant's Clinic, where she worked until 1917, when she volunteered to join the American Red Cross unit of the U.S. Army Hospital, Number 4. Even before becoming active in wartime nursing, Leete had been a Red Cross volunteer and was number 159 of the original enrollees of Red Cross nurses.

Her unit was the first American unit to sail for Europe (May 7, 1917). When she reached the Continent, her duties and responsibilities were expanded. She served for a brief period with the Bureau of Tuberculosis of the Red Cross, then coordinated efforts of the Rockefeller Commission for the Prevention of Tuberculosis to work with French sanatoria and hospitals. On September 5, 1917, she was appointed chief nurse with the American Red Cross Children's Bureau of the Department of Civil Affairs, Red Cross Commission for France. In this capacity she began training French women to serve as home visitors in Paris.

Transferred to military duty after the United States entered the war, she served as chief nurse of the American Red Cross Military Hospital, Number 5, Auteuil Tent Hospital. After being released from this responsibility at the beginning of 1919, the Red Cross assigned her to the Balkan Commission as chief nurse for northern Serbia, attached to Palanba Hospital. During her stay there the Serbian government recognized her for her wartime services. While serving in Serbia, she contracted typhus and returned to the United States on July 15, 1919.

She again took up child-health nursing, accepting a position in 1920 as field director for the American Child Hygiene Association. This entailed overseeing the adoption and implementation of the standards of child care that she had developed in Cleveland. When the American Child Hygiene Association joined with the American Child Health Association, her concepts were broadened to an older group of children. Her next position was as director of the Brooklyn (N.Y.) Maternity Center Association and its free clinics for prenatal and postnatal care. It was here in the summer of 1924 that she organized a Mothercraft Club through which

women were provided prenatal care and instruction, the first such club of its kind in the United States.

The typhus she had contracted in Europe permanently affected her health and forced her retirement from the Maternity Center shortly after to a somewhat less demanding position as director of Wavecrest, a convalescent home for children in Far Rockaway, Long Island. She died November 9, 1927, in Brooklyn of an acute mastoid infection. She was buried at Hartfield, near Jamestown, N.Y., with full military honors.

BIBLIOGRAPHY

Dock, L.L., et al. *History of American Red Cross Nursing.* New York: Macmillan, 1922.

Fitzpatrick, M.L. *The National Organization for Public Health Nursing 1912–1952.* New York: National League for Nursing, 1975.

"Harriet L. Leete." *American Journal of Nursing* 28 (January 1928): 71–72, 95.

Hawkins, J.W. "Harriet L. Leete." In *Dictionary of American Nursing Biography.* M. Kaufman, ed. Westport, Conn.: Greenwood, 1988. Pp. 225–27.

Kernodle, P.B. *The Red Cross Nurse in Action, 1882–1948.* New York: Harper, 1949.

Pennock, M.R., ed. *Makers of Nursing History.* New York: Lakeside, 1928. Pp. 62–63.

Vern L. Bullough

Lucile Petry Leone
b. 1902

One of America's most outstanding nurses is Lucile Petry Leone. She possessed leadership skills and versatile talents that made her most suited to assume the responsibilities of assistant surgeon general, United States Public Health Service. She also served as chief nurse officer of the Public Health Service of the Department of Health, Education and Welfare. It is historically significant that Leone also held the rank of admiral, the first woman to become an assistant surgeon general in the Public Health Service as well as the nation's first woman entitled to wear the gold braid of an admiral. A most capable, innovative nurse educator, administrator, and perceptive writer, her contributions influenced the advancement of the nursing profession on a national and international level.

Born in Lewisburg, Ohio, January 23, 1902, Leone was the daughter of David D. and Dora B. (Murray) Petry. A petite, attractive, and energetic young woman, she was brought up to assume responsibility. Her summers were spent working in a cannery, a dry goods store, and a broker's office.

She attended the University of Delaware, from which she graduated with honors and a bachelor of arts degree. In 1927 she entered the Johns Hopkins School of Nursing, completing that program in 1929. She then went to Yale University as a clinical instructor. In 1929 she moved to the University of Minnesota and remained there until 1940, moving from a position as clinical instructor to associate professor and assistant director of the School of Nursing. She then went to Teachers College, Columbia University, to complete study for an advanced degree but this was interrupted when she accepted an appointment to the United States Public Health Service as its first woman administrator. She served for two years before moving to Cornell University as Dean of the New York Hospital School of Nursing. She continued to gain credits at Columbia, and though she earned a master's degree there, she never completed the doctorate. Increasingly she turned to government service.

As the demands for nurses grew during World War II, the U.S. Army and Navy demanded more and more nurses. War had broken down many of the employment barriers for women, and nursing education was finding it difficult to recruit students. This situation motivated nurses, hospital administrators, and educators to organize and develop recruitment plans.

It is interesting to note that when the United States entered World War I in April 1917, the government identified an acute shortage of nursing personnel. To meet the demand for nurses then, a revolutionary concept was put forth to establish an Army School of Nursing to meet the national emergency. The school opened May 1918 and closed October 1931. Economy was the major factor as the war had ended and the cost of operating the school was excessive. When the school closed, assurance was given that it would be reopened if there were another war. However, the War Department reneged and suggested that civilian schools of nursing should meet this responsibility.

After the United States entered World War II, the government again recognized the threat to public health and created the Student War Nurse Reserve, which later became known as the Cadet Nurse Corps. Spearheaded by the provocative representative from the 22nd Ohio district, Frances P. Bolton, President Roosevelt on June 16, 1943, approved a limited federal subsidy for civilian schools of nursing. The Bolton Act, as it became known, was designed to meet both military and essential civilian nursing needs. Established July 1, 1943, and unanimously approved by the 78th Congress, it offered high-school graduates an education and career in nursing at no expense to the individual.

It was recognized that a Division of Nurse Education should be established in the office of the surgeon general, at the United States Public Health Service to administer the act. Dr. Thomas Parran, surgeon general, established the division and selected Lucile Petry Leone, then dean of Cornell School of Nursing, to administer the program. One month after her appointment as dean of Cornell she was granted a leave of absence to assume these new responsibilities. Leone began her recruitment effort by sending telegrams to 1,294 nursing schools inviting them to participate in the program. She believed that by increasing enrollment and assigning cadet nurses to civilian as well as military hospitals, experienced graduate nurses could be released to meet the nursing needs of the army and navy. Leone spearheaded an intensive recruitment campaign on a local and national level. The provisions of the act offered high-school graduates an all-expense scholarship, an education in nursing, and an opportunity to contribute to the war effort. A monthly stipend of $15 to $30 and an attractive grey uniform with scarlet epaulets were provided. Approximately 49,000 students were immediately recruited, 6,000 short of the overall goal. However, over a three-year period approximately 180,000 students were recruited nationally for schools of nursing. This was a successful endeavor although it was designed primarily to meet wartime needs. One of the most beneficial effects of this program was that the public was well informed on the essential need for nurses and the valuable services they rendered. It also provided the needed public support for the advancement of nursing and insight into the costs of educating nurses. In addition, this program provided an opportunity to assess these costs and to study how they should be met.

In June 1949, she was appointed Assistant Surgeon General, USDHS, with the rank of admiral, a rank she held until her retirement. Leone's career was multifaceted in that she was a prolific writer, lecturer, and researcher, as well as an educator. Her writings primarily concentrated on improving the effectiveness of nursing programs, upgrading the nurses's skills and proficiency, and promoting the value of public-health work. She was keenly interested in international health programs and was a member of the United States Delegation to the first World Health Assembly of the World Health Organization held in Geneva, Switzerland, in 1948. Later she became a member of the World Health Organization's Expert Committee on Nursing. Her philosophy on human welfare included sharing of knowledge, cooperation, and respect for nations. She believed that acts of kindness, altruism, and the desire to help others to help themselves was a humanitarian ideal. As a spokesman for world health, she believed nurses working in vastly separated sections of the world brought hope, health, and strength to the people. She felt strongly about nurses working with various member nations of the World Health Organization helped to improve their lifestyle and better prepared them to handle famine, poverty, and recurring illnesses in their native lands.

On October 21, 1954, the Mayo Memorial Building at the University of Minnesota, Minneapolis, was dedicated. Leone presented a paper that explored a range of values related to the nursing care of patients. She emphasized preventive principles and the teaching of health concepts to patients and their families. She suggested that nursing care should be organized in terms of individual patient care rather than in an assembly-line of procedures for groups of patients. She found it paradoxical that in an era when the nurse–patient relationship was considered to be therapeutic, nurses were spending less time with patients. Hospital designs that provided rooms with two-way communications lessened patient contact. This system inhibited vital and direct communication with patients. "Reverence for Life," a theme of Albert Schweitzer was quoted frequently by Leone throughout her presentation as a valued goal for nursing.

Leone was honored by a member of Congress on August 10, 1954. J. Vaughan Gary, Congressman from Virginia, addressed the House of Representatives and extended his remarks to include the address of Leone delivered for the anniversary of the founding of Westhampton College of the University of Richmond. This address entitled "Today's Challenge to the College Women in the Professions" was placed in the *Congressional Record* so that all women could understand the benefits and challenges for women entering the professions. In her presentation the values she emphasized are reflected in the following statements:

> Professional education also prepares for living over and beyond professional living. Disciplined thinking in the analysis of professional problems can create a pattern for solving family and citizenship problems, can increase the objectivity with which issues are dealt and the skepticism about superficial answers and demagoguery. . . .

> The challenge to the college woman in the professions lies in something more than the urge to develop new technical knowledge

and skill. The challenge lies in examining the values of what we do, in developing the human-relations potential in our fields, and in relating these larger goals of the evolving American culture.

Leone was active in many professional organizations and served in the capacity of president, chairperson, member or advisor. She was a charter member of the Board of Medicine, National Academy of Sciences. Other affiliations include member, Board on Medical Education and Research; member, W.K. Kellogg Foundation; editorial board member, *American Journal of Public Health*; chairperson, Advisory Committee Sealantic Fund Program for Disadvantaged Youth in Nursing; chairperson, Board of Directors American Journal of Nursing Inc.; chairperson, National Nursing Accrediting Service; president, National League for Nursing; fellow, American College Hospital Administrators; editorial advisor on nursing, McGraw-Hill Book Company.

After 25 years of public service, Lucile Petry Leone retired from her position as the Public Health Service's chief nurse officer, February 1966. She returned to her home in Dallas, Texas, with her husband, Dr. Nicholas C. Leone, a Public Health Service researcher, whom she married on June 1, 1952. On her retirement 2,500 nurses of the Public Health Service established in her honor the Lucile Petry Leone Award to encourage nursing leadership. The award, administered by the National League for Nursing, is given biennially to an outstanding nurse-instructor. Additional awards that she has received include the American Legion Auxiliary Award 1955, the Lasker Award 1957, the Florence Nightingale Medal of the International Committee by the Red Cross, the Annie Jump Cannon Centennial Medal, and the Distinguished Service Medal from the United States Public Health Service 1966. Leone has also been awarded several honorary degrees including doctorates from University of Delaware, Boston University, Alfred University, Hood College, Adelphi College, Keuka College, Wagner College, and a special citation from the University of Buffalo.

Throughout her career Leone encouraged families and communities to utilize and capitalize on the humanistic services of nurses as valuable and vital in meeting the health needs of society.

Leone, who retired from the Public Health Service, February 1, 1966, is a remarkable talented woman whose contributions are valued and appreciated by the nursing community worldwide.

PUBLICATIONS BY LUCILE PETRY LEONE

"Basic Professional Curricula in Nursing Leading to Degrees." *American Journal of Nursing* 37 (March 1937): 286–97

"Nursing Education in Higher Institutions of the North Central Association." *North Central Association Quarterly* (April 1940): 401–14.

"The United States Cadet Nurse Corps." *American Journal of Nursing* 45 (December 1945): 12.

"Expand the Nursing Curriculum." *Modern Hospital* (September 1947): 75–76.

"Professional Education for Nursing of the Future." *Ohio Nurses' Review.* (July 1948): 115–23.

"We Hail an Important 'First.'" *American Journal of Nursing* 49 (October 1949): 630–33.

"Statewide Planning for Nurse Training." *Hospitals* 23 (November 1949): 61–62.

"Planning Nursing Education for Present-Day Needs." *Ohio Nurses' Review* (October 1951): 158–63.

"The Art of Nursing." *Journal of the American Medical Association* 157 (April 1955): 1381–83.

With M. Arnstein et al. "Surveys Measure Nursing Resources." *American Journal of Nursing* 49 (December 1949): 770–72.

With T. Dodds et al. "Simplifying Hypodermic Injections." *American Journal of Nursing* 40 (December 1940): 1345.

With J.V. Gary. "Today's Challenge to the College Woman in the Professions." *Congressional Record* (August 10, 1954): A5910–20.

With E. Spalding. "The Production Front in Nursing." *American Journal of Nursing* 43 (October 1943): 900–01.

With E.M. Vreeland, "Nursing Education." *Higher Education.* 8 (April 1952): 181–86.

BIBLIOGRAPHY

Bolton, F. P. "The Author of the Bolton Act Explains Its Implications for the Future." *Modern Hospital* 61 (September 1943): 59–61.

Conde, M. *The Lamp and the Caduceus.* Washington, D.C.: Army School of Nursing Alumnae Association, 1975. P. 9.

Personal Interviews by the author, undated.

Delores J. Haritos

Edith Patton Lewis

b. 1914

Edith Patton Lewis was a journalist who worked for the American Journal of Nursing Company from 1945 to 1980, serving as an editor of the journals owned by the company during that time span. She was managing editor of *Nursing Research,* 1952–57; editor of the *American Journal of Nursing,* 1957–59; contributing editor of the *American Journal of Nursing,* 1963–70; and editor of *Nursing Outlook,* 1970–80.

Lewis was born in Philadelphia on August 27, 1914, to Anna May (Insertell) and William Harrison Patton. She graduated from Smith College with a baccalaureate in psychology and spent a year as a psychological intern at the Worcester State Hospital, Massachusetts. She then entered the Frances Payne Bolton School of Nursing at Western Reserve University, Cleveland, earning a master's degree in 1939.

She worked for a year as a psychiatric staff nurse at the New York Hospital in Weschester County; then from 1940–42 she was at the Massachusetts General Hospital in Boston, serving as a head nurse, supervisor, and instructor. From 1942–45 she worked as director of nursing education at the Norwich State Hospital in Connecticut, where she was responsible for the educational program of students who were affiliated with the hospital from area nursing schools. Since these were the war years, Patton was also involved with recruiting students into the U.S. Cadet Nurse Corps. She often visited colleges to speak about the opportunities offered by a career in nursing. In 1945 she became a full-time journalist as a member of the editorial staff of the *American Journal of Nursing.*

She married Leon Phillips Lewis on January 10, 1948, and although she reduced her commitment to the journal to part time to raise a family, she never really quit her work as a writer and editor.

Building on her wartime experiences as a nurse recruiter, Lewis wrote two short books focused on nursing as a career. The first titled *Opportunities in Nursing* was published in 1952 and the second in 1962 titled *Nurse: Careers Within a Career in Professional Nursing.* In these works Lewis argued that nursing is a desirable field because it is so varied, and she considered her own developing career in journalism a part of the field of nursing.

Her name first appeared on the masthead of *Nursing Research* as managing editor in October 1953. The journal was new, having been established at the time the nursing organizations were restructured in 1952. There were no other research-oriented nursing journals at the time. A committee of nurse researchers headed by a faculty member directed the activities of the journal for the first year. Lewis was added to bring the skills of a professional journalist to the task. She continued in this role until 1957, she then served as acting editor of the *American Journal of Nursing* 1957–59.

Following this term of editorial duties, Lewis again reduced her commitment to the journal company and spent more time at her home in Norwich, Connecticut. This gave her the opportunity to take on special assignments as contributing editor. A major focus of her writing during the decade of the sixties was on the growing tide of discontent among nurses over their low salaries and poor working conditions. In 1962 the *American Journal of Nursing* sent her to Bradenton, Florida, to cover the story of five nurses who were fired from the county hospitals because they tried to organize to improve working conditions. The group sought assistance from the Florida Nurses' Association, but the association could not deliver much help because the 1947 Taft-Hartley Labor

Relations Act had exempted nonprofit hospitals from the necessity of collective bargaining. This law was buttressed by Florida statutes and by the 1946 pledge of the American Nurses' Association not to strike.

In 1966 Lewis wrote about a power struggle in a California psychiatric hospital. Nurses were kept out of certain wards where technicians were supervisors. The nurses charged abuse and neglect of patients and wanted access to all of the hospitalized patients. The California Nurses' Association supported them and eventually reform came to the hospital. Later that year in another report, Lewis focused on the more traditional aspects of collective bargaining for wages and benefits. The nurses of the nineteen City of New York hospitals, with the support of the New York State Nurses' Association, decided they would resign en masse if demands for increased salaries and improved working conditions were not met. This action violated the ANA no-strike pledge; so the situation was tense. Lewis covered it in detail, rejoicing with the nurses when the city agreed to submit the issue for arbitration. Lewis's support for the nurses was reemphasized in a letter she wrote to the editor of the *Nursing Times* praising the nurses for their collective actions.

In 1968 the American Nurses' Association repealed its no-strike pledge, and in 1969 Lewis covered the Cedars of Lebanon Hospital strike in Los Angeles. Her series of articles undoubtedly contributed to the changing climate of opinion among nurses about collective-bargaining activities.

Her articles about the changing educational system for nursing in the United States tended to be more cautious and analytical. She often wrote about the three competing systems of education: diploma, the community college associate of arts program, and baccalaureate education.

In December 1970 Lewis was appointed acting editor of *Nursing Outlook*, with a full appointment following shortly. In addition to being an American Journal of Nursing publication, *Nursing Outlook* was also the official voice of the National League for Nursing. Since the league re-

flected all three types of nursing programs all were given coverage. Lewis's editorials often focused on issues of the day, and her position was pro-nursing, but she was also willing to remind nurses of their duty to the public. Lewis developed the American Journal of Nursing Company's Contemporary Nursing Series. She edited two of the books in the series, using articles from the company's journals focused on the new roles for nurses and the issues related to these roles. Her support for the clinical-nurse specialist was unequivocal, but support for the nurse practitioners was tempered with concern because nurse practitioners were so closely allied with medicine.

In the June 1980 issue of *Nursing Outlook* Lewis wrote her farewell editorial. In reflecting on her 35 years in nursing publication, she indicated that her major satisfaction had come from working with nurses who wanted to write. She gave personal attention to writers and potential writers, critiquing and encouraging them. She was particularly proud of the fact that she had never sent a writer a form letter.

After retirement Lewis continued to cover ANA conventions. The reports in *Nursing Outlook* for 1983–86 were done by her. She was finally forced to stop writing when her failing eyesight made it too difficult.

Lewis received the Distinguished Alumna Award for the Francis Payne Bolton School of Nursing in 1975. She was given Honorary Recognition by the Connecticut Nurses' Association in 1978 for Distinguished Service to the Profession and in 1982 for Outstanding Contribution to Nursing Education. She was made a fellow of the American Academy of Nursing in 1977. She continues to make her home in Connecticut.

PUBLICATIONS BY EDITH PATTON LEWIS

BOOKS

Opportunities in Nursing. New York: Vocational Guidance Manuals, 1952.

Nurse: Careers Within a Career in Professional Nursing. New York: Macmillan, 1962.

Editor. *The Clinical Nurse Specialist.* New

York: American Journal of Nursing Company, Contemporary Nursing Series, 1970.

With M.H. Browing, and E.P. Lewis, eds. *The Expanded Role of the Nurse.* New York: American Journal of Nursing Company, 1973.

ARTICLES

"Fire on the Ninth Floor." *American Journal of Nursing* 62 (February 1962): 50–55.

"The Bradenton Story: A Community Crisis." *American Journal of Nursing* 62 (October 1962): 58–63.

"Night Boat from Havana." *American Journal of Nursing* 63 (April 1963): 70–74.

"The Fairview Story." *American Journal of Nursing* 66 (January 1966): 64–70.

"The New York City Hospital Story." *American Journal of Nursing* 66 (July 1966): 1526–35.

"Transatlantic Nursing." Letter to the Editor. *Nursing Times* (February 17, 1967).

"USA: Nursing Education in Ferment." *International Nursing Review* 15, No. 1 (1968): Part I, 50–60; 15, No. 2, (April 1968): Part II, 122–33.

"The Cedars of Lebanon Story." *American Journal of Nursing* 69 (November 1969): 2385–90.

"The More Things Change." *American Journal of Nursing* 85 (February 1985): 220.

SELECTED EDITORIALS

"A Nurse is a Nurse—or Is She." *Nursing Outlook* (January 20, 1972): 21.

"The Health Care Consumer: Compliant Captive." *Nursing Outlook* (January 23, 1975): 20.

"Proof of the Pudding." *Nursing Outlook* (November 23, 1975): 683.

"Small Expectations." *Nursing Outlook* (September 26, 1978): 553.

"The Professionally Uncommitted." *Nursing Outlook*, (May 27, 1979): 323.

"A Profession in Search of a Definition." *Nursing Outlook*, (May 28, 1980): 289.

"Reflections on an Editorial Career." *Nursing Outlook*, (June 28, 1980), 351.

BIBLIOGRAPHY

Lewis, E.P. Front Matter (biographical material). *Opportunities in Nursing.* New York, Vocational Guidance Manuals, 1952. P. iii.

Kelly, L.Y. "An Editor's Salute to an Editor." *Image* 12 (June 1980).

Lewis, E.P. *Who's Who in America*, 45th ed. Chicago: Marquis, 1988.

Bonnie Bullough

Harriet (Camp) Lounsbery
1851–1946

Harriet Camp Lounsbery served as a nurse in the Spanish-American War, was a pioneer in school nursing, and was a significant figure in the development of nursing in West Virginia.

She was born in Indianapolis, Indiana, on November 3, 1851. The family moved to her parents' native Vermont when she was still an infant. Lounsbery graduated from Temple Grove Seminary, Saratoga Springs (now Skidmore College), New York, and then went to nursing school at the Brooklyn Homeopathic Hospital School for Nurses in Brooklyn, from which she graduated in 1881. She did private-duty nursing in New York City from 1881 to 1885, at which time she became superintendent of the school of nursing from which she had graduated. She served as superintendent until 1892, when she left to marry Dr. Lounsbery (1893). In 1898 at the outbreak of the Spanish-American War she volunteered as nurse and succeeded Anna C. Maxwell as chief nurse of Sternberg Hospital at Chickamauga Park, Georgia. It was the largest facility for troops from the northern states, and her staff of 160 nurses provided desperately needed nursing care for the disproportionately large number of soldiers who became ill from typhoid fever, malaria, and dysentery, diseases brought on by the inadequate sanitary facilities. She kept careful records of the progress of each case of typhoid fever both among the soldiers and the nurses, and her statistics proved helpful in establishing the epidemiology of the disease. They were used in investigations of the prevalence of typhoid fever in other army camps. After the war she was president and then secretary of the Organization of Spanish-American War Nurses. She volunteered to be listed as a member of the nursing service of the American Red Cross following the war and was the 1,050th nurse to be enrolled. After the war she and her husband settled in Charleston, West Virginia, where from 1907 to 1924 she worked as a school nurse, including a four-year stint as supervisor.

She was very active in the organization of the West Virginia State Nurses' Association in 1905 and served as that organization's president from 1905 to 1918. Lounsbery prepared the bill for the association calling for registration of nurses. First introduced in 1905, it was defeated in that year but passed in essentially the same form in 1907. West Virginia, however, posed a unique problem for nurses since even with the passage of the bill there was a regulation in the state constitution prohibiting women from holding office. Since appointees to the Board of Nursing were considered public officials, all the original members were men, including Lounsbery's husband, who served as secretary.

Lounsbery was a pioneer in school nursing and helped initiate the West Virginia program just five years after the first had started in New York City. She also followed the example of other school nurses in giving lectures on practical hygiene. During the 1918 influenza epidemic she was in charge of an emergency hospital in West Virginia.

Probably, Lounsbery is best known to other nurses for her books, the first of which appeared only under her initials H.C.C. in 1889 and was one of the earliest books on ethics for nurses. She died March 24, 1946, in Huntington, West Virginia.

PUBLICATIONS BY
HARRIET (CAMP) LOUNSBERY

BOOKS

A Reference Book for Trained Nurses. Buffalo, N.Y.: Lakeside, 1889.

Making Good on Private Duty: Practical Hints to Graduate Nurses. Philadelphia: Lippincott, 1912.

A Syllabus of Hygiene for Lower Grades of the Public Schools; A Guide for the Teacher. Charleston, W. Va.: Lovett, n.d., 192 pp.

ARTICLES

"Some Reminiscences of Sternberg Hospital." *American Journal of Nursing* 2 (October 1902): 1–5; 2 (November 1902): 81–84.

BIBLIOGRAPHY

Kalisch, P. "Heroine of '98." *Nursing Research* (1975): 411–29.

Lounsbery, H.C. *American Journal of Nursing* 27 (March 1927): 197; 46 (June 1946): 431.

Lounsbery, H.C. Personal Summary. American Journal of Nursing Collection, Nursing Archives, Mugar Library, Boston University.

Vern L. Bullough

Emily Lemoine Loveridge
1860–1941

Nurse administrator and teacher Emily Lemoine Loveridge founded the Good Samaritan Hospital School of Nursing in Portland, Oregon, and influenced nursing education and hospital administration in the region.

Loveridge was born on August 28, 1860, in Hammondsport, New York, the daughter of the Reverend Daniel Loveridge and Marie Lemoine (Wolfolk) Loveridge. She graduated from Norwich Academy and taught primary school for six years in order to earn money to attend nursing school. She received her nursing education at Bellevue Hospital Training School in New York City. During her senior year the superintendent of Good Samaritan Hospital wrote her a letter urging her to come to Portland to organize a nurse training school.

The School of Nursing at Good Samaritan Hospital was founded in June 1890, the first school of nursing in the Northwest, and Loveridge served as its head for 15 years. In her reminiscences published in the *American Journal of Nursing* in 1930 she describes her workday of 12 to 16 hours. In addition to being superintendent, she was also floor nurse and operating-room supervisor, and in her leisure moments she performed tasks of sewing, cleaning, and painting. In 1905 she became superintendent of the Good Samaritan Hospital, a position that she held until her retirement in 1930. She was a member of a small group of nursing administrators who initiated the organization of the present Oregon Board of Nursing in 1910, and four years later the nursing graduates took the first licensure examination administered in Oregon.

Loveridge was active in the American Hospital Association, and at the National Convention in 1941 she was honored by the association for her contribution to hospital administration and nursing education.

Known as Aunt Emily and as a compassionate friend to countless nursing students, she raised a niece, a nephew, and a young girl orphaned during the flu epidemic of 1919. She died in Portland, on April 26, 1941. In 1966 Loveridge Hall, a nine-story residence for 200 student nurses, was dedicated in her memory at Good Samaritan Hospital.

PUBLICATIONS BY EMILY LEMOINE LOVERIDGE

"Providing a Substitute for the Special Nurse." *Modern Hospital* 29 (August 1927): 75–77.

"Reminiscences of Forty Years in Hospital Work." *American Journal of Nursing* 30 (June 1930): 777–78; also *Bulletin of the American Hospital Association* 4 (April 1930): 48–52.

BIBLIOGRAPHY

"Bellevue Alumnae Honor Miss Loveridge." *Modern Hospital* 27 (November 1926): 85–86.

Good Samaritan Hospital School of Nursing Since 1890. Portland: Good Samaritan Hospital and Medical Center, 1966.

Kalisch, P., and B. Kalisch. *The Advance of American Nursing.* Boston: Little, Brown, 1978.

Pennock, M.R. *Makers of Nursing History.* New York: Lakeside, 1940.

Lilli Sentz

Isabel Wetmore Lowman

1865–1954

Associate editor of the *Visiting Nurse Quarterly of Cleveland*, Isabel Wetmore Lowman was a nonnurse who had a profound influence on public-health nursing in Cleveland as well as throughout the country.

Lowman was born in Cuyahoga Falls, Ohio, on August 3, 1865, the daugther of Henry S. and Louise Wetmore. Largely educated in Europe, she married John Henry Lowman, by whom she had three sons. Dr. Lowman was one of the city's foremost physicians. He served on the faculty of the School of Medicine at Western Reserve University for more than 40 years and was founder of the Tuberculosis Dispensary and the Anti-Tuberculosis League of Cleveland. He died in 1918 while returning from Europe.

Isabel Lowman's active connection with nursing began in 1902 with the formation of the Visiting Nurse Association, and she later became chair of the committee that published the *Visiting Nurse Quarterly.* Other associates were Isabel Hampton Robb, Mathilda Johnson, and Annie M. Brainard, and it was in Robb's sitting room that these women worked out the practical details of the journal.

Cleveland was very active in promoting the idea of a national association to coordinate visiting nursing groups all over the country, and when the National Organization for Public Health Nursing was born in Chicago in 1912, the *Quarterly* became its official organ. Annie M. Brainard was the editor with Lowman as associate editor. In 1918 it became a monthly publication, the *Public Health Nurse.* The goal of the editorial committee was to provide information, encouragement, and warning to help solve the many problems of the nursing shortage, priority of service, protection of nursing standards, as well as consider many other wartime issues.

Active in many organizations, Lowman was influential in founding the Cleveland Infants' Clinic, which developed into the Babies' Dispensary and Hospital, and she helped establish the first Red Cross teaching center in the city. Lakeside Hospital School of Nursing was for many years a particular interest of Lowman's. Influenced by her husband's work to place medical colleges under the aegis of a university, Lowman wanted nurses to place their professional preparation on the highest possible basis, and she lent her considerable influence to the fight. The Lowman Dormitory of the Frances Payne

Bolton School of Nursing at Western Reserve University was named in her honor for her contributions to the hospitals.

When District No. 4 of the Ohio State Nurses' Association wanted to raise funds for a Florence Nightingale Centenary Foundation, Lowman was asked to write the interpretative sketch of Nightingale and to visit the 13 districts to present the purpose of the campaign. The funds were raised, and Lowman appreciated the trust shown her as a lay woman by the nurses of Ohio.

Concerned with the professional isolation of nurses in the field, Lowman also headed the scholarship committee of St. Barnabas Guild for Nurses of the Episcopal Church, an organization that brought missionary nurses from many parts of the world to Cleveland for training.

Lowman died in Tampa, Florida, on May 8, 1954.

PUBLICATIONS BY ISABEL WETMORE LOWMAN

Editorials. *Visiting Nurse Quarterly of Cleveland* (1909-1923).

"The Need of a Standard for Visiting Nursing." *Visiting Nurse Quarterly* 4 (January 1912): 8-16.

"A Cameo Out of the Past." *Public Health Nursing* 29 (July 1939): 411-12.

"Annie M. Brainard." *Public Health Nursing* 34 (1942): 322-24, 329.

BIBLIOGRAPHY

Brainard, A.M. *The Evolution of Public Health Nursing*. Philadelphia: Saunders, 1922.

Bower, I.M. *Public Health Nursing in Cleveland 1895-1928.* Cleveland: Western Reserve University, 1930.

Fitzpatrick, M.L. *The National Organization for Public Health Nursing, 1912-1952: Development of a Practice Field.* New York: National League for Nursing, 1975.

Howell, M.G. "Isabel Wetmore Lowman." *Nursing Outlook* 3 (February 1855): 79-80.

Obituary. *Cleveland Plain Dealer*, May 11, 1954, 10 University Hospitals of Cleveland. Archives. Cleveland, Ohio.

Lilli Sentz

Theresa Inez Lynch
b. 1896

Theresa Inez Lynch was an innovative pioneer nursing leader who sought to move basic nursing education from hospital control to a university setting. She was the first dean of the School of Nursing at the University of Pennsylvania. One of the first nurses in the country to receive a doctoral degree (1940), she strongly advocated high standards for nurses both academically and in clinical practice. She believed in a close link between nursing education and nursing service.

Lynch was born on August 9, 1896, in Winchester, Virginia, the fourth of five children. Her father, Maurice M. Lynch, was a lawyer, and her mother, Theresa B. Ahern Lynch, was active as a civic leader in Virginia. Southern graciousness and proper manners were an integral part of her family life.

Lynch had a happy childhood and traveled to Europe several times. After graduating from Winchester High School, she attended the Mary Washington College in Fredericksburg, Virginia, 1914-16, and Marymount College, Tarrytown, New York, 1916-17. Through her uncle, Michael Ahern, a Latin scholar and teacher, Lynch learned Latin at an early age. She majored in Latin at college and later taught Latin, history, and English at Handley High School in Winchester.

About 1916-17, while Lynch was at a house party of a friend whose father was on the Supreme Court of Pennsylvania, several attending the party thought it would be patriotic to go into nursing because there was a war (World War I) going on, and they felt they would be needed. Until this time, Lynch had no attraction toward any particular profession.

As a result, Lynch entered the University of Pennsylvania Training School for Nurses in Philadelphia in 1917. Only two years of high school were required but several in her immediate group had between one and two years of college—one close classmate and lifelong friend was Gladys Marter, who had attended Vassar. Lynch's father did not approve of her going into nursing, saying repeatedly, "It took the bloom off the rose." While at school, Lynch became editor-in-chief of her class yearbook. She also was active in sports, playing tennis, hockey, and basketball, but her favorite activities were ice skating and dancing.

As a nursing student, Lynch was inspired by Mary Virginia Stephenson, a Virginian who took particular interest in her. Stephenson was educational director and later became the administrative (nurse) director of the Hospital of the University of Pennsylvania. M. Louise Snyder, the director of nursing at the hospital, was another role model.

Lynch completed the three-year program in 1920 at age 24, worked as a head nurse, and took the state board examinations. She then taught Latin and English at Handley High School in Winchester, Virginia, from 1923–27. This was followed by her becoming a laboratory assistant in bacteriology and biochemistry at George Washington Medical School, 1927–29. Combining her interest in science and nursing, she became an instructor of nursing arts and bacteriology at Sydenham Hospital, New York City, 1929–30. This was followed by six years at Willard Parker Hospital in New York City: three as education director and three as director of nursing (1930–36). While here she worked with many outstanding physicians and researchers. She participated in early research in identifying and treating poliomyelitis and diphtheria. Her experience at Willard Parker Hospital prompted her to write *Communicable Disease Nursing*, published in 1942, which came out as a second edition in 1950.

Lynch interspersed clinical teaching, practice, and administration with academic studies at Teachers College, Columbia University, where she acquired a master of arts degree in 1934. She received a doctorate in education from New York University in 1940.

In her graduate studies, Lynch concentrated on sociology, and being in New York City, she was able to observe the sociopolitical system firsthand inasmuch as she was associated with a city and state department of nursing. This experience, including six years as a faculty member at New York University, provided the skills she needed when invited by the board of trustees at the Hospital of the University of Pennsylvania in Philadelphia to take charge of nursing education and administration. Her accomplishments during her tenure at the University of Pennsylvania, 1942–47, included the initiation of two-year, four-year, and five-year nursing education programs, the latter two leading to the baccalaureate degree in nursing. During this time, about 600 Cadet Corps nurses were educated at this university school. Lynch emphasized nursing research while eliminating the many menial duties of nurses.

While at the University of Pennsylvania, Lynch recruited additional faculty members as many had gone with Hospital Base Unit No. 20 to the China-Burma-India war zone. She also developed curricula, taught classes, and established new clinical affiliations for the students. Her ultimate goal was to set up a nursing school at the University of Pennsylvania separate from the control of the University Hospital. During this time, she also commuted to Hunter College in New York City, where she taught two classes.

In 1944 the five-year basic program leading to the degree of bachelor of science in nursing was established at Pennsylvania. In 1947 she returned to New York City, where she continued the development of a nursing program she had begun. In 1949 she returned to the University of Pennsylvania to become professor of nursing and dean of the School of Nursing and to establish the degree program. During this time Lynch chaired the first Committee on Careers of the National Recruitment Committee of the National League of Nursing Education.

In 1950 the School of Nursing at the University of Pennsylvania was established by the board of trustees in the Division of Medical Affairs. It included the five-year program leading to the bachelor of science in nursing degree and programs leading to the B.S. degree in nursing education. Lynch was appointed the first dean of the school.

She is credited as well with guiding the early stages of development of the baccalaureate program in nursing at the Thomas Jefferson University in Philadelphia. She also organized the program and then became acting dean and professor in the College of Nursing of Crozer Foundation in 1965 (later this became the College of Nursing at Widener University, Chester, Pennsylvania.)

Lynch was cofounder with Lillian S. Brunner of the History of Nursing Museum in Philadelphia in May 1974. In 1975 the collection was moved to the Pennsylvania Hospital, Philadelphia, the oldest hospital in the United States.

In her late 80s Lynch cared for an older sister and lived in Washington, D.C., to be near her. Later she moved to Saunders House near the Lankenau Hospital in Philadelphia. In spite of physical difficulties due to a fractured hip and cataract eye surgery, she attended the fiftieth anniversary celebration of the School of Nursing at the University of Pennsylvania in September 1985.

Lynch was a member of Pi Lambda Theta, National Honor Society in Education, and of Sigma Theta Tau, National Honor Society in Nursing. She received honorary recognition from the Pennsylvania Nurses Association, the Philadelphia District of the Pennsylvania Nurses Association, and the Pennsylvania League for Nursing. She was made an honorary citizen of New Orleans for her contributions to nursing education. She received the Distinguished Alumnus Award from the Nurses' Alumni Association of the Hospital of the University of Pennsylvania. In 1980 she was elected an honorary fellow in the American Academy of Nursing. Lynch is listed in *Who's Who of American Women* (1958, 1961, 1964, 1966, 1968, 1970).

PUBLICATIONS BY THERESA INEZ LYNCH

BOOKS

Communicable Disease Nursing. St. Louis: Mosby, 1942, 1959.

With J.F. Landon and L.W. Smith. *Poliomyelitis* New York: Macmillan, 1934.

ARTICLES

"Approaches to Integration. The Administrator's Role." In *Concepts of the Behavioral Sciences in Basic Nursing.* New York: National League for Nursing, 1958. Pp. 108–10.

"From Hospital to Home Nursing: A Referral System Facilitates the Patient's Transition from a Hospital to a Community Service." *American Journal of Nursing* 48 (November 1948): 684–86.

"Nursing Profession Moves toward Equality." *Woman's Press* 44 (1950): 18–19.

"The Committee on Careers in Nursing Offers Some Hints on Community Planning for Student Recruitment Programs," *American Journal of Nursing* 50 (January 1950): 51–52.

"The Continuing Development of the Nurse Practitioner." In *Improvement of Nursing Practices.* New York: American Nurses Association 1961.

"There's Nothing Like Nursing for Adventure in a Career." *Woman's Press* 44 (1950): 12–13.

"Recruitment–1951. The Committee on Careers in Nursing Reports Its Activities During the Past Year." *American Journal of Nursing* 52 (March 1952): 301–03.

BIBLIOGRAPHY

Alumni Newsletter (School of Nursing, Hospital of the University of Pennsylvania) 12 (Winter 1981).

Lynch, T.L. Interviews (taped) with the author, Philadelphia, December 11, 1985, and May 13, 1986.

Lynch, T.L. Personal correspondence with the author, 1980–85.

Main Line Times (Wayne, Pennsylvania). October 10, 1985.

Lillian Brunner

Nancy A. Lytle

1924–1987

Nancy A. Lytle was an educator, writer, and innovator in the field of health care for women. She is regarded as one of the leaders of the women's health movement that evolved in the 1970s from the clinical specialties of obstetric and gynecologic nursing.

Lytle's family lived in Fredericksburg, Ohio, where she was born on October 14, 1924, the daughter of George B. and Bertha G. Lytle. Her father was a plumber, electrician, and hardware dealer. She had two brothers, Carl G. and John B. Her childhood and youth were spent in Fredericksburg, and she graduated from Fredericksburg High School in 1942. Throughout her life she maintained an interest in books and music, especially opera.

Lytle completed her basic nursing training at Fairview General Hospital School of Nursing, Cleveland, and earned a B.S. in nursing from the University of Pittsburgh. She completed her M.A. degree and her Ed.D. in nursing education at Teachers College, Columbia University.

Before joining the faculty at Case-Western Reserve University in 1968, Lytle was director of the graduate program in maternal health nursing at the State University of New York at Buffalo. Before that she was an assistant professor of obstetrical nursing at Ohio State University School of Nursing. At the time of her death she was professor and chairman of maternity and gynecologic nursing at Frances Payne Bolton School of Nursing and chairwoman and administrative associate of maternity and gynecologic nursing at University Hospitals, Cleveland.

As an instructor of student nurses, Lytle introduced innovative ways of teaching family-centered nursing in a maternity setting by having new parents address the students, sharing their needs and experiences. In 1969 she led a pilot project at University Hospitals to expand the role of the father in the childbirth experience. Her efforts involved both graduate students and staff nurses in furthering family-centered care. She was also a leader in the development of programs for childbirth preparation, for sibling visitation in maternity settings, and for "high-risk" mothers and newborns. Her endeavors reached into the community and included helping secondary-school administrators to develop a demonstration project enabling pregnant adolescents to remain in school and receive prenatal and postpartum health care. She also consulted with the Ohio and Virgin Islands Departments of Health and served as a consultant for several universities— the University of Virginia, Emory University, University of Wisconsin, University of Illinois, and Virginia Commonwealth University.

Lytle influenced her students and colleagues to look ahead, to think analytically and in innovative ways; she envisioned nurses as researchers in clinical and applied areas and encouraged her students to prepare for this role through disciplined study. *Nursing of Women in the Age of Liberation*, published in 1977, set forth her belief in nursing's role in assisting women to be responsible for their own health needs and goals.

Lytle was a charter member of the American Academy of Nursing and a member of the Sigma Theta Tau. In 1980 the Ohio Senate awarded her the Outstanding Service in Health Care Award. The Ohio Nurses' Association and the National Foundation-March of Dimes named her March of Dimes Nurse of the Year in 1984. She was honored by Cleveland's University Hospitals for her leadership in nursing at the McDonald Hospital for Women. A plaque of dedication in her name was placed in the hospital in 1986.

Nancy Lytle died in Cleveland on August 24, 1987, of cancer. Her contribution to nursing can be summarized in her own words as helping to promote "an awareness of new and heretofore essentially unrecognized needs of the female population."

PUBLICATIONS BY NANCY A. LYTLE

BOOKS

Nursing of Women in the Age of Liberation. Dubuque, IA: W.C. Brown Inc., 1977.

ARTICLES

"Faculty Involvement in Quality Assurance Programs." Publication 15-1611. New York: National League for Nursing, 1976. P. 45.

"Jurisdiction of Nursing: Areas of Control and Accountability in Delivery of Primary Health Care Services" in *Primary Care by Nurses: Sphere of Responsibility and Accountability.* Publication G-127. Kansas City, MO.: American Nurses Association, March 1977. Pp. 20–28.

With R.M. Vrbanac. "New Parents are the Teachers" *Nursing Outlook* 4 (April 1956): 221–22.

BIBLIOGRAPHY

Lytle, C., and J. Lytle. Personal communication with the author, 1989.

"Nancy A. Lytle." Obituary. *Cleveland Plain Dealer*, August 29, 1987.

Schlotfeldt, R., M.L. Wykle, L.J. Nosek, K.M., Budd, and F.R. Young, *Frances Payne Bolton School of Nursing*, Case Western Reserve University, Cleveland, 1987.

Marianne Brook

Sarah Aloysius McCarron

1879–1964

Sarah Aloysius McCarron served as a Red Cross nurse on the front in World War I and in the Balkans, where she was awarded the Serbian Cross of Mercy for her work in public health and child welfare.

McCarron was born on October 13, 1879, the daughter of Charles and Catherine (Duffy) McCarron. She graduated from Williamsburg Hospital School of Nursing in New York City in 1909 and was certified as a registered nurse by the State of New York in 1910. She entered the field of public-health nursing in New York City, working as a school nurse, and in April 1911 enrolled with the Red Cross Nursing Service. Prior to the outbreak of World War I, she also served as a public-health nurse in Mexico.

On September 8, 1914, McCarron sailed on the historic *Ship of Mercy* as a Red Cross nurse. She was one of 120 trained nurses who were selected with special regard to physical fitness for service as well as previous training. Only those without close home connections were chosen. Each nurse promised to remain in Europe for six months and was allowed only the luggage that she could carry herself. If the war lasted longer than six months, those who desired would be replaced and sent home. The nurses and 30 physicians and surgeons embarked for Falmouth, England. Helen Scott Hay, who had been chosen by Queen Elinora of Bulgaria to oversee the building of a hospital in that country, was in charge of the nurses. McCarron was assigned to a military hospital in Cosel, a town near the Russian border, where many of the seriously wounded soldiers were treated. She returned to the United States in April, 1915.

In 1917 McCarron was reassigned to Base Hospital No. 2 at Fort Bliss, Texas, and served in the Army Reserve Corps for six months before returning to Europe, where she was stationed at hospitals in Neuilly and Chateau Theirry, France. She was assigned to the surgical ward, her hours of duty from 7:30 A.M. to 7:00 P.M. with three hours off during the day if time permitted. On December 18, 1918, she was released from the hospital at Chateau Thierry to join the Balkan Commission. She traveled to Podgoritza, Montenegro, where she worked as a public-health nurse. There was much poverty in Podgoritza, the inhabitants were poorly clothed, food was scarce, and there was no means of heating in many homes or in the elementary school. At the end of her tour of duty, McCarron received a citation from the Serbian Red Cross and was awarded the Serbian Cross of Mercy. She was also commended by the Red Cross for her devoted service and remarkable work among the poor.

McCarron returned to the United States on August 2, 1919, and was employed by the Public Health Service in New York until her retirement in 1942. During the term of Governor Alfred E. Smith she worked with him to win higher pay for nurses. A member of the Brooklyn Local Committee on Red Cross Nursing Service, she chaired the committee from 1932 to 1941. She was an American Legion member for 43 years and at one time was commander of Brooklyn Post 967. In 1927 she was elected delegate to the American Legion convention in France.

McCarron died at the Veterans Administration Hospital in New York City on January 8, 1964, at the age of 84.

BIBLIOGRAPHY

American National Red Cross. *History of American Red Cross Nursing*. New York: Macmillan, 1922.

American Red Cross Archives. American Red Cross National Headquarters, Washington, D.C.

Comet. P.S. No. 73, Brooklyn, June 1918.

Matthews, I. Interview with the author, 1989.

Obituary. *New York Times*, January 10, 1964, 43:3.

Lilli Sentz

Ada Belle McCleery

dates unknown

Ada Belle McCleery was a nursing administrator and educator who served as secretary of the National League of Nursing Education in the 1920s.

She graduated in 1910 from the nursing program of Wesley Memorial Hospital in Chicago and studied for one year at the School for Civics and Philanthropy there. She also attended a summer session at Teachers College, Columbia University.

She did private-duty and tuberculosis nursing. From 1913–14 she was business manager of the Cook County Tuberculosis Hospital at Dunning, Illinois, and then of the tuberculosis division of the Cook County Institution in Oak Forest. Early in 1915 she spent two months touring schools of nursing in the eastern United States.

On May 1, 1915, she was named director of nurses at Evanston Hospital, Evanston, Illinois. During her first year she enacted several improvements, including making high-school graduation a requirement for entrance, admitting probationers in groups, increasing the probationary period from two to three months, and upgrading recreational activities and uniforms. Under her tenure enrollments grew, affiliations with other institutions were expanded, and the contagious-disease unit of the hospital improved. In 1919 she completed arrangements for a combined course with Northwestern University. She was named superintendent of the hospital in 1921.

She was president of the Illinois State Nurses Association for two years and treasurer of the Illinois State League of Nursing Education for three years. In 1912 she was named to the board of directors of the Illinois State Association of Graduate Nurses. She also served as a member of the board of the National League of Nursing Education and a trustee of the American Hospital Association. In the 1930s she was a member of the Council of Administrative Practice of the American Hospital Association, the first woman to serve on that body. She was active in several other national and state nursing organizations, and authored several papers on nursing education and hospital management.

PUBLICATIONS BY ADA BELLE MCCLEERY

"Cost of Nursing School." *American Journal of Nursing* 23 (December 1922): 201–05.

"Hospital and Training School Administration. The Relation of the Superintendent of Nurses to the Superintendent of the Hospital." *American Journal of Nursing* 23 (November 1923): 124–27.

"The Rise of Educational Standards for Schools of Nursing." *Modern Hospital* 33 (September 1929): 49–53.

BIBLIOGRAPHY

"Ada Belle McCleery, R.N., Secretary, National League of Nursing Education." *Pacific Coast Journal of Nursing* 23 (April 1927): 204.

"Our Contributors." *American Journal of Nursing* 23 (November 1923): 115.

Smith, C.L. *The Evanston Hospital School of Nursing: 1898–1948.* Chicago: Evanston Hospital School of Nursing, 1948.

"Some Leaders along the Way, Miss Ada Belle McCleery." *Trained Nurse and Hospital Review* (April 1938): 413.

Alice P. Stein

Helen Grace McClelland

1887–1984

Helen Grace McClelland directed the School of Nursing at Pennsylvania Hospital and instituted many changes and innovations that influenced the development of the nursing profession. She was one of three women to be awarded the Distinguished Service Cross for bravery during World War I.

McClelland was born in Austinberg, Ohio, on July 25, 1887, the daughter of Raymond G. and Harriet Lee (Cooper) McClelland. Her father was a Presbyterian minister. She was educated at Shepardson Preparatory School in Granville, Ohio, and entered Denison University planning to study medicine. While she was recuperating from an acute attack of appendicitis, two of her attending nurses suggested that she study nursing since they felt that women did not have any future in medicine, save for missionary work. She followed their advice, applied for admission to the Pennsylvania Hospital in Philadelphia, and entered the School of Nursing on October 31, 1908. The training normally lasted three years, but due to a bout of typhoid fever and diphtheria, McClelland did not graduate until May 1, 1912.

At the suggestion of friends she accepted a post at a hospital in Weiser, Idaho, following her graduation, and in 1913 she moved to Virginia, where she served as head nurse at the Norfolk General Hospital. Two years later she joined the American Ambulance Hospital Service and was sent to France for six months. Upon her return she worked briefly in Norfolk and in Easton, Maryland. In 1917 she joined the Pennsylvania Base Hospital No. 10, which was being assembled for duty in France. From May 7, 1917, until May 25, 1919, she served with the Casualty Clearing Station at Le Treport, France, as a member of the U.S. Army Nurse Corps. During an air raid she saved the life of her tentmate and was awarded America's Distinguished Service Cross. She is one of only three women to hold this medal. She was also awarded the British Royal Red Cross, First Class.

After her discharge she returned to the hospital in Easton, Maryland. In 1926 she went again to Pennsylvania Hospital and was appointed director of nursing in 1933. During World War II she organized the nursing component of Pennsylvania Hospitals's 52nd Evacuation Hospital.

During her professional career McClelland played an important role in changing the nursing profession. She instituted a shorter work day for nurses, encouraged faculty and nurses to seek additional education, and offered leaves of absence. She also solicited friends of the hospital to endow scholarships. After World War II McClelland studied ways to solve the postwar nursing shortage, implemented a two-year program to prepare nurses for bedside care, and designed a four-year college nursing course.

On June 30, 1956, after 23 years at the hospital, McClelland retired from Pennsylvania Hospital to a farm near Reading, Pennsylvania, where she pursued her interests in gardening, fishing, and hunting. In 1973 she moved to Frederickstown, Ohio, near her birthplace. Five years later she was inducted into the Ohio Women's Hall of Fame and in 1980 into the Ohio Senior Citizen's Hall of Fame.

McClelland died December 20, 1984, at the age of 97 at Columbus University Hospital in Columbus, Ohio.

BIBLIOGRAPHY

Kalisch, P., and B. Kalisch. *The Advance of American Nursing.* Boston: Little, Brown, 1978.

Matthews, I. Interview with the author, 1989.

West, R.M. *History of Nursing in Pennsylvania.* Philadelphia: Pennsylvania State Nurses' Association, 1926.

Lilli Sentz

Annabella McCrae
1863–1948

In her role as a nurse educator Annabella McCrae made significant contributions to the nursing profession. A teacher of nursing students for 39 years, she helped shape the careers of over 2,000 nurses. Her book *Procedures in Nursing* provided one of the first structured, standardized texts for nursing students, with an emphasis on patient care.

Born in 1863 in St. Louis, Quebec, McCrae was the daughter of John McCrae, a farmer, and Anne McCallum McCrae. Her mother died three days after Annabella's birth, and the baby was sent to live with her devoted, elderly Aunt Mary. Her father died seven years later. McCrae received her primary education from a tutor and at a private girls' school. However, as she was raised in a strict Victorian atmosphere, which did not recognize the importance of higher education for females, McCrae's studies and her desire to become a teacher were interrupted. She moved to Montreal with her aunt, who died when McCrae was 18 years old.

Determined to continue her education, McCrae entered the McLean Hospital School of Nursing in Somerville, Massachusetts, in 1890. Thus began her lifelong pursuit of knowledge in the field of nursing. After graduating from McLean in 1892, she began postgraduate work at a private school in Montreal. She soon returned to Massachusetts, where, in 1895, she graduated from the Massachusetts General Hospital Training School for Nurses in Boston. It is with this school that she had a long and prestigious association.

McCrae's professional career began with her appointment as assistant superintendent of the Quincy Hospital in Quincy, Massachusetts, a position she held for seven years. In 1902 she was appointed second assistant of nurses at Massachusetts General Hospital, with an eventual promotion to first assistant. In 1912 McCrae was assigned to the position of full-time instructor of nursing, a responsibility she held until her resignation in 1934. Dedicated and uncompromising, she was described by Dr. N.W. Faxon, former director of Strong Memorial Hospital in Rochester, New York, as "a determined spirit, sustaining high ideals of conduct, service, achievement throughout many years; a great teacher of nurses."

Throughout her career, McCrae was active in both the pursuit of knowledge and the sharing of that information with her students and peers. In 1916 she attended Teachers College at Columbia University in New York City to enhance her skills as an educator. She continued taking such courses until 1933. During World War I she took a leave of absence to teach a course on nursing practice at the Army School of Nursing, Camp Devens, Massachusetts. One of her most noteworthy accomplishments was the publication of her book *Procedures in Nursing: Preliminary and Advanced.* While maintaining a full-time teaching position, McCrae wrote this two-volume text between 1920 and 1925. The book was combined into one volume in 1927 and subsequently revised. Reprinted nine times and translated into several foreign languages, it represents a significant achievement in the history of nursing education.

Beginning in 1903, when she attended an organizational meeting of the Massachusetts State Nurses Association, and throughout her career, McCrae was an active participant in professional nursing organizations. She served as chair of the Census Committee of the Massachusetts State Nurses Association for nine years, helping to compile credentials from schools whose alumni associations wished to join that organization. McCrae was an early member of the Massachusetts League of Nursing Education and, in 1924, an organizer of the Anne Strong Club for instructors of nursing. She was a founding member of the Suffolk County Nurses Central Directory, which served as a registry service for private-duty nurses. In addition, she served as president of the Sick Relief Committee of Massachusetts General Hospital for nine years.

In 1934, in recognition of her numerous achievements in nursing education, McCrae was awarded the Walter Burns Saunders Memorial Medal, given to the nurse who "has made to the profession or to the public some outstanding contribution either in personal service or in the discovery of some nursing technique that may be to the advantage of the patient and of the profession."

Annabella McCrae died in February 1948.

PUBLICATIONS BY ANNABELLA MCCRAE

BOOKS

Procedures in Nursing. 2 vols. Boston: Whitcomb & Barrow, 1923–25.

ARTICLES

"Planning for Communicable Diseases." *Hospitals* 12 (February 1938): 84–86.

BIBLIOGRAPHY

Friedman, A. Howell. "McCrae, Annabella." In *Dictionary of American Nursing Biography.* M. Kaufman, ed. Pp. 241–42. Westport, Conn.: Greenwood, 1988.

Parsons, S.E. "Annabella McCrae." In *National League of Nursing Education: Biographic Sketches, 1937–1940.* New York: The League, 1940.

"The Saunders Memorial Award." *Public Health Nursing* 26 (June 1934): 282.

Linda Karch

Mary Eleanor McGarvah

1886–1979

Mary Eleanor McGarvah was the first nurse attorney. She was an expert in public-health law and regulation.

McGarvah was born on June 15, 1886, in Windsor, Ontario, Canada, to James and Mary Lanspeary McGarvah. Her father was an engineer on the Grand Central Railroad; she had three brothers and three sisters. The family moved to Detroit in 1900, where Eleanor lived for the rest of her life. She was a citizen of the United States. All of the McGarvah children were well educated (physicians and teachers) and involved with their church. McGarvah was a member of the Plymouth Brethren Church, where she taught Sunday school and participated in Bible study.

McGarvah graduated from Farrand Training School for Nurses, Harper Hospital in Detroit, on April 27, 1911. In December she was registered as number 2114 with the Michigan State Board of Registration of Nurses. In June 1925 McGarvah completed the requirements for graduation from Detroit Central High School. This was accomplished so that she could enroll in the law school of the University of Detroit. In June 1929 she was awarded the bachelor of law degree and was issued a certificate of admission as an attorney in the state of Michigan on September 30, 1929. She was admitted to the Michigan Supreme Court in October 1929, and in August 1931 she was admitted to the District Court of the United States for the Eastern District of Michigan as an attorney and counselor, soliciter advocate, and proctor of the court.

After graduating from nursing school, McGarvah worked as a private-duty nurse until July 1, 1914, when she joined the Detroit Health Department as a school nurse. She held badge number 2. She decided public-health nursing would be her field; she liked the preventive accomplishments of that aspect of nursing. During the summer McGarvah was given the task of investigating the high infant-mortality rate. Her investigation led her into immigrant neighborhoods, where the use of midwives was prevalent. She discovered the midwives were not reporting the births, so the statistics were inaccurate. By 1918 prenatal clinics were established in Detroit, and most midwives were registered. After a year, Eleanor became a supervisor in the new special investigation division of the Detroit Health Department.

This new division monitored the registration of midwives, violations of the medical-practice act, day nurseries and boarding homes for children, and orphanages. Her trips into court made it apparent that the Health Department needed legal/legislative clout to make progress. This greatly influenced her decision to go to law school. In 1946 McGarvah was promoted to be director of the Division of Special Investigation. She retired from that position in 1955, having served the Detroit Health Department for 41 years. She also maintained an independent law practice with evening and Saturday hours.

During her public-health practice in Detroit, McGarvah is credited with getting licensure for midwives and massage parlors, setting up the court procedures for dealing with communicable disease (mainly tuberculosis), authoring the original Michigan regulations for convalescent homes and homes for the aged, and making regular inspections of the boarding homes for children. At the national level, McGarvah's major contribution was writing the second and third editions of *Jurisprudence for Nurses* with Carl Scheffel (1939, 1945). This book is believed to be the first book on nursing and the law.

The first edition published in 1931 led to considerable discussion by nursing leaders. The case examples were criticized as outside the range of nursing experience. In the preface to the second edition, Scheffel defended his work and announced a collaborator for that edition (McGarvah). She referred to studying carefully "the reaction of the nursing profession to the first edition in order to select with intelligence additional subject matter." An important issue discussed in these two editions is specialties in nursing or the legal responsibility of "special nurses."

McGarvah was known as a kind person with a good sense of humor. She was devoted to public service and her church and family. She was supportive of public-health nurses and defended them in their cases.

Mary Eleanor McGarvah died on April 3, 1979, in Grand Rapids, Michigan, from arteriosclerotic heart disease. Her personal papers were donated to the Detroit Main Library, Personal Historical Section. In 1987 the Mary Eleanor McGarvah Humanitarian Award was established by the American Association of Nurse Attorneys Foundation. The awardee is expected to demonstrate significant public service and involvement in health law or policy issues.

PUBLICATIONS BY
MARY ELEANOR MCGARVAH

With C. Scheffel. *Jurisprudence for Nurses.* New York: Lakeside, 2nd ed. 1939; 3rd ed. 1945.

BIBLIOGRAPHY

Citation for Mary Eleanor McGarvah Humanitarian Award, May 15, 1987 (written by C.E. Northrop).

Correspondence by the author with two friends of McGarvah and E.M. Cordell (niece), Franklin, Michigan, 1986–88.

Green, B. "In Memory of Mary Eleanor McGarvah: A Key Role Model in Our Nation's History of Health Care." *Congressional Record* (June 16, 1988): E2021.

Northrop, C.E. Personal files on McGarvah.

Northrop, C.E. and M.E. Kelly. "First Nurse Attorney, Mary Eleanor McGarvah." *Legal Issues in Nursing.* Pp. vii–viii. St. Louis: Mosby, 1987.

Laurie K. Glass

Charlotte Macleod

1852–1950

Charlotte Macleod was principal of the Waltham (Mass.) Training School for Nurses, which offered an alternative to the conventional hospital training in the 1890s. She was a nursing education leader in both the United States and Canada.

Macleod was born in New Brunswick, Canada, on November 11, 1852. Soon orphaned, she was raised by an uncle. Before beginning her nursing career, she taught school in Canada for 15 years.

She graduated from the Waltham Training School for Nurses in 1891 and then took courses at the Long Island College Hospital in Brooklyn (N.Y.) and the McLean Insane Hospital (Mass.).

She returned to the Waltham Training School as principal in 1892 and served there until 1898. Waltham students got most of their training in physicians' offices and by doing visiting nursing. They attended daily lectures given by cooperating physicians. During the final terms they spent most of their time nursing in homes, returning to the school for review and final examinations. Macleod extended the course to two and one half years in 1894 and to three years in 1895.

On a five-month leave in 1896, Macleod met with Florence Nightingale and other nursing leaders and studied methods of training nurses for both hospital and district nursing in England. As a result of this trip, the Waltham Training School became the first school in the United States and the second in the English-speaking world to offer a preparatory course for probationary nurses.

Macleod returned to Canada in 1898 to become chief superintendent of the Victorian Order of Nurses, then being founded by Lady Aberdeen to commemorate Queen Victoria's diamond jubilee. The order was a professional organization for district visiting nurses, and Macleod's appointment was based partly on the fact that the Waltham Training School was the only one in the United States to teach visiting nursing. Macleod traveled all over Canada on behalf of the order until ill health forced her resignation after six and a half years.

She traveled in Scotland and France from May 1904 to May 1905 and then started and headed the Training School for Visiting Nurses of the Boston Instructive Visiting Nurses Association. From 1909–12 she performed similar functions for the Training School for Attendants being set up by the Brattleboro (Vt.) Mutual Aid Association.

Over the next four years she held a series of temporary appointments. In 1913 she was superintendent of nursing services at Miradero Sanitarium, Santa Barbara, California, and later temporary superintendent of Waltham Hospital. In 1914 she was acting matron of the Roxbury House of Mercy in Boston and taught at the Garland School in Boston and in Dublin, New Hampshire. From 1915–17 she did parish and social service work at Christ Church, New York City.

In 1917 she semiretired to Winchendon, Massachusetts, where a sister lived. She returned to Waltham briefly in 1921 to administer the home-nursing course at the Waltham Training School. She died October 21, 1950.

PUBLICATIONS BY CHARLOTTE MACLEOD

"District Nursing." *Trained Nurse* 25 (September 1900): 177–78.

"Nursing Education in Canada." *Canadian Nurse* 36 (October 1940): 664–68.

"The Victorian Order [of Nurses] in Canada. Proceedings Third International Congress of Nurses*, September 18–21, 1901, Buffalo, N.Y. Cleveland: Savage, 1901.

BIBLIOGRAPHY

Charlotte Macleod. Undated pamphlet. Waltham Training School. Waltham Training School Archive, Mugar Memorial Library, Boston University, Boston.

Pennoch, M.R., ed. *Makers of Nursing History.* New York: Lakeside, 1940.

"The Waltham Training School for Nurses." *Trained Nurse* 12 (January 1894): 1.

Alice P. Stein

Clara Barton McMillen

1869–1957

Clara Barton McMillen was a crusader for improved standards of nursing practice and a leader in promoting enactment of the New York State Nurse Practice Act of 1903. For many years she was director of District 13 of the New York State Nurses Association, which covers Manhattan, the Bronx, and Staten Island. She was founder and a member of the board of directors of the Alumnae Association of St. Luke's Hospital Training School for Nurses and for more than 30 years served as chairman of the St. Luke's Hospital registry committee.

McMillen was born in Lebanon, Ohio, and was named for Clara Barton, a friend of her father, Dr. Alexander McMillen. She attended Bishop Bowman College in Pittsburgh, Pennsylvania, and was graduated from St. Luke's in 1899.

McMillen began doing private-duty nursing immediately after graduation and continued until her retirement in 1927. She was a home-defense nurse from 1918–19.

She was active in the St. Luke's Alumnae Association throughout her career. After successfully lobbying for the Nurse Practice Act, she served as chair of the association's Legislative Committee for several years. For 14 years she chaired the committee to provide Christmas greetings and boxes for alumnae shut-ins. She also helped to raise funds and govern two rooms at the hospital that were endowed and set aside for use of graduates of the school. In 1938 she chaired the Alumnae Association committee that organized the fiftieth anniversary celebration of the founding of the school.

Concerned with the housing problems of nurses, she served in 1921 on a committee to raise funds for the Central Club for Nurses, a residence for nurses operated by the YWCA. After the building was dedicated, she continued on the committee, which managed it until its reorganization in the 1940s.

Even her hobbies were devoted to serving the cause of nursing. As a member of the Navy Comfort League, she contributed more than 1,500 hand-knitted articles during World War I.

McMillen died April 30, 1957, at St. Luke's Hospital.

PUBLICATIONS BY CLARA BARTON MCMILLEN

"Private Duty Nursing." *American Journal of Nursing* 19 (October 1918): 7–8.

BIBLIOGRAPHY

Cleveland, Mrs. W., J. Tuell, Mrs. C. Ott. "Miss Clara Barton McMillen." *St. Luke's Alumnae Bulletin* (Summer 1957): 26–28.

"Clara B. McMillen, Nursing Leader, 88." Obituary. *New York Times*, May 3, 1957.

Alice P. Stein

Mary G. McPherson

d. 1956

For a quarter century, beginning in 1920, Mary G. McPherson served, first as superintendent of nurses and principal of the school of nursing at Ellis Hospital, Schenectady, New York, and later as the hospital's administrator. She also was widely recognized for her work in child welfare.

McPherson was graduated from the Samaritan Hospital School of Nursing, Troy, New York, in October 1913. She immediately was named assistant to the superintendent and instructor in nursing there, thus becoming one of the first nursing instructors in northeastern New York.

In the spring of 1917 she joined the Army Nurse Corps. She was in the first convoy of the American Expeditionary Forces to go to France and served at St. Nazaire from June 1917 to January 1919. She completed her military service by teaching at the Army School of Nursing at Camp Upton, Long Island, until it closed in August of that year.

A civilian again, McPherson became a nursing instructor at Burnett Hospital, Fresno, California. In June 1920 she returned to Schenectady to become superintendent of nurses and principal of the school of nursing at Ellis Hospital. In her four years in that post, the school more than doubled its enrollment. When she became acting administrator of the hospital on January 1, 1925, it averaged 158 patients a day. During her tenure that figure rose to 400.

McPherson did child-welfare work with the American Legion for several years. She was chairman of the Fourth District of American Legion Welfare Committee and a member of the Legion's state and county child-welfare committees. She was honored several times by the New York State Department of the Legion.

McPherson held several posts in professional organizations. From 1923–31 she was a member of the New York State Board of Nurse Examiners and for several years also served on its advisory council. For one year she was secretary of the New York State League of Nursing Education. She also was president of the Hospital Association of Northern New York and a trustee of the New York State Hospital Association. She was a fellow of the American College of Hospital Administrators and a member of the national and state hospital associations. She served Zonta International as a district chairperson and board member and also was a member of the American Legion.

She retired from Ellis in April 1946 and

lived in Niskayuna and Menands, New York, until 1952, when she moved to Hollis, New Hampshire. She became a semi-invalid in 1950 and died at the home of a sister, Mrs. R. David Savall, in Hollis, on April 5, 1956.

BIBLIOGRAPHY

"Long-Time Administrator at Ellis Dies." *Schenectady Union-Star*, April 9, 1956.

"Miss Mary G. McPherson." Undated typescript, Archives of Ellis Hospital, Schenectady, New York.

"Miss McPherson Dies; Headed Ellis 21 Years." *Schenectady Gazette*, April 9, 1956.

Alice P. Stein

Florence A. McQuillen
1903–1982

In 1948 Florence A. McQuillen was appointed executive director of the American Association of Nurse Anesthetists. McQuillen held the office for 22 years, exercising an already legendary control over all facets of its business. In addition she was responsible for the editing of *Anesthesia Abstracts* from shortly after its inception in 1937 until its cessation in 1965. This massive scholarly undertaking made her, according to Dr. John S. Lundy, "very likely the best-read person on the literature of the anesthesia." A brilliant and powerful personality, McQuillen was uniquely suited to lead nurse anesthetists through years of turbulent change and growth.

McQuillen was born in 1903 in Mahtwa, Minnesota. She entered the Central School of Nursing at the University of Minnesota in 1922 and graduated in 1925. She then received her anesthesia education at the Minneapolis General Hospital. She served as superintendent of nurses at Frances Mahon Memorial Hospital in Glasgow, Montana, a position that also made her the sole anesthetist for the hospital. Her next position was at St. John's Hospital in Fargo, North Dakota.

It was there that she met Dr. John S. Lundy, the chief of the anesthesia department at the Mayo Clinic in Rochester, Minnesota. Upon his invitation, she joined his staff in 1927 and for the next 21 years worked closely with him as chief nurse anesthetist and as a clinical instructor. It was at Mayo Clinic that she began her editorship of *Anesthesia Abstracts*, which for decades served the field by offering summaries of the most significant research developments. Lundy later recalled the origin of this enterprise:

> In 1937 I started the practice of holding weekly meetings of members of the Section of Anesthesiology of the Mayo Clinic. We each read papers on anesthesia as we found them in the current medical literature, prepared abstracts of the papers and discussed the papers within the group. Later, by means of an arrangement with the Burgess Publishing Company of Minneapolis, a publication named *Anesthesia Abstracts* was made available.

The first volume included 207 abstracts from 68 journals by 35 abstractors, both physician and nurse anesthetists. The formidable scope of the project remained the same, but the group effort soon became a solo one. As Lundy noted, "meetings of this group did not persist very long," and "soon [McQuillen] took over all the work involved in the preparation of material for this publication, and she alone produced *Anesthesia Abstracts* from then [on]."

This endeavor, as Lunday pointed out in 1965, made McQuillen's position unique. "Her contribution to the development of the literature on anesthesia is not excelled and probably will not be." Lundy then stated: "Continuation of her efforts in this respect is very important to the field of anesthesia: I hope that on the day she relinquishes her salient labors another person imbued with her dedication to anesthesia will be on hand to carry on the task of preparing the material for more issues of *Anesthesia Abstracts*." But there would be no successor to McQuillen. She retired from the project, and 1965 was the last volume of the series.

Lundy's acknowledgement of McQuillen's role is especially important because throughout the life of the project, authorship on the title page was credited to both "John S. Lundy, M.D. and F.A. McQuillen" (later, the gender specific "Florence A. McQuillen" was used), with the doctor's name given precedence.

In 1948 McQuillen left the Mayo Clinic for Chicago to become executive director of the American Association of Nurse Anesthetists (AANA). She arrived at an especially challenging time for the association and the profession. Founded in 1931 with 40 members, AANA membership had grown to 3,200. The burden of daily business had proven too great for the incumbent lay executive secretary.

There were also pressing professional issues. For example, during World War II many nurses received emergency training in anesthesia. A significant number of them now had to be brought into the profession without sacrificing the educational standards that the association had labored so hard to establish.

In addition, there was a renewal of anti-nurse anesthetist activity on the part of anesthesiologists hostile to nurses in the field. Anesthesia as a medical specialty was given great impetus from World War II. It resulted not only from the increased complexity of anesthetics, but also from a military structure that encouraged medical specialization and a GI Bill that supported medical residencies. With this newly strengthened position, some anesthesiologists launched a vigorous national public relations campaign that was anti-nurse anesthetist. Their message to the country was that anesthesia was safe only when administered by a physician. (The word "anesthesiologist" was a 1930s' coinage of American physician anesthetists who wanted to distinguish their work from that of nurses.) In another postwar action the board of directors of the American Society of Anesthesiologists in 1947 "adopted a statement in its bylaws to the effect that it was unethical for an anesthesiologist to participate in the training of nurses"; it also "precluded giving lectures at the annual meeting for the American Association of Nurse Anesthetists."

Into this situation stepped the paradoxical and indefatigable McQuillen. At the time of her appointment, AANA President Lucy E. Richards expressed the belief that "Miss McQuillen will be able to give more efficient attention to both state and national affairs than has hitherto been possible." This faith did not go unrewarded. No association leader before or after McQuillen would exercise comparable control over all facets of its business.

McQuillen's style of leadership is best described as one of "benevolent dictatorship." In her first year as executive director, she reminded members that "we [in the executive office] do not set policies; that is done for us by you and your duly elected Board of Trustees. We do hope to carry out your assignments." Yet, at the same time, McQuillen in fact controlled the flow of information in the association.

Under McQuillen the association publications ceased to communicate, much less discuss, controversial, critical issues. She prepared the agenda of meetings of the board of trustees. Mary Alice Costello (AANA president, 1963–64) recalled: "She wouldn't give us the agenda beforehand. So, when you were president, an issue would come up, and you would have to say, 'Miss McQuillen, would you explain it to the Board?' because you didn't know about it. And she didn't want anybody to know about it." Similarly, McQuillen herself produced the minutes of the meetings of the board of trustees, thus controlling the record of business.

For her part, McQuillen had discovered in her first year in office that various important committees had labored for years on issues such as accreditation of schools. She said, "It was tragic to me to find out that the entire work, long hard hours of work with one of the Committees this year, [duplicated] the same work that had been done as long as seven years ago. There has been no continuity of committee activity. That, I think, is tragic, and I do think we can remedy it, I hope." When one considers that all the work was done by nurses employed full time as anesthetists, without the benefit of staff support or strong executive coordinator, it is not surprising that some progress came slowly.

McQuillen remedied the situation by taking control.

At the end of her career McQuillen sketched a brief review of her 22-year tenure as executive director. She highlighted the achievement of the AANA's accreditation program for schools of anesthesia for nurses and the recognition of the AANA by the U.S. Department of Health, Education and Welfare as the proper agency for accreditation and certification. The title "Certified Registered Nurse Anesthetist" (CRNA), used to identify members of the profession, was adopted in 1957. There was also the creation of the association's Council, which increased the participation of state affiliates and was the forerunner of the Assembly of States. In 1969 an optional continuing-education program (made mandatory in 1977) was adopted, making the AANA the first professional nursing group to institute a continuing-education policy. A history of the profession, written by Virginia S. Thatcher, was published in 1953. AANA membership had grown from 3,200 to 14,539.

In 1965 McQuillen was named Health Association Executive of the Year by *Hospital Management*. In announcing its award, the editorial noted:

> The phenomenal growth of this professional association is mainly due to the organizational genius of Miss McQuillen, who provided the leadership to pilot this group of specialized registered nurses to the national status of a recognized profession in the United States of America. . . . Although the burden of direction of the American Association of Nurse Anesthetists weighs heavily on her shoulders, Miss McQuillen is a person of never-failing good humor who answers her own telephone and has a *bon mot* for everyone whom she meets. She contributes generously of her time and effort to the work of the hospital and health agencies whenever she is requested to do so and her skillful grasp of current problems is without parallel in the field. She is truly the leader in her profession and her authority in the health field is undisputed.

Unfortunately, McQuillen was reluctant to release the reins of power, and, though talking of retirement for years, it became a reality only when the board decided in 1970 that the time had come. Her style of leadership had lost its effectiveness. The health-care scene had changed dramatically since 1948.

In 1981, on the occasion of the fiftieth anniversary of the AANA, McQuillen was honored with the Agatha Hodgins Award for Outstanding Accomplishment. Marie A. Bader (AANA president 1968–69) voiced the consensus of the membership in acknowledging, "Mack was the right person at a time when we needed someone to take over the pressing needs of the Association. She was a dedicated woman whose life was the Association. I sincerely believe we would not be here celebrating our fiftieth anniversary if it had not been for the careful charting of our course by this lady."

McQuillen died December 19, 1981, in her Minneapolis home.

PUBLICATIONS BY FLORENCE A. McQUILLEN (SELECTED)

"Cerebral Manifestations of Anoxia: A Review of the Literature." Parts 1 and 2. *Journal of the American Association of Nurse Anesthetists* 17 (May 1949): 137–67; (August 1949): 256–65.

"Cerebral Manifestations of Anoxia." Part 3. *Journal of the American Association of Nurse Anesthetists* 18 (May 1950): 84–86, 97.

"Nurse Anesthetist Education." *Accreditation in Higher Education*, Lloyd C. Blanch, ed., Chapt. 27. Washington D. C.: U. S. Government Printing Office, 1959.

"Postanesthesia Observation Room." *Journal of the American Association of Nurse Anesthetists* 16 (February 1948): 20–24.

Editor and chief contributor. *Anesthesia Abstracts*. 1937–1965.

BIBLIOGRAPHY

Bankert, M. *Watchful Care, A History of America's Nurse Anesthetists*. New York: Continuum, 1989.

"Florence A. McQuillen named recipient of Hodgins Award." *AANA News Bulletin* (November 1981).

"Former AANA executive director Florence A. McQuillen dies," *AANA News Bulletin* (March 1982).

"Health Association Executive of the Year." *Hospital Management* 100 (August 1965): 28.

Marianne Bankert

Ann Kathryn Magnussen

1899–1975

Ann Magnussen served as the national director of the American Red Cross nursing and health programs from 1950 to 1964. An internationally acclaimed nursing leader, she was recognized for outstanding and meritorious service with the Red Cross.

A native of Clinton, Iowa, Magnussen was born on February 24, 1899, to Christian and Laura Ingwersen Magnussen. She was the second born of six children and the only girl. Her brothers were Hans, Carl, Ernst, Harro, and Marcus.

After graduating from the Clinton High School, Magnussen enrolled in the LaCrosse Hospital School of Nursing in LaCrosse, Wisconsin, where her aunt, Ella Ingwersen, was superintendent of the hospital. She received her nursing diploma in 1924. She later attended the University of Minnesota and received a B.S. degree.

Magnussen began her Red Cross career as a public-health nurse for the Plymouth County, Iowa, chapter in 1930, at a time when many county public-health services were funded by the American Red Cross (ARC). During the next eight years she was county nurse and senior nurse for Woodbury County, Iowa, with her office located in Sioux City.

In 1939 she rejoined the Red Cross as a nursing field representative for the organization's midwestern area office in St. Louis, and from 1940 to 1943 she served as assistant director of nursing for the area office. She then transferred to the ARC southeastern area office in Atlanta, where she served first as deputy director and then director of nursing services.

Magnussen came to Red Cross national headquarters in Washington, D.C., in 1947, as director of disaster nursing and nurse enrollment. The next year she was named deputy national director of ARC nursing services and two years later was appointed director.

Active in a number of nursing organizations, she served on the board of directors of the American Nurses' Association (1958–62) and as its first vice-president (1962–64). She also served six years on the board of directors of the American Journal of Nursing Company, including one year as first vice-president (1966). She was on the board of directors of the National Health Council and was president of the District of Columbia League for Nursing (1955–57). She chaired the Nursing Advisory Committee of the League of Red Cross Societies, Geneva, Switzerland.

In May 1963 Magnussen was awarded the Florence Nightingale medal, the highest international nursing honor. The gold medal is awarded biennially by the Red Cross International Committee in recognition of exceptional service.

After her retirement from the Red Cross in 1964, she was appointed to a newly created role of nursing consultant to the Division of Medical Care Standards, Bureau of Family Welfare, U.S. Department of Health, Education, and Welfare. In this position her responsibilities included making recommendations to the bureau on matters relating to nursing care as part of the medical care provided by public assistance and preparing guidelines for nursing care for use by state agencies.

In 1967 she retired to Omaha, Nebraska, where she lived until 1974, when she moved to Fort Worth, Texas, to live with her brother, Harro A. Magnussen. She died on July 4, 1975.

The Magnussen Award, named in her honor, was established by the ARC in 1968. It recognizes outstanding nurses who, through their resourcefulness and dedication, help to accomplish the mission of the ARC nursing and health program by extending health education or service to those most in need.

PUBLICATIONS BY
ANN MAGNUSSEN

"The Teaching Procedures Used in Red Cross Home Nursing." *Public Health Nursing* 44 (January 1952): 21–24.

"Nursing in Disaster. 1. Red Cross Service." *American Journal of Nursing* 56 (October 1956): 1290–91.

"Nursing Under the Red Cross Today." *Nursing Outlook* 9 (March 1958): 158–60.

"This I Believe . . . About Nursing's Responsibility to Interpret Nursing." *Nursing Outlook* 13 (February 1965): 51.

"Who Does What—in Defense, in Natural Disaster." *American Journal of Nursing* 65 (March 1965): 118–21.

With R.S. Boyer, "Polio is a Community Problem." *Nursing Outlook* 3 (March 1955): 135–38.

BIBLIOGRAPHY

"Ann Magnussen Dies at 76, Red Cross Nursing Official." *Washington Post,* July 9, 1975.

"Ex-Red Cross Official to be Buried in Iowa." *Fort Worth (TX) Star Telegram,* July 6, 1975.

"Florence Nightingale Medal Winners." *Nursing Outlook* 11 (July 1963): 533.

"Former Nursing Director at ARC Dies." Obituary. *American Journal of Nursing* 75 (September 1975): 1434.

"LORCS (League of Red Cross Societies) Meets in Greece." *American Journal of Nursing* 60 (March 1960): 388.

Magnussen, A. Papers. American Red Cross, National Archives, Washington, D.C.

Magnussen, H. Letter to the author, January 8, 1989.

"National Director of American Red Cross Retires." *Nursing Outlook* 12 (March 1964): 16.

Signe S. Cooper

Mary Ann Maher

1902–1982

Mary Ann Maher served as the first dean of two schools of nursing: she was the founding dean of the Boston College School of Nursing and later the founding dean of the University of Massachusetts School of Nursing. She was instrumental in incorporating concepts of mental hygiene and influence of the family into nursing practice.

Born on March 12, 1902, in Exeter, New Hampshire, she was the daughter of Ellen Sheehan and William Maher. A graduate of Robinson's Seminary, Exeter, New Hampshire, in 1920, she received a diploma from the Rhode Island Hospital School of Nursing in Providence in 1930. In addition, she later received a certificate in public-health nursing from Simmons College, Boston, after which she went on to attend Teachers College, Columbia University, receiving a B.S. in 1941 and an M.A. in 1949.

After receiving her diploma in nursing in Providence, she moved to Rochester, New York, where for a year she served as a teacher and supervisor in the School of Nursing of Strong Memorial Hospital. She returned to Providence to become an instructor in the Rhode Island Hospital School, 1931–36, after which she became a staff nurse and special project director for the Visiting Nurse Association of Boston. From 1938–40 she served as a public-health nursing instructor at Massachusetts General Hospital School of Nursing in Boston. After attending Teachers College (1940–41), she joined the Board of Registration in Nursing of the Commonwealth of Massachusetts as supervisor of schools of nursing, a position she left in 1946 to become a regional public-health consultant for the U.S. Children's Bureau in New York City. In 1947 she became founding dean of the Boston College School of Nursing, a position she held for only a brief time before returning to get her master's degree from Columbia University.

After receiving this degree, she was appointed associate professor of the Boston University School of Nursing, and in 1953 she was appointed the first dean of the new University of Massachusetts School of Nursing in Amherst, where she served as dean until 1970.

One of Maher's major concerns as dean was to raise the level of faculty in collegiate nursing schools. She was instrumental in securing federal funding for a successful seven years of summer workshops for the continuing education of nursing faculty from a variety of schools in New England. Focus of the summer courses was on the arts, sciences, and humanities. From her original work at Rochester's Strong Memorial Hospital where she had been introduced to a multidisciplinary approach to health, she emphasized the importance of understanding family setting and mental hygiene in nursing practice. She was also an advocate of nurses working with other professionals in social work, nutrition, and early childhood. To put these concepts into practice, she received grants to demonstrate the importance of this concept of health care to residents of housing projects.

Maher was active in various nursing organizations. She was president of the Massachusetts League for Nursing (1960–61) and served for a time as a member of the State Board of Registration in Nursing, as well as the executive committee of the Massachusetts Committee on Children and Youth and the Governor's Advisory Committee for Planning for Mental Health. During its founding years she was on the executive committee of the New England Council on Higher Education for Nurses and was active in the Department of Baccalaureate and Higher Degree Programs of the National League for Nursing. In recognition of her role as a "distinguished nursing educator," she received an honorary doctor of science degree from Boston University in 1969. A scholarship fund in her name was set up at the University of Massachusetts at the time of her retirement. Her alma mater, on June 16, 1973, gave her the Nurses' Alumnae Association Award to honor her outstanding contribution to nursing, and she was noted as an outstanding graduate in 1980, marking her 50 years as a graduate of that school. She died February 11, 1982, in Amherst, Massachusetts.

BIBLIOGRAPHY

Friedman, A.H. "Mary Ann Maher." *Dictionary of American Nursing Biography*. M. Kaufman, ed. Pp. 253–55. Westport, Conn.: Greenwood, 1988.

Friedman, A.H. "Nursing Revisited: Oral History and Mary A. Maher." *Massachusetts Nurse* (May 19, 1984).

"Mary Ann Maher." *American Journal of Nursing* 82 (June 1982): 998.

Nursing Archives, Mugar Library, Boston University.

Vern L. Bullough

Marguerite Lucy Manfreda
b. 1910

The professional career of Marguerite Lucy Manfreda has been stamped with two hallmarks: esteemed psychiatric-nursing educator and influential author of three psychiatric-nursing books, one of which she authored through seven editions.

Manfreda, the seventh daughter in a family of nine girls and two boys, was born to Frank and Felicia Tomasiello Manfreda on November 13, 1910, in rural Wallingford, Connecticut, 13 miles north of New Haven and Yale University. Both parents came from Italy—her mother as an infant and her father as a young man, who, after having served in Garibaldi's army and then having made two attempts to reach the United States in ships that developed leaks, finally landed at Sandy Hook, New Jersey. Initially, he settled in Meriden, Connecticut, but shortly thereafter moved to Wallingford, where he operated a shoe-shine and confectionery store across from the railroad station.

When Manfreda was 10 years old, her mother died. Despite the tragedy, Manfreda recalled a happy childhood that was strongly influenced by her older sisters and father. It included piano lessons for all the children, sing-alongs accompanied by their father playing the accordion, and summer vacations at the family property near the Quinnipiac River. Reading was encouraged for knowledge and enjoyment. Self-discipline and education were promoted to develop self-sufficiency.

In 1928 Manfreda graduated from Lyman Hall High School in Wallingford. Shortly thereafter she entered the Hartford (Conn.) Hospital Training School for Nurses (HHTS), a career choice that was influenced by a visiting nurse who had treated Manfreda when she was a young teenager. Manfreda graduated in 1933.

While Manfreda was working as a new staff nurse on the surgical service of the New Haven Hospital, Evelyn Sturmer, the head nurse of the Yale Institute of Human Relations asked Manfreda to consider joining the institute's staff. Manfreda's decision to accept a position introduced her to the clinical specialty that she was to pursue for the remainder of her professional career. Manfreda recalled that, unlike most other nursing settings of the time, "freedom of thought" prevailed at the institute. Further, despite the fact that nurses were not allowed to read patients' records because that was considered a breach of the patients' privacy, the focus of nursing was truly the nurse-patient relationship.

In 1940 Manfreda joined the staff of the New York State Psychiatric Institute in New York City for a five-year period. There Florence Newell, nursing director of the institute, became a lifelong colleague. A highlight of Manfreda's experience at the institute was her first publication, "The Electroencephalogram," which appeared in the *American Journal of Nursing*. The article, which was written at the prompting of a physician who had heard Manfreda lecture and demonstrate to Columbia University medical students about the new diagnostic technique for neuropsychiatric examinations, is even more notable for the inclusion of suggestions for psychological support for patients undergoing the procedure.

In 1947 Manfreda received a bachelor of science degree from the New York University School of Education. She then returned to HHTS for a year, where, as an assistant nursing arts instructor, she integrated the emotional aspects of illness and health teaching principles in the course content. She then assumed the position of chief night supervisor and then the director of nursing education

at the Institute of Living (formerly known as the Hartford Retreat) in Connecticut. While in the supervisory position, Manfreda, at the request of the F.A. Davis Company, undertook the revision of Katharine McLean Steele's *Psychiatric Nursing*, becoming the coauthor for the fourth through sixth editions, sole author for the seventh, eighth, and ninth editions, and then coauthor again for the tenth and last edition in 1977. Emphasized in each edition was the nursing approach, the therapeutic influence of the environment, and social and educational activities upon the patients' recovery.

By now recognized as both an educator and a specialist in psychiatric nursing, Manfreda was sought by Florence Newell, then consultant to the Illinois Department of Mental Health, to be the director of the psychiatric nursing affiliation program at the 6,500-bed Elgin State Hospital. The year—1952—was critical for that was the year that the National League for Nursing determined that psychiatric nursing become a mandatory curriculum subject in schools of nursing. Manfreda established the Elgin program and remained there for 10 years. Simultaneously, she completed the requirements for a master of arts degree, with a major in teaching psychiatric and mental-health nursing, from Teachers College, Columbia University, in 1961. In the same year that she received her advanced degree, her book entitled *Teaching Psychiatric and Mental Health Nursing* was published. It was described by Sturmer as "the first text designed for the use of teachers of psychiatric nursing and for those concerned with the integration of sociopsychosomatic concepts in all areas of nursing." In 1962 Manfreda returned to the East, first to Greystone Park State Hospital in New Jerey and then to the Essex County (N.J.) Hospital, where she held positions similar to those she had held in Illinois.

In 1968 Manfreda returned to Illinois as the director of the Swedish-American Hospital School of Nursing in Rockford. There Manfreda developed a psychiatric-nursing component that allowed students to have both theortical instruction and clinical experience in their home hospital, as well as in the newly built mental-health center in Rockford, rather than at the Anna State Hospital, which was 500 miles away. That change was also advanced by the availability of federal grants that encouraged diploma school faculty members to become prepared as psychiatric-nursing instructors and by the fact that student affiliations with state mental hospitals were being discontinued.

From 1972 to 1976, when she retired as emeritus professor of nursing, Manfreda was an associate professor at Black Hawk College in Moline, Illinois. There she had further developed and coordinated a program in psychiatric nursing for three Moline diploma schools of nursing in conjunction with the program being conducted by the college for its own students.

Throughout her professional career, Manfreda was active in nursing organizations on both the local and state levels. Further, while on summer vacations during the latter part of her career, she planned and participated in programs, funded by a federal mental-health grant, for graduate professional nurses employed in mental hospitals and allied health agencies in Little Rock, Arkansas. For that work she was recognized by both the state of Arkansas and the Arkansas League for Nursing.

As a result of her widely read publications, her effective leadership in private and public psychiatric institutions in various geographical locations, her work with professional organizations, and her experience in both diploma and collegiate educational settings, Manfreda's life has been touched by many nursing leaders. Among them were Elizabeth Bixler, Annie W. Goodrich, Effie Taylor, Kathleen Black, Agnes Ohlson, and Janet Geister. Now, back in Wallingford, Connecticut, the energy, perseverance, dedication, and concern that Manfreda showed throughout her active professional career are being directed toward leadership in community, hospital, and church activities, the writing of psychiatric-nursing history, and frequent contact with her family and associations of long-standing.

PUBLICATIONS BY MARGUERITE LUCY MANFREDA

BOOKS

Steele, K., and M. Manfreda. *Psychiatric Nursing*. Philadelphia: Davis, 4th ed. 1950; 5th ed. 1954; 6th ed. 1959.

Teaching Psychiatric and Mental Health Nursing. Philadelphia: Davis, 1961.

Psychiatric Nursing. Philadelphia: Davis, 7th ed. 1964.

Gibson, A., and M. Manfreda, eds. *The Remotivator's Guide Book*. Philadelphia: Davis, 1967.

Psychiatric Nursing. Philadelphia: Davis, 8th ed. 1968; 9th ed. 1973.

And S. Krampitz. *Psychiatric Nursing*. Philadelphia: Davis, 10th ed. 1977.

The Roots of Interpersonal Nursing. Wallingford, Conn.: The author, 1982.

ARTICLES

"The Electroencephalogram." *American Journal of Nursing* 44 (December 1944): 1144–49.

"Money Isn't Everything." *American Journal of Nursing* 47 (February 1947): 80–82.

"From Out of Antiquity: Personal Reflections." Privately published by author, 1983.

"A Half Century of Nursing: Personal Reflections." *Society for Nursing History Gazette* (Spring 1985): 1–7.

"Annie Goodrich's Psychiatric Nursing Program." *American Association for the History of Nursing Bulletin* 22 (Spring 1989): 3–7.

With M. Stormer. "Fenestration for Hearing Impairment." *Trained Nurse & Hospital Review* (December 1945): 408–10.

BIBLIOGRAPHY

Battle, E. Review of *Psychiatric Nursing*, 9th ed. by M. Manfreda. *Nursing Outlook* 21 (November 1973): 689.

Cohelan, E. Review of *Psychiatric Nursing*, 7th ed. by M. Manfreda. *American Journal of Nursing* 64 (October 1964): 165.

Manfreda, M. Private papers. Personal interviews with the author, July–August 1990.

"Professional Literature: Teaching Psychiatric and Mental Health Nursing." *Journal of Psychiatric Nursing* 1 (January 1963): 65.

Smoyak, S., and S. Rouslin, eds. *A Collection of Classics in Psychiatric Nursing Literature*. Pp. ix–x. Thorofare, N.J.: Stack, 1982.

Eleanor Krohn Herrmann

Bernice D. Mansfield

1879–1971

Bernice Mansfield was one of the group of nurses who pushed for the legislative action leading to the organization and incorporation of the Maine State Nurses Association (MSNA) on December 10, 1914, and became one of its founding members. She served as the first treasurer and on its first Executive Committee.

Born in Orono, Maine, Mansfield attended the local schools and the Castine (Maine) Normal School. She then graduated from the Eastern Maine General Hospital School of Nursing in Bangor in 1904. For a period of time she served as staff nurse at that institution, advancing to the position of hospital nurse supervisor (comparable to a director of nursing service).

With the entrance of the United States into World War I in 1917, she enlisted in the U.S. Navy Nurse Corps and became chief nurse at the Great Lakes Naval Training Center Hospital. Transferred to the Pacific, she helped to establish a naval hospital in Samoa in 1918. After the war Mansfield served as chief nurse at the Brooklyn (N.Y.) Naval Hospital. She retired in 1939 with the rank of lieutenant, the highest rank then accorded to nurses.

Best known for her administrative and organizational abilities, Mansfield worked as a volunteer with the Red Cross and Civil Defense Agency in Bangor during World War II. She was active in the MSNA for many years, serving in various capacities.

She moved to Florida and resided at the Maranatha Retirement Home in Lake Alfred, Florida, until her death on October 22, 1971, at the age of 92.

PUBLICATIONS BY BERNICE D. MANSFIELD

"Nursing in American Samoa." *International Nursing Review* 8 (1933): 73–79.

BIBLIOGRAPHY

Philbrick, J.C. "In Memoriam: Bernice D. Mansfield, R.N." *Maine Nurse* 3 (January 1972): 6–7.

Marianne Brook

Sister Amy Margaret

ca. 1869–1941

Sister Amy Margaret was a nursing educator whose specialty area was pediatrics. Her nursing activities were a component of her religious vocation in the Sisters of St. Margaret (Episcopalian). Sister Amy's career was cut short by ill health. The 25 years she spent in nursing established her as "one of the great educators in pediatric nursing and a leader in the profession."

Little is known about Sister Amy's early life. She was born in England to parents of both American and English heritage; one source indicated that she was privately educated. At about age 17, she migrated to the United States and entered the novitiate of the Sisters of St. Margaret in Boston. At the time she joined the order, Sister Amy had no formal education or training in nursing.

The Sisters of St. Margaret in the United States were an offshoot of the English order, St. Margaret's Sisterhood, which had been founded by the Reverend Dr. John Mason Neale in 1854. The order had established itself as a provider of nursing care and arranged for its probationers to have training at Westminster. The English order provided Florence Nightingale with nurses to serve in Crimea. Dock (1931) credited the Anglican orders with moving nursing from the "depths into which it had fallen" because the women of culture and refinement who entered these religious communities set high standards for performance.

The Sisters of St. Margaret were invited to Boston to establish a children's hospital managed by sisters similar to Children's Hospital in Washington, D.C. In 1871, Mother Alice, the superior of the Sisters of St. Margaret in East Grinstead, England, came to the United States bringing with her Sister Theresa to serve as superintendent of the hospital. The first few years were devoted to developing the community and arranging for training of sisters at Boston City Hospital. St. Margaret's Infirmary, Boston's first private hospital, opened in 1877. It consisted of two rooms in the convent. Later the infirmary moved to larger quarters and became the Children's Hospital of Boston. Children's Hospital was managed by the Sisters of St. Margaret, and Sister Amy began her nursing career after entering the novitiate in 1896.

Although she had no formal nursing education, Sister Amy Margaret was involved not only with instructing nursing students, but also nursing sick infants at Boston's Seashore Home (later to become the Boston Floating Hospital) during the summer months. In 1889 she was sent to St. Barnabas Hospital in Newark, New Jersey, also managed by her order. While there, Sister Amy provided both general and maternity nursing care to patients. After a year at St. Barnabas she and another sister were sent to organize Christ Hospital in Jersey City, New Jersey. Circa 1890–91, she did private nursing in Halifax, Nova Scotia. After her return from Canada she became the superintendent of nurses at St. Barnabas but was forced by illness to take a year's leave of absence.

In 1894 Sister Amy returned to Children's Hospital of Boston as instructress of nurses and remained there for the rest of her nursing career. Since she lacked formal nursing education, she decided to take the nursing courses provided for members of the order at Children's Hospital. She had been offered a diploma but refused to accept it until she had completed all course work and passed all examinations. Her diploma was conferred in 1902.

From 1903 until 1906 Sister Amy was the assistant superintendent of nurses at Children's Hospital and became superintendent of the training school. In 1907 the hospital expanded its nursing education program to include a secular training school. The school was later described as being one of a select group with excellent standards and a model training school. Sister Amy's innovations in American nursing education were, in large part, responsible for the success of the school.

Even prior to becoming superintendent of the Training School, Sister Amy had been involved with formulating educational strategies for the school. In 1897 the student's workday had been limited to eight hours, and, by 1900, students were no longer paid for their work. The money saved was used to pay graduate nurses to serve as instructors. Later, the school charged tuition in order to avoid the need for apprenticeship-type education. In 1901 the program was lengthened to three years and a high-school diploma was required for admission. It was found that, despite tuition charges and greater selectivity, the school was able to increase enrollment.

Sister Amy had also been involved in increasing the clinical opportunities for the student nurses. Affiliations were actively sought to expand their knowledge and experiences. In 1904 affiliation agreements with Boston Lying-in and Corey Hill hospitals provided maternal and private adult nursing experience. One particularly innovative affiliation was with the Social Services Department at Massachusetts General Hospital. In the 1909 school report Sister Amy stated that, to her knowledge, such an experience was the first attempt in the United States to provide instruction for nurses in medical social work.

Sister Amy had also been instrumental in obtaining an agreement between Simmons College of Boston and Children's Hospital School of Nursing. In 1904 students were given four months of instruction at the college in anatomy, physiology, chemistry, bacteriology, and sanitation prior to any other training from Children's Hospital. It was felt that the students would best learn this content if they were not tired and distracted from ward work. After completion of these courses, the students were given two more months of study at the hospital in domestic science, cooking, and essentials of practical hospital work. This six months constituted the probationary period. Theoretical content was considered to enhance the practical instruction as students were grounded in the essentials of science and would have "correct habits of observation and orderly methods of thought."

In addition to her organizational abilities and innovations in education, Sister Amy was noted as an excellent teacher. Goostray (1940), writing the history of

Children's Hospital, called her "one of the most outstanding teachers that The Children's Hospital has had." Goostray also quoted a 1900 graduate of the training school: "I was so thoroughly grounded [by Sister Amy] in the carefulness of the details of nursing that I have been able to do much for the sick poor and student nurses also." Lucas (1938) noted that physicians also learned from and appreciated Sister Amy "whose fine spirit permeated every detail of a most vigorous training . . . [and who] taught many an interne more about the diseases of children than he would ever have learned without her."

Sister Amy also involved herself with the needs of the profession in general. She was the first, and for some time the only, religious member of the National League of Nursing Education. She had joined this organization when it was still the American Society of Superintendents of Training Schools for Nurses (ASSTSN) and was the first nurse of a religious order to serve as a counselor for that organization. She served on various committees of these organizations and attended conventions when possible. At the Fourteenth Annual Meeting of the ASSTSN in 1908, she presented a program on the specialized care of the pediatric patient, including content on normal growth and development.

Ill health again became a problem for Sister Amy. In late 1911 she was unable to continue her position at Children's Hospital. Sara Rice took over in her absence, but Sister Amy's recuperation was slow and she formally resigned in 1913.

The Sisters of St. Margaret relinquished responsibility for the administration of Children's Hospital in 1917. Although Sister Amy recovered, she did not return to Children's Hospital. She served her order as mistress of novices at the Mother House in Boston and was later infirmarian. After spending some years as an invalid, Sister Amy died at St. Margaret's Convent in Boston on March 6, 1941.

Sister Amy's ideas on nursing education were beyond those generally held by the public. Her insistence on earning her diploma when it was not considered necessary showed a commitment to nursing education rather than strictly training. The development of the affiliation with Simmons College also indicated that she valued education. Sister Amy retired from nursing before there was wide acceptance of her ideas (e.g., an eight-hour day for students, college courses as preparation for clinical practice), but the school she had helped develop was a source of ideas and a model for nursing educators who would follow.

PUBLICATION BY SISTER AMY MARGARET

"Artificial Feeding." *American Journal of Nursing* 7 (April 1907): 521–24.

BIBLIOGRAPHY

Dock, L., and I. Stewart. *A Short History of Nursing*, 3rd ed. Pp. 113–14. New York: Putnam, 1931.

Dolin, J. *Nursing in Society: a Historical Perspective*, 14th ed. P. 361. Philadelphia: Saunders, 1978.

Doyle, A. "Nursing by Religious Orders in the United States: Part VI—Episcopal Sisterhoods." *American Journal of Nursing* 30 (December 1929): 1466–83.

Goodnow, M. *Nursing History*, 7th ed. P. 216. Philadelphia: Saunders, 1944.

Goostray, S. *Fifty Years: a History of the School of Nursing, The Children's Hospital, Boston.* Boston: Alumna Association of the Children's Hospital School of Nursing, 1940.

Lucas, W. *Children's Diseases for Nurses.* P. 13. New York: Macmillan, 1938.

Sellew, G., and Sr. M. Ebel. *A History of Nursing*, 3rd ed. P. 278. St. Louis: Mosby, 1955.

"Sister Amy Margaret." Biographical sketch. Veronica M. Driscoll Center, Guilderland, New York. Photocopy.

"Sister Amy Margaret." Obituary. *American Journal of Nursing* 41 (April 1941): 509.

Leslie M. Thom

Mother Marianne of Molokai

1836–1918

Mother Marianne of Molokai began her career as an educator and administrator, but she made her major contribution to nursing as a pioneer in the care of patients suffering with leprosy. For almost 35 years she practiced nursing and directed the Sisters of Saint Francis as they served patients at several leprosy centers in the Hawaiian Islands in the closing years of the nineteenth century. Her religious calling, combined with a strong sense of cleanliness and hygiene, enabled Mother Marianne to direct her sisters in the care of hundreds of patients without any of these nurses contracting the disease.

She was born Barbara Kopp, the first child of Peter and Barbara Witzenbacher Kopp, in 1836 in Heppenheim of Hesse (modern-day Germany). When Barbara was just over a year old, the family migrated to Utica, New York. Early in her life, she felt a strong calling to enter religious life. Her mother died at an early age, leaving six children and a grief-stricken husband. Barbara took charge of the home until the family had grown and scattered. She then entered St. Anthony's Convent in Syracuse, New York, and on November 19, 1862, at the age of 26, joined the Sisters of the Third Order of St. Francis. She completed her novitiate and became Sister Marianne on November 19, 1863. She began her work as a teacher in the school of the Church of the Assumption in Syracuse.

She proved to be a gifted leader and administrator, and by August 1875 she had become superior of St. Joseph's Hospital in Syracuse. When the call to go to Hawaii came, Mother Marianne was serving at the hospital and as the provincial superior for her order.

In 1883 Mother Marianne led a group of six Franciscan sisters to the Hawaiian Islands to work with Father Damien in a hospital mission serving lepers. Leprosy first appeared in the islands in the 1850s. Father Damien had gone to Molokai in 1873 where 809 lepers were isolated and had pioneered as a missionary among these people with the feared disease. The sisters were assigned initially to the Kakaako Branch Hospital near Honolulu, caring for the lepers isolated there. In 1889, after Father Damien's death from leprosy and many improvements were achieved on Molokai, the sisters were allowed to move to the larger leper colony. They began work in the Bishop Home for Girls and Women on the island. Mother Marianne was 45 when her most challenging job began in Hawaii.

The Kakaako Branch Hospital was a crude collection of primitive buildings set close to the sea a mile from Honolulu. Sanitation and housekeeping standards were appalling for the 200 inpatients. After working in the hospital without any amenities or adequate supplies, three of the sisters, including Mother Marianne, moved to the Malulani Hospital on Maui. The sisters' days in both hospitals consisted of cooking, cleaning, and disinfecting as well as bedside care.

Mother Marianne directed the mission work of the sisters on Molokai and Maui until her death. None of her sisters ever contracted leprosy. Mother Marianne believed God would protect those doing His work. She also attributed freedom from infection to scrupulous cleanliness, care with dressings, and good hygiene practices within the order.

Mother Marianne undermined her usual robust health with an exhausting workload, which demanded 18–20-hour days and few respite breaks. She coped with chronic pain and complications of tuberculosis until her death at the age of 83. Mother Marianne's efforts and those of the many sisters who joined her left several institutions for lepers, including the largest sanctuary on Molokai, in exemplary condition.

BIBLIOGRAPHY

Cardwell, I. *Damien the Leper*. London: Allan, 1931.

Dutton, C. *The Samaritans of Molokai*. New York: Dodd, Mead, 1932.

Farrow, T. *Damien the Leper*. New York: Image Books, 1963.

Halsermenn, C., ed. *Catholic Encyclopedia*. Vol. X, pp. 444–45. New York: Appleton, 1911.

Jacks, L.V. *Mother Marianne of Molokai*. New York: Macmillan, 1935.

Quinlan, T. *Damien of Molokai*. New York: Appleton, 1903.

Linda Sabin

Julia St. Lo Mellichamp

1877–1939

Julia St. Lo Mellichamp gave 30 years of service to nursing as a private-duty and institutional nurse. An active participant in professional associations, Mellichamp was an articulate advocate of standards for the profession, including the creation of a national registry for nurses, and devoted much of her career to the improvement of nurses' working conditions.

Julia Alberta (later St. Lo) Mellichamp was born on April 13, 1877, in Florence, South Carolina. She was the first of eleven children, five boys and six girls, born to Edward Henry Mellichamp II and Evelyn Pierce Loper Mellichamp. Four sisters and one brother survived past infancy. Edward Mellichamp was active in the Episcopal Church in North Carolina and South Carolina, but he was not an Episcopal minister, as stated in some biographical articles on Mellichamp.

Mellichamp received most of her early education at home due to an attack of infantile paralysis. She eventually graduated from college and became a school teacher. After a few years of teaching, she returned to school for a business course and became a legal secretary. She then decided to pursue a career in nursing and enrolled at Sarah Leigh Hospital School of Nursing in Norfolk, Virginia, graduating with honors in 1906.

From 1906 to 1911 Mellichamp worked as a private-duty nurse. Her involvement with professional associations began in 1909 when she served as treasurer of the Virginia State Nurses Association. She eventually found private-duty nursing too physically demanding and became the first school nurse in Norfolk, Virginia, in 1911, serving in the position until 1917. While employed as a school nurse, she served as state chairman of the Red Cross Nursing Service in Virginia (1911–17) and also spent time as president of the Sarah Leigh Alumnae Association and president of the Norfolk Division of the Virginia State Nurses Association.

In 1914 Mellichamp became the executive secretary and treasurer of the Virginia State Board of Examiners of Nurses, a po-sition she held until 1920. An early advocate of a national nursing registry, she articulated her vision in a speech she gave at the 1915 Graduate Nurses' Association Convention in Roanoke, Virginia. In this speech Mellichamp noted the benefits of a registry, stating that "to the community the registry affords ready access to all classes of nursing service and vouches for the moral and professional fitness of each of its members. . . . Furthermore it affords financial protection by its regular tariff of fees for various branches of work. . . ."

From 1917 to 1920 Mellichamp served as inspector of hospital training schools. As inspector, she advocated a number of reforms that are now standard in the profession. The use of graduate nurses as night supervisors, a standard training program for student nurses, certification requirements for nursing teachers, and standard outlines for nursing courses.

Also at this time, she began her national professional involvement. In 1917 she was appointed to the board of directors of the National Organization for Public Health Nursing. In 1919 Mellichamp became a charter member of the Virginia State League of Nursing Education and then moved to West Virginia, where she became chairperson of the Public Health Nursing Section of the West Virginia Nursing Association. From 1920 to 1927 she served as school nurse and social worker in Greenbrier County, West Virginia. In 1927 she returned to South Carolina to work as supervising nurse and social worker in Dorchester County. Continuing her work in South Carolina, Mellichamp was director of the Bureau of Social Service in Jasper County (1933–34) and school nurse in Jasper and Colleton counties (1934–35).

From 1935 until her death in 1939 Mellichamp was the librarian at the Charleston, South Carolina, County Health Department. She also began work at this time on a genealogical history of the Mellichamp family. When a tornado struck Charleston in 1938, Mellichamp assisted with disaster relief. At the time of her death, she was corresponding secretary of the South Carolina State Nurses Association, District I.

Julia St. Lo Mellichamp died of a malignancy in the Riverside Infirmary, Charleston, South Carolina on November 24, 1939, at the age of 62.

PUBLICATIONS BY
JULIA ST. LO MELLICHAMP

"The Development and Value of a Nurses' Registry." *American Journal of Nursing* 17 (October 1916): 24–28.

BIBLIOGRAPHY

"Julia St. Jo [sic] Mellichamp." Obituary. *American Journal of Nursing* 40 (January 1940): 106–07.

"Miss Julia Mellichamp." Obituary. *Charleston* (S.C.) *News and Courier*, November 26, 1939.

Pennock, M.R., ed. *Makers of Nursing History.* Pp. 96–97. New York: Lakeside, 1940.

"Sketch Given of Miss Mellichamp." Undated clipping. *Charleston News and Courier* (Charleston, South Carolina), 1943.

Mellichamp, E.H. IV. Correspondence with the author, 1989–90.

Margaret R. Wells

Lucy Jane Rider Meyer
1849–1922

Lucy Jane Rider Meyer contributed in many ways to the deaconess movement in the Methodist Church in the late-nineteenth century. Although her primary goal was to prepare women for professional service in the church, her strong support of nursing education promoted the development of nursing in Chicago during a critical period of development. Meyer was uniquely educated in science, medicine, and theology, which enabled her to begin a training school for nurses at Wesley Hospital in Chicago as a major part of her program for deaconesses. She viewed nursing as a ministry just as appropriate as many other fields for women to study in order to serve the church. She played a significant role in the promotion of nursing, like other women physicians of the period, by providing the necessary theoretical instruction and clinical supervision to prepare practitioners for this emerging field.

Meyer was born in New Haven, Vermont, the first child of Jane (Child) and Richard Rider. The prosperous Rider family grew to nine children and lived a very deep religious life together. At the age of 13 Meyer was confirmed in the Methodist Church.

She attended the local elementary school and graduated from the New Hampton Literary Institution in Fairfax, Vermont, in 1867. She then spent two years teaching in Canada and South Carolina. While in South Carolina, she taught for Quakers, running a freedmen's school. She then enrolled at Oberlin and in just two years received her bachelor's degree. She became engaged to a medical student who planned to become a missionary, so in 1873 she entered the Woman's Medical College of Pennsylvania in Philadelphia in order to equip herself to serve as a missionary. Her fiancé died in 1875, and Meyer lost heart to complete her studies. She returned to Vermont, cared for her aging parents, and turned to writing for Methodist Church papers and publications.

In 1876 she returned to work as the principal of the Troy Conference Academy in Poultney. After just a year, she entered the Massachusetts Institute of Technology to study chemistry. She then moved to Chicago to teach chemistry and continue her education. In 1881 she accepted a position as a field secretary for the Illinois State Sunday School Association for the Methodist Church. During this period her commitment to church work in society grew steadily.

On May 23, 1885, she married Reverend Josiah Shelly Meyer, a former theological student and businessman who was deeply committed to the church's role in social work. One son, Shelly Rider, was born two years later. In 1887 Meyer received her M.D. degree from the Woman's Medical College of Chicago.

In October 1885 she and her husband opened a Bible normal school to provide training for women entering religious, particularly missionary, careers. The school's program expanded from visiting the poor to overseeing the Methodist philanthropic institutions in Chicago, including Wesley Memorial Hospital.

In 1887 Dr. Isaac Danforth, who was to be Wesley Hospital's first chief of staff, was given three rooms in Meyer's training school. The pair began teaching students the basics of nursing. As space for providing care to patients became available, nursing was added to the formal school curriculum. The hospital opened officially on Christmas Day, 1888. In 1892 a non-deaconess training school for nurses was begun at the hospital, but it became more deaconess-oriented by 1899.

Meyer devoted the remainder of her life to the deaconess movement and conducting her educational program at the Chicago Training School. She used her broad educational background to prepare social workers, nurses, and teachers for full-time church service. Over 40 philanthropic institutions, including hospitals, orphanages, and homes for the elderly, were begun by her and the graduates of the Chicago Training School during the first 30 years of the program's existence.

The diaconate encouraged by Meyer was deeply influenced by the German deaconess movement begun by Pastor Theodore Fliedner. This same movement had greatly affected Florence Nightingale as well. Meyer, however, viewed deaconesses as neither clergy nor laity in the church, but as professional religious workers set apart with a distinct character and functions. Meyer viewed nursing as one of several "callings" women could fulfill in society, and she was uniquely prepared to help educate all of the various students in the training school.

Sadly, Meyer never saw the Methodist Church recognize and organize deaconesses into a single organization. Throughout her lifetime she was embroiled in jurisdictional conflicts over the organization of the many deaconess groups throughout the country.

In her later years, Meyer developed Bright's disease and heart trouble and moved to California in search of health in the milder climate. She continued to grow weaker and returned to Chicago, where she died at Wesley Hospital at the age of 72.

PUBLICATIONS BY
LUCY RIDER MEYER

BOOKS

Real Fairy Folks: Explorations with the World of Atoms. Boston: Lathrop, 1887.

Deaconesses: Biblical, Early Church, European and American. Chicago: The Message, 1889. Cincinnati: Cranston and Stowe, 1892.

The Shorter Bible. New York: Hunt and Eaton, 1895.

Deaconess Stories. Chicago: Hope Publishing, 1900.

Mary North. Chicago: Revell, 1903.

ARTICLES

"The Mother in the Church." *Methodist Review* (September–October 1901).

Extensive additional contributions to Methodist publications, 1895–1917.

BIBLIOGRAPHY

Golder, G. *History of the Deaconess Movement in the Christian Church.* Cincinnati: Jennings and Pye, 1903.

Harmon, N., ed. *The Encyclopedia of World Methodism.* Vol. I, pp. 469–70. Nashville: United Methodist Publishing House, 1974.

Horton, I. *High Adventure: Life of Lucy Rider Meyer.* New York: Methodist Book Concern, 1928.

Keller, R., et al. *Called to Serve: The United Methodist Diaconate.* Nashville: United Methodist General Board of Higher Education and Ministry, 1987.

Miller, R. "Lucy Rider Meyer." In *Notable American Women 1607–1950.* E.J. James, ed. Vol. 2, pp. 534–36. Cambridge, Mass.: Belknap Press, 1971.

Price, C. *Who's Who in American Methodism.* New York: Treat, 1916.

Linda Sabin

Mary Annice Miller
1910–1962

Mary Annice Miller was an early leader in the development of in-service education in hospitals. Her book *In-Service Education for Hospital Personnel*, was the first definitive work on the subject and is a nursing classic.

Miller was born on June 27, 1910, in Creswell, Oregon, to James Roy Miller and Liva Dora Alexander Miller. Both parents were born in this country. Her father was a blacksmith and her mother a seamstress. She was the oldest of four children, the others being Melvin, Nadine, and LaVerna.

Miller grew up in Creswell and was graduated from the Creswell High School. She enrolled in the Good Samaritan Hospital School of Nursing in Portland, Oregon, receiving her diploma in 1934. Later she completed requirements for a B.S. degree in nursing education from the University of Washington.

Miller's first employment was at the Good Samaritan Hospital as a general-duty nurse. She was then appointed night supervisor and later assistant supervisor of the outpatient department, Harborview Hospital, Seattle, and after that served as a supervisory nurse with the Thurston-Mason-Olympic Health Department. During World War II she was a member of the Army Nurse Corps for three and a half years, stationed in England for a time.

In the early 1950s Miller was a hospital nursing consultant with the Washington State Department of Health. During this time she chaired a committee of the Washington State Nurses Association responsible for a study of nursing functions. Approved and funded by the American Nurses' Association (ANA), the study was an investigation of nursing activities in two urban hospitals and one small community facility in Washington. Miller analyzed the data and wrote the final report. As one of the studies sponsored by the ANA, frequent references are made to it in the book *Twenty Thousand Nurses Tell Their Story*.

In 1954 Miller left Washington and joined the staff of the National League for Nursing (NLN) in New York City, where she was employed until her death eight years later. Her work with the NLN began with the Nursing Aide Training Project, a nationwide effort conducted between 1954

and 1956. The program was a "train-the-trainer" effort, designed to strengthen the teaching skills of nurses responsible for aide training programs in hospitals and nursing homes. This was at a time when increasing numbers of nursing assistants were employed in hospitals, with minimal training for their job responsibilities.

Miller's later responsibilities as assistant director of the NLN's Department of Hospital Nursing were providing consultant services to hospitals in initiating or improving their staff education programs. Shortly before she died, she began a monthly column on in-service education in *Nursing Outlook*; two articles were published posthumously.

Undoubtedly, Miller's most important contribution to the profession was the manual *In-Service Education for Hospital Personnel*, published in 1958 by the NLN and cosponsored by the American Hospital Association. It was urgently needed at the time it was published, as many hospitals were just beginning to initiate in-service education programs. It was widely used in hospitals and health agencies throughout the country, not only because little else was available, but also because of the soundness and clarity of the content. The book reflects Miller's belief that effective nursing care was related to the knowledge and skills of providers of that care.

In addition to memberships and participation in professional nursing organizations, Miller was a member of the American Society of Training Directors. She was instrumental in organizing the first hospital and health agency group within that organization.

Miller died at the age of 52 on October 24, 1962, at Grand Central Hospital in New York City.

Dramatic changes in nursing practice and the increased mobility of nurses following World War II created a demand for hospital in-service education, but hospitals were ill prepared to meet it. Miller believed that hospitals and other health agencies had a responsibility for on-the-job training of their personnel, and she pioneered ways of helping institutions meet the learning needs of the nursing staff.

PUBLICATIONS BY
MARY ANNICE MILLER

BOOKS

In-Service Education for Hospital Nursing Personnel. New York: National League for Nursing and the American Hospital Association, 1958.

ARTICLES

"The Hospital Nursing Consultant Goes Consulting." *American Journal of Nursing* 52 (December 1952): 1486–88.

"Nursing Functions Study Completed." *Washington State Journal of Nursing* 26 (January 1954): 2–5.

"The Nursing Aide Project Re-evaluated." *Nursing Outlook* 3 (February 1955): 80–82.

"The Nursing Procedure Breakdown as a Teaching Tool." *Nursing Outlook* 3 (April 1955): 199–200.

"In-Service Education" and "The Needs in Hospital Nursing Service Administration." In *The Yearbook of Modern Nursing, 1957–1958.* M.C. Cowan, ed. Pp. 310–13; 197–200. New York: Putnam, 1958.

"Transition: Student to Employee." *Nursing Outlook* 10 (February 1962): 84–87.

"Inservice Education—What Why Where How When." *Nursing Outlook* 10 (August 1962): 541–43.

"Inservice Education—Staff Development versus 'Inservice Education Programs.'" *Nursing Outlook* 10 (September 1962): 610.

"Inservice Education—Conceptual Handicaps (Part One)." *Nursing Outlook* 10 (October 1962): 691.

"Inservice Education—Conceptual Handicaps (Part Two)." *Nursing Outlook* 10 (November 1962): 753.

"Inservice Education—Are Orientation and Skill Training True Inservice Education?" *Nursing Outlook* 10 (December 1962): 787.

BIBLIOGRAPHY

Hughes, E.C., H.M. Hughes, and I. Deutscher. *Twenty Thousand Nurses Tell Their Story.* Philadelphia: Lippincott, 1958.

"Mary A. Miller." Obituary. *American Journal of Nursing* 62 (December 1962): 125.

"Mary A. Miller, '52, Nursing Consultant." Obituary. *New York Times,* October 25, 1962.

Mary Annice Miller. File, National League for Nursing, New York, New York.

"Mary Annice Miller Dead." Obituary. *Nursing Outlook* 10 (November 1962): 759.

"Mary Miller to Work for NLN." *Washington State Journal of Nursing* 26 (April–May, 1954): 10.

Miller, M. Letter from brother to the author, February 10, 1989.

Signe S. Cooper

Nannie Jacquelin Minor
1871–1934

Nannie Minor was one of the founders of public-health nursing in Virginia. She helped found a nurses' settlement and devoted her off-duty hours to providing services to the poor of Richmond. In 1902 the settlement nurses joined in founding the instructive Visiting Nurse Association, which began to organize the care of the sick throughout the city. Tuberculosis patients received services through the dispensary or were cared for at the Pine Camp Sanitarium, available to the indigent. The association, which preceded the founding of the city's health department, was the only organized source of social and health services during its first six years of its existence.

Born in Charlottesville, Virginia, on June 15, 1871, Minor was the daughter of Ann Fisher Colstan and John B. Minor. Her father was a professor of law at the University of Virginia. She graduated from the nursing school of Old Dominion Hospital in Richmond in 1900 and went on to do postgraduate studies at Johns Hopkins Hospital in Baltimore, as well as the Thomas Wilson Sanitarium in Pikesville, Maryland. For the first two years after her graduation, she supported herself by private-duty nursing while she did her volunteer work, and then from 1902 to 1922 she was affiliated with the Visiting Nurse Association, most of the time as the head of its nursing staff.

In 1922 Minor became director of public-health nursing in the Bureau of Child Welfare for the Virginia State Board of Health. In this capacity she was responsible for organizing public-health nursing throughout the state, particularly in rural areas that previously had lacked such services. She established 45 public-health nursing services.

Instrumental in securing the nurses' registration law in Virginia, Minor also served for ten years on the Board of Nurses Examiners. After her death in Lewisburg, West Virginia, on January 30, 1934, she was memorialized by the nursing section of the Medical College of Virginia Alumni Association.

PUBLICATIONS BY
NANNIE JACQUELIN MINOR

"The Status of the Colored Public Health Nurse in Virginia." *Public Health Nurse* 16 (May 1924): 243–44.

BIBLIOGRAPHY

"Deaths: Nannie Jaquelin Minor." *American Journal of Nursing* 34 (March 1934): 303–04.

Fairs, W. "Two Hundred Years of Nursing in Richmond." *American Journal of Nursing* 37 (August 1937): 847–49.

Unpublished material. American Journal of Nursing Collection, Nursing Archives, Mugar Memorial Library, Boston University.

"Who's Who in the Nursing World, Nannie Jaquelin Minor." *American Journal of Nursing* 25 (February 1925): 116.

Vern L. Bullough

Mildred L. Montag

b. 1908

Mildred L. Montag is known as a preeminent nurse educator whose envisioning a new type of health-care worker—the technical nurse—proved to be the inception of an innovative type of nursing education program. In 1963 Montag received the first Linda Richards Award presented by the National League for Nursing in recognition of the meritorious nature of her unique, pioneering contributions to nursing.

The prototype educational program that Montag originally presented in her doctoral dissertation published in 1951 became the foundation for the associate-degree nursing programs based in junior and community colleges, which continue to prepare nursing students for a career in nursing today. The two-year, accelerated educational preparation that she proposed deviated markedly from the hospital and baccalaureate programs already in existence before the 1950s. Montag's proposals initially caused great concern and controversy among nurse educators but swiftly proved to be a viable educational alternative.

Mildred Louise Montag was born on August 10, 1908, in Struble, Iowa, the eldest of three children. When the children were very young, their father died, and following their mother's death when Mildred was 16, the three were adopted by their uncle, a successful businessman, who supplied a secure financial environment where both encouragement and the monetary means to pursue a college education were provided.

Montag was influenced to pursue a degree in nursing through her association with several family friends who were nurses. She received a B.A. from Hamline University in St. Paul, Minnesota, in 1930, and a B.S. in nursing from the University of Minnesota in 1933. She was subsequently employed as instructor at the University of Minnesota School of Nursing and then was instructor of nursing arts, at St. Luke's Hospital in New York City before becoming the first director of the Adelphi College School of Nursing, Garden City, New York, in 1943.

A critical shortage of nurses and subsequent short staffing in hospitals, caused in part by the previous closing of many nursing schools in the 1930s, was made more acute because of the demands for medical personnel in the armed services during World War II. This situation led to the establishment of many new schools of nursing in the mid-1940s to alleviate the shortage of nurses. The nursing program at Adelphi College was initiated under the direction of Montag in January 1943, supported by a grant from the U.S. Public Health Service, and was afterward almost completely funded through the U.S. Cadet Nurse Corps. Although the Adelphi nursing program retained some of the characteristics of the hospital-school educational programs, under Montag's direction it broke with many of the old educational traditions that prevailed in the hospital schools. The program was organized to ensure that all nursing classes were held on campus rather than in the surrounding hospitals. The area hospitals were used only for clinical experience, the student work week was reduced, and nursing students at Adelphi had more time and the opportunity to become integrated into the college environment on campus. Dormitories for nursing students were built on the campus. Nursing students were admitted to the program under the general admissions procedures of the college and had to maintain academic standing that met the required standards of the college as a whole. These changes, considered innovative and significant deviations from past practice, are credited to Montag's leadership and direction. During the years that Montag served as director, over 500 students graduated from the program at Adelphi.

In 1948 Montag pursued doctoral studies at Teachers College, Columbia University. To finance her tuition, she initially taught on a part-time basis, but was quickly persuaded to become a full-time instructor there. Pursuit of her doctoral degree was slowed by the additional responsibilities, but the encouragement given by such noted nursing leaders as Katherine Densford, Lucille Petry (Leone), and Isabel Stewart convinced Montag that she should continue beyond the master's level at Teachers College. She applied for, and was a recipient of, an Isabel Hampton-Robb Scholarship. This scholarship allowed her to return to full-time student status and to work on her doctoral dissertation, which quickly was to become the cornerstone for associate-degree nursing education after it was published in 1951. During her doctoral studies Montag became interested in vocational education, and some of her later educational proposals were influenced by vocational concepts to which she was exposed in several courses taken at Teachers College.

In addition to her innovative doctoral thesis, Montag has authored a variety of textbooks for nurses that deal with topics ranging from pharmacology to basic nursing techniques. Notably, these textbooks are concerned with the total care of the patient and stress the role of the nurse as health teacher. Additionally, Montag has written journal articles and project reports that have influenced the direction of nursing education, especially the evolution of associate-degree programs.

The Division of Nursing Education of Teachers College at Columbia University, initiated and sponsored the Cooperative Research Project in Junior and Community College Education for Nursing and placed the project under the direction of Montag (1952–57) while she was assistant professor and later advanced to professor of nursing education at the college. This cooperative project was the first major research undertaking of the Institute of Research and Service in Nursing Education of Teachers College, spanned five years, and ultimately provided statistical and descriptive data that proved invaluable in the evaluation of associate-degree nursing programs and the performance of associate-degree graduates in the workplace.

Montag's final report on the project, *Community College Education for Nursing*, fulfilled three purposes: it provided a description of how the experimental associate degree program was developed; it provided a systematic evaluation of the graduates of the new program; and it attempted to draw implications for the profession of nursing about issues related to the differentiation of professional and technical preparation for nursing. Montag's conclusions remain at the center of some of the controversial issues discussed in nursing education and practice at the current time.

Montag served as a professor of nursing education at Teachers College for over 20 years before her retirement in the 1970s when she became Professor Emeritus there. Throughout her career in nursing education, she has provided original ideas that continue to influence the preparation of associate-degree nurses, and through her leadership has assured that associate-degree programs have been grounded in rigorous evaluative procedures. Few books on nursing education written by a nurse have so rapidly and thoroughly revolutionized nursing education and impacted so directly on nursing service as Montag's published dissertation and subsequent work in nursing education.

PUBLICATIONS BY MILDRED L. MONTAG

BOOKS

The Education of Nursing Technicians. New York: Putnam, 1951, reprinted 1971.

The Evaluation of Graduates of Associate Degree Programs. New York: Teachers College Press, Columbia University, 1972.

With M. Filson. *Nursing Arts.* Philadelphia: Saunders, 1948, 1953.

With L.G. Gotkin. *Community College Education for Nursing: An Experiment in Technical Education for Nursing.* New York: McGraw-Hill, 1959.

With Sister A. Rihm and H.K. Mock. "A Transition in Nursing Education: Guidelines Resulting from the Phasing Out of a Diploma Nursing Program and the Establishment of an Associate Degree Program. University of Albuquerque, Division of Nursing, Regina School of Nursing." Santa Fe: Research Coordinating Unit, State Department of Education, 1967.

With A.R. Rines. *Handbook of Fundamental Nursing Techniques.* New York: Wiley, 1976.

With A.R. Rines. *Nursing Concepts and Nursing Care.* New York: Wiley, 1976.

With R.P.S. Swenson. *Fundamentals of Nursing Care,* 3rd ed. Philadelphia: Saunders, 1959.

With H.N.G. Wright. *A Textbook of Pharmacology and Therapeutics.* Philadelphia: Saunders, 1939, 1942, 1944, 1948, 1951, 1955, 1959. Title varies slightly in earlier editions.

With H.N.G. Wright. *Drugs and Solutions.* Philadelphia: Saunders, 1952.

ARTICLES

"Integral Nursing School: One College, One Health Agency, and Four Hospitals Pool Facilities." *Hospitals* 17 (October 1943): 56–58.

"Technical Education in Nursing." *American Journal of Nursing* 63 (May 1963): 100–03.

"Nurse Faculty in Associate Degree Programs." *Nursing Outlook* 12 (July 1964): 40–42.

"Where Is Nursing Going?" The Ruth V. Matheney Memorial Lecture, presented at the 1975 NLN Convention, New Orleans. NLN Publication 23-1585. New York: National League for Nursing, 1975.

"The External Degree." *Imprint* 29 (October–November 1982), 25–26.

"The Associate Degree Nurse: Technical or Professional. An Honest Difference and a Real Concern." NLN Publication 23-1946. Pp. 1–4, 17–18. New York: National League for Nursing, 1983.

BIBLIOGRAPHY

Anderson, B.E. *Nursing Education in Community Junior Colleges.* Philadelphia: Lippincott, 1966.

DeLoughery, G.L. *History and Trends of Professional Nursing,* 8th ed. New York: Mosby, 1977.

Lawrence, K.E., and H.S. Rowland, eds. *The National Nursing Directory.* Rockville, Md.: Aspen, 1982.

Safier, G. *Contemporary American Leaders in Nursing: An Oral History.* Chap. 9. New York: McGraw-Hill, 1977.

Karen L. Buchinger

Willie Carhart Morehead

1900?–?

Willie Carhart Morehead had a varied career as a nurse, but is primarily known through her reminiscences published by a vanity press in 1953. She served as a tuberculosis control nurse in some of the mountain country of the South, where often her car was the first automobile the children of the area had ever seen. Later she worked as a nurse on various government projects during the Depression, moved on to become a nurse in a woman's penitentiary, and for a time was a supervisor of nursing for a 600-bed state tuberculosis hospital located next to a state mental hospital. She also worked with the Margaret Sanger Foundation as a sort of free-lance family planner. She interrupted her career for a time to get married and have three children, Patsy, Clyde, and Nancy.

A southerner by birth she was born on the family plantation in Virginia, had an official coming out party, and in spite of the fact that nursing was considered un-ladylike went into nursing. Very little is known of her personal and private life now, even the hospital training school at which she acquired her nursing degree.

PUBLICATION BY
WILLIE CARHART MOREHEAD

The Saving Grace. New York: Vantage Press, 1953.

Vern L. Bullough

Elba Lila Morse

1882–1975

A registered nurse, Elba Lila Morse de-voted her entire professional career of over 50 years to the public health and welfare of the people of Michigan, particularly mothers and children. She was one of Michigan's first rural public-health nurses under the Red Cross, and from 1919 to 1931 it is estimated that she traveled over 300,000 miles to deliver care to her pa-tients. As a county nurse, she demon-strated home care of people with commu-nicable diseases and maternity and infant care in the home. Because of her ability, qualities of leadership, and her ardent in-terest in public health, the Red Cross ap-pointed her the regional nursing director for the state of Michigan. This role in-cluded serving as a nursing consultant to the 30 Red Cross county nurses (prior to the establishment of the Division of Nuring in the Michigan Department of Health) and organizing Red Cross relief to people following several regional disasters.

In 1931 she assumed the nursing su-perintendent role of the Northern Michi-gan Children's Clinic, which was estab-lished by the Children's Health Fund. Under her directorship the clinic became the focal point of health activity and con-structive community service for the Upper Peninsula of Michigan. She was a co-founder in 1934 of the Bay Cliff Health Camp for children (in the Upper Penin-sula) and served as its director until 1964.

For her dedicated service and leadership in the care of youth she received honorary degrees from the University of Michigan (master of science, 1953) and Northern Michigan University (doctor of science, 1955). She was a delegate to the Midcen-tury White House Conference on Children and Youth (1950), honored as Nurse of the Year by the Michigan Nursing Center As-sociation (1952), and was the third recip-ient of the Senator Charles Potter Award for aiding the handicapped (1954).

Elba Lila Morse was born on May 13, 1882, on a farm near Sandusky, Michigan, to Dilas P. Morse and Nancy Sophia Hall Morse. She had a twin sister Eva, and two brothers, Hiram Beach Morse (a physi-cian) and Olney Ray Morse (a pharmacist). She graduated from Sandusky High School in 1899 and then from Spring Arbor Seminary Junior College, a paro-chial Free Methodist girls' school. On Sep-tember 18, 1909, she graduated from the Peterson's Training School for Nurses in Ann Arbor, Michigan, and then served as an undergraduate assistant at the school. After receiving instruction in anesthetics, she administered all of the anesthetics in the hospital.

In 1910 Morse took a 10-month leave of absence from Peterson's Hospital in order to travel to Europe with a cousin who was one of the early woman graduates from the medical school at the University of Michi-gan. During this trip she purportedly studied at the Allgemeine Krankenhaus in Vienna (accounts of this study range from the study of education to midwifery to labo-ratory techniques and anesthesia). In Au-gust 1911 she resumed her assistant du-ties at Peterson's, and she held this position until 1914, when she resigned to take charge of the Maternity Department at University Hospital, Ann Arbor, Michi-gan. During this time she taught nursing students in the University of Michigan Training School for Nurses. On July 15, 1915, she returned to Peterson's to become the superintendent of nurses.

In 1918 Morse resigned from Peter-son's Hospital expecting to enter military service, but due to the signing of the Ar-mistice she entered public-health nursing under the Red Cross. She recruited nurses for the U.S. Army, Navy, and the Red Cross out of the Chicago regional offices. In 1921 she was employed by the American Red Cross to work in her home county of Sanilac as one of Michigan's first rural public-health nurses. Because of her ability, qualities of leadership, and her ardent interest in public health, the Red Cross appointed her regional nursing director for the state of Michigan. Part of her job was to serve as nursing consultant to the 25 or 30 Red Cross county nurses in the state. During these years she organized Red Cross relief for several regional disasters.

Then in 1923 and 1925 (while still with the Red Cross) she was employed by the University of Michigan as a lecturer in public-health nursing and was instrumental in helping to develop the public-health nursing program at the University. In 1927 she became a district supervising nurse of the Detroit Visiting Nurse Association (VNA) and in this role she endeared herself to the VNA, its patients, its board, and all of its cooperative relationships with other agencies.

As a result of her work in the community, first through the Red Cross and then with the VNA, she became involved with the Children's Fund of Michigan (a $10-million fund established in 1929 by Senator James Couzens, which was given for the welfare of children in Michigan and to be used over a 25-year time period).

One of the first proposed ventures of the Children's Fund was the establishment of a clinic at St. Luke's Hospital in Marquette (later named the Northern Michigan Children's Clinic). Morse performed the preliminary field work for this clinic, and, as a result, she was appointed as the nursing superintendent of the clinic. She served in this role for the next 23 years of the clinic's life. In 1954 when the Children's Fund ended, according to the original directives mandated by Senator Couzens, the clinic was incorporated into St. Luke's Hospital. Morse was directly involved in organizing the county nurse system for the entire Upper Peninsula of Michigan as well as overseeing the building of the clinic and its work in caring for children of the Upper Peninsula.

In 1934 she and Dr. Goldie Corneliuson (a pediatrician) combined forces to establish the Bay Cliff Health Camp, which initially was directed at combating the severe malnutrition that existed in the children of the region. Later it expanded to include children with many different health problems—diabetes, rheumatic fever, cardiac disease, orthopedic problems, stuttering, hearing impairment, blindness, and polio. The organizational work and fund raising were undertaken by Morse, and through her continuing efforts she generated support from the city, county, and Upper Peninsula organizations. She was the director of the camp from its inception until 1964.

In 1965 she went to Iron River, Michigan, to live with a longtime friend. In 1970 she entered an extended-care facility, and on July 3, 1975, she died at the age of 93 in Iron River, Michigan.

Throughout her nursing career Morse took an active role in professional and community organizations. She was president of the Michigan State Nurses Association, 1934–36, and in 1934 she attended the Biennial ANA convention in Washington D.C. She served as president of the Marquette District Nurses Association (1941), assisted in the establishment of the Northern Michigan School of Practical Nursing, served as chairman of the Business and Professional Women's Club for the Upper Peninsula district, served on the Board of Directors of the Upper Peninsula Conference of Social Welfare, served on the board of directors of the VNA in Marquette, served as chair of war work (1942) for the Upper Peninsula, and was active in numerous other community organizations, such as the Girl Scouts, Boy Scouts, and the Maternal Health League of Michigan, an early chapter of Planned Parenthood.

Besides the honors she was accorded, as previously described, she was honored posthumously in 1986 at the dedication of a $250,000 therapy center (occupational and physical therapy) that was named in her honor at the Bay Cliff Health Camp. In 1990 she was inducted into the historical division of the Michigan Women's Hall of Fame, the first nurse to receive the honor.

As was typical of the women who pursued a nursing career in the early 1900s, Morse forfeited the traditional role of a woman, which included marriage, children, and devotion to a husband and family. Besides raising 6 of her sister's 12 children (she assumed guardianship when her sister died of typhoid in 1932), "her family" in a larger context were the children of Bay Cliff Health Camp and the whole Upper Peninsula. In 1991 she is still frequently referred to as "Aunt Elba" by those who knew her and has been labeled as an "universal aunt" to many nurses to whom she was a moral supporter.

Besides her work she also enjoyed music, attending conferences, travel, and an appreciation for art. She particularly enjoyed collecting antique glass.

BIBLIOGRAPHY

Unpublished materials. Archives, Nursing History Society of the University of Michigan, Ann Arbor; Archives, Bentley Historical Library, Ann Arbor, Michigan; J.M. Longyear Research Library, Marquette County Historical Society, Marquette, Michigan.

Linda K. Strodtman

Mary Kelly Mullane

b. 1909

With a strong commitment for the establishment of nursing education in institutions of higher learning, Mary Kelly Mullane has stood at the forefront in local, state, and national arenas as a proponent for the highest standards in curriculum, research, and service. As a practitioner, author, educator, and administrator, she strove for excellence in nursing and was nationally recognized as "the statesman" of the nursing profession during her career. She has made outstanding contributions to the profession and to health care in the country.

Mary Elizabeth Kelly Mullane was born on September 25, 1909, in New York City to Irish Catholic parents, Ann Nilan and Thomas J. Kelly. She is the oldest of three siblings, a sister Dorothy and a brother Thomas. Her sister Dorothy also became a well-known nurse. Mullane grew up in a multigenerational household where "children were to be seen and not heard and where politics was a constant topic." Her continued interest in politics was probably influenced by her father and grandfather, who were businessmen in New York City and were active in local politics.

Mullane received her diploma in nursing in 1931 from Holy Name Hospital School of Nursing in Teaneck, New Jersey. She became interested in this school of nursing because her mother and father had been involved in the establishment of the hospital. Her father had been on one of the committees responsible for the building of the hospital and her mother helped organize the auxiliary at the hospital. Her sister Dorothy attended the nursing program with her, fostering their long-standing close professional and personal relationship. Mullane obtained a bachelor of science degree in 1935 and a master of arts degree in 1942 from Teachers College, Columbia University. She achieved her Ph.D., with a major in administration in higher education at the University of Chicago in 1957.

After graduation from the diploma program, she worked as a private-duty nurse for six months until she was recruited back to Holy Name Hospital to become the assistant supervisor of the operating room. Her interest in nursing education was fostered at this time since she had responsibility for overseeing the work of nursing students. She then became an instructor in nursing arts at St. Joseph Hospital in Paterson, New Jersey, and later an instructor in science at St. Francis Hospital in Jersey City. During this time, she began taking night classes at Columbia University in New York.

After receiving her B.S. degree, Mullance moved to Detroit, where she soon became one of the founders of the department of nursing at Mercy College of Detroit. She next became the assistant director of nursing services at Detroit's Receiving Hospital and became an associate professor and later assistant to the dean of nursing at Wayne State University, where she helped create an autonomous school of nursing within the university. She has cited the experience of working with Dean Katherine Faville as one of her happiest times. Together they helped open the opportunities for black nursing students in Detroit because many of the hospitals prior to their efforts had not allowed black nurses to receive their clinical training in their hospitals.

In the summer of 1950 Mullane enrolled in doctoral studies at Columbia University. When she was invited to join a seminar group for nursing-service administration sponsored by the W.K. Kellogg Foundation at the University of Chicago, she transferred there and combined the seminar work with course work for the Ph.D. Mullane described the seminar program as a milestone of development in the nursing profession. Fourteen university graduate programs stemmed from it. She also wrote the evaluation report of this seminar program, *Education for Nursing Service Administration.*

She returned to Wayne State University and organized the nursing-service administration major in the master's program. In 1952 she married John Thompson Mullane, an accountant and business executive, and resigned as assistant to the dean to become a part-time faculty member. During the next seven years, she also was director of programs for the Cunningham Drug Company Foundation, a charitable organization.

She was recruited as dean of the School of Nursing at the University of Iowa, where during her three-and-a-half-year tenure she brought about the transition of the undergraduate clinical curriculum in nursing, which was primarily under control of University Hospital, into a program under the control of the college faculty and financially supported by the university. Typical of the schools during that period, students had manned the University Hospital, were housed in its nurses' home, and were not charged tuition during their junior and senior years. Using the students for service, the hospital actually had been in major control over the clinical aspects of the nursing major.

In 1962 Mullane went to the University of Illinois, where under her leadership as dean the college moved from a small program offering only baccalaureate preparation for nursing to a nationally recognized college offering the gamut of preparation for nursing careers. Under her dynamic leadership the college experienced a period of extensive growth and development. Mullane was responsible for planning of the 11-story College of Nursing building and successfully secured funding for that building not only from the university, but also from state and federal sources. She was skilled in faculty development. Convinced that nursing education must meet the standards of other disicplines, she insisted that nursing faculty must have appropriate preparation. Recognizing the leadership potential for nursing, she encouraged able faculty to enroll for doctoral education, while planning and laying the groundwork for the doctoral program at the college. She brilliantly defended to the university's governing bodies the need for research in nursing and the granting of the Ph.D. degree in nursing.

Mullane retired as dean in 1971 and took a six-month sabbatical leave. To learn the modern technological applications of management, she studied in the Department of Systems Engineering at the Circle Campus of the University of Illinois, later incorporating these concepts into the major courses in nursing-service administration. She did extensive research on the management and direction of nursing services in hospitals and other health-care facilities. She was concerned about the lack of comparable attention to the problems of nursing service and the need for analysis and improvement of nursing service, and she returned to the College of Nursing in the spring of 1972 to inaugurate the nursing-service administration major. She retired from the university in 1975 but continues as professor emerita and is active in fund raising and support of the College of Nursing.

In 1976 Mullane was recruited to be the executive director of the American Association of Colleges of Nursing and worked half time in this position until 1978, when she retired from her nursing career.

In addition to serving as a leader in four collegiate nursing programs, she served as a leader in professional organizations. Early in her career, she was elected to be the first president of the National Council of Catholic Nurses (1940–44) and then served as a member of the board of directors (1944–52). In Michigan she served on various committees as member and as chair from 1936–59 in the Michigan State Nurses Association and in the Michigan League for Nursing. She served as vice-president in the Detroit District of the state association (1955–57). On the national level, she served on several committees between 1950 and 1976 and chaired the ANA Committee on Research (1965–69), and the Council of Member Agencies' Baccalaureate and Higher Degree Programs of the National League for Nursing (1961–65).

From 1965–70, while dean at the University of Illinois, she was the chairperson of the Illinois League for Nursing and Illinois Nurses Association Study Commission on Nursing. This landmark study was the impetus for the organized development of nursing education in the state of Illinois. Because it was one of the most comprehensive studies of nursing and needs and resources, the study became a role model for studies in other states. While in Illinois, Mullane also served as a member of the Chicago Board of Health and as a member of the board of directors of the Infant Welfare Society.

As a member of the board of directors of the Association of Collegiate Schools of Nursing, she participated on the Committee on the Structure of National Nursing Organizations (1946–50). This committee, which included representatives from the major six national nursing organizations in the country, recommended the two-organization plan, namely the American Nurses' Association for nurse members only and the National League for Nursing for nurses, nonnurses, schools of nursing, and nursing services. As vice-president of the Deans of Collegiate Schools of Nursing, she helped design the dean's action program in support of the Nurse Training Act from 1969–71. She was a member of several federal review panels at the National Institutes of Health and was appointed a member of the National Advisory Council for Nurse Training for the United States Public Health Service (USPHS). She also served as a consultant to the U.S. Air Force.

Early in her career Mullane was honored for her contributions to nursing. In 1958 she was the Detroit "Nurse of the Year" and was the recipient of a Special Service Award from the Michigan State Pharmaceutical Association. In 1960 Providence Hospital of Detroit endowed the Mary Kelly Mullane Scholarship in the School of Nursing. She was elected into membership in Pi Lambda Theta (national education honor society) in 1951 to the Lambda Chapter at the University of Chicago, in the Gamma Chapter of Sigma Theta Tau at the University of Iowa in 1960, and into Phi Kappa Phi in the University of Illinois chapter in Urbana in 1962. She was awarded honorary membership in the Institute of Medicine of Chicago in 1970 and the Chicago Pediatric Society in May 1971. The University of Illinois College of Nursing Alumni Association and Alpha Lambda Chapter of Sigma Theta Tau voted to sponsor an annual Mary Kelly Mullane Clinical Nursing Symposium. This symposium has continued annually, and the 24th symposium was held in 1991. She continues to be a participant in activities of the Alpha Lambda chapter, where she continues her membership in Sigma Theta Tau.

In 1972 Mullane received the Distinguished Honorary Award from the ANA in Recognition for Professional Achievement. Particularly noted was

> her keen vision and her appreciation of the contributions that nursing can make have led her to promote excellence in nursing, with the knowledge that nursing must expand to meet the needs of a changing society. The example she has set in her own career will serve to remind others that the pursuit of excellence is in the true service of a profession.

She was also cited in the General Assembly of the state of Illinois House of Representatives with a resolution of commendation for professional achievement in June 1972 for "her monumental contributions to the profession of nursing and to the improvement of the health care delivery system to the people of Illinois."

She received an honorary doctor of science degree from Southern Illinois University in Carbondale in 1971 and from the University of Illinois in 1980. She also received an honorary doctor of humane letters degree from Loyola University in 1973. Among her national awards, she received the M. Adelaide Nutting Award from the National League for Nursing in June 1975, the R. Louise McManus Medal for Outstanding Contributions to Nursing from Teachers College, Columbia University Nursing Education Alumni Association in April 1977, and the Founder's Award from Sigma Theta Tau in November 1978. The University of Illinois Alumni Association conferred the Distinguished Service Award in June 1976, and in 1977 she was elected into membership in the American Academy of Nursing.

After her retirement from the University of Illinois, Mullane served as half-time executive director of the American Association of Colleges of Nursing in Washington, D.C. (1976–78). She chaired the American Pharmaceutical Association's Task Force on Women and continued to speak at commencements and at various meetings. She was the keynote speaker at the thirty-fifth anniversary of the College of Nursing at the University of Illinois in May 1990.

A prolific writer, Mullane has left her mark on the profession in a variety of journals, always emphasizing excellence in practice, teaching, and administration. Her impact as a "leader of leaders, a scholar, an eminent nurse educator, and educational administrator and a tireless champion of quality health care and educational standards for the health professions" (as cited on the conferring of her honorary degree at the University of Illinois) continues on those faculty and students she mentored and in the students and faculty she helped to develop.

Mullane currently resides in Naples, Florida, with her sister Dorothy, also a nationally recognized nurse leader who was the editor of *Supervisor Nurse* (later named *Nursing Management*) before her retirement.

PUBLICATIONS BY MARY KELLY MULLANE

BOOKS

Education for Nursing Service Administration. An Experience in Program Development by Fourteen Universities. Battle Creek, Mich.: W.K. Kellogg Foundation, 1958.

DISSERTATION

"Identification and Validation of Criteria of Excellence for Nursing Service Administration." Ph.D. dissertation, University of Chicago, March 1957.

ARTICLES (SELECTED)

"From Blueprint to Bedside." *American Journal of Nursing* 52 (July 1952): 875–76.

"The New Employee." *Catholic Nurse* 5 (June 1957): 17–30.

"What is Administration?" *Michigan Nurse* 30 (December 1957): 1965–67.

"Social Values of Catholic Nursing." *Biennial Report and Proceedings of the National Council of Catholic Nurses* (1958): 62–66.

"Validation of Criteria for Nursing Service Administration: Report of a Study." *Proceedings of the Forty-first Biennial Convention of the American Nurses' Association* (June 1958).

"Proposals for the Future of Nursing." *Nursing Forum* 1 (Fall 1962): 73–84.

"Care Systems and Nursing Education." *Nursing Outlook* 2 (October 1963): 74–82.

"Nursing Service and Patient Care." *Hospital Progress* (November 1963): 85–88.

"Modern Nursing and Education for It." *New York State Journal of Medicine* 65 (March 1965): 690–94.

"Today's New Nurses: What Can They Do As Graduates of Collegiate Schools?" *Military Medicine* 130 (July 1965): 703–06.

"Nursing Faculty Roles and Functions in the Large University Setting." Memo to Members, Council of Baccalaureate and Higher Degree Programs. Pp. 1–4. New York: National League for Nursing, February 1969.

"Nursing and the Health Problems of Our Times." *Supervisor Nurse* (January 1971): 74–78.

"The Spirit of '76; Involvement and Commitment." *People, Power, and Politics for Health Care.* Pp. 81–88. New York: National League for Nursing, 1976.

"Nursing Care and the Political Arena." *Nursing Outlook* 23 (November 1975): 669–701.

"Politics at Work." *RN* (July 1976): 45–51.

"The Role of the Dean: State of the Art." *Proceedings of the Deans' Seminar, Jackson Hole, Wyoming,—July 21–23, 1980.* Washington, D.C.: Association of Colleges of Nursing, 1980.

"The Nature of the University or College and the Mission of the School of Nursing . . . Classics from Our Heritage. *Journal of Professional Nursing* 1 (September–October, 1985): 315–16.

BIBLIOGRAPHY

"Dr. Mary Mullane Will Retire as Dean of Nursing." *Medical Center News* (University of Illinois, Chicago) 26 (December 1970).

"A Great University Reports on Quality in Higher Education. The Education of the Professional Nurse." *Illinois Alumni News* 45 (April 1966): 16.

"An Interview with Mary Kelly Mullane." Videotaped interview by M.E. Whalen, curator, Midwest Nursing History Resource Center, with M.K. Mullane and E. Anderson. University of Illinois College of Nursing, May 1990.

Mary Kelly Mullane Materials. Archives, University of Illinois College of Nursing, Chicago.

Mullane, M.K. Personal communication with the author, August 29, 1990.

Nelson, J., and Committee on the Structure of National Nursing Organizations and Structure Steering Committee. *New Horizons in Nursing.* New York: Macmillan, 1950.

Safier, G. *Contemporary American Leaders in Nursing. An Oral History.* Pp. 234–53. New York: McGraw-Hill, 1977.

"70+ and Going Strong. Dorothy Kelly and Mary Mullane; Footloose and Fancy Free." *Geriatric Nursing* 3 (May/June 1982): 196–97.

Susan Dudas

Tressie Virginia Myers

1903–1988

Tressie Virginia Myers was a pioneer in total patient care. Long before most nurses thought it was proper to delve into the emotional and spiritual aspects of patient care, Tressie was teaching and modeling its importance. She was the second national director of Nurses Christian Fellowship. In that position she planted a vision for the spiritual dimension of nursing, which today has blossomed into a major nursing concern.

Myers was born at home on a farm near Kinross, Iowa, on May 28, 1903. She was the third child of Charles and Mary Snell Myers. Her mother died of spinal meningitis in 1918, so Tressie took over the duties of mother to her two older brothers and two younger sisters at the age of 15. The strong leadership skills she developed during that time of hardship were evident. She continued to be a nurturer with a strong practical bent throughout her nursing career.

During the Depression Myers enrolled in Manchester College in Indiana, but financial pressures led her to begin teaching elementary school before completing her studies. In 1929 she graduated from Mt. Morris College in Illinois and continued her teaching career in public schools in Iowa and Illinois.

After 10 years of teaching elementary school, she enrolled in Michael Reese Hospital School of Nursing in Chicago. She graduated in 1938 and continued at Michael Reese Hospital as head nurse and instructor. While she was teaching there, a small group of students asked her to become the faculty advisor for their Bible study group. That was the beginning of her association with Nurses Christian Fellowship (NCF). In 1948 Myers left her teaching job to join the staff of NCF. Two years later she succeeded Alvira Anderson as director, becoming NCF's second national director. She continued to serve in that position until 1968.

In the time that she served as NCF director, the organization grew from being a handful of nurses and nursing students in a few hospitals to a major influence in the area of spiritual care and nursing ethics. Myers was also a major influence in the lives of NCF staff workers. She expected excellence in their work as she did in her own. Her example was often hard to live up to. She traveled extensively and showed deep personal interest in the nurses she served. She never seemed to forget a name, probably because she prayed intensely for everyone she met.

Myers set high standards for the NCF

staff. Nurses whom she recruited for NCF had to have two years of clinical experience and a deep commitment to nursing, as well as a strong Christian commitment. If she met students who in her opinion would make good NCF staff workers, she began grooming them for the job. She encouraged them to serve in leadership positions, to study the Bible and to pray, and to be the very best nurses they could be.

Her high standards had much to do with the credibility NCF earned within the nursing community. Colleagues remember Myers as a highly professional person who wanted to have a dynamic impact on nursing, but who acted with care and caution. She could be strongly assertive without forcing people to think her way.

Myers insisted that NCF work in the heart of professional nursing, not on the fringes. She encouraged nurses in NCF to become active in professional organizations. Under her leadership NCF organized a booth, special speakers, and, eventually, professional sessions at state, national, and international nursing conventions.

She had a global vision for nursing. She inspired dozens of nurses to go overseas as missionaries, and through her influence, Christian nurse movements developed in numerous other countries. Myers had a special part in encouraging the establishment of the Evangelical Nurses Fellowship of India.

Her retirement as director of NCF was followed by three years of development work for the organization. Even after her retirement and death, her influence continues. The growing interest in the spiritual dimension of nursing was largely the result of Myers's vision and the nurses who have written, conducted research, and taught concepts of spiritual care to colleagues throughout the United States and the world.

As already noted, Myers expected a lot of others, and they usually met her expectations, but she also had high standards for herself. She was a "workaholic" who loved her work because she loved God and loved people, especially nurses. Following her retirement to Keokuk, Iowa, she remarked, "I have found retirement is not a time to sit on the front porch and rock in your rocker. There is no such thing as retirement for the Christian; only a change of work location."

During her retirement she continued to work with people, organizing and teaching Bible studies for the First Baptist Church in Keokuk and praying diligently for her friends in NCF. She died on October 29, 1988, in Keokuk, of a cardiac and pulmonary arrest. It followed several years of illness with Parkinson's disease.

Tressie Myers could not boast of a string of advanced degrees or a long list of publications, but her influence will be felt in nursing for years to come. She believed in "total patient care," beginning with the heart. She believed in competence and commitment—as a nurse and as a Christian—and she modeled what she believed.

BIBLIOGRAPHY

Corcoran, K. "McMurtry Remembers Tressie Myers." *InterVarsity* (Winter 1988): 17.

Myers, I. Phone conversations by the author with Myers's sister, May 1989.

Obituary. *Journal of Christian Nursing* 6 (Winter 1989:) 35.

Judith Allen Shelley

Helen Nahm

b. 1901

During her active professional career, Helen Nahm was regarded as one of the most influential American nurse educators of the mid-twentieth century. Her academic career as well as her tenure at the National League for Nursing have provided the profession of nursing with a legacy of growth and development that continues to this day. Her vision of nursing education is particularly exemplified by her commitment to the education of nurses in the social sciences.

Nahm was born in Augusta, Missouri, in 1901. She credits her father's strong belief in the importance of education with her own academic pursuits and with the fact that four of his five children, all daughters, received baccalaureate degrees; two of them also completed doctoral degrees, one of whom was she.

In a short autobiography that Nahm wrote in the 1960s at the request of a young college student, she recalled how even as a child she had thought of becoming a nurse. She entered the University of Missouri at Columbia intending to study home economics. When she was hospitalized for a minor illness during that first year, she was so impressed by the nurses that she decided to pursue a diploma in nursing. Because so few institutions awarded baccalaureate degrees in nursing, after receiving her diploma in 1924 she completed a bachelor's degree in zoology and graduated in 1926.

After graduation, Nahm worked for a year at the University Hospital in Columbia, but in 1927 she accepted a teaching position at Scott and White Hospital in Temple, Texas, where she was the only full-time instructor. She taught nursing arts, anatomy, physiology, and pharmacology; at that time most of the teaching of nurses was done by physicians.

In 1930 she returned to Missouri, where she worked for a time as a surgical and maternity nurse at the Washington University Hospitals in St. Louis. She then returned to the University of Missouri as an instructor at the School of Nursing and, in 1935, assumed the position of director of the School of Nursing at her alma mater. During a one-year leave of absence, she completed a master's degree in psychology at the University of Minnesota. She left the directorship in 1941 and enrolled in a doctoral program at the University of Minnesota. When World War II began in December of that year, she felt she should return to work and accepted a position as director of the Hamline University School of Nursing in St. Paul, Minnesota. From 1941–46 she balanced an academic and working life while completing her doctorate in educational psychology and general education. She then accepted a position as director of the Division of Nursing Education at Duke University in Durham, North Carolina. Her

influence was significant in the institutions that she served.

In 1950 she moved into the world of national nursing education with her appointment as director of the National Nursing Accrediting Service. In 1952 she assumed the position of director of the Department of Baccalaureate and Higher Degree Programs at the newly established National League for Nursing (NLN) and in 1953 was appointed director of the Division of Nursing Education for the organization.

These were very important years not only for the NLN but also for nursing education. Establishing a single nursing accreditation service was in itself a Herculean effort. When Nahm became director of the Division of Nursing Education, she had to gain acceptance for the accrediting program from outside groups. When, soon after she became the director, the league denied accreditation to 278 schools, Nahm faced substantial criticism, anger, and opposition from the schools and some outside organizations. Her commitment to rigorous accreditation standards remained steadfast, however, and the NLN was eventually recognized as the official accrediting agency for nursing. In recognition of her distinguished achievements during the formative years of the NLN, that organization awarded Nahm the Mary Adelaide Nutting Award in 1967.

In 1958 Nahm began an 11-year tenure as the dean of the School of Nursing at the University of California, San Francisco (UCSF). During that time the school grew in size from a student body of 250 to 450, with a corresponding faculty increase from 25 to 60. Nahm introduced an experimental undergraduate program leading to a baccalaureate degree, an expanded clinical specialty program terminating in a master's of science degree, and a visionary doctoral program, one of the few in the country at that time and the only one in the West, enabling students to study for a doctorate of nursing science. Because she believed that there is an explicit difference between medicine and nursing, she defined professional nursing as an independent and interdependent practice, in addition to its dependent functions. To this end, she created a department within the UCSF School of Nursing devoted entirely to the social and behavioral sciences. This was the first basic science department within a school of nursing and has served as a prototype since its inception.

Throughout her professional career and into her retirement, Nahm served all of nursing through her contributions to various commissions, committees, task forces, etc. She masterminded a consortium nursing education program (COGEN) and succeeded in persuading 11 schools of nursing to work cooperatively to improve the instruction of graduate students in California and Nevada. She was a member of the American Medical Association Advisory Group to the AMA Committee on Nursing, served as a member of the NLN board of directors for several years, and was a member of the ANA Committee for the Study of Credentialing in Nursing.

Although Nahm retired from the University of California in 1969, she did not retire from her interest in and enthusiasm for nursing. In her early retirement years she organized directors of schools of nursing and health-care agencies in San Francisco to work together to facilitate the professional role of the new graduate nurse and thus improve the quality of care. She shared research findings, innovative ideas, and her vision with the community, the nation, and the world through her publications, travels, and numerous addresses.

Nahm has received many well-deserved awards. In addition to the Mary Adelaide Nutting Award, she has been awarded honorary doctorate degrees by the Universities of Missouri, Cincinnati, and Florida. In 1977 she received the Distinguished Service Award from the University of Minnesota Alumni Association and was inducted as an honorary fellow of the American Academy of Nursing in 1978. In 1981 the School of Nursing at UCSF inaugurated the annual Helen Nahm Research Lecture honoring excellence of scholarship and dedication of purpose as exemplified by Nahm herself. She presently resides in Washington, Missouri.

Over the years, Nahm has been highly praised by her colleagues. One considered her to be possibly *the* leading academician in nursing in the entire world. Another characterized her leadership style as being one of "pride in achievement as opposed to vanity of ambition." Yet another described her as exemplifying excellence and an enviable dedication to the nursing profession and the quality of scholarship.

PUBLICATIONS BY HELEN NAHM

BOOKS AND MONOGRAPHS

An Evaluation of Selected Schools of Nursing. Monograph, American Psychological Association. Stanford, Calif.: Stanford University Press, 1948.

With C.W. Taylor, M. Harms, M. Quinn, and S. and J. Mulaik. *Measurement and Prediction of Nursing Performance.* Parts I and II. Salt Lake City: University of Utah, 1965.

ARTICLES (SELECTED)

"Job Satisfaction in Nursing." *American Journal of Nursing* 40 (December 1940): 1389–92.

"Mental Hygiene Knowledge of Senior Students in Schools of Nursing." *Journal of Educational Research* 41 (November 1947): 193–203.

"Autocratic Versus Democratic Beliefs and Practices of Senior Students in Schools of Nursing." *Journal of Social Psychology* 27 (May 1948): 229–40.

"What Makes Student Nurses Unhappy." *Hospitals* 22 (June 1948): 51–54.

"Satisfaction With Nursing." *Journal of Applied Psychology* 32 (August 1948): 335–43.

"A Follow-up Study on Satisfaction with Nursing." *Journal of Applied Psychology* 34 (October 1950): 343–46.

"Accreditation Now!" *American Journal of Nursing* 51 (August 1951): 523–26.

"Continuity and Progression in Nursing Education." *American Journal of Nursing* 58 (June 1953): 845–47.

"Nursing Education Today: Its Advantages." *Nursing World* 127 (August 1953): 16–18.

"Psychology Instruction in Nursing Schools." *Nursing Outlook* 2 (April 1954): 188–90.

"Trends in Nursing Education as Seen from a National Organization Point of View." *Teachers College Record* 55 (May 1954): 438–55.

"Research in Psychiatric Nursing." *Nursing Outlook* 5 (February 1957): 89–91.

"Annual Administrative Reviews, Nursing Education." *Journal of American Hospital Association* 32 (April 16, 1958): 61–69.

"Planning for the Future of Education in Nursing." *The League Exchange*. New York: National League for Nursing, 1959.

"Generalized Versus Specialized Baccalaureate Degree Programs in Nursing." *American Journal of Nursing* 59 (November 1959).

"Planning for the Future of Education in Nursing." *Canadian Nurse* 56 (December 1960): 1073–78.

"The Pursuit of Excellence in the West—Five Years of WCHEN." *The Pursuit of Excellence in Nursing*. Report of the Fifth Annual Western Conference on Nursing Education, March 22–23, 1962, Denver Colorado.

Interviews with the publishers of the *Japanese Journal of Nurses' Education* and the *Japanese Journal of Nursing*. Tokyo, 1962. Reports published in August 1962 issues.

"Expectations of Students in Graduate Education." *Nursing Forum* 1 (Fall 1962): 19–27.

"Trends in Nursing in the United States." *Nursing Journal of Singapore* 3 (January 1963).

"Further Education of Professional Nurses." Chap. VIII. *The Surgeon General's Report and Collegiate Nursing Education*. New York: National League for Nursing, 1963.

"Nursing Education, Responsibility for Preparation of Leadership Personnel." *International Journal of Nursing Studies* 2 (1965): 95–103.

"Nursing Dimensions and Realities." *American Journal of Nursing* 65 (June 1965): 96–99.

"Tribute to the Past—Prelude to the Future." *International Nursing Review* 13 (July–August 1966): 14–23.

"The Registered Nurse and Baccalaureate Education." *Nursing Forum* 1 (1967).

With D.I. Miller. "Relationships Between Medical and Nursing Education." *Journal of Medical Education* 35 (August 1961): 849–51.

With D.M. Smith and R.E. Hunter. "Evaluating Student Progress in Clinical Experience." *American Journal of Nursing* 50 (May 1950): 343–46.

BIBLIOGRAPHY

Archives. Dean's office, School of Nursing, University of California, San Francisco.

Personal communications with the authors by UCSF School of Nursing faculty, 1990.

Patricia Struckman
Margretta M. Styles

Lalu Nathoy (Polly Bemis)
1853–1933

While known as the "Angel of Salmon River," a woman who could cure people with Chinese herbs, Lalu Nathoy, later called Polly Bemis, is best known for her place in the folklore of the American West as the bride who was won in a poker game. Nathoy was eventually freed by the man who won her and later earned the love and respect of the people of Grangeville, Idaho, through her industry, her sweet nature, and her outstanding nursing talents.

Nathoy was born in Northern China on September 11, 1853. Her mother and father were farmers. There were several children in the family—at least two younger brothers and Nathoy. In China male children were traditionally highly valued, whereas female children were sometimes regarded as chattel. But Nathoy's father favored her and called her his "thousand pieces of gold," vowing that he would never sell her to raise cash in hard times, a common practice of the day. In fact, to forestall this prospect, when crops were poor, to save the family farm from the tax collector, Nathoy's father allowed her to work by his side in the fields, which was then unheard of and caused him much ridicule from his neighbors. But in 1871 when a drought had stretched to five years and caused famine, Nathoy's desperate parents were forced to sell her, reputedly for two bags of soybeans, to bandits who threatened the family's lives. The bandits in turn sold her to a procurer in Hong Kong, who brought her to America. Once in America she was sold at auction to a Chinese merchant named Hong King for $2,500. She was 16 years old. Nathoy was then transported to the mining town of Warren's Meadows, Idaho, where she worked in Hong King's saloon, washed and mended clothes, and nursed miners who were sick. It was in the saloon that Charlie Bemis, a man who had often protected Nathoy from boisterous miners, won her in a poker game from Hong King. Later Bemis was shot in the head in a barroom brawl. When the doctor had given up hope for him, Nathoy removed the bullet from Bemis's face with a crochet hook. When slivers that remained became critically infected, she extracted the splinters with a razor and bathed the wound continually with medicinal herbs she had gathered from the mountains. Bemis recovered. In 1894, after living together in a common-law marriage for over 18 years, Nathoy and Bemis were legally married. Nathoy came to be called Polly Bemis.

After their marriage, Nathoy and Bemis moved from Warrens Meadow to Salmon Canyon. There Nathoy farmed, growing vegetables, fruit, and Chinese herbs for the Chinese herbalist, Li Dick, who had prescribed herbs for Nathoy's patients. Bemis staked a gold claim during the Buffalo Hump Rush of 1901, and Nathoy and Bemis became accepted members of the community, although by that time the gold rush was over and most Chinese had left or been run out of the area.

In Warren, Nathoy was the "official nurse" for anyone who was sick. It did not matter if the patient could not pay. Nathoy splinted and nursed a young man who was brought to her with broken legs. She again saved Bemis's life by nursing him back from near death from pneumonia, and she saved a baby who had been brought to her by hollowing out a reed, putting it down the baby's throat, and sucking out the mucus. R.G. Bailey called her the "Angel of Salmon River."

Yet Nathoy's skills were not enough to save Charlie Bemis from tuberculosis. Bemis died in 1922 at the age of 70. Thereafter Nathoy grew somewhat withdrawn. The myth about her had begun to grow. She was interviewed by the Idaho County Free Press, and an article mentioning her appeared in *National Geographic* in the 1930s. Eventually she returned to Grangeville, Idaho, lived on her land in a small cabin, and had the land homesteaded by family friends, Charles Shep and Pete Klinkhammer, to whom she deeded her property upon her death.

Lalu Nathoy died at the Idaho County Hospital, Grangeville, Idaho, on November 6, 1933. The city council of Grangeville acted as her pallbearers. Although she had wanted to be buried next to her husband at Salmon Canyon, Nathoy was buried at Prairie View Cemetery, Grangeville. The creek that ran through her property is called Polly Creek. In a time when Chinese in the United States had limited opportunities, Lalu Nathoy earned her freedom from slavery and helped her family, friends, and neighbors by nursing them in traditional Chinese ways. It was as a nurse she endeared herself to her fellow Idahoans, but she is most remembered as a character from the Old West—the bride who was won in a poker game.

BIBLIOGRAPHY

Bailey, R.G. *River of No Return.* Lewiston, Idaho: Bailey-Blake Printing, 1935.

Drago, H.S. *Notorious Ladies of the Frontier.* New York: Dodd, 1969.

Elsensohn, M.A. *Idaho County's Most Romantic Character, Polly Bemis.* Cottonwood: Idaho Corporation of Benedictine Sisters, 1979.

Horan, J.D. *Desperate Women.* New York: Putnam, 1952.

Lalu Nathoy Papers. Idaho State Library, Boise.

McCunn, R.L. *Thousand Pieces of Gold.* New York: Dell, 1981.

Memorabilia. St. Gertrude's Convent, Cottonwood, Idaho.

Miller, H.M. *Westering Women.* Garden City, N.Y.: Doubleday, 1961.

Tinling, M. *Women Remembered.* Westport, Conn.: Greenwood, 1986.

Yung, J. *Chinese Women of America.* Seattle: University of Washington Press, for Chinese Culture Foundation of San Francisco, 1986.

Dorothy Tao

Sophie Caroline Nelson
1886–1964

A pioneer in the field of public-health nursing, Sophie Caroline Nelson gave 40 years of service to the nursing profession. She was instrumental in setting standards for public-health nursing and gaining acceptance of public-health nursing as part of the total health-care effort. Nelson also contributed to the articulation of standards for Visiting Nurse associations through her 28 years of service with the John Hancock Mutual Life Insurance Company.

Sophie Caroline Nelson was born September 4, 1886, in Denmark. She was the younger of two daughters in a family of five children. Her family moved to America when she was young, and she grew up in Watertown, Massachusetts. The Nelson family physician, Dr. Alfred Worcester, founded the Waltham Training School for Nurses (Waltham, Mass.) and often told the young Nelson that he expected her to graduate from the school.

In 1912 Nelson did graduate from the four-year program at the Waltham Training School for Nurses. Throughout her nursing career she continued to take postgraduate courses in public-health nursing administration and social and health problems, including a course in public-health nursing at Teachers College, Columbia University, in New York City (1924).

Following her graduation, Nelson spent two to three years as a private-duty nurse in Massachusetts. Her interests soon turned to public health, however, and in 1915 she became the first infant welfare nurse on the Cambridge Board of Health, a position she held until 1916. In 1917 and 1918 she served in the Pediatric Nursing Service of the American Red Cross in Belgium and France. As chief nurse of the Children's Bureau headquartered in Lyons, France, she developed hospitals for repatriated children and refugees and also organized a course for visiting health professionals.

From 1919 to 1921 Nelson was superintendent of the Babies' Milk Fund of the District Nurses Association in Louisville, Kentucky, and also spent some time as superintendent of the Louisville Public Health Nursing Association. Nelson left Kentucky in 1921 to assist the American Red Cross with the development of nursing services and relief programs for children. Serving as field director for nursing

services in Central Europe and the Balkans, she oversaw the organization's activities in Austria, Hungary, Serbia, and Bulgaria. This project brought her to Greece in 1922 to provide relief services after a disastrous fire in Smyrna, where she organized a public-health nursing course at the American Hospital in Constantinople (now Istanbul, Turkey).

In 1923 Nelson returned to the United States and became director of nursing for the Boston Health League. She moved to Missouri in 1924 to serve as director of the Visiting Nurse Association in St. Louis. Nelson returned to Massachusetts in 1925 to begin employment with the John Hancock Mutual Life Insurance Company, a position that would dominate 28 years of her nursing career.

As the director of the John Hancock Visiting Nurse Service, Nelson developed the Life Conservation Service. This innovative service, established long before prepaid health insurance benefits were common, provided home nursing services and health education activities for the company's policyholders. The primary purpose of the service was to combat the high maternity mortality and general mortality rates among many of the company's industrial policyholders, a group characterized by low incomes and a lack of access to quality health care and health information.

The service contracted with Visiting Nurse associations across the country to provide home nursing care and educational services for policyholders with acute illnesses and those requiring all phases of maternity care. It was eventually expanded to cover individuals with chronic illnesses. Existing health-care programs were not duplicated by the service; instead, policyholders were referred to the appropriate health-care provider.

Information booklets on health explained illnesses and medical information in simple terms and also assisted in educating policyholders. Over the course of its 28 years, the program produced 75 million booklets and provided nursing service to 2 million policyholders in 27 states. The program was eventually discontinued as health-care benefit programs, hospital services, and health education programs for the public improved and expanded. In her article, "Twenty-Eight Years and Eleven Million Visits," Nelson described this innovative program in detail.

While employed at John Hancock, Nelson continued her service to the nursing profession. From 1930 to 1934 Nelson was president of the National Organization for Public Health Nursing. In 1931 she took a four-month leave of absence to serve as special consultant to the surgeon general of the United States Public Health Service. Nelson served as chairperson of the Public Health Nursing Section of the International Council of Nurses in 1937.

During World War II she served as vice-chairperson of the National Nursing Council for War Service (1944). This organization became the National Nursing Council after the war, and Nelson was its chair for two years (1946–48). The council focused on the economic status of nurses, education within the profession, and the continuing education needs of nurses. It made many important contributions to the profession during its eight and one-quarter years of existence. While on the council, Nelson was appointed to a council of consultants to the Nursing Service of the Veterans Administration, focusing her efforts on community nursing.

Nelson's additional professional service included terms as president, Massachusetts Central Health Council; vice-president, Massachusetts Organization of Public Health Nursing; president, Greater Boston Nursing Council; member of the executive committee, Boston Health League; and first nurse member of the Committee on Administrative Practice of the American Public Health Association. She also assisted in organizing many community nursing councils and was instrumental in establishing the Nursing Council of United Community Services in Boston.

In 1950 Nelson was elected assistant secretary of the John Hancock Mutual Life Insurance Company. She was the first woman to be elected an officer of the company and remained in the position until her retirement to Newton, Massachusetts, in 1953.

While retired, she continued her active involvement with nursing as a public-health volunteer and a member of professional committees and through work with the local Red Cross, the Nursing Council of United Community Services, and social and health agencies in Newton.

Nelson received many honors acknowledging her contributions to nursing. In 1951 she received the Florence Nightingale Medal of the International Red Cross, the twenty-first nurse to receive the honor. In 1955 Nelson was the first woman to be awarded the Lemuel Shattuck Award of the Massachusetts Public Health Association in recognition of her service to public-health nursing. Also in 1955 the Massachusetts State Nursing League awarded Nelson and Stella Goostray, another nursing leader, honorary memberships in the Massachusetts League for Nursing and the National League for Nursing. In 1956 Nelson was appointed a consultant to the North Atlantic Region of the National League of Nursing Committee on Early Nursing Source Materials. France, Serbia, Austria, and Hungary also honored her with medals.

Sophie Caroline Nelson died on February 10, 1964, in Boston, Massachusetts.

PUBLICATIONS BY SOPHIE CAROLINE NELSON

ARTICLES (SELECTED)

"Work with Children in Lyons, France." *Public Health Nurse* 11 (September 1919): 722–28.

"Nursing in Relation to the Three Plans for Municipal Health Departments." *American Journal of Public Health* 17 (March 1927): 239–46.

"Study of Chronic Cases." *Public Health Nurse* 21 (November 1929): 577–78.

"How Public Health Nursing Can Best Serve the Community." *Modern Hospital* 37 (September 1931): 128.

"The Survey of Public Health Nursing." *Public Health Nursing* 26 (May 1934): 227–28.

"Elinor D. Gregg." In *National League of Nursing Education: Biographic Sketches, 1937–1940.* New York: The League, 1940.

"The National Nursing Council Reports." *American Journal of Nursing* 46 (December 1946): 816–19; 48 (December 1948): 756–58.

"Tasks Accomplished." Final report, National Nursing Council. *American Journal of Nursing* 48 (December 1948): 756–58.

"Mary Seawall Gardner." *Nursing Outlook* 1 (December 1953): 668–70.

"Twenty-Eight Years and Eleven Million Visits." *American Journal of Nursing* 53 (December 1953): 1469–70.

"Mary Seawall Gardner." *Nursing Outlook* 2 (January 1954): 37–39.

"A Retirement Income Plan." *American Journal of Nursing* 58 (November 1958): 1555.

With M.L.K. Hall. "Cost of Nursing Service." *Public Health Nursing* 31 (October 1939): 573–77.

BIBLIOGRAPHY

"Florence Nightingale Medals Awarded." *American Journal of Nursing* 51 (August 1951): 20 adv., 24 adv.

Friedman, A.H. "Nelson, Sophie Caroline." In *Dictionary of American Nursing Biography*, M. Kaufmann, ed. Pp. 267–69. Westport, Conn.: Greenwood, 1988.

Goostray, S. "Sophie Nelson: Public Health Statesman." *American Journal of Nursing* 60 (September 1960): 1268–69.

"Ladies with Lamps." Editorial. *New England Journal of Medicine* 253 (December 1955): 989–90.

"Miss Nelson Retires." *Nursing Outlook* 1 (September 1953): 534, 536.

Papers. Nursing Archives, Mugar Memorial Library, Boston University, Boston.

"Sophie Nelson." Obituary. *American Journal of Nursing* 64 (April 1964): 150–51.

Margaret R. Wells

(Annie) Ethel Northam

1894–1968

Ethel Northam was a pioneer nursing theorist although her work was not really recognized and appreciated until after her death.

She was born in Atlantic, Virginia, on December 9, 1894. She attended high school in Snow Hill, Worcester County, Maryland, graduating in 1913. She then worked as a substitute teacher in Worcester County until 1917, when she was appointed principal of the primary school in Snow Hill. She left that post in 1918 to attend the Johns Hopkins Hospital School of Nursing in Baltimore, from which she graduated in 1921. After graduation she worked as a head nurse on the medical and obstetrical wards at Hopkins, a position she left to become head nurse at Mountainside Hospital in Montclair, New Jersey, in 1923. In 1926 she returned to Johns Hopkins Hospital, first as a head nurse of a medical ward and then in the delivery room. She became an instructor of obstetrical nursing in the Hopkins School of Nursing in 1926 and in 1929 became director of nursing arts. From 1938 to 1944 she was superintendent of nurses in the Baltimore Hospital for Women; this was followed by a stint as superintendent of nurses at Syndeham Hospital in Baltimore, and then in 1946 she became superintendent of nurses at Frederick City Hospital at Frederick, Maryland.

She is best known as the coauthor with Hester Frederick of *A Textbook of Nursing Practice*, published in 1928. The text was one of the earliest to adopt a theoretical basis for practice and to describe the recipients of nursing services as care agents. Nursing activities are seen as focusing on the promotion of the care agent. From these assumptions it is possible to trace the evolution of ideas to contemporary models and theories.

Northam was also involved in pioneering work in nursing research illustrating the nursing time required for care of the mother and infant and what the nurse does in caring for the sick.

Throughout her life she remained an active alumna of the Johns Hopkins Hospital School of Nursing, as well as a member of the American Nurses' Association, and the National League of Nursing Education. In 1961 she retired to Snow Hill, Maryland, to live with her sister and brother, and she died there on November 23, 1968.

PUBLICATIONS BY (ANNIE) ETHEL NORMAN

BOOKS

With H. Frederick. *Textbook of Nursing Practice*. New York: Macmillan, 1928, 2nd ed. 1938.

ARTICLES

With A.T. Beckworth. "Temperature of Fluids for Infusion." *American Journal of Nursing* 31 (February 1931): 179–81.

With A.B. Mortensen, "Public Health Nursing: The Nurse as a Supervisor of Attendance." *Pacific Coast Journal of Nursing* 35 (December 1939): 719–21.

With C. Wasserberg et al. "Some Time Studies in Obstetrical Nursing." *American Journal of Nursing* 27 (July 1927): 543–44.

BIBLIOGRAPHY

Alan Mason Chesney Medical Archives. Johns Hopkins Medical Institutions, Baltimore. Included is a manuscript biography located with records of the Johns Hopkins Alumni Association.

"Ethel Norman." *Johns Hopkins Nurses' Alumnae Magazine* (July 1958).

Vern L. Bullough

Lucille E. Notter

b. 1907

In 1981, Teachers College, Columbia University, presented Lucille Elizabeth Notter with the Medal for Distinguished Service, and in 1985 she was elected as an honorary fellow of the American Academy of Nursing. Both of these honors acknowledge the esteem with which she is held in the nursing profession for her many contributions to nursing education and for her noted expertise and leadership in nursing research.

Notter was born on July 13, 1907, in Frankfort, Kentucky. She was the eldest of five children. Her father was a public utilities salesman. She attended Catholic parochial schools through high school. The monetary constraints related to being the member of a large family delayed the possibility of attending college for several years after graduation from high school, and Notter initially worked as a record-room clerk in a local hospital. Although she had not earlier envisioned nursing as her chosen career, she was influenced to enter nursing school through her expo-

sure to the nursing profession while working in the hospital and through her friendship with Mabel McCracken, a graduate of Saints Mary and Elizabeth Hospital School of Nursing in Louisville, Kentucky.

Notter graduated from Saints Mary and Elizabeth Hospital School of Nursing in 1931. During the following eight years (1932–40) she held positions as head nurse, supervisor, and instructor at Michael Reese Hospital School of Nursing in Chicago.

In 1941 she obtained a B.S. in nursing education from Teachers College, Columbia University, and was employed for the next nine years by the Visiting Nurse Service of New York (1941–50), where she held successive positions as staff nurse, supervisor, administrative assistant, and educational director. In 1946, during her employment at the Visiting Nurse Service of New York, she earned an M.A. in supervision in public-health nursing from Teachers College.

She became the director of the Joint Education Program, Visiting Nurse Service of New York and Visiting Nurse Association of Brooklyn (1950–54). She received an Ed.D. in administration of educational programs also from Teachers College in 1956 and then served as the assistant executive director of the Visiting Nurse Association of Brooklyn (1956–60).

She held faculty positions at Hunter College of the City University of New York, Department of Nursing Education, from 1960–63, where she was adjunct assistant professor, and was on the faculty of the Writers' Workshops, Boston University School of Nursing from 1963–66.

Notter authored a number of books, several of which have had successive editions and all of which have become standards of nursing literature. The most recent edition of one prototype research text (*Essentials of Nursing Research*) was published in 1988; the fact that the first edition of this text was published in 1974 gives credit to its continued relevancy of content.

After serving on the editorial board from 1957 until 1961, Notter served as the first full-time editor of the journal, *Nursing Re-*

search, for 12 years (1961–73). During her tenure as editor, she worked vigorously to increase the frequency and expand the length of this publication while consistently encouraging nursing researchers to apply rigorous scientific methods of inquiry to research projects and communicate the results through publication.

In years overlapping with the editorship of *Nursing Research*, she served as the editor of the *International Nursing Index* (1965–73), a bibliographic tool linking health professionals with the wealth of nursing literature worldwide. She subsequently held a three-year appointment as co-editor of the journal *Cardiovascular Nursing*, beginning in 1973.

Concurrent with these editing responsibilities, she was project director of the American Nurses' Association Annual Nurse Research Conferences (1965–73). These meetings provided an annual forum for the exchange of knowledge gained through research, enabling nurse-investigators to share information about their scientific inquiries during an important period in the development of research in nursing.

In answer to the increasing need for provision of educational opportunities for registered nurses who were graduates of associate degree and diploma programs to obtain a baccalaureate education, many nursing programs began to expand independently or alter their curriculum in the 1960s to offer what became known as open curriculum in addition to their generic nursing curriculum. As director of the National League for Nursing, Division of Research Open-Curriculum Project, Notter was originally responsible for the four Open-Curriculum Conferences held as part of the "action" phase of the open-curriculum project. Her role was expanded to include the directorship of the project, "An Evaluation of Open-Curriculum Projects and Open-Curriculum Students in Nursing Education," part of the "study phase" of the project, which carried out an in-depth examination of the results elicited during a longitudinal study of nursing programs offering nontraditional curricula for nursing students. Under Notter's leadership, this project spearheaded dissemination of information about open curriculum programs, examined career mobility opportunities available through nursing education, and developed guidelines to govern the vital development and refinement of quality open-curriculum systems that continue to offer nurses educational opportunities for advancement in the profession of nursing today.

PUBLICATIONS BY LUCILLE E. NOTTER

BOOKS

Essentials of Nursing Research. New York: Springer, 1974, 1978, 1983, 1988 with J.R. Hott.

With A.M. Robinson. *Clinical Writing for Health Professionals.* Bowie, Md.: Brady, 1982.

With E.K. Spaulding. *Professional Nursing: Foundations, Perspectives, and Relationships.* Philadelphia: Lippincott, 1939, 1941, 1946, 1950, 1954, 1965, 1968, 1970, 1976. Title varies in some editions.

ARTICLES AND REPORTS (SELECTED)

"Coordinating Home Health Care for Persons with Long-Term Illness." *Public Health Nursing* 39 (December 1937): 602–05, 608.

"Disinfection of Clinical Thermometers." *Nursing Outlook* 1 (October 1953): 569–71.

"Visitors Are Important People." *Nursing Outlook* 3 (July 1955): 372.

"Proposals for the Use and Training of Public Health Nurses' Aides." Ed.D. dissertation, Teachers College, Columbia University, New York, 1956.

"The Vital Significance of Clinical Nursing Research." *Cardiovascular Nursing* 8 (September–October 1972): 19–22.

"The Case for Historical Research in Nursing." *Nursing Research* 21 (November–December 1972): 483.

"Twelve Years and Sixty Editorials Later." *Nursing Research* 22 (September–October 1973): 387.

With W.L. Johnson and M. Robey. "Selected Readings from Open-Curriculum Literature; an Annotated Bibliography." NLN Publication 19-1525. New York: National League for Nursing, 1974.

With M. Robey and M.H. Weinstein. "Guidelines for Implementation of Open-Curriculum Practices in Nursing Education." NLN Publication 19-1701. New York: National League for Nursing, 1978.

With M. Robey. "The Open Curriculum in Nursing Education. Final Report of the NLN

Open-Curriculum Study." NLN Publication 19-1799. New York: National League for Nursing, 1979.

With A.F. Spector. "Nursing Research in the South: A Survey." Atlanta, Ga.: Southern Regional Educational Board, May 1974.

Edited with M. Robey. "Proceedings, 1st Open-Curriculum Conference in Nursing." National League for Nursing, Division of Research, November 27-28, 1973, St. Louis. NLN Publication 19-1534. New York: National League for Nursing, 1974.

Edited with M. Robey. "Proceedings, 2nd Open-Curriculum Conference." National League for Nursing, Division of Research, November 6-7, 1974, New York. NLN Publication 19-1559. New York: National League for Nursing, 1975.

Edited with M. Robey. "Proceedings, 3rd Open-Curriculum Conference." National League for Nursing, Division of Research, November 7-8, 1975, New York. NLN Publication 19-1586. New York: National League for Nursing, 1975.

BIBLIOGRAPHY

Notter, L.E. Biographical material in *Essentials of Nursing Research*. New York: Springer, 1988.

Safier, G. *Contemporary American Leaders in Nursing: An Oral History*. Chap. 12. New York: McGraw-Hill, 1977.

Karen L. Buchinger

Dorothy Jean Novello

1925-1984

The contributions of Dorothy Jean Novello to the nursing profession covered all facets of nursing education, as well as the political and legislative arenas. Her tremendous influence on nurses and nonnurses will be remembered for decades to come.

Novello was born on July 19, 1925, to Eugene and Josephine LaFace in Pittsburgh, Pennsylvania, the youngest child in a family of four daughters. She graduated from Holy Rosary School in 1943. During high school she was a member of the debate team, a member of the Senate Council, editor of the yearbook, and an honor student. Following graduation from

St. Joseph's Hospital School of Nursing (Pittsburgh) in 1946, she married Paul Dobruschien, a musician who died in 1949. Later she married Frank Novello, who died in 1983.

After nursing school Novello was employed as a staff nurse, head nurse, supervisor, and assistant director in the Pittsburgh area. In 1949 she became an instructor at the Allegheny General Hospital School of Nursing and was appointed educational director of the program in 1953, where she remained for the next four years. During this period she obtained a bachelor of science in nursing and a master's degree from Duquesne University, where she also was an instructor in the graduate school.

In 1957 Novello moved to Erie, Pennsylvania, to work as an assistant professor at Villa Maria College. She commuted to Boston and obtained her Ph.D. in clinical psychology from Harvard University. She remained at Villa Maria until her death. During those 27 years she served the college as a professor with the administrative appointments of chairperson of the Department of Nursing, dean of the Erie Institute for Nursing, and vice-president of academic affairs. She was also the recipient of honorary degrees from Villa Maria College (L.L.D.) and from Villanova University (S.Sc.D.).

Her other awards were many. They included being a charter fellow of the American Academy of Nursing; one of the first 100 Distinguished Alumni, Duquesne University; fellow, National League for Nursing; the Pennsylvania League for Nursing's first annual award recipient for Outstanding Contributions to Nursing in Pennsylvania; Pennsylvania Nurses Association's Honorary Recognition for Continuing Efforts to Elevate the Profession; and member of the honorary society Eta Chapter, Sigma Theta Tau.

Novello was an outstanding scholar as evidenced by the more than 30 publications published during the last 15 years of her life on such topics as health care, credentialing, consumerism, and nursing education. She presented more than 50 papers in the Commonwealth of Pennvania during her last decade and over

25 papers nationally. She did a comparative study of health-care delivery systems in Japan, Hong Kong, and the People's Republic of China and served on the editorial boards of *Nursing Outlook* and *Nursing and Health Care.*

Novello provided outstanding leadership to nurses in Pennsylvania through a variety of activities. She was the chairperson, vice-chairperson, and member of several statewide committees and commissions, including the Governor's Committee on Personnel Needs for New Modes and Methods of Health-Care Delivery, the executive committee of the Health Coordinating Council, and the Pennsylvania Master Plan for Higher Education. She was active in many community and governmental organizations in Erie and the surrounding counties. In 1983 Novello was honored for her 25 years of service to Villa Maria College and the nursing community of Erie by the establishment of the Dorothy Jean Novello Scholarship Fund. Nationally, she made a significant contribution as a member of the National Academy of Science's Institute of Medicine Committee to Implement the Study on Nursing and Nursing Education.

Her political expertise was also evidenced by the leadership she gave to the Pennsylvania State Board of Nurse Examiners. She became a member in 1967 and then chairperson in 1969, a position she held at the time of her death. Her commitment to the board and through it to nursing and nurses will be hard to equal.

Novello's contributions to nursing organizations were multifold. She was a member of the board of directors of the American Association of Colleges of Nursing. She held many offices in the Pennsylvania Nurses Association at the state and district levels. The PNA's Foundation has named, in her honor, the library of the Kathryn J. Grove Center for Nursing in Harrisburg. She was president, member of the board of directors, and chairperson of many committees for the Pennsylvania League for Nursing. She served as president, a member of the board, first vice-president, and an accreditation visitor for the Council of Baccalaureate and Higher Degree Programs.

Novello was a highly skilled politician, sensitive and compassionate, an individual who was wise and who displayed that wisdom through a variety of activities. She never lost touch with her students and valued being a mentor.

A quote taken from her 1984 annual report describes her visions:

> Only as high as I reach can I grow.
> Only as far as I seek can I go.
> Only as deep as I look can I see.
> Only as much as I dream can I be.

Novello died in Erie, Pennsylvania, on September 5, 1984.

PUBLICATIONS BY DOROTHY JEAN NOVELLO

ARTICLES (SELECTED)

"Disphragmatic Hernia–Nursing Care." *American Journal of Nursing* 56 (1956): 185–87.

"A Process Theory of Administration." *Counselor Education and Supervision* 1 (1961): 90–96.

"Regionalization—The Core of the Revamped NLN Structure." *Nursing Outlook* 17 (1969): 16–20.

"Nursing Service and Nursing Education Work Together—Contributions of Programs in Liberal Arts College," *Proceedings*, Council of Baccalaureate and Higher Degree Programs, National League for Nursing, 1970.

"National Health Insurance—Implications for Nursing." *Proceedings*, Council of Baccalaureate and Higher Degree Programs, National League for Nursing, 1971.

"The Health of Americans—A Nursing Affair." *Proceedings*, Council of Baccalaureate and Higher Degree Programs, National League for Nursing, 1972.

"The National Health Planning and Resources Development Act—What It Is and How It Works." *Nursing Outlook* 24 (1976): 354–58.

"Licensure and Credentialing: Purposes, Problems and Implications." In *Licensure and Credentialing.* Pp. 1–12. New York: National League for Nursing, 1978.

"The Consumer's Role in Health Care." In *Consumerism and Health Care.* Pp. 1–6. New York: National League for Nursing, 1978.

"Report on Credentialing Health Manpower: A Nurse's Perspective." Pp. 16–20. New York: National Health Council, 1978.

"Focus for Forecasting: Organizational Issues." Prospectives for Nursing: A Symposium. Pp. 20–40. Washington, D.C.: U.S. Department of Health and Human Services, Public Health Service Division of Nursing, 1980.

"Concepts of Care—From Here to There." In *Future Encounters in Health Care*. New York: National League for Nursing, 1980.

BIBLIOGRAPHY

Antoun, L.M., S.S.J. Letter to the author from the president, Villa Maria College, December 10, 1984.

Carlson, K., Legislative program director, Pennsylvania Nurses Association, telephone interview with the author, February 1989.

Gorny, D.A. Letter to the author from the dean, Erie Institute for Nursing, October 29, 1984.

Smith, M.S. Faculty member of Villa Maria College interview with the author, February 1989.

Enid Goldberg

Sylveen V. Nye

1860–1936

A pioneer in the organization of New York's nurses at both the local and state levels, Sylveen V. Nye was one of the founders of the Buffalo Nurses Association (BNA) in 1895 and the New York State Nurses Association in 1901.

Born in 1860 in the town of Hector, Schuyler County, New York, Nye was the fifth of eight children born to Ebenezer Meltiah William and Margaret (Sharp) Nye. She was a ninth-generation American, descended from Benjamin Nye, who settled in Massachusetts in 1636. The Nye family was well known in New York State because of the many jurists and public servants among its members.

Nye received her early education in private schools and in 1888 entered the Indianapolis City Hospital Training School for Nurses. After completing the program, Nye went to Philadelphia, where she worked as a head nurse and later as night supervisor at the Hospital of the University of Pennsylvania. Serious illness forced her to resign. Following a recuperation period, she accepted a position as superintendent of the Lexington Heights Hospital in Buffalo, New York. In 1896 Nye was employed by the Buffalo branch of the Women's Department of the New York Life Insurance Company, a position she held for 30 years.

Early in her career, Nye recognized that unity among nurses was essential for the advancement of the profession. During her tenure as superintendent of Lexington Heights Hospital, she was instrumental in founding an association representative of the hospitals and training schools in the Buffalo area. The first meeting was held in February 1895, and Nye was elected president by the 11 charter members who attended. Incorporated as the Nurses Association of Buffalo in 1899, its goals included implementation of a benefit fund for members and establishment of libraries in local nurse training schools.

During the 1890s nursing's leaders were becoming increasingly disturbed about the proliferation of training schools whose programs did not adhere to acceptable standards for the preparation of nurses. Concerned about the effects of inadequate education on the future of nursing and the welfare of society, Nye advocated uniform standards and qualifications for nurse training and the enactment of legislation that would regulate and protect the title of nurse. To that end she supported the establishment in New York of a state association for nurses. That association would provide the vehicle for attaining the necessary laws. She envisioned as requisite a standardized curriculum, uniform entrance requirements, and a testing mechanism for validating competence.

In the spring of 1900 an informal meeting was held for the purpose of exploring mechanisms for founding a state association in New York. A committee comprised of Nye (as chairperson), Isabel Merritt, Lavinia Dock, Annie Damer, and Eva Allerton was formed and assigned the task of planning a statewide meeting to be held in Albany.

The meeting was scheduled for April 16 and 17, 1901, and publicized to all nursing clubs, alumnae associations, and training schools in the state. Fifty-six nurses attended the meeting, which was held at the city hall in Albany on the designated dates. The New York State Nurses

Association (NYSNA) was established by those in attendance, and Nye was elected president. NYSNA was the first state association organized in this country and included among its members many of the most distinguished nurse leaders of the time.

At the meeting a constitution was adopted and goals were defined. Much discussion focused on membership requirements, but no consensus was reached. Thus, the development of by-laws had to be postponed. Those present, however, were inducted as charter members upon payment of one dollar.

A second meeting of NYSNA scheduled for September, 1901 was postponed because it conflicted with the International Congress of Nurses (ICN) meeting planned in conjunction with the World's Pan-American Exposition in Buffalo. Nye was a highly visible participant in the proceedings of the ICN and, as president of NYSNA, presented a paper supportive of strategies leading to state registration for nurses. During the ICN meeting Nye's Buffalo colleagues served as hostesses for the delegates from the many nursing organizations represented.

On January 21, 1902, a second NYSNA meeting was held, and membership requirements were established (only graduates of general hospitals and state hospitals for the insane were eligible). This was unacceptable to Nye and the BNA. A resolution not to affiliate with NYSNA was adopted by BNA, and Nye publicized her opposition to the membership by-law, calling it restrictive and unfair to the majority of nurses in New York.

At the conclusion of her term as president of NYSNA in April 1902, Nye was once again elected president of BNA, an office she held until 1906. She was also one of three members of BNA's legislative committee appointed to monitor legislative action affecting nursing in New York State.

In the fall of 1902, NYSNA's proposed nurse registration bill (Armstrong-Davis Bill) was publicized to the nursing community in New York in an effort to generate support. Nye was outspoken in her opposition to several provisions in the bill.

She objected to the composition of the Board of Examiners, which excluded physician participation, and to the title "registered nurse" as the credential for nurses meeting the specified requirements. However, the bill was approved by the members of NYSNA and submitted to the legislature in February 1903.

Nye enlisted the aid of her brother, State Assemblyman Olin T. Nye, who prepared a substitute bill and submitted it to the state Assembly one week earlier than the nurses' proposal. A bitter, prolonged debate ensued, but the Nye Bill was finally amended to conform with the Armstrong-Davis Bill. Approved by both houses of the New York State Legislature, the bill was signed into law on April 27, 1903.

Irrespective of the law's enactment, Nye continued to voice her dissatisfaction with the legislation and monitored its effects over time. She stayed actively involved in nursing affairs in Buffalo throughout the remainder of her career and was presented with a diamond and ruby ring by the members of BNA when she completed her term as president in 1906.

In 1926 Nye retired to her family home (Nyeholme) in Schuyler County, where she enjoyed entertaining her many friends. Jane Delano, a lifelong friend from their early childhood days had died in 1919 and bequeathed to Nye such items as fine china, art, and linens, which Nye took pride in displaying to visitors.

Nye died on August 16, 1936, at Reading, New York, having earned the distinction of being the first president of the first state nurses' association in the United States.

PUBLICATIONS BY SYLVEEN V. NYE

ARTICLES

"The Proposed New York State Nurses Association." *Trained Nurse and Hospital Review* 25 (December 1900): 397–400.

"Official Reports of Societies." *American Journal of Nursing* 1 (September 1901): 932–34.

"Organization and Legislation for Nurses." *Third International Congress of Nurses.* Cleveland: Savage, 1901.

"The Bill of the New York State Nurses Association." *Trained Nurse and Hospital Review* 30 (January 1903): 24–28.

BIBLIOGRAPHY

Birnbach, N. "The Genesis of the Nurse Registration Movement in the United States, 1893–1903." Unpublished doctoral dissertation, Teachers College, Columbia University, 1982.

Breay, M., and E. Fenwick. *History of the International Council of Nurses 1899–1925.* Geneva: The Council, 1931.

"Buffalo Associaton Not to Affiliate." *American Journal of Nursing* 2 (June 1902): 699–700.

Buffalo City Directory. 1894–1901 editions, Buffalo, New York.

"The Buffalo Nurses Association." *American Journal of Nursing* 1 (September 1901): 910–11.

Clarke, M. *Memories of Jane A. Delano.* New York: Lakeside, 1934.

Driscoll, V. *Legitimizing the Profession of Nursing: The Distinct Mission of the New York State Nurses Association.* New York: Foundation of NYSNA, 1976.

"Editor's Letter-Box." *Trained Nurse and Hospital Review* 30 (April 1903): 250–51.

"Editor's Miscellany." *American Journal of Nursing* 1 (October 1900): 59–60.

"In the Nursing World." *Trained Nurse and Hospital Review* 30 (March 1903): 179–80.

"The New York State Nurses Convention." *American Journal of Nursing* 1 (May 1901): 594–97.

"Nursing Legislation News." *Trained Nurse and Hospital Review* 30 (March 1903): 173.

"Nursing News from Buffalo, N.Y." *Trained Nurse and Hospital Review* 29 (November 1902): 370–71.

Records of the Schuyler County Historical Society. Montour Falls, New York.

Report of the New York State Nurses Association 1901–1906. New York: Irving Press, 1907.

"State Legislation." *Trained Nurse and Hospital Review* 27 (November 1901): 282.

"Sylveen V. Nye." *American Journal of Nursing* 36 (November 1936): 1173.

"Sylveen V. Nye." *Quarterly News* 9 (January 1937): 19.

"To New York State Nurses." *Trained Nurse and Hospital Review* 26 (April 1901): 220–21.

Nettie Birnbach

Ethel Janette Odegard
1891–1977

Almost all of Ethel Odegard's 45-year nursing career was devoted to the improvement of nursing education and was closely tied to her belief in the value of college courses for nursing students. After 25 years of teaching, she changed career tracks to administer the board of nursing of the District of Columbia, where she continued her efforts to upgrade nursing education.

Odegard was born December 16, 1891, in Merrill (Lincoln County), Wisconsin, the youngest child of Olaus Pederson Oegard and Helle Nilson Grelland Odegard. Both parents were born in Norway, as were their two oldest children, Johanna and Peter. After the family migrated to Wisconsin in 1882, Nels, Sigurd, and Ethel (christened Edel) were born. Her father worked in saw mills and lumber yards and was engaged in lumbering during the winter months. The family attended the Norwegian Evangelical Lutheran Church.

Odegard graduated from the Merrill High School in 1910. She then enrolled in Dr. Ravn's Hospital School of Nursing in Merrill, from which she graduated in 1912. The school existed only a few years, and its two-year program was typical of schools of nursing at the time.

Odegard began her professional career as a private-duty nurse in Merrill and served as a head nurse in Dr. Ravn's Hospital for a short time. In 1913–14 she took a six-month postgraduate course in pediatrics, obstetrics, and gynecology at the Michael Reese Hospital in Chicago. Soon after that she enrolled in the University of Wisconsin in Madison and received her B.A. degree in 1919, with a major in bacteriology and a minor in sociology. At the time nurses' salaries were low, and her savings were not adequate to support Odegard in school, but her Uncle Erik Odegard assisted her financially, and part of the time that she was enrolled at the university she lived with her brother Sigurd and his wife.

In 1919 Odegard was appointed superintendent and instructor of nurses at the

Mary Lanning Memorial Hospital School of Nursing in Hastings, Nebraska. In this position she arranged for students to take courses at Hastings College. This led to her lifelong interest in the use of college facilities for nursing education.

In 1921 she returned to her native state to become assistant superintendent of nurses and educational director at Madison General Hospital School of Nursing in Madison. She was the first full-time nurse instructor to be employed at the school, established 17 years earlier.

After three years in Madison Odegard was appointed the first director of the Central School of Nursing associated with the Milwaukee Vocational School (now the Milwaukee Area Technical College). Under this arrangement students from four hospital schools in the city were given instruction in the basic sciences. Later the number of course offerings was increased; this arrangement lasted over 40 years. Odegard administered the program and taught anatomy, physiology, and bacteriology. During the summer she enrolled at Teachers College, Columbia University, in New York, and received her master's degree in nursing education in 1929.

In 1930 she resigned her position and spent several months traveling in Norway, Denmark, and Sweden. Then, because of illness in the family, she held only temporary positions for the next two years. For a few months she worked with Nina Gage at the newly organized nursing program at Hampton Institute, Hampton, Virginia. She then accepted a year's appointment at Highland Hospital School of Nursing, Oakland, California, replacing a faculty member on leave of absence. In 1933 she was appointed assistant superintendent of nurses at Miami Valley Hospital School of Nursing, Dayton, Ohio, where she taught the basic sciences and directed the ward teaching program.

In 1937 Odegard went to St. Mary's Hospital School of Nursing, Rochester, Minnesota, as science instructor, and that fall joined the faculty of the College of St. Theresa, Winona, Minnesota. She was employed there until 1943, when she joined the faculty of St. Louis City Hospital School of Nursing, St. Louis, Missouri,

where she was assistant director and taught the basic sciences.

After an extensive career in nursing education, on April 1, 1944, Odegard was appointed executive secretary of the Nurses' Examining Board of the District of Columbia, where she remained until her retirement in 1957. In this position she was responsible for the registration of nurses in the District, as well as supervision of the schools and programs in basic nursing. In her 13-year tenure she saw the establishment of the National State Board Test Pool Examination and the National Accreditation Service of the National League for Nursing.

Odegard took a year's leave of absence (1952–53) as a Fulbright scholar and served as nursing advisor to the medical faculty at the University of Alexandria, in Alexandria, Egypt. Here she assisted in curriculum revision, gave lectures on nursing education, and helped plan the nursing library.

On her retirement in April 1957, Odegard was presented a Distinguished Service Award presented by the Graduate Nurses' Association of the District of Columbia, the D.C. League for Nursing, and the Nurses' Examining Board. After retirement, she went to Rome to attend the Congress of the International Council of Nurses, followed by several months in Europe, visiting schools of nursing, licensing agencies, and nursing organizations in France, Germany, and England.

The author of a number of professional publications, Odegard also wrote numerous travel, genealogical, and historical articles and several translations of Norwegian publications. She was proud of her Norwegian heritage and spoke the language fluently.

She was interested in travel, music, and art. In 1949 she and her sister Johanna Torkelson of Merrill presented two oil paintings by Wisconsin artists to the Merrill High School in honor of their mother.

Odegard lived in Washington, D.C., for several years after her retirement, but in 1973 she moved to Fairhaven, a retirement center in Whitewater, Wisconsin. She died February 28, 1977, at the Fort Atkinson Community Hospital.

The University of Wisconsin—Madison was the recipient of her legacy, and each year several nursing students are awarded Ethel Odegard Scholarships.

PUBLICATIONS BY ETHEL JANETTE ODEGARD

BOOKS

Microbiology Laboratory Manual. St. Louis: Mosby, 1944.

A Norwegian Family Transplanted: The Genealogical Writings of Ethel J. Odegard. Decorah, Iowa: Anundsen, 1974.

With F.E. Colien. *Principles of Microbiology.* St. Louis: Mosby, 1941.

ARTICLES

"Preparing the Nurses for Professional Life." *Modern Hospital* 28 (February 1927): 132, 134, 136.

"Why the State Should Support Schools of Nursing." *Modern Hospital* 44 (April 1935): 75–76.

"The Nurses State Their Case." *Medical Annals of the District of Columbia* 16 (July 1947): 394–96.

With R.B. Scott. "Help with Licensure Problems." *American Journal of Nursing* 57 (October 1957): 1297–98.

BIBLIOGRAPHY

"About People You Know: Ethel J. Odegard." *American Journal of Nursing* 44 (May 1944): 499.

Ackley, S. "Eminent Teachers: Ethel J. Odegard." *American Journal of Nursing* 29 (July 1929): 843–44.

Ethel Odegard Papers. Archives, State Historical Society of Wisconsin, Madison.

Evans, L.T. "A Chronological Description of Miss Odegard's Experience and Accomplishments." In *A Norwegian Family Transplanted.* Ethel Odegard. Decorah, Iowa: Anundsen, 1974.

"Miss Ethel J. Odegard." Obituary. *Capital Times* (Madison, Wisconsin), March, 1977.

"Program Given at Presentation of Two Paintings." *Merrill* (Wisconsin) *Daily Herald,* December 7, 1949.

Signe S. Cooper

Mary Agnes O'Donnell

d. 1938

Mary Agnes O'Donnell played a prominent role as a nurse educator in the southern United States and Cuba at the turn of the century. Her nursing and administrative skills led to the establishment of schools of nursing in New Orleans, Louisiana, and Havana, Cuba. She received high commendation from the Cuban government for her 34 years of service in elevating the standard of nursing care provided to the Cuban people.

Although little information is available about O'Donnell's early years, it is known that she had a sister, Anna Esther O'Donnell, who also became a nurse. She was a native of Saugerties, New York, and received her nursing education at the Bellevue School of Nursing in New York City, graduating in either 1891 or 1892. In 1893 at the request of Sister Agnes, superioress of the Sisters of Charity in New Orleans, O'Donnell arrived in that city to establish a school of nursing at Charity Hospital. At the time, Charity Hospital accommodated 800 patients, including the poor and needy. In this setting O'Donnell gained experience in treating a wide range of disorders, including the tropical diseases that she would later encounter while working in Cuba. The first nursing class at Charity Hospital, including Agnes's sister, Anna O'Donnell, was accepted in January 1894 and graduated on December 11, 1895. For their efforts, these dedicated nurses were paid $8 during their first year of service and $12 for their second year! O'Donnell later moved to New York City with her sister.

At the outbreak of the Spanish-American War, she moved south to nurse soldiers in Jacksonville, Florida, where a typhoid epidemic was taking its toll. In 1899 O'Donnell was requested by General Leonard Wood, governor of Cuba, to establish a school of nursing in that country. Working with her sister and a group of graduate nurses from Bellevue, she organized a school of nursing at Nuestra Señora de las Mercedes in Havana. Having no standardized text to use with her nursing students, O'Donnell translated into Spanish the teachings of Isabel Hampton Robb. Among the graduates of the first class in 1902 was Martina Guerva, who later became president of the Cuban Nurses Association.

In addition to her role as educator, O'Donnell spent many years serving patients in outlying areas of Cuba. In 1909 she began her work in public-health nursing through the Visiting Nurses of Furbush, eventually serving as head nurse at a tuberculosis sanitarium.

O'Donnell's many contributions to nursing in Cuba did not go unrecognized. In 1928 the Cuban government awarded her a gold medal for her 25 years of service. She was presented the Cross of the Order of Dr. Carlos J. Finlay in 1930. Dr. Finlay was an illustrious member of the Mercedes Hospital staff and her staunch supporter. On July 23, 1938, two months after her death, the nursing school at Mercedes Hospital was renamed for her.

O'Donnell was thought of with fondness and respect by her students and peers. With a viewpoint considered liberal at that time, she believed that nursing and medical students should be treated on the same social and intellectual level, as their common goal was the care of the patient. Addressing the First Conference of Welfare and Correction in 1902, she urged the recognition of nursing as a "profession for women which made it unnecessary for them to be supported by anyone." She was described by a successor as "a beautiful character. In her were combined the rare qualities of a good administrator and a kindly humane personality." In 1930 she was awarded a diploma and gold medal by the Cuban Nurses Association in recognition of her "untiring zeal on behalf of nurses and of nursing."

Mary Agnes O'Donnell died on May 23, 1938, aboard the steamship S.S. *Dixie*, while returning to New York from a vacation in New Orleans.

BIBLIOGRAPHY

Ireland, N.O. *Index to Women of the World from Ancient to Modern Times: Biographies and Portraits.* Westwood, Mass.: Faxon, 1970.

"Mary Agnes O'Donnell: Pioneer Educator in the South." *Trained Nurse and Hospital Review* 101 (August 1938): 136–39.

"Mary Agnes O'Donnell." *New York Times*, May 27, 1938, 17.

Nursing Studies Index, 1930–49. Vol. II, p. 57. Philadelphia: Lippincott, 1970.

Pennock, M.R., ed. *Makers of Nursing History.* New York: Lakeside, 1940.

Linda Karch

Agnes K. Ohlson
b. 1902

During the active years of her professional career, Agnes K. Ohlson committed herself with vigor to the nursing profession as the chief examiner for the Connecticut State Board of Nurse Examiners and, simultaneously, as a committee member and officer of state, national, and international nursing organizations.

Ohlson was born in New Britain, Connecticut, on February 20, 1902, the second of four children and only daughter of Johannes and Karlina (Nelson) Ohlson. Her parents, who had emigrated from Sweden as teenagers, met and married in New Britain. Her father was a cabinet maker who eventually had his own business, and her mother was a homemaker. Ohlson was educated in New Britain, graduating from New Britain High School in 1919. Her parents were opposed to her desire to enter nursing, believing that she should follow the traditional pattern of marriage and homemaking. Her father said if she was still intent on nursing when she was 21, then he would voice no further objection. She went to work as a secretary to the vice-president of Landers, Ferry, and Clark, a large manufacturing company in New Britain. Although she found the work interesting and exciting, she retained her desire to be a nurse and graduated from the Peter Bent Brigham School of Nursing in Boston in 1926.

Her first position, in 1926, was as a supervisor at Wesson Maternity Hospital in Springfield, Massachusetts. After nine months, recognizing that she needed more education in order to feel more competent in these positions, she entered Teachers College, Columbia University, in New York City. During the time she was a student she took a position as assistant director of nursing at Truesdale Hospital in Fall River, Massachusetts, and was back and forth between Truesdale and Teachers College, receiving a bachelor of science degree in 1931. In the same year, at age 29, she assumed the position of director of nursing at Waterbury Hospital, Waterbury, Connecticut, which she held until 1936.

During her tenure at Waterbury she was elected to the board of directors of the Connecticut Nurses Association, and CNA suggested her name to the governor for appointment to the State Board of Nurse Examiners. She was appointed as a board member in 1935 and assumed the permanent post of secretary in 1936, resigning from her directorship at Waterbury. She served in this capacity for more than a quarter of a century, until her retirement in 1963.

Strongly influenced by Carrie Hall, the superintendent of nurses and principal of the school of nursing at her alma mater Brigham and a woman actively involved in speaking on nursing issues through professional organizations, Ohlson joined the American Nurses' Association (ANA) soon after her graduation, first in Massachusetts, then in Connecticut after she left her position at Wesson. This organization became the platform through which she began to exert some influence on the profession. One of her important contributions was the establishment of a group at ANA for nurses who were members of state boards of nurse examiners.

Ohlson had been deeply disturbed at the process of testing for licensure that was used in Connecticut as well as across the country. In Connecticut the board members, sometimes aided by faculty who taught a specialty, wrote essay questions that were administered to graduate nurses seeking licensure. These exams were then read and graded by the board. Ohlson was appalled by the limitations of the process, realizing that the obligation of the board to protect the citizens of the state by assuring competence on the part

of registered nurses was very hard to assure by such an examination. At ANA meetings, where she had the opportunity to talk with members of state boards across the country, she realized that the process was similar everywhere. She asked ANA to sponsor a meeting for state board people that became an ANA committee. Eventually, both ANA and the NLN (National League for Nursing) formed committees to address concerns of state board members that ultimately led to the development of the State Board Test Pool exams. Evidence of her leadership can be seen in her service as chair of the ANA Bureau of State Boards of Nurse Examiners and chair of the Committee on State Board Problems of the National League of Nursing Education (NLNE).

Her record of service to nursing through offices in professional organizations is extensive. In 1948 she ran for the office of ANA treasurer but lost to Lucy Germain. By that time her record showed that she had been a consultant to the U.S. Cadet Nurse Corps, part-time assistant executive secretary of ANA, chair of the ANA Bureau of State Boards of Nurse Examiners, and chair of the education section and president of the Connecticut Nurses Association. When she ran for secretary of ANA in 1950, she had added chairman of the NLNE Committee on State Board Problems and the presidency of the Connecticut League for Nursing to the record. She won that election. She continued to further her education during this time, completing a master of arts degree in 1951 at Trinity College, Hartford, Connecticut, with a major in government.

During her term as secretary she chaired the ANA Committee on Legislation as well as the Committee on State Boards of Nursing. She served as secretary until 1954, when she was elected president of ANA, an office she held for two terms until 1958. In January 1955 the American Nurses' Foundation was officially established with Agnes Ohlson as the first president. Later that year as president she represented the ANA at the biennial meeting of the ICN board of directors. While she was serving her second term as ANA president, in 1957 she was elected to a four-year term as president of the International Council of Nurses (ICN). This was followed by a four-year term as vice-president (1961–65). Despite this uninterrupted record of service in major elected posts, Ohlson retained her position as chief examiner for the state board in Connecticut and fulfilled the responsibilities of that job. One example of the intensity of her time commitment was in 1944 when she was consultant to the U.S. Public Health Service for the Cadet Nurse Corps. In order to fulfill her state board obligations she stayed in Washington, D.C., during the week, returned to Connecticut on Friday night, did state board business on the weekend, and returned to Washington on Sunday evening. Another example is when she was president of ICN. After completing her day in Connecticut, she would go to New York to get an evening flight to London. She slept on the plane, arrived in London in time to start an ICN board meeting at 11 A.M., and, when the meeting was over, returned to New York, then on to Connecticut, to resume her state board duties.

Ohlson was held in high esteem by colleagues and associates. When she resigned from Waterbury Hospital to take the permanent position at the state board, the headline on the front page of the *Waterbury American*, April 13, 1936, read "Miss Agnes Ohlson Resigns Post at Waterbury." While she was ANA president, she was honored at a testimonial dinner in Connecticut attended by nurse colleagues, representatives of other health groups, and members of the state government. Resolutions were written into the record of the Connecticut Legislature and the *Congressional Record* on the occasion of her election to the presidency of ICN. In 1959 she was granted life membership in the Foundation of the Women's Auxiliary of the American Swedish Historical Museum in Philadelphia. This award is given to a woman of Swedish background who has made an outstanding contribution in her field, as well as in service to others. On the occasion of its Diamond Jubilee the Connecticut Nurses Association established awards in the names of five distinguished Connecticut nurses. Ohlson was the first recipient of the Agnes Ohlson Award, given nurses who have been outstanding advocates for the public good and the nursing profession through political action.

Ohlson currently resides in Clearwater, Florida, and maintains an active interest in the development of the nursing profession.

PUBLICATIONS BY AGNES K. OHLSON

"Eight-hour Plan for Private Duty Nurses." *American Journal of Nursing* 32 (December 1932): 1275–76.

BIBLIOGRAPHY

"About People You Know." *American Journal of Nursing* 44 (November 1944): 1092.

"Candidates for ANA Election." *American Journal of Nursing* 48 (April 1948): 268.

"Candidates for ANA Election." *American Journal of Nursing* 50 (April 1950): 254.

Connecticut Board of Examiners for Nursing. Board Minutes. Hartford: The Board, 1905–1970.

"News About Nursing." *American Journal of Nursing* 54 (August 1954): 999–1000.

Nursing Outlook 7 (June 1959): 373.

Ohlson, A. Interviews (taped and transcribed) with the author, June 21–23, 1989; March 15, 1990, Clearwater, Florida.

Who's Who in America, A Biographical Dictionary of Notable Living Men and Women, 1958–59. Vol. 60, p. 2085. Chicago: Marquis, 1958.

Carol A. Daisy

Virginia Mae Ohlson

b. 1914

Virginia Mae Ohlson's interest in international public-health nursing has always been the driving force behind her work. She served as public-health nursing consultant and later as chief nurse of the Public Health and Welfare Section of General MacArthur's headquarters in U.S.-occupied Japan after World War II. On her return to the United States she was invited back to the Orient as a nurse consultant with the Atomic Bomb Casualty Commission in Hiroshima, Japan. A year later, after the United States had signed the peace treaty with Japan, she was appointed nurse representative of the Rockefeller Foundation in Japan. She used these experiences later to help design the first program of international studies at the College of Nursing, University of Illinois at Chicago. It was largely through her influence that in 1986 the school became the first U.S. World Health Organization (WHO) Collaborating Center for Nursing, which concurrently serves as the Secretariat (executive director) of the Global Network of WHO Collaborating Centers for Nursing, situated in 19 areas of the world.

One of three sisters, Ohlson was born in Chicago on October 31, 1914. As a young girl, she was fascinated by the stories of the foreign missionaries of her church and those of a local public-health nurse. Determined to become a public-health nurse, in 1933 she graduated from North Park Junior College, Chicago, and received her diploma in nursing in 1937 from the Swedish Covenant Hospital School of Nursing, Chicago. After a brief experience as an operating-room nurse at the Swedish Covenant Hospital, she was offered a staff position as a public-health nurse at the Department of Health in Evanston, Illinois. In 1943 she became director of nursing at the Evanston department. During her years there she had a firsthand introduction to research as she assisted Dr. Louis Sauer in his work in the development of the DPT vaccine. She enrolled part time at the University of Chicago while working full time at Evanston. In 1946 she received the bachelor of science degree and, by examination, the public-health nursing certificate from the state of Illinois.

Ohlson's career in international nursing began in 1947 during the U.S. occupation of Japan following World War II. She was one of a group of Americans employed as civilian nurses by the U.S. Army of Occupation. Each American nurse had a Japanese nurse counterpart, who was to hold a position similar to her own at the end of the U.S. occupation. Together, they worked side by side with Japanese nurses,

physicians, and government officials to reestablish organized nursing education and practice in Japan. Their work included the development of the Japanese National Nursing Law, which regulated the education, registration, and practice of nurses, public-health nurses, and midwives. With the help of the American nurses, the Japanese Nursing Association, which had lost its membership in the International Council of Nursing (ICN) during the war years, was reorganized and readmitted into the ICN in 1949.

When initially assigned to the Public Health and Welfare Section of General MacArthur's headquarters, the Supreme Command of Allied Powers (SCAP), Ohlson functioned as the public-health nursing consultant. Her primary Japanese nursing counterpart was the chief public-health nurse of the Japanese Ministry of Health and Welfare. Ohlson was promoted rapidly; after two years her civilian rank became equal to that of an army colonel. In 1949 she was appointed chief nurse of the Public Health and Welfare Section, SCAP, when the previous chief, Major Grace Alt, left Japan for graduate study in the United States.

Ohlson returned to the United States at the close of the U.S. occupation of Japan (1951). Six months later she was appointed by the U.S. Energy Commission to work with the Atomic Bomb Casualty Commission (ABCC) in Hiroshima, Japan. Her first position with the ABCC was as a public-health nurse consultant. Two months later she was promoted to be director of nursing. The ABCC was an organization of the U.S. Energy Commission set up to study the effects of the atomic bomb on the populations of Hiroshima and Nagasaki. Ohlson and her Japanese nurse counterpart supervised 25–30 Japanese nurses in assisting in the care and study of patients who were the atomic bomb casualties and in documenting injuries, illnesses, and anomalies resulting from radiation.

Following a year in Hiroshima, the Ministry of Health and Welfare of the Japanese government invited Ohlson to return to Tokyo under the employment of the Rockefeller Foundation. In this capacity she worked closely with Japanese nursing leaders in implementing systems for the accreditation of schools of nursing and refining processes for examination and licensure of nurses as set up by the new national nursing law. While a nurse with the Rockefeller Foundation, she also worked with Japanese nurses and university faculties in the initiation of their first baccalaureate programs in nursing at the University of Tokyo and the Women's University in Kochi. Ohlson returned to the United States in December 1954 after a total of eight years in Japan.

She received the master of science degree in nursing education (public-health nursing administration) from the University of Chicago in 1955. From 1956 to 1960 she was one of eight full-time faculty members in the Department of Nursing Education at the University of Chicago. In 1961 she enrolled in the doctoral program there and received her Ph.D. in 1969.

In 1963, while a part-time doctoral student at the University of Chicago, Ohlson joined the faculty at the University of Illinois College of Nursing as associate professor and director of public-health nursing. Although the college already had a National League for Nursing accredited baccalaureate nursing program, it had not been designated as an approved institution offering preparation for public-health nursing. The attainment of that approval for the college became Ohlson's initial goal, and in 1964 the college received full approval for its program offering preparation for public-health nursing. Ohlson was appointed to full professorship and the first head of the Department of Public Health Nursing in 1970. In the same year, she was instrumental in formulating the first master's program in public-health nursing at the college and in the state of Illinois.

When Dr. Mary Kelly Mullane, dean of the College of Nursing, retired in 1971, Ohlson was appointed acting dean. During her years as acting dean the college's first off-campus programs for nursing were established in Peoria and Urbana. Because of her devotion to the newly developing master's program in public-health nursing, Ohlson returned as head of that department in 1973 and remained in that position until her resignation as department head in 1980.

Throughout her years at the University of Illinois, College of Nursing, Ohlson had always placed an emphasis on international nursing. On resignation as head of the Department of Public Health Nursing, she was appointed to a new position in the college—assistant dean and director of the Office for International Studies. In 1980 the graduate courses in public-health nursing came to the attention of Amelia Maglacas, then the chief nurse officer of the World Health Organization (WHO) in Geneva, Switzerland. Consequently, Ohlson was invited to Geneva to work with Maglacas in the preparation of a guide for reviewing nursing-education curricula for content in primary health care. This work and other consultation appointments with WHO strengthened the university's ties to the international organization. In 1986 the College of Nursing became the first WHO Collaborating Center for International Development in Primary Health Care. Today Ohlson is professor emerita and consultant in International Health at the University of Illinois, College of Nursing at Chicago, where she is employed on a part-time basis. She teaches international courses, works with international students, and assists the college in its roles as a WHO Collaborating Center and as Secretariat of the Global Network of WHO Collaborating Centers for Nursing Development.

Ohlson has received many honors and awards during her professional career. One that she prizes highly is the Pearl McIver Award for Distinguished Service in Public Health Nursing, presented to her by the American Nurses' Association. She has been honored by the Japanese Ministry of Health on two occasions, and in 1982 the Japanese Nursing Association (JNA) awarded her its First International Honorary Membership Award. In 1990 she was elected honorary member of the Global Network of WHO Collaborating Centers.

Her work has taken her around the world. She has been invited by universities in Japan, Taiwan, the Philippines,

Saudi Arabia, Bahrain, and Egypt to evaluate plans for nursing curriculum. The friends that she has made in Japan and the work that she did there have drawn her back many times, such as on vacation with Rosemary Ellis in 1968, on sabbatical in 1974 and to the ICN Congress hosted by the JNA in 1977.

Ohlson's deep-seated commitment to God has guided her through her life as a nurse. She believes in the caring dimension of nursing, the dimension that places love for all of God's life as the top priority. This belief is reflected in her views on the professional obligations of nurses. She believes that nurses have a responsibility to those they serve as well as a responsibility to their profession. She believes in teamwork among health professionals and that people cannot be served effectively in a health-care system where its practitioners are divided. It is clear from her work overseas, her emphasis on international studies, and her ties with the World Health Organization that she views nursing from a global perspective that transcends cultural and geographical, as well as generational, boundaries.

PUBLICATIONS BY VIRGINIA MAE OHLSON

BOOKS

With J. Kaser. *Guidelines for Public Health Nurses in Health Centers.* Tokyo: Medical Friend Publishing, 1954.

CHAPTERS IN BOOKS

"Reflections in Nursing." In *History of Japanese Nursing.* Pp. 200–05. Tokyo: Japanese Nurses Association, 1967.

"Graduate Preparation for Community Health Nursing Practice." In *Current Perspectives in Nursing, Social Issues and Trends.* B. Flynn, ed. St. Louis: Mosby, 1977.

"International Nursing: Role of the ICN and WHO." In *Current Issues in Nursing,* 2nd ed. J. McCloskey and G. Mosby, eds. Boston: Blackwell, 1985.

"International Nursing: The WHO and ICN." In *Current Issues of Nursing,* 3rd ed. St. Louis: Mosby, 1990.

PAMPHLETS

Tuberculosis: The Patient and You. Tokyo: Medical Friend Publishing, 1954.

"An International View." Monograph. In *Issues of Nursing Practice* (American Nurses' Association) (1985).

ARTICLES (SELECTED)

"Profile of the Public Health Nurse." *Journal of the American Medical Association* 198 (October 1966): 326–27.

"Nurse Education as a Form of Adult Socialization." Doctoral dissertation, Microfilm, University of Chicago, 1969.

"Baccalaureate Nursing Education in the United States." *International Nursing Review* 24 (November/December 1977).

"Japanese Nursing Association: Memories and Expectations." *KANGO (Japanese Journal of Nursing)* 8 (1982).

"Primary Health Care: A Conceptual Framework." *Journal of Nursing Science* (Taiwan, ROC) (1987).

"Primary Health Care in the USA: Its Strategies." *Journal of Nursing Science* (Taiwan, ROC) (1987).

BIBLIOGRAPHY

Ohlson, V. "Virginia M. Ohlson." In *Making Choices, Taking Chances: Nurse Leaders Tell Their Stories.* T.M. Schorr and A. Zimmerman, eds. St. Louis: Mosby, 1988.

Polly Belcher
Mary Brey-Schneider

Marion Gemeth Parsons

1871–1968

Marion Gemeth Parsons was best known for her services during World War I, first with the Harvard Unit, a volunteer medical unit that was based at a British Hospital in Camiers, France, and then after the United States entered the war, with the Boston City Hospital Unit, which served with the American forces and was based at Base Hospital Number 7 in Tours, France. At the end of the war she established the Czechoslovakia State School of Nursing in Prague and served as its director from 1919–1923.

Born in Fort Fairfield, Maine, August 28, 1871, Parsons was the daughter of Horatio M. and Mary Humphrey Parsons. She attended school in Fort Fairfield and in 1902 enrolled in the Boston City Hospital Training School for Nurses, from which she graduated in 1905. She also attended Teachers College, Columbia University. From 1905–09 she was employed as head nurse at the Boston City Hospital. In 1909 she moved to San Francisco to become superintendent of the City and County Hospital, later known as the San Francisco Hospital. In 1913 she moved to New York City to be an instructor in the New York Hospital, and she left this position in 1914 to join the Harvard Unit in support of the Allied cause. In 1917 she transferred from the Harvard Unit to the Boston City Hospital Unit in Tours. After her return from Prague in 1923, she became an instructor at Boston City Hospital, a position she held until her retirement to Fryeburg, Maine, in 1940.

For her wartime service with the British, she was decorated at Buckingham Palace by King George V. In 1923 the Czechoslovakian government awarded her the Order of the White Lion along with a citation personally presented by President Thomas Masaryk. She was one of the few women ever to receive such an award. The American Red Cross also gave her an award as did the London Committee of the Czechoslovakia State School of Nursing.

She died Augsut 29, 1968, in Norway, Maine.

BIBLIOGRAPHY

Friedman, A.H. "Marion Gemeth Parsons." *Dictionary of American Nursing Biography.* M. Kaufman, ed. Westport, Conn.: Greenwood, 1988.

Obituary. *Portland* (Maine) *Press Herald,* August 31, 1968.

Vern L. Bullough

Phoebe Yates Pember

1823–1913

Phoebe Yates Pember served as chief matron for a division of Chimborazo Hospital in Richmond, Virginia, during the Civil War. She is best remembered for the humorous and realistic accounts of life in a Confederate hospital published in her diary, *A Southern Woman's Story.* This work has been judged by historians as one of the finest Civil War memoirs for its insights into conditions in a major Confederate hospital.

Pember was born in Charleston, South Carolina, on August 18, 1823, to a wealthy and cultured Jewish family. She was the fourth of seven children of Jacob Clavius Levy and Fanny Yates Levy. The family moved to Savannah, Georgia, around 1850.

Little is known of Pember's early life and schooling, although she may have been privately educated by tutors. Her diary and letters, written with style and grace, indicate that she was a well-educated woman. She married Thomas Pember of Boston prior to the Civil War. Shortly after the wedding, her husband contracted tuberculosis and died in Aiken, South Carolina, on July 9, 1861, at the age of 36. After his death, Pember returned to her parents' home in Savannah.

In 1862 the family moved to Marietta, Georgia. Pember was bored and restless there and yearned for an interesting and challenging life. In November 1862 she received a correspondence from Mrs. George W. Randolph, wife of the Confederate secretary of war, offering her the post of matron at Chimborazo Hospital in Richmond, Virginia. Pember accepted the post.

Chimborazo Hospital was the largest hospital in Confederacy and for its time the largest in the world. It served over 76,000 patients. Pember's main responsibility was to preside over a large division of the hospital, but her supervisory duties extended throughout the entire institution. Her tasks as matron included supervising hospital workers, carrying out the surgeons' orders, supervising sanitation, and overseeing food preparation for the soldiers. Pember met considerable opposition in the discharge of her duties. Although an act of the Confederate Congress clearly prescribed the responsibilities of hospital matron, most of the medical and nursing care was provided by men during the war. The male employees at

Chimborazo resented being supervised by a woman and felt that Pember was invading their territory. In spite of those prejudices, Pember concentrated on providing high-quality nursing care for all patients.

She attended carefully to the dietary needs of the soldiers. She tried to procure foods patients craved and liberally dispensed her specialty, chicken soup. Whiskey, however, had to be rationed. Pember took this responsibility seriously and doled out only the liquor that was medically prescribed. When hospital employees tried to steal liquor for their own consumption, she guarded the whiskey barrel with a gun.

Pember nursed her patients with courage and diligence. She wrote letters for the soldiers and comforted the dying. One soldier's final request was to see his best friend before he died. After an extended search, Pember found the friend and brought him to the dying soldier's bedside. Her compassionate care of the terminally ill served as a model for future generations of nurses.

When the war was over, Pember remained at her post after the hospital was invaded by Federal troops. She continued to care for Federal and Confederate soldiers, refusing to have them transferred when they were too sick to travel.

Pember returned home to Savannah with only a silver dime and a box of Confederate money. She devoted the balance of her life to writing and travel. She died in Pittsburgh, Pennsylvania, on March 4, 1913, at the age of 89.

Pember's diary has provided a model of compassion, resourcefulness, and courage in the face of prejudices against women. Her writings are one of the best first-person accounts of life inside a Confederate hospital.

PUBLICATIONS BY PHOEBE YATES PEMBER

A Southern Woman's Story. New York: Trow, 1879.

BIBLIOGRAPHY

Pember, P.Y. *A Southern Woman's Story: Life in Confederate Richmond.* B.I. Wiley, ed. St, Simon's Island, Ga.: Mockingbird Books, 1959.

Hannah Williamson

Hildegard E. Peplau

b. 1909

Defining nursing in general as "a significant therapeutic interpersonal process," Hildegard E. Peplau provided the leadership in developing the significance of interpersonal relationships in the development of psychiatric nursing in particular. Her landmark book, *Interpersonal Relations in Nursing*, published in 1952 integrated theories into her model at a time when nursing theory development was relatively new. She has also contributed to the profession through her work with the national organizations of nursing—the American Nurses' Association and the National League for Nursing.

Born on September 1, 1909, in Reading, Pennsylvania, Peplau was the second of six children of Gustav and Ottylie (Elgert) Peplau. Both parents emigrated from Germany to the United States, but they were originally from the same village in Poland. Peplau had two sisters and three brothers.

Peplau's father worked as a fireman on the Reading Railroad, and her mother was a homemaker, although she did work in a factory when her husband was on strike. Peplau chose nursing at a time when choices for women were limited, but she did not decide to go into nursing until she was a teenager. Having received her diploma in 1928 from the Reading Evening High School, in Reading, Pennsylvania, she entered the Pottstown Hospital School of Nursing in nearby Pottstown and graduated with a diploma in nursing in 1931.

It has been suggested that Peplau's first student experience in psychiatry, in 1930 at the Norristown State Hospital, may have influenced her interest in psychiatric care. While still a student, she was assigned by the nursing superintendent to play tennis with the only woman physician on the staff. This inauspicious arrangement led to a position as camp nurse at New York University's summer camp for physical education. This, in turn, opened up an unexpected opportunity, as she was recommended for the position of school nurse at Bennington College, Vermont, by the camp director. While serving as nurse at the College Health Service, she was offered and accepted a full scholarship by the president of Bennington.

During her years at Bennington College (1936–43), her work in the College Health Service, as well as her student experiences, provided her with opportunities to meet and work with well-known theorists and therapists, such as Erich Fromm, Freda Fromm-Reichman, and Harry Stack Sullivan. Influenced by Sullivan's lectures, Peplau has been engaged in interpreting and extending his theories into the realm of nursing education and practice ever since. She received her B.A. in interpersonal psychology in 1943 from Bennington College.

During World War II (specifically, 1943–45), Peplau served as a first lieutenant in the U.S. Army Nurse Corps and was assigned to the School of Military Neuropsychiatry in England.

In 1945 she enrolled as a graduate student at Teachers College, Columbia University, in New York City, where her clinical placement was at the New York State Psychiatric Institute. She received her M.A. in teaching and supervision of psychiatric nursing in 1947. By 1948 she had completed her manuscript for the book *Interpersonal Relations in Nursing*, which was not published until 1952. That same year, she worked as educational director of the postgraduate program in psychiatric nursing at Highland Hospital in Ashville, North Carolina. Returning to New York and to Teachers College in 1948, she served as instructor and director in the advanced program in psychiatric nursing and instructor in nursing education for the next five years.

Peplau then worked as a private-duty psychiatric nurse in New York City, 1953–54. By 1954 she was employed by Rutgers, the State University of New Jersey, College of Nursing. She remained at Rutgers for 20 years, beginning as a part-time instructor and working her way through the ranks to chairperson and then director of psychiatric nursing and upon her retirement to professor emerita. During this time she also maintained a part-time psychotherapy practice.

During the 1950s and 1960s Peplau conducted numerous workshops for nurses so she could share her knowledge and clinical expertise. In these workshops she redefined and pioneered the development of psychiatric nursing as a clinical specialty.

Hildegard Peplau's international prominence is well earned. From her appointment in 1948 as a member of the first expert advisory committee to the World Health Organization to board member of the International Council of Nurses, her contributions to a global perspective on health and nursing have been acknowledged. From 1973–79, she was third vice-president of the International Council of Nurses. She has served as consultant to the surgeon general of the air forces of Turkey and Labrador and has lectured extensively in Canada, Africa, and South America. These lectures were compiled by a student of Peplau's and published in a book entitled *The Psychotherapy of Hildegard E. Peplau* (by William E. Field, Jr.) in 1979.

Peplau also has numerous other accomplishments to her credit. She is the recipient of several honorary doctorates, served as interim executive director of the ANA in 1970, and was elected president of the ANA for 1970–72. She also served as second vice-president of the ANA from 1972–74. Other appointments include director of the New Jersey State Nurses Association, national nurse consultant to the surgeon general of the air force, nursing consultant to the U.S. Public Health Services, and nursing consultant to the National Institute of Mental Health.

In 1980 the ANA published a document entitled *Nursing: A Social Policy Statement.* Peplau made significant contributions to the development of this landmark paper. From 1963 through 1987 she held many national and international visiting university professorships. Her writings have been broadly disseminated, and she continues to publish and present her ideas, sharing her expertise through presentations and consultations both at home and abroad.

In 1990 the ANA board of directors, at the request of the Council of Psychiatric Mental Health Nursing, established the Hildegard E. Peplau Award, with Peplau as the first recipient. This is the only ANA national award that specifically recognizes the outstanding contributions of a psychiatric mental-health nurse.

Hildegard Peplau has consistently spoken with clarity and urgency of the need for the profession to assume full responsibility for its advancement. She has been a voice of reason and vision, maintaining a humanistic perspective throughout her career.

Peplau maintains that nursing's mission is "to manifest tenderness and to nurture human capacities and bring them to full fruition" and sees this as "basic to developing nursing practice that fosters favorable change in the living of troubled people." Her humanitarian concerns have not gone unnoticed. When asked how she would like to be remembered, she responded by saying: "As a responsible citizen and a nurse and leave the rest to history."

In 1991 Hildegard Peplau lived in Sherman Oaks, California.

PUBLICATIONS BY HILDEGARD E. PEPLAU

BOOKS, MONOGRAPHS, CHAPTERS, AND PROCEEDINGS (SELECTED)

Interpersonal Relations in Nursing. New York: Putnam, 1952, 1988. London: Macmillan, 1976, translated into Japanese.

"Educating the Nurse to Function in Psychiatric Services." In *Nursing Personnel for Mental Health Programs.* Pp. 37–42. Atlanta: Southern Regional Education Board, 1958.

"Principles of Psychiatric Nursing." In *American Handbook of Psychiatry.* S. Arieti, ed. Vol. 2, 1840–56. New York: Basic Books, 1959.

"An Approach to Research in Psychiatric Nursing." In *Training for Clinical Research in Psychiatric Mental Health Nursing.* Pp. 5–44. Washington, D.C.: Catholic University of America, 1963.

"Counseling in Nursing Practice." In *Handbook of Counseling Techniques.* E. Harms and P. Schrieber, eds. Pp. 382–93. New York: Pergamon, 1963.

"A Working Definition of Anxiety." In *Some Clinical Approaches to Psychiatric Nursing.* S. Burd and M. Marshall, eds. Pp. 333–36. New York: Macmillan, 1963.

Basic Principles of Patient Counseling. Philadelphia: Smith, Kline & French Laborato-

ries, 1964, 4th printing 1969. Spanish edition, 1968.

"Theory: The Professional Dimension." In *Proceedings of the First Nursing Theory Conference.* C. Norris, ed. Pp. 33–46. Kansas City: University of Kansas Medical Center, 1969.

"Historical Development of Psychiatric Nursing"; "Interpersonal Techniques: The Crux of Psychiatric Nursing"; "Loneliness"; "Therapeutic Concepts"; "The Work of Clinical Nurse Specialists in Psychiatric Nursing." Reprinted in *A Collection of Classics in Psychiatric Nursing Literature.* S.A. Smoyak and S. Rouslin, eds. Pp. 10–46, 47–49, 88–108, 244–50, 276–81. Thorofare, N.J.: Slack, 1982.

"Nursing Science: A Historical Perspective." In *Nursing Science: Major Paradigms, Theories, and Critiques.* R.R. Parse, ed. Pp. 13–29. Philadelphia: Saunders, 1987.

"Theoretical Constructs and Applications in Psychiatric Nursing Practice." In *Psychiatric and Mental Health Nursing: Theory and Practice.* W. Reynolds and D. Coombs, eds. London: Croom-Helms, in press.

With S.A. Smoyak. "Pattern Perpetuation in Schizophrenia." In *Schizophrenia: Current Concepts and Research.* S. Sankar, ed. Pp. 125–32. Hicksville, N.Y.: RJD, 1969.

ARTICLES (SELECTED)

"Present Day Trends in Psychiatric Nursing." *Neuropsychiatry* 3, No. 4 (1956): 190–204.

"An Undergraduate Program in Psychiatric Nursing." *Nursing Outlook* 21, No. 4 (July 1956): 400–10.

"Must Laboring Together Be Called Teamwork? Problems in Team Treatment of Adults in State Mental Hospitals." *American Journal of Orthopsychiatry* 30 (January 1960): 103–08.

"Interpersonal Relations and the Process of Adaptation." *Nursing Science* 1, No. 4 (1963): 272–79.

"Professional and Social Behavior: Some Differences Worth the Notice of Professional Nurses." *Quarterly Magazine* (Columbia University, Presbyterian Hospital School of Nursing Alumni Association) 50, No. 4 (November 1964): 23–33.

"Psychiatric Nursing Skills and the General Hospital Patient." *Nursing Forum* 3, No. 2 (1964): 28–37.

"Nurse-Doctor Relationships." *Nursing Forum* 5, No. 1 (1966): 60–75.

"Nursing's Two Routes to Doctoral Degrees." *Nursing Forum* 5, No. 2 (1966): 57–67.

"Interpersonal Relations and the Work of the Industrial Nurse." *Industrial Nurses Journal* 15, No. 10 (1967): 7–12.

"Professional Closeness, a Special Kind of Involvement with Patient, Client, or Family Group." *Nursing Forum* 8, No. 4 (1969): 342–60.

"Communication in Crisis Intervention." *Psychiatric Forum* 2 (Winter 1971): 1–7.

"Creativity and Commitment in Nursing." *Image: Journal of Nursing Scholarship* 6 (1974): 3–5.

"Is Health Care a Right? Affirmative Response." *Image: Journal of Nursing Scholarship* 7 (1974): 4–10.

"Talking with Patients." *Comprehensive Nursing Quarterly* 9, No. 3 (1974): 30–39.

"Midlife Crisis." *American Journal of Nursing* 75 (1975): 1761–65.

"Psychiatric Nursing: Role of Nurses and Psychiatric Nurses." *International Nursing Review* 25, No. 2 (1978): 41–47.

"A New Statement Defines Scope of Practice." *American Nurse* 12, No. 4 (1980): 1, 8, 24.

"The Psychiatric Nurses: Accountable? To Whom? For What? *Perspectives in Psychiatric Care* 18 (1980): 128–34.

"Some Reflections on Earlier Days in Psychiatric Nursing." *Journal of Psychosocial Nursing Mental Health Services* 20 (1982): 17–24.

"Interpersonal Constructs for Nursing Practice." *Nursing Education Today* 7, No. 5 (1987): 201–08.

"Tomorrow's World." *Nursing Times* (January 1987): 29–32.

"The Art and Science of Nursing: Similarities, Differences, and Relations." *Nursing Science Quarterly* 1, No. 1 (1988): 8–15.

"Future Directions in Psychiatric Nursing from the Perspective of History." *Psychosocial Nursing and Mental Health Services* 27, No. 2 (1989): 18–21, 25–28.

OTHER

"Interview with Dr. Peplau: Future of Nursing." *Japanese Journal of Nursing* 39, No. 10 (1975): 1046–50.

Marshall, Jr. "Dr. Peplau's Strong Medicine for Psychiatric Nurses." *Smith, Kline & French Reporter* 7 (March–April 1963): 7, 11–14.

O'Toole, A.W., and S.R. Welt, eds. *Interpersonal Theory in Nursing Practice: Selected Works of Hildegard E. Peplau.* New York: Springer, 1959.

BIBLIOGRAPHY

American Nurses' Association. "Hildegard E. Peplau." *One Strong Voice.* Pp. 583–92. Kansas City: ANA Press, 1976.

Carey, E.T., L. Rasmussen, B. Searcy, and N.L. Stark. "Hildegard E. Peplau: Psychodynamic Nursing." In *Nursing Theorists and Their Work,* A. Marriner, ed. Pp. 181–95, 203–17. St. Louis: Mosby, 1986.

Fitzpatrick, J.J., and B. Evans. "Honorary Doctorates Awarded to Nurses: A 51-Year Review." *Journal of Professional Nursing* 5, No. 3 (1984): 159–63.

Franz, J. "70+ and Going Strong: Hildegard E. Peplau: Grand Dame of Psychiatric Nursing." *Geriatric Nursing* (November/December 1986): 328–40.

Gregg, D.E. "Hildegard E. Peplau: Her Contributions." *Perspectives in Psychiatric Care* 3 No. 16 (1978): 118–21.

Helene Fuld Health Trust (producer) and D. Wallace (director). *Portraits of Excellence: Hildegard Peplau.* Videorecording. Oakland, Calif.: Studio Three, 1988.

Peplau, H.E. "A Personal Challenge for Immediate Action." In *Facing up to Changing Responsibilities: An Institute Sponsored by the Conference Group on Psychiatric Nursing Practice of the American Nurses' Association.* New York: ANA, 1964.

"Profile." *Nursing* 74, No. 4 (1974): 13.

Rouslin, S.W., and A.W. O'Toole. "Hildegard E. Peplau: Observations in Brief." *Archives of Psychiatric Nursing* 111, No. 5 (1989): 254–64.

Sills, G.M. "Hildegard E. Peplau: Leader, Practitioner, Academician, Scholar, and Theorist." *Perspectives in Psychiatric Care* 16, No. 3 (1978): 122–28.

Elizabeth M.B. Visone
Olga Maranjian Church

Maria Celina Phaneuf

b. 1907

Maria Celina Phaneuf was a pioneering leader in the development of methods for evaluating quality of care. She is best known for her work with the nursing audit and quality assurance, but her contributions to health care extend much further. She directed a five-year demonstration and evaluation study by the Associated Hospital Service of New York that resulted in changes in New York State insurance law to permit insurance plans to pay for home care. Related outcomes were widening of Blue Cross coverage to extended-care facilities and inclusion in the initial Medicare rules of coverage for continuing care outside acute-care hospitals. She was responsible for the development of the National League for Nursing's *Criteria for Evaluating the Administration of a Public Health Nursing Service* and was a member of the American Nurses' Association task force that wrote the landmark declaration *Nursing: A Social Policy Statement.* The continual impetus for her activities has been her ethically based conviction that health-care providers have an obligation to assure that quality health care is available to those who need it.

Born in Richford, Vermont, on April 14, 1907, Phaneuf was the daughter of Eugene Phaneuf and Mary Boulanger Phaneuf. A younger brother, Edward B. Armour, was born of her widowed mother's later marriage. She was educated in the Richford schools and graduated in 1924 from Richford High School as valedictorian and class poet. Near the time she graduated from nursing school, she found herself responsible for the support of her mother and young brother. This responsibility continued until about 1942.

Phaneuf graduated in 1928 from Grace Hospital School of Nursing in New Haven, Connecticut. This school had Yale University affiliations for psychiatry and communicable-disease training as well as a visiting-nurse service affiliation. She received a bachelor of arts in nursing education from Teachers College at Columbia University in 1949 and a master of arts in nursing education from the same institution in 1954. Because the bachelor's and master's curricula were being revised throughout this time, she was able to pursue public-health nursing in considerable depth. She started coursework toward a doctoral degree but felt that her work at the Associated Hospital Service had such importance for future patients and their families that she should not allow her attention to be diverted even slightly.

Marion Whitmore, chief clinical nursing instructor at Grace Hospital and recognized in the hospital for her clinical expertise, exerted a strong influence on Phaneuf as a student, making her eager to pursue further education in nursing.

From the time she graduated in 1928 until 1935, Phaneuf held positions at Grace Hospital, starting as head nurse on the male surgical ward while a senior student and progressing to supervisor, night superintendent, and finally assistant director of nursing.

In 1935 she joined the staff of the Putney School, located in Putney Vermont, to establish a health program for students and faculty. A new and progressive secondary residential school for children from privileged families, the school was located on 600 acres in rural Vermont, some 20 miles from the nearest hospital or physician. The health program that Phaneuf designed provided a variety of services, ranging from accident prevention and health promotion to infirmary care. Phaneuf recalls that the faculty and students were "intellectually stimulating" and that she rapidly acquired much public-health knowledge.

Her experiences at the Putney School provided an education that was foundational to her subsequent work. She recalls two valuable life lessons. One, "never underestimate people's capacities," came from observing the way in which young students accepted responsibility and functioned with "firmness and skill" when accidents occurred. The second, "never assume acceptance in the absence of evidence that it exists," came from a more unique circumstance. At the end of her first year she was astonished to learn that her return to the school for the next year (as well as that of faculty members) was dependent on student approval. She learned of this system of evaluation only after she was asked to stay the second year. She recalls, "While I had resisted the authoritarian regime of the hospital, I had not thought about having my employment depend on lay persons, let alone adolescent ones. Upon reflection, I realized that had students not accepted me as nurse, I could not have been effective in continued work with them."

In 1942 Phaneuf left the Putney School for New York City in order to pursue the formal education she had so long desired. While she attended Teachers College, she also worked as a visiting nurse. She lived in International House and worked in its health service the first year she was in New York. She then joined the Henry Street Settlement Nursing Service, which shortly thereafter became the Visiting Nurse Service of New York. During the 10 years she was there, she progressed from staff nurse to supervisor. She gained considerable experience with people from a variety of cultures and economic backgrounds in Queens, Manhattan, and the Bronx, including persons in industry who were covered by the Metropolitan Life Insurance Company. An experience invaluable to her future direction was participation in the early days of the Montefiore Hospital Home-Care Program, which was designed to provide continuity of care at home for chronically ill patients recently discharged from the hospital. The Visiting Nurse Service of New York provided the nursing care, while the Montefiore program provided all other services.

In 1952 the director of the service, Marion G. Randall, proposed to Phaneuf and the Associated Hospital Service of New York that Phaneuf conduct a study on the feasibility of providing visiting nurse service to Blue Cross subscribers. Phaneuf was willing but also requested she be given additional responsibilities in the office of the medical director of Associated Hospital Service. This move to be a part of the operations of the service aside from the feasibility study was based on her recognition that she must establish her credibility and be accepted as valuable in order for the study to succeed. The responsibilities she assumed included utilization review and moot case review, and they continued throughout her employment with the Associated Hospital Service.

Feasibility of funding visiting nurse services by Blue Cross subscribers was established through a carefully conducted demonstration and evaluation project that extended from 1952 to 1957. This research in health-care organization was the first participation of a Blue Cross Plan in studying either home care or a mechanism for evaluating cost effectiveness of care given. It was also the first evaluation study that appraised the quality of nursing care provided. In addition to devising the necessary study evaluation procedures, Phaneuf created a hospital-based, nurse-directed organizational structure with a mechanism for payment for providing continuity of care for those who wanted home care instead of continued hospital stay.

An important general outcome of this study was an understanding of the kind of structure, standards, and controls needed for an effective permanent program of post hospital care at home for large numbers of patients. Consequently, in 1959 (after previous attempts by Blue Cross in 1955 and 1956), the New York State insurance law was revised to permit insurance plans to pay for home care. Phaneuf was appointed director of the new Associated Hospital Service Home-Care Program in 1960. The organizational structure of the program and patient outcomes are outlined in journal articles and Blue Cross publications describing the program. Nursing service in the home was provided exclusively by Visiting Nurse associations and public-health agencies. Each hospital's home-care program was directed by an appropriately qualified nurse on the hospital staff. To this day, some Blue Cross plans continue to provide some elements of this service. A related outcome of the evaluation project was the widening of Blue Cross coverage to extended-care facilities; the trial for this program was conducted in collaboration with Lydia Hall at the Loeb Center for Nursing and Rehabilitation at Montefiore Medical Center.

As a necessary part of assuring quality home care, Phaneuf promoted development of the National League for Nursing "Criteria for Evaluating the Administration of Public Health Nursing Service," published in June 1961. This was the first articulation of standards for the administration of home-care programs, and they were used to appraise the administration of agencies used by the Home-Care Program. It is on record in Blue Cross documents that the program helped bring about the adoption of the NLN criteria. Phaneuf's insistence that a nursing organization assume the leadership in establishing these guidelines came at a time when the role of nurses in Blue Cross and other payment organizations was not accepted by those in traditional nursing positions or organizations. By achieving the promulgation of home-care program standards by the NLN, she was able to broaden the influence of nursing to new arenas in health care. Phaneuf believed this was essential because nurses have the greatest involvement with patients. These standards were the forerunner of the current Community Health Accreditation Program (CHAP) operated by the NLN.

If the years at Grace Hospital, Putney School, and the Visiting Nurse Service could be termed foundational years in which Miss Phaneuf acquired a broad and solid grounding in a variety of areas, the Blue Cross years (1952–66) can be cast as a developmental time in which her evaluation vision formed, grew, and bore fruit. Over a period of seven years (1953–60) Phaneuf developed a formalized pattern for auditing nursing care, using the first set of data from the Blue Cross feasibility study. Because this work was conducted within the context of the Blue Cross home-nursing study, corporate considerations prevented publication until after the insurance laws were changed and the Home-Care Program was established.

The Phaneuf Nursing Audit format and pattern, based on components of care derived from seven nursing functions, was the first articulation of a systematic method for evaluating the process of nursing care. This system has been useful in the United States and Canada in many different types of agencies, and it has been used by other health-care professionals besides nurses. The method for evaluation of care involves the people providing the care, with the intent of accountability for care given.

The Great Society legislation of Lyndon Johnson's presidency included health-care benefits for the elderly. Because of her experience with Blue Cross, and more specifically the Home-Care Program, Phaneuf was asked to serve on a small medical group that worked with the Social Security Administration. This group assisted with the implementation of the 1965 Medicare law, providing guidance for rules and regulations. Her participation was influential in establishment of Medicare coverage for continued care outside acute-care hospitals.

In 1967 Phaneuf joined the faculty of Wayne State University College of Nursing as chair of the Public Health Nursing Department. She believed a faculty position would allow her to continue her work in health-care organization. What she did not realize was that her basic sense of ethics and social accountability to people requiring health care would be multiplied and brought to the fore by the events in which she became involved. As a university located in inner-city Detroit, Wayne State was particularly involved in the recovery from the Detroit race riots of 1967.

Before she left New York, Phaneuf had joined the Medical Committee for Human Rights, a national committee that provided medical support during civil-rights demonstrations. Other activities of the committee were to support opportunities for minorities in health professions education and to provide nonviolent civil-rights leadership in health care. Members of the Detroit Committee (including Phaneuf) were active during and after the riots. At a time when communication from traditional sources with troubled segments of the Detroit community was viewed with suspicion, the committee provided a mechanism for access and acceptance. Phaneuf's activities included some underground work directed toward helping specific persons as well as extensive participation in the formation of an Inner-City Health Care Clinic after the riots.

Phaneuf held a joint appointment on the Wayne State University School of Medicine faculty in community health and engaged in collaborative practice with some physicians of the faculty. She cochaired with a professor of medicine a multidisciplinary committee established by the dean of the School of Medicine that focused on the development of a plan and curriculum for courses to be shared by students from the Schools of Medicine, Nursing, Pharmacy, and Social Work. Ethics was the focus of one of the newly developed courses.

Phaneuf retired from Wayne State in 1972, the same year in which her book,

The Nursing Audit, was published. Retirement brought new activities. She spoke frequently to various groups about the nursing audit and served as a visiting professor in the School of Nursing at the University of Texas at Austin and at the University of Texas Health Science Center at San Antonio, teaching about health-care organization, development, and financing. She also served as a member of the American Nurses' Association Task Force on the Nature and Scope of Nursing and Characteristics of Specialization in Nursing, which produced the ANA Social Policy Statement in 1980.

For her work on the feasibility of home care, in 1959 Phaneuf received the Award for Merit for Research in Medical Care Organization from the Public Health Association of New York City. In 1973 Wayne State University, where she holds professor emeritus status, honored her with the Maria C. Phaneuf Quality Assurance Symposium Series, and in 1977 she received the Award for Distinguished Achievement in Nursing Practice from the Nursing Education Association of Teachers College, Columbia University. In 1987 she was awarded the Marie Hippensteel Lingeman Founders' Award for Excellence in Nursing Practice by Sigma Theta Tau International. She is a fellow in both the American Academy of Nursing and the American Public Health Association.

Until his death in 1990 at the age of 63, Phaneuf maintained a close and loving relationship with her brother. Currently residing in San Diego, California, she is sustained by a faithful reliance on her God. Although the number of activities in which she is involved have decreased, her commitment to nursing remains undiminished. Her apartment home is filled with books, magazines, and journals representing a wide variety of topics, many far removed from the health-care field. She has agreed to place her professional papers in the archives of the Southwest Center for Nursing History, located at the University of Texas at Austin School of Nursing. When asked to reflect on her professional career, Phaneuf commented, "I learned more from the successes than I

did the failures." Phaneuf believes an excerpt from "Ulysses" by Alfred Tennyson best describes her journey through this life.

"I am part of all that I have met,
Yet all experience is an arch where-
thro'
Gleams that untraveled world
whose margins fade
For ever and for ever when I move."

PUBLICATIONS BY
MARIA CELINA PHANEUF

BOOKS

The Nursing Audit: Profile for Excellence. New York: Appleton-Century-Crofts, 1972.

The Nursing Audit: Self Regulation in Nursing Practice, 2nd ed. New York: Appleton-Century-Crofts, 1976.

MONOGRAPHS (SELECTED)

Visiting Nurse Study: Interim Report. New York: Associated Hospital Service of New York, 1955.

Report of a Study Concerning the Feasibility of Providing Visiting Nurse Service Following Hospitalization for Blue Cross Subscribers. New York: Associated Hospital Service of New York, 1957.

Home Care Reports. New York: Associated Hospital Service of New York, 1961, 1962, 1963, 1964.

"Home Nursing Services." In *Textbook for Welfare, Pension Trustees and Administrators,* Vol. V. 9th Annual Conference. Elm Grove, Wis.: National Foundation of Health, Welfare and Pension Plans, 1963.

"Quality Assurance: A Nursing View." In *Quality Assurance of Medical Care.* Conference on Quality Assurance of Medical Care. DHEW Pub. (HSM) 73-7021. Rockville, Md.: U.S. Department of Health, Education and Welfare, Health Services and Mental Health Administration, Regional Medical Programs Service, 1973.

"A Concluding Paper." In *Issues in Evaluation Research.* Pp. 137–48. Kansas City, Mo.: American Nurses' Association, 1976.

With A. Donabedian. "Evaluating the Quality of Medical Care." In *Institute on Planning and Administration of Nursing Service in Medical Care Programs.* Ann Arbor: University of Michigan School of Public Health Continuing Education Service, 1968.

With N.M. Lang. "Issues in Professional Nursing Practice: Standards of Nursing Practice." *ANA Monographs.* Kansas City, Mo.: American Nurses' Association, 1985.

ARTICLES (SELECTED)

"Nursing Services in the Home." *Academy of Medicine of New Jersey Bulletin* 8 (June 1962): 94–99.

"Home Care Following Hospitalization." *Journal of Health and Human Behavior* 4 (Spring 1963): 22–28.

"Quality of Care: Problems of Measurement, Part I: How One Public Health Nursing Agency Is Using the Nursing Audit." *American Journal of Public Health* 59 (October 1969): 1827–32.

"Quality of Care: Problems of Measurement, Part II: Some Issues in Evaluating the Quality of Nursing Care." With Avedis Donabedian. *American Journal of Public Health* 59 (October 1969): 1833–36.

"Consumer Participation in Health Care Planning: Some Reflections." *Michigan Nurse* 46 (January 1973): 8–9.

"Model for Quality: A Matric." *AORN Journal* 23 (April 1976): 759–65.

"Future Directions for Health Care: The Nursing Perspective in Evaluation and Evaluation Research." *Nursing Research* 29 (March–April 1980): 123–26.

"Occupational Health Nursing: A Perspective for 1980." *Occupational Health Nursing* 28 (July 1980): 9–13.

With M. Wandelt. "Three Instruments for Measuring the Quality of Nursing Care." *Hospital Topics* 50 (August 1972): 20–23, 29. Reprinted by National League for Nursing, Pub. 15-611, 1975.

With M. Wandelt. "Quality Assurance in Nursing." *Nursing Forum* 13 (1974): 328–59. Reprinted in *Nursing Digest* 4 (Summer 1976): 32–35.

With M. Wandelt. "Obstacles to and Potentials for Nursing Quality Appraisal." *Quality Review Bulletin* 7 (April 1981): 2–5.

With M. Wandelt. "Three Methods of Process-Oriented Nursing Evaluation." *Quality Review Bulletin* 7 (August 1981): 20–26. Reprinted in *Quality Review Bulletin* Special Edition 1982.

BIBLIOGRAPHY

Founders' Award Nomination. Sigma Theta Tau International, Indianapolis, Indiana, April 1987.

Phaneuf, M.C. Private papers, personal letters to, and conversations with the author, 1980–90.

Alice Redland

Lisbeth D. Price

d. 1891?

Lisbeth D. Price was the author of one of the early textbooks in nursing, advocating more district nursing. She also saw a hierarchical order in the health-care system with physicians at the top, followed by nurses, and then patients. She considered patients inferior to nurses and urged nurses to get help from the patients in cleaning and dusting the wards. Though she urged nurses to achieve the "keenest sympathy for all" patients, she also held that nurses should retain strong self-discipline and always seize the opportunity to "sow seeds of morality" among her patients.

Little is known about Price's personal life. She graduated as a member of the third class of the Philadelphia General Hospital training school in 1888. The school had been established by Alice Fisher, who had been recommended for the post by Florence Nightingale. Price dedicated her book to Alice Fisher "my friend and teacher." She worked in the Philadelphia Hospital and the Medico-Chirugical Hospital of Philadelphia as well as serving as a private-duty nurse. Between 1889 and 1891 Price was manager of the nursing school at Meadville City Hospital in Meadville, Pennsylvania, and it was there that she wrote her book. Though the text was published by a local Meadville publisher, it was distributed by the Lakeside Publishing Company of Buffalo, which also published the journal *Trained Nurse and Hospital Review*, which gave the book national circulation. The magazine promoted Price's book in 1893, but by 1896 it was no longer listed, and no more is known about Price. She had left Meadville in August 1891 because of health problems and went to Providence, Rhode Island, for the sea air. She apparently died there, probably in 1891.

PUBLICATIONS BY LISBETH D. PRICE

Nurses and Nursing. Meadville, Pa.: Flood and Vincent, 1892.

BIBLIOGRAPHY

Flaumenhaft, E., and C. Flaumenhaft. "American Nursing and the Road Not Taken." *Journal of the History of Medicine and Allied Sciences* 44 (1989): 72–89.

Lippman, D.T. *The Evolution of the Nursing Textbook in the United States from 1873 to 1953: A Preliminary Survey.* Ann Arbor, Mich.: University Microfilms, 1980.

Vern L. Bullough

Anne Prochazka

b. 1897

A pioneer in physiotherapy when it was still part of nursing, Anne Prochazka made her reputation as a nurse physiotherapist with the Visiting Nurse Association in Chicago. The handicaps she had to overcome to become a nurse are also indicative of the struggle that many nurses of the past went through to succeed in their chosen profession.

Prochazka was born in Zaluzi in what is now Czechoslovakia in 1897. Her father was a small-town merchant. The family consisted of five children, four girls and a boy (the youngest child). Prochazka's older sister, who had attended the university for two years, went to Oklahoma to work as a governess. When an aunt and uncle decided to go to Oklahoma and buy a farm, they invited one of the older girls to accompany them. When at the last minute she decided to get married instead, Prochazka was invited in her place. She was then 15 years old. After living in Oklahoma for a year, she moved to Cleveland, where she supported herself as a maid.

When her older sister moved to Chicago, Prochazka decided to follow her and enter nurse training. Though she had been in the United States for some four years, she still spoke little English since she had lived in an immigrant community where it was not necessary for her to learn it. When she tried to go into nursing, she found that she had both to speak better English and have a high-school diploma.

To support herself, she became a live-in light housekeeper at fifty cents (later $2) a week, plus her room and board. She was also allowed to go to high school, from which she graduated at age 23. Prochazka then entered the Cook County Hospital Nurses' Training School, from which she received her diploma some three years later. She applied to the Visiting Nurse Association of Chicago for a job and was put on their list but requested to get additional experience first. She then served as a private-duty nurse for a brief time before joining the VNA, starting her career at the age of 27.

Prochazka became interested in the problems of crippled children and received a VNA scholarship to attend an eight-week course in physiotherapy from the Harvard Medical School in 1928. The next year she went back for more training, and when Northwestern University began to offer work in physiotherapy went there as well. She worked with polio victims and became affiliated with programs run by the National Foundation for Infantile Paralysis. Feeling the need to upgrade herself further, she accepted a scholarship from the National Foundation for Infantile Paralysis to take a year's course in public-health nursing at Western Reserve University in Cleveland, where she received her bachelor's degree. She continued to be a visiting nurse in Chicago but as a physiotherapist-orthopedic specialist.

BIBLIOGRAPHY

Yost, E. *American Women of Nursing.* Pp. 135–54. Philadelphia: Lippincott, 1947.

Vern L. Bullough

Elizabeth Mills Reid

1858–1931

Elizabeth Mills Reid was a philanthropist, Red Cross worker and supporter, and a social leader who was primarily interested in hospitals and nursing. She was a leader of international society, possessing initiative, constructive ability, foresight, and a great measure of tact. Whatever captured her interest benefitted immeasurably from her attention, wisdom, and financial generosity. She exhibited throughout her life a sympathy for the poor and the sick of all races and all countries and contributed in many ways toward the alleviation of their suffering.

Reid was born in New York City on January 6, 1858, the only daughter and second child of Darius Ogden Mills and Jane Templeton (Cunningham) Mills. Her mother was the daughter of James Cunningham of Irvington, New York, a prominent shipowner and shipbuilder. Her father was a distinguished capitalist and philanthropist, whose family was of English descent, having emigrated from northern England to America in colonial days and settled in New York City. Reid's father went to California in 1849, where he became part owner and developer of the famous Comstock gold lode. In the next 30 years he built a fortune in mining and banking, organizing the Bank of California, of which he was president for 30 years. Elizabeth and her brother, Ogden, spent their early years in California, in either Sacramento or at their country home in San Mateo. They also spent much time at the Hudson Valley home of their maternal grandparents, for the family frequently traveled east.

Reid's education was initially supervised by governesses and then was continued at Mlle. Vallette's School in Paris and Anna C. Brackett's School in New York City. But perhaps more important to her spirit of philanthropy than formal education were the times in which she grew up and the social position and wealth of her family. Reid was a beautiful child, and she lived her life as a beautiful girl and woman. With her wit and high spirits, she could have easily lived a full life as a social leader. But the assassination of Abraham Lincoln, the bitter and destructive Civil War with its attendant frightfully poor and inadequate care for the sick and wounded, and the lack of adequate medical care for the poor in America left a deep impression on her. She became convinced that something must be done to alleviate

such suffering and that she had the ability, vitality, and courage to bring about changes in these areas.

On April 26, 1881, she married Whitelaw Reid of New York City, editor and chief owner of the *New York Tribune*. He was 20 years her senior. The wealthy and socially prominent Reid, an Ohioan who had been a famous Civil War reporter, had succeeded Horace Greeley as editor of the *Tribune* in 1872. The couple had three children, two of whom survived. The Reids were a very happy couple, supplementing financially and emotionally each other's ambitions and aspirations so that each of them would be able to lead a full and useful life.

Soon after her marriage, Elizabeth Reid became interested in the achievements of Florence Nightingale, who was a pioneer for clean hospitals and for schools to train nurses. Philanthropy soon became the dominating activity of Reid's life, and she was to contribute large sums of money and support actively and personally the institutions to which she contributed.

In 1883, Reid became a member of the board of managers of the Bellevue Training School for nurses, to which board she gave 48 years of service without a break. For ten years she served as vice-president of the board. Even later in life when she was living abroad, she would take a ship to New York to be able to sit with the board when important matters were to be considered. She also helped to ease the plight of the babies of the poor on New York's East Side. She did this through the Sunnyside Day Nursery, of which she became president, and by contributing 1,000 complete sets of garments each year for the babies of the East Side. Also, seeing that blacks in the South had no hospitals to go to and that there were no trained black nurses, Reid established a public hospital for black patients and a training school for black nurses in Charlie Hope, Virginia. In 1886 she established a medical department at the Church of the Incarnation in New York—the first agency of its kind—as a memorial to her mother. Its function was to provide the services of a doctor and nurse to care for the sick in the neighborhood.

Her interest in hospitals and nursing led to her involvement with the American Red Cross, to which organization she contributed great sums of money and her social and political influence until her death. Her first involvement was following the outbreak of the Spanish-American War in 1898, when she became a member of Auxiliary No. 3 (the Red Cross Society for the Maintenance of Trained Nurses), using her expertise and social skills to raise money for the training of nurses. Her group was quite successful at fund raising and under her leadership persuaded President McKinley to accept over 600 of the society's trained nurses for service in military hospitals in the United States, Cuba, and the Philippines.

Nursing service to the armed forces had proven so successful during the Spanish-American War that the establishment of an army nurse corps seemed logical and inevitable, and the women of Auxiliary No. 3 worked to bring it about. Provision for a U.S. Army Nurse Corps was included in the Army Reorganization Bill of 1901.

In 1905 the charter meeting of the New York chapter of the American Red Cross was held at Reid's home. That same year she supported and cooperated with Mabel Boardman in reorganizing the Red Cross following Clara Barton's retirement, and Reid became an active director. In 1912 she contributed generously to help establish the Red Cross Rural Nursing Service, later renamed the Town and Country nursing service, and served as chair of this committee from 1913–15.

The outbreak of World War I absorbed Reid's attention. During the war she served as chair of the American Red Cross in London and deputy commissioner of the Red Cross for Great Britain. She contributed funding to support Paignton House in London for wounded soldiers and converted the American Art Students' Club in Paris, which she had founded while her husband had been minister to France, into a hospital for officers and the American Red Cross headquarters. In France she endowed hospital rooms, outfitted ambulances, and helped organize the American Hospital at Neuilly.

It must be noted that from 1889–92,

Whitelaw Reid served as minister to France and as ambassador to Great Britain from 1905 until his death in 1912. Elizabeth Reid was extremely well received in these countries, and she contributed both money and time to their charitable and social service organizations. She established the Barnesby Boys' and Girls' Club for underprivileged children in London and an institution for British workmen in that city's Islington district. For her many benefactions to France she was awarded the Cross of Chevalier in the Legion of Honor in 1922.

For many years she served on the board of the Mills Training School for Male Nurses in New York. In memory of her father, she built the Mills Memorial Hospital in San Mateo, California, and, with her brother and sister, built St. Luke's Hospital in San Francisco. She contributed funds for the Edward L. Trudeau Sanatorium at Saranac Lake, New York, one of the donors to the D.O. Mills Training School for Nurses and Reid House, a home for nurses.

While traveling in France in 1931, Elizabeth Reid contracted pneumonia. She died at her daughter's villa at St. Jean, Cap Ferrat, near Nice in France on April 29, 1931. A memorial service was held in the American Cathedral of Paris. Her funeral was held at the Cathedral of St. John the Divine in New York, with burial at Sleepy Hollow Cemetery in Tarrytown, New York. As the *New York Times* commented in its editorial of April 30, 1931: "In a day when 'society' had lost its moorings, and even its compass, she carried on the fine old tradition."

Not a single one of the institutions that she founded or worked for was forgotten by Elizabeth Mills Reid. Every one of them, and many more, were remembered in her will, which contained bequests for their support amounting to $750,000.

BIBLIOGRAPHY

Art Treasures and Furnishings of Ophir Hall. New York: Bradford, 1935.

Baehr, H.W., Jr. *The New York Tribune Since the Civil War.* New York: Dodd, Mead, 1936.

Cortissoz, R. *The Life of Whitelaw Reid.* New York: Scribner, 1921.

Dock, L.L., et al. *History of American Red Cross Nursing.* New York: Macmillan, 1922.

Kernodle, P.B. *The Red Cross Nurse in Action, 1882–1948.* New York: Harper, 1949.

McGovern, J.T. *Diogenes Discovers Us.* Pp. 89–102. Freeport, N.Y.: Books for Libraries Press, 1933.

National Cyclopedia of American Biography. Vol. XXII, pp. 2–3. New York: White, 1898–   .

Notable American Women, 1607–1950; A Biographical Dictionary. Vol. 3, pp. 132–33. Cambridge, Mass.: Belknap Press of Harvard University Press, 1971.

Marilyn C. Kihl

Mary Margaret Riddle

1856–1936

Mary Margaret Riddle was a nationally recognized nursing leader and administrator. The significant positions she held in many nursing organizations and her vigorous and long-standing participation helped to shape and elevate the profession.

A descendent of Pennsylvania Dutch stock, Riddle was born on June 6, 1856, on a farm in Turbotville, near Muncy, Pennsylvania, to John Riddle and Elizabeth (Bieber) Riddle. After her mother died when she was a small child, her father, a farmer, moved her and her two older sisters to Constantine, Michigan. There Riddle received her education in the public school, graduated in 1875, and stayed to teach mathematics for 11 years. Her first two years as a teacher were spent in the district school; as was the custom, she "boarded" throughout the school years, spending one week with the family of a school member before moving on to the next. For the following 9 years of her teaching career she held a high-school position. Riddle changed careers in her early thirties and entered the 11-year-old Boston City Hospital Training School for Nurses in Massachusetts on January 1, 1887. The Constantine School Board, so

sure she would drop out and return to teaching, employed a temporary person for four months to fill Riddle's position. Riddle persevered in her desire to be a nurse and graduated from the training school in 1889.

Riddle remained at Boston City Hospital until 1904. She held positions as night superintendent, matron of the convalescent home, matron of the contagious-diseases department, and assistant superintendent of nurses to Lucy Lincoln Drown. While in Boston, Riddle began a lifelong pattern of strong involvement with professional nursing organizations and efforts to promote the advancement of nursing. She served as president of the Boston City Hospital Nurses' Alumnae Association for 15 years beginning in 1897. For the years 1900–04 Riddle commuted to New York City to lecture on hospital administration in the hospital economics course at Teachers College, Columbia University. One of the founders of the Associated Alumnae of Trained Nurses of the United States, forerunner of the American Nurses' Association, Riddle served as president 1902–05. In 1903 she began a fruitful 30-year association with the American Journal of Nursing Company, serving as treasurer until 1932, editor with the Department of Hospital and Training School Administration (1912–19), and as a board member for many years. Her contributions and direction assisted in the development and success of the *American Journal of Nursing.* Riddle also served as editor for *Modern Hospital Magazine* in the Department of Nursing, 1914–16. Riddle assisted in the organization of the Red Cross in Massachusetts and contributed many papers for nursing conventions and professional meetings.

Riddle assumed the position of superintendent of the hospital, training school, and nurses at the Newton Hospital, Newton Lower Falls, Massachusetts, in 1904. During her 17-year tenure her considerable efforts and foresight helped the institution to become an exemplary model. She taught nursing of infectious diseases and offered a short course in psychology and lectures on ethics. Public-health nursing experience was offered to selected students through an arrangement with the Henry Street Settlement and Teachers College in New York City and to others through the Newton District Nursing Association. In the interest of both patients and nurses, the nurses' work day was shortened under her to eight hours. Riddle witnessed the graduation of over 300 nurses from the Newton Hospital Training School during her time there.

Riddle was instrumental in the movement to establish nursing standards by state registration and licensure. She helped form the Massachusetts State Nurses Association and served as the first president, 1903–10, leading the movement toward registration of nurses in her state. Despite bitter opposition and deflating setbacks during those years, a bill was signed into law on April 29, 1910, largely as a result of her efforts. Riddle was the recipient of Massachusetts Registered Nurse License No. 1, issued to her on November 15, 1910. That year she was also elected president of the American Society of Superintendents of Training Schools for Nurses, the forerunner of the National League of Nursing Education. Riddle served as first chairperson of the Massachusetts Board of Registration in Nursing until 1926. She was made an honorary member of the Massachusetts State Nurses Association in 1931 and also served as the second historian. Riddle was treasurer of the Isabel Hampton Robb Memorial Fund (1911–32) and treasurer of the McIssac Loan Fund for Nurses for 15 years.

During World War I Riddle answered the call to nursing leaders to help enroll nurses for war service. She organized 55 nurses for the first Harvard Unit sent overseas in 1915. At age 62, Riddle spent the last six months of 1918 as superintendent of nurses at the Army School of Nursing, Camp Devens. There she helped organize an Army Nurse Corps nurse-induction system.

Riddle retired from the Newton Hospital in 1922 at the age of 65. The Newton nurses presented her with a $1,000 purse, and the Mary M. Riddle Scholar Award was begun. The award was presented annually to the outstanding student of a group of selected students consisting of Mary M. Riddle Scholars until the close of the school on August 5, 1986. Riddle moved back to her hometown but continued to attend every commencement of the Newton Hospital training school until the year of her death. On June 4, 1926, the Massachusetts State Nurses Association honored her with a reception and banquet. During her retirement she wrote a historical sketch of the Boston City Hospital, published in 1928.

Riddle's health declined rapidly after returning from a Florida trip in the spring of 1936. The older sister with whom she lived died also that spring. By summer Riddle suffered from severe facial pain and was hospitalized for an arteriosclerotic condition that resulted first in blindness of her right eye, then total blindness. Riddle died on November 19, 1936, at the age of 80. The following year a memorial service was held for her at Trinity Church, Copley Square, Boston, on May 12, 1937, the date commemorating the birthday of Florence Nightingale.

PUBLICATIONS BY MARY MARGARET RIDDLE

BOOKS

Boston City Hospital Training School for Nurses: Historical Sketch, 1878–1928. Boston: Boston City Hospital Nurses' Alumnae Association, 1928.

ARTICLES (SELECTED)

"The Relations of Training-Schools to Hospital Administration." Read at the International Congress of Nurses, September 1901. *American Journal of Nursing* 2 (May 1902): 576–82.

"Presidential Address." To the Nurses' Associated Alumnae of the United States. *American Journal of Nursing* 3 (August 1903): 838–46.

"Presidential Address." To the Nurses' Associated Alumnae of the United States. *American Journal of Nursing* 4 (July 1904): 753–60.

"The Present Status of Educational Methods." *American Journal of Nursing* 5 (June 1905): 604–10.

"Presidential Address." To the Nurses' Associated Alumnae of the United States." *American Journal of Nursing* 5 (August 1905): 731–36.

"Why We Should Have State Registration for Nurses." *American Journal of Nursing* 7 (January 1907): 240–44.

"Presidential Address." To the American Society of Superintendents of Training Schools for Nurses." *American Journal of Nursing* 12 (December 1911): 180–84.

"Grading of Nurses." In American Hospital Association. *Transactions of the Fifteenth Annual Conference.* Pp. 130–41. Kingston, Ontario: AHA, 1913.

"Hourly Nursing." Read at the Eighteenth Annual Convention of the American Nurses' Association, June 1915. *American Journal of Nursing* 15 (August 1915): 962–68.

"Reminiscences of Early Days of the *American Journal of Nursing.*" *American Journal of Nursing* 25 (October 1925): 838–41.

BIBLIOGRAPHY

Dock, L.L., et al. *History of American Red Cross Nursing.* New York: Macmillan, 1922.

Doona, M.E. "Nursing Revisited: Mary M. Riddle (1856–1936)." *Massachusetts Nurse* 52 (October 1983): 4.

Downes, K.M. *A Tradition of Excellence: A Centennial Review of the Newton-Wellesley Hospital School of Nursing, 1886–1986* (1986). Archives, Paul Talbot Babson Memorial Library, Newton-Wellesley Hospital, Newton, Massachusetts.

Flanagan, L. *One Strong Voice: The Story of the American Nurses' Association.* Kansas City, Mo.: American Nurses' Association, 1976.

"In Memoriam." *American Journal of Nursing* 37 (June 1937): 677.

"Mary M. Riddle: An Appreciation." *Bulletin* (Massachusetts State Nurses Association) 6 (January 1937): 2–3.

"Mary M. Riddle: In Memory." *Trained Nurse and Hospital Review* 98 (June 1937): 617.

"Mary M. Riddle, R.N.: Treasurer American Journal of Nursing Company." *Pacific Coast Journal of Nursing* (June 1915): 258–59.

"Miss Riddle Broadens Her Field of Work." *American Journal of Nursing* 14 (February 1914): 333–34.

Newton Nurses' Alumnae Bulletin 8 (January 1937): 1–6. "Issue dedicated to the memory of Mary M. Riddle." Contains multiple short essays outlining contributions and offering reminiscences of Riddle.

"Nurses of Note." *British Journal of Nursing* 52 (January 31, 1914): 83.

Obituary. *American Journal of Nursing* 37 (January 1937): 112–13.

Riddle, M.M. Papers. Nursing Archives, Boston University, Mugar Memorial Library, Boston.

Watson, S.A. "Mary M. Riddle." *Newton Nurses' Alumnae Bulletin* 8 (January 1937): 2–3.

"Who's Who in the Nursing World: Mary M. Riddle." *American Journal of Nursing* 21 (June 1921): 619.

Sharon Murphy

Alice M. Robinson

1920–1983

Alice M. Robinson was a leader in psychiatric nursing, a nurse author, and an editor.

Born December 4, 1920, in Islip, New York, Robinson was the daughter of William Beverly Robinson and Le Van (Cowell) Robinson. She graduated from the Duke University School of Nursing in Durham, North Carolina, in 1944. Upon receipt of a diploma in nursing, Robinson enlisted in the Army Nurse Corps, serving as a staff nurse. Following her separation from service, she took a position as a coordinator of psychiatric nursing at George Washington University Hospital in Washington, D.C. In that position she was responsible for the organization and supervision of a psychiatric-neurosurgical unit in what was then a new hospital. While employed there, she completed a baccalaureate in nursing at Catholic University of America.

Having completed her degree, Robinson entered the VA Hospital system, accepting a supervisory position in psychiatric nursing in Little Rock, Arkansas. A year later she accepted the director of nursing service and education position at the Menninger Foundation, Topeka, Kansas. Following this experience, the opportunity for a teaching fellowship in psychiatric-nursing education at Boston University School of Nursing presented itself. She accepted the post, remaining there for two years, during which time she earned a master of science degree in nursing education.

Following the completion of graduate study in 1950, Robinson became the director of nursing and nursing education at Boston State Hospital, Dorchester, Massachusetts. This was an extremely challenging experience in that she was responsible for the nursing care of 3,000 psychiatric patients. She supervised more than 600 nursing personnel and assisted with the in-service education programs for all staff. At the time of her tenure, the hospital provided clinical experience for nursing students. Robinson assumed responsibility for the clinical rotation of approximately 250 students each year.

Always looking for a new challenge, in 1956 Robinson accepted the position of director of nursing education at Vermont State Hospital in Waterbury. In that role she was responsible for the in-service education program for all nursing personnel. It was through her efforts that the affiliate program in psychiatric-nursing education for diploma and associate-degree programs in the state was established.

Her editorial career began in 1963 when she became the associate editor of *Nursing Outlook*. In 1966 she became senior editor and in 1967 editor-in-chief, a position she held until October 1970. Feeling the need for change, she left *Nursing Outlook* to accept the post of senior nursing editor of *RN* magazine. She remained there until 1975.

A gifted writer and teacher, Robinson decided to try her entrepreneurial skills and established her own business. Her enterprise was known as Specialized Consultants in Nursing. The company provided educational programs in nursing administration, psychiatric nursing, clinical writing, communication skills, and human relations. Among the most popular of her offerings were her courses in clinical professional writing. Many nurses published following her expert teaching. Her background in editing, psychiatric nursing, nursing administration, teaching, and writing served as an invaluable tool for her in the conduct of nursing management and writing courses, as well as clinical nursing workshops. She remained active in her business until her death on March 18, 1983.

Robinson was a prolific writer. She contributed heavily to the nursing litera-ture during her professional career. She published numerous articles, was a contributing author, and authored or co-authored five books. She was called upon frequently as a speaker and workshop leader. Robinson's contributions as a spokesperson, editor, and writer have provided a rich legacy for nursing.

PUBLICATIONS BY ALICE M. ROBINSON

BOOKS

The Psychiatric Aide. Philadelphia: Lippincott, 1954.

The Unbelonging. New York: Macmillan, 1958.

Working with the Mentally Ill. Philadelphia: Lippincott, 1971. Also published in Swedish and Finnish.

With L.E. Notter. *Clinical Writing for Health Professionals.* Bowie, Md.: Brady, 1982.

With M.E. Reres. *Your Future in Nursing Careers.* New York: Rosen, 1972.

ARTICLES (SELECTED)

"The R.N.: Without Her, No ICUs." *RN* 35 (March 1972): 46–51.

"Ongoing Inservice Programs Are a Must." *RN* 35 (July 1972): 50–56.

"Men in Nursing. Their Career Goals and Image Are Changing." *RN* 36 (August 1973): 36–41.

"Problem-oriented Record: Uniting the Team for Total Care." *RN* 38 (June 1975): 23–28.

"Making a Career Choice: Think Twice." *Imprint* 22 (October 1975): 24–26.

"Want to Get Your Message Across? Write About It!" *Imprint* 23 (October 1976): 45.

BIBLIOGRAPHY

Dictionary of American Nursing Biography. M. Kaufman, ed. Westport, Conn.: Greenwood, 1988.

"In the Tradition of Excellence." *Nursing Outlook* 30 (May 1982): 291.

Memorabilia of Alice M. Robinson in the custody of Mary Ann Tuft, Chicago, 1989.

"New Chief Editor named for Nursing Outlook." *American Journal of Nursing* 67 (January 1967): 47.

Robert V. Piemonte

Martha E. Rogers

b. 1914

Nationally renowned nurse theoretician, educator, author, lecturer, and consultant, Martha Elizabeth Rogers has contributed original theoretical concepts and been a strong force in American nursing throughout a career that spans more than 50 years.

Rogers was born in Dallas, Texas, on May 12, 1914, the eldest of the four children of Bruce Taylor Rogers and Lucy Mulholland Keener Rogers. Her father was employed in the insurance business, and the family heritage included a number of relatives who were active women suffragists. A strong family conviction about the value of a college education and an interest in social welfare were early influences which affected Martha's educational pursuits. An educational trust established by an uncle for his grandnieces and grandnephews assisted Martha and her siblings in obtaining a post-secondary school education.

Rogers attended the University of Knoxville (Tennessee) from 1931–33, where she studied the sciences while considering what specific area of study to select as a major. Medicine or law were alternative careers that were under consideration during that period. When a friend decided to attend the local hospital school of nursing in Knoxville, Rogers also applied to the Knoxville General Hospital School of Nursing and was accepted. She graduated from the diploma program in 1936 and obtained her B.S.N. in public-health nursing from George Peabody College, Nashville, in 1937. Her first job was as a rural public-health nurse for the Children's Fund of Michigan, Clare, from 1937–39. During the years 1940–45 she held various positions with the Visiting Nurses Association in Hartford, Connecticut, where she was successively promoted from staff member to assistant supervisor, then to a position as assistant education director, and finally to acting education director.

In 1945 she received an M.A. in public-health nursing supervision, from Teachers College, Columbia University. She subsequently relocated to Phoenix, Arizona, where she held the position of executive director of the Visiting Nurses Association from 1945–51.

She was a visiting lecturer at Catholic University of America, Washington, D.C., for 1951–52 and obtained an M.P.H. from Johns Hopkins University in 1952.

In 1953 she was a research associate at Johns Hopkins and obtained her Sc.D. from that institution in 1954. Her doctoral thesis examined the association of prenatal maternal and fetal factors with later development of childhood behavior problems.

From 1954 until 1975 she was professor and head of the Division of Nurse Education, New York University. Following her retirement in 1975, she has continued to teach at New York University and is professor emeritus there.

Martha Rogers has contributed a large body of theoretical concepts to the expanding body of nursing-science literature. Additionally, she frequently has expounded on the need to forego what she identifies as anti-educational archaisms found in nursing education. As the author of numerous journal articles and papers delivered at professional meetings, presented in forthright language, she consistently urged nursing educators and researchers to focus their attention on such issues as the need to professionalize nursing through emphasis on the formulation and implementation of baccalaureate and higher degree education curricula in nursing, the need to elaborate the scientific basis of nursing practice as a basis of professional education, and differentiation of professional and technical careers in nursing. As editor of the *Journal of Nursing Science* for the years 1963–65, when the journal ceased publication, Rogers's editorials unceasingly focused attention on these issues, and she continues to contribute actively in this arena as lecturer, author, and consultant.

The theoretical framework that she developed and that is expounded in her books, journal articles, and papers encompasses a complex interrelated conceptual knowledge base. Often shorthandedly referred to as the "Science of Unitary Human Beings," or more encompassing as "Rogerian Science," Rogers' attempts to look at synergistic man within an organized conceptual system and parallels some of the concepts found in general system theory. Since its original publication in 1970, this nursing theory, based on Martha Rogers's synthesis of her knowledge of anthropology, sociology, astronomy, philosophy, mythology, history, and religion, has been a controversial issue in nursing.

Rogers has been an energetic leader and consultant in many professional organizations and has received numerous awards and honors in recognition of her contributions to nursing. She served as consultant to the U.S. surgeon general and the U.S. Air Force from 1969–73. She is a past president of the New York State League for Nursing, and is a member of the National League for Nursing and the American Nurses' Association, where she has served on a variety of committees. Additionally, she has been a member and president of the Society for the Advancement in Nursing, the American Association for Higher Education, the American Association of University Professors, Sigma Theta Tau, Kappa Delta Phi and is a fellow of the American Academy of Nursing. She holds numerous honorary degrees from educational institutions in the United States and is a recipient of many awards and honors, such as the Mary Tolle Wright Leadership Award; an award and citation from Chi Eta Phi Sorority, Omicron Chapter (1960) for Inspiring Leadership in the Field of Intergroup Relation; and an award and citation from New York University, Division of Nurse Education, faculty and alumni (1965), in recognition of her outstanding contributions to nursing.

She continues to sound a reveille in both nursing education and practice by elucidating a visionary view of today's so-called crisis in nursing as an opportunity for further evolution of the profession of nursing if nurses are willing to seize the day.

PUBLICATIONS BY MARTHA E. ROGERS

BOOKS

Educational Revolution in Nursing. New York: Macmillan, 1961.

Reveille in Nursing. Philadelphia: Davis, 1964.

An Introduction to the Theoretical Basis of Nursing. Philadelphia: Davis, 1970.

ARTICLES

"Responses to Talks on Menstrual Health." *Nursing Outlook* 1 (May 1953): 272–74.

"The Association of Maternal and Fetal Factors with the Development of Behavior Problems among the Elementary School Children." D.Sc. dissertation, Johns Hopkins University, Baltimore, 1954.

"Viewpoints—Critical Areas for Nursing Education in Baccalaureate and Higher Degree Programs." An address given at the meeting of the Council Member Agencies of the Department of Baccalaureate and Higher Degree Programs, Williamsburg, Virginia, March 26, 1962.

"Some Comments on the Theoretical Basis of Nursing Practice." *Nursing Science* (April 1963): 11–13, 60–61.

"Nursing: A Science of Unitary Man." In *Conceptual Models for Nursing Practice*, 2nd ed., J.P. and R.C. Riehl, eds. Pp. 329–37. New York: Appleton-Century-Crofts, 1980.

"Beyond the Horizon." In *The Nursing Profession: A Time to Speak.* N.L. Chaska, ed. New York: McGraw-Hill, 1983.

"Science of Unitary Human Beings: A Paradigm for Nursing." A paper presented at the International Nurse Theorist Conference, Edmonton, Alberta, May 2, 1984.

"The Nature and Characteristics of Professional Education for Nursing . . . (Classics from Our Heritage)." *Journal of Professional Nursing* 1 (November–December 1985): 381–83.

"High Touch in a High-Tech Future." *NLN Publication* 41-1985 (1985): 25–31.

"Nursing Science and Art: A Prospective." *Nursing Science Quarterly* 1 (August 1988): 99–102.

"Creating a Climate for the Implementation of a Nursing Conceptual Framework." *Journal of Continuing Education in Nursing* 20 (May–June 1989): 112–16.

"Visions of Rogers Science-based Nursing. A Conversation with Martha Rogers on Nursing in Space." NLN Publication 15-2285. Pp. 375–86. New York: National League for Nursing, 1990.

"Visions of Rogers Science-Based Nursing. Nursing: Science of Unitary, Irreducible, Human Beings: Update 1990." NLN Publication 15-2285. Pp. 5–11. New York: National League for Nursing, 1990.

With A.M. Lilienfeld and B. Pasamanick. "Prenatal and Paranatal Factors in the Development of Childhood Behavior Disorders. *Acta Psychiatrica et Neurologica Scandinavica* Suppl. 102 (1955).

BIBLIOGRAPHY

George, J.B. *Nursing Theories: The Base for Professional Nursing Practice*, 3rd ed. Pp. 211–30. Norwalk, Conn.: Appleton & Lange, 1990.

Hektor, L.M. "Martha E. Rogers: A Life History." *Nursing Science Quarterly* 2 (Summer 1989): 63–73.

Malinski, V. *Explorations on Martha Rogers' Science of Unitary Human Beings*. Norwalk, Conn.: Appleton-Century-Crofts, 1986.

Parse, R.R. "Martha E. Rogers: A Birthday Celebration." editorial, *Nursing Science Quarterly* 2 (Summer 1989): 55.

Safier, G. *Contemporary American Leaders in Nursing: An Oral History*. Chap. 14. New York: McGraw-Hill, 1977.

Sanford, R. "The SAIN Alternative: An Interview with Martha Rogers." *Journal of Nursing Care* 11 (July 1978): 20–23.

Sarter, B. *The Steam of Becoming: A Study of Martha Rogers' Theory*. NLN Publication 15-2205. New York: National League for Nursing, 1988.

Society of Nursing Professionals. *Who's Who in American Nursing*. Society of Nursing Professionals, 1984.

Karen L. Buchinger

Hannah Anderson (Chandler) Ropes

1809–1863

An articulate New England reformer before the Civil War, Hannah Ropes served as matron of the Union Hotel Hospital in Georgetown, D.C., during the war. She used her prominent social position and acquaintance with political leaders to induce improvements in the care of wounded soldiers. She felt that nurses empathized with the soldiers' suffering, whereas physicians tended to view them more as "cases." She promoted the philosophy that nurturing and compassion are as important as scientific procedures in professional nursing.

Ropes' bold example gave other women courage in their efforts to make a difference in a male-dominated society. Her recently published diary and letters have enhanced public understanding of the conditions Civil War soldiers faced and the role of nursing in a wartime society.

The seventh of 10 children, Hannah Anderson Chandler was born to Peleg and Esther Parsons Chandler in New Gloucester, Maine, on June 13, 1809. Her father was a prominent lawyer. An older brother, Theophilus Parsons Chandler, became assistant U.S. treasurer for Boston, and a younger brother, Peleg, was a leading Boston lawyer and politician.

There is no record of her early education, but it appears likely that she attended public schools. The home environment fostered learning through frequent family discussions about social issues.

She married an educator and farmer, William Henry Ropes, in Bangor, Maine, in February 1834. He held a number of posts in teaching and school administration, and they settled eventually in Waltham, Massachusetts. Of their four children, only Edward, born in 1837, and Alice, born in 1841, survived to adulthood. Overworked and beset by health problems, William moved to Florida sometime after 1847 and never returned. Hannah Ropes filed for divorce in later years, and he died in 1864.

Ropes became interested in abolition and the free-soil movement and in 1855 moved with her daughter Alice to Leavenworth, Kansas, where Edward, only 18, had taken a homestead. During their brief stay there, Ropes did private-duty nursing and began to see nursing in the context of political struggle. Devoted to the ideals of motherhood, she felt that the most effective nurses were, in part, surrogate mothers.

Fearing for their personal safety amid the growing turmoil on the frontier, she and Alice returned to the East in April 1856 and settled in Massachusetts. Ropes nursed sick friends, but her main interest was social issues. Her activities brought her the friendship of leaders such as Congressman and General Nathaniel P. Banks and Senator Charles Summer. She also wrote a novel, *Cranston House*, and a book of memoirs, *Six Months in Kansas, by a Lady*.

When a nephew, Charles Peleg Chandler, sent her a copy of Florence Nightingale's *Notes on Nursing: What It Is and What It Is Not,* Ropes felt an immediate empathy with Nightingale's ideals. Nightingale's example, plus the desire to serve Edward if he were to be a soldier and be wounded, moved Ropes to volunteer as a nurse when the war broke out.

She was appointed matron of the Union Hotel Hospital in Washington, D.C., in July 1862. There she found unsanitary conditions, with latrines next to the kitchen, no morgue, and poor ventilation. Calling the hospital, "a perfect pestilence box," she went directly to Secretary of War Edwin M. Stanton, who had it inspected and improved and delinquent administrators removed. This was the first of many such encounters by which Ropes sought to improve the lot of both the enlisted men and the nurses who served them.

Her own first nursing case at the hospital was General Henry Wilson, a former Massachusetts senator, who had collapsed at the entrance of the hospital. On her staff was Louisa Alcott, who had taken time out from full-time writing to work there. Following the arrival of wounded from the Battle of Fredericksburg, Alcott wrote of her: "The hall was full of these wrecks of humanity, . . . and in the midst of it all, the matron's motherly face brought more comfort to many a poor soul than the cordial draughts she administered, or the cheery words that welcomed all, making of the hospital a home." Alcott's references to Ropes have been instrumental in keeping Ropes's memory alive.

During this time Ropes kept a diary and wrote many letters, apparently intending to publish them. However, she contracted typhoid pneumonia in December 1862, and, in a letter to Edward dated January 9, 1863, observed: "I have been sick. . . . I am doing my last work now." She died on January 20 and was buried near her father in the cemetery in New Gloucester, Maine. In her mother's spirit, Alice became a teacher of emancipated slaves in New Bern, North Carolina. Edward continued as a private in the Union Army until the end of the war.

Ropes's diaries and letters remained in private possession until 1957, when they began arriving in the Special Collections Division of the University of California at Riverside. Edited and published in 1980, they depict many of the leaders of the time from a personal perspective. For example, while Secretary of War Stanton had a reputation for being gruff and distant, Ropes saw him as caring deeply for the suffering of his men.

Hannah Ropes's writings provide new insights, not only into the human side of the Civil War, but also the emergence of nursing as a profession that plays a vital role in the welfare of human society.

PUBLICATIONS BY HANNAH ANDERSON (CHANDLER) ROPES

BOOKS

Six Months in Kansas, by a Lady. Boston: Jewett, 1856.

Cranston House, a Novel. Boston: Clapp, 1859.

Civil War Nurse, The Diary and Letters of Hannah Ropes. J.R. Brumgardt, ed. Knoxville: University of Tennessee Press, 1980.

BIBLIOGRAPHY

Alcott, Louisa. *Hospital Sketches and Camp and Fireside Stories.* Boston: Roberts, 1869.

Alice P. Stein

Martha Montague Russell
1867–1961

Nurse administrator and Red Cross nurse in France during World War I, Martha Montague Russell was awarded the Florence Nightingale Medal for distinguished service.

Russell was born on September 18, 1867, in Pittsfield, Massachusetts, to John Wiley and Mary (Montague) Russell. She spent her childhood in Sunderland, Massachusetts, graduated from Amherst High School, and attended Mt. Holyoke College, 1887–89. She entered the New York Hospital School of Nursing in 1892, receiving her diploma two years later.

Russell served as assistant superintendent at the Providence Lying-In Hospital (Rhode Island), 1897–1900; as director of nursing at West Penn Hospital, Pittsburgh, Pennsylvania, 1901–03; and as superintendent of nursing at Sloane Hospital, 1904–17. In July 1917 she was sent overseas as the first representative of the Red Cross Nursing Service to France, where she organized the nursing activities that would care for almost 3 million soldiers. One of her first actions was to distribute winter equipment to the lightly clad nurses of the base hospitals. She also organized a local committee to enroll American nurses overseas into the American Red Cross Nursing Service.

Discouraged by organizational difficulties and in almost complete physical exhaustion, she returned to the United States in 1918. She was awarded the Florence Nightingale Medal for distinguished service during the war, an honor bestowed annually only upon one nurse of any nation.

After her return she accepted the position of superintendent of the School of Nursing at the University of Colorado, a post she held until 1926 when she moved back East. Until her retirement, she served in various nursing positions in West Virginia, New Jersey, and New York City.

Russell was elected to a number of offices, including secretary and director of the National League of Nursing Education. She was also the author of several papers on nursing topics.

Russell retired in 1940 but returned later to duty at the Providence Hospital. She spent the last ten years of her life in Florida and died on July 16, 1961, in Front Royal, Virginia.

PUBLICATIONS BY MARTHA MONTAGUE RUSSELL

"Club-Houses, Hostelries, and Directories for Nurses." *American Journal of Nursing* 5 (August 1905): 802–07.

"Hospital Furnishings." *American Journal of Nursing* 26 (November 1926): 841–46.

"Report of the Committee on Health Insurance." *American Journal of Nursing* 17 (July 1917): 864–66.

"Training for Obstetrical Nursing." In *Annual Report*, 1909, and *Proceedings of the 15th Convention Including Report of Second Meeting of American Federation of Nurses.* Baltimore, 1910.

"What Social Insurance Will Mean to Nurses." *American Journal of Nursing* 17 (February 1917): 388–93.

BIBLIOGRAPHY

Archives, American Red Cross, Washington, D.C.

College History and Archives. Mount Holyoke College, Williston Memorial Library, South Hadley, Massachusetts.

Daughters of the American Revolution Magazine (November 1921): 644–45.

Dock, L.L., et al. *History of American Red Cross Nursing.* New York: Macmillan, 1922.

Kernodle, P.B. *The Red Cross Nurse in Action 1882–1948.* New York: Harper, 1949.

One Hundred Year Biographical Directory of Mount Holyoke College 1817–1937. South Hadley, Mass.: Alumni Association of Mount Holyoke College, 1937.

Russell, Martha Montague. Correspondence. Nutting Collection, Columbia University, New York.

"Who's Who in the Nursing World." *American Journal of Nursing* 23 (1923): 938.

Lilli Sentz

Katharine Anne Alexis Sanborn
1859–1941

A leader in nursing education, Katharine Anne Alexis Sanborn organized the St. Vincent's Hospital Training School for Nurses, New York City, in 1892 and served as superintendent for 42 years (1892–34). Under her skilled direction the school achieved accreditation by the Board of Regents of the University of the State of New York, one of the earliest to be so recognized. Sanborn's work was often acknowledged in reports of the New York State Department of Education. As a vital member of several instrumental nursing organizations, her contributions helped advance pioneering efforts toward the professionalization of nursing.

Sanborn was born on October 16, 1859, in Sharon, Vermont, the daughter of Ebenezer Sanborn and Clara Gould (Stevens) (Nute) Sanborn. Her father's occupation has been listed as both mechanical engineer and farmer. Sanborn had an older brother, Edward, and a younger brother, William. She also had a stepsister, Clara, and a step-brother, John, the children from her mother's previous marriage. The family moved to South Berwick, Maine, shortly after Sanborn was born. Her father died there in 1863, leaving a young family. Sanborn's mother then relocated the family to Boston, where her sister, Kate Stevens, joined them. Sanborn was greatly influenced toward Catholicism and nursing by her aunt, who was a nurse. Sanborn attended Villa Anna Academy in Rachine, Quebec, and the Convent of Our Lady of Mercy in Newburgh, New York. She contracted typhoid fever but recovered completely. The family moved to Jersey City, New Jersey, where she pursued her studies in music and the German and French languages. She played the organ and taught music in Jersey City and New York for five years. She also served as a companion to her stepsister. At this time she resided in Nyack, New York.

In 1888, at the age of 28, Sanborn enrolled in the New York Hospital Training School for Nurses, New York City, which was under the direction of Irene Sutliffe, superintendent of nurses. After graduating in 1890, Sanborn performed one year of private-duty nursing. She then accepted the position of matron and head nurse of the Country Branch of the Skin and Cancer Hospital, overlooking the Hudson River on Fordham Heights, in New York City. In May 1892, Sanborn, who had been highly recommended by Sutliffe, was asked to become director of nurses and establish a training school at St. Vincent's Hospital. The Sisters of Charity had carried total responsibility for the provision of nursing care since the hospital's opening in 1849. An attempt had been made to organize a training school by a graduate nurse from Bellevue but failed. Sanborn, who described herself as an "organizer," was only two years out of train-

ing school when offered the opportunity, but she took up the challenge. She came to St. Vincent's Hospital in July 1892, and she proved to be the capable and competent organizer that was needed. The following year she declined the position of head of nurses at the Sloane Maternity Hospital in New York City, choosing instead to immerse herself in her role as educator at St. Vincent's. It was to become her life's work. On October 15, 1892, the St. Vincent's Hospital Training School for Nurses opened under Sanborn's direction. The first class completed training in October 1894 and commencement exercises were held May 9, 1895, at the Chamber Music Hall of Carnegie Institute. Sanborn was eventually to see 1,063 nurses graduate during her long and remarkable tenure with the school. Among them was her niece Kathryn Walsh Sanborn, a graduate of the class of 1929.

Sanborn worked diligently throughout her career to develop and refine the educational component of the training school. Upon her arrival she began planning to institute an organized plan of instruction. Initially, Sanborn instructed students at the bedside, as did the hospital physicians and the ward sisters. By the next year, 1893, Sanborn had arranged with the attending physicians to provide lecture courses to the nurses in surgical nursing, general medicine, and gynecology. Sanborn recognized early on that her students needed educational experiences not readily available at St. Vincent's Hospital. Therefore, she arranged numerous affiliations to provide experiences in obstetrical nursing, invalid cooking, and pediatric nursing. Later, an affiliation with the Henry Street Settlement House and Teachers College at Columbia University provided public-health nursing experience.

In September 1898, during the Spanish-American War, Sanborn traveled to Camp Black in Long Island for two weeks to care for army recruits stricken by a raging typhoid epidemic. She supervised the removal of the patients to various hospitals when the camp was dispersed.

The training school at St. Vincent's offered a two-year course until September

1902, when it was lengthened to three years. That same year Sanborn succeeded in having a separate residence built for the nurses. In January 1905 the school received its certification of registration from the Board of Regents of the University of the State of New York. Sanborn now required her applicants to have at least one year of high school or the equivalent. The number of hours worked by a student was reduced from 12 hours to 9½ hours per day. When the Committee on Education of the National League of Nursing Education set forth *The Standard Curriculum for Schools of Nursing* in 1917, Sanborn quickly adopted the proposals and revised the curriculum. By 1926 the Committee on the Grading of Nursing Schools had begun its work. The training school at St. Vincent's Hospital was among the nation's state-approved schools to participate. Meanwhile, Sanborn managed to continue her own education. She took courses in hospital and training school administration and in teaching at Teachers College, Columbia University. She subscribed to the *American Journal of Nursing* from its first issue in 1900. Throughout her career she proved herself to be receptive to change and was progressive in her vision of nursing.

Memberships in professional nursing organizations were of prime importance to Sanborn. She maintained a high degree of involvement and held several offices. She attended the first convention of the American Society of Superintendents of Training Schools for Nurses, which was held in New York City in January 1894. She enrolled as a member at that time, and at the sixth annual convention, in May 1899, she presented a paper on the care of patients with infectious diseases at the Willard and Minturn hospitals. She remained active in this organization, which was the forerunner of the National League of Nursing Education, for the rest of her professional life. She was also a member of the Nurses Associated Alumnae of the United States from its inception until her death. In 1902 Sanborn was elected first vice-president of the Alumnae Association of the New York Hospital Training School for Nurses. She was a vigorous participant in the Alumnae Association of St. Vincent's Hospital Training School for Nurses from its organization in 1897. On October 25, 1917, as a measure of the members' esteem, the association presented her with a gift of $1,057.28 on the twenty-fifth anniversary of her position as superintendent. On December 6, 1923, Sanborn was made an honorary member.

Sanborn retired on September 1, 1934, at the age of 74. Her successor was Sister Mary Ursula, one of her students and a graduate of St. Vincent's and of Teachers College. The Alumnae Association of St. Vincent's Training School for Nurses, on the event of her retirement, established the Katharine A. Sanborn Scholarship Fund for advanced study to be given annually to a graduate of the School. The initial amount of the award was $600. The scholarship is still awarded annually, but, the usual amount now is $2,000.

Sanborn resided at the nurses' residence connected with the school until her death. On May 7, 1937, Sanborn was forced to decline an invitation to the celebration of the sixtieth anniversary of the founding of the New York Hospital School of Nursing, her alma mater, due to a persistent attack of sciatica, which fatigued her greatly. She died on Sunday, February 23, 1941, at St. Vincent's Hospital at the age of 81. Had she lived another year, she would have witnessed the celebration of the golden anniversary of the School of Nursing at St. Vincent's Hospital.

Sanborn kept many handwritten records and was a faithful letter writer. During World War I she corresponded with many of her former students. The unique role she played in their lives and the meaning that they brought to her life may be gleaned from 52 letters she received during the war and saved. Those letters documented her correspondents' adventures and fears and illuminated their special link to her. Now preserved as part of the archives of St. Vincent's Hospital, they serve as testimony to Sanborn as mentor and friend and allude to her qualities of compassion and leadership.

BIBLIOGRAPHY

Baer, E.D. "Letters to Miss Sanborn: St. Vincent's Hospital Nurses' Accounts of World War I." *Journal of Nursing History* 2 (April 1987): 17–32.

Byrne, M.L. "A History of St. Vincent's Hospital School of Nursing." Master's thesis, Catholic University of America, 1941. Microfiche.

Hodson, J., ed. *How to Become a Trained Nurse.* New York: Abbatt, 1898.

"Katharine A. Sanborn." Obituary. *American Journal of Nursing* 41 (April 1941): 509.

"Katharine A. Sanborn." Obituary. *New York Times*, February 25, 1941.

"Katharine A. Sanborn Retires." *American Journal of Nursing* 34 (November 1934): 1065.

"Miss Sanborn of St. Vincent's Hospital, New York, Dies." Obituary. *Trained Nurse and Hospital Review* (April 1941): 284.

Nagle, M.R. "Life of Katharine Sanborn." Teachers College, Columbia University, New York, May 1967. Photocopy.

Sanborn, K. Papers. Archives, St. Vincent's Hospital School of Nursing, New York.

Sanborn, V.C. *Genealogy of the Family of Sanborne or Sanborn in England and America 1194–1898.* Concord, N.H.: Rumford Press, 1899.

Walsh, M. *With a Great Heart: The Story of St. Vincent's Hospital and Medical Center of New York 1849–1964.* New York: St. Vincent's Hospital and Medical Center of New York, 1965.

Sharon Murphy

Marjorie E. Sanderson

b. 1911

Marjorie E. Sanderson made numerous contributions to nursing education during a career that spanned over 50 years. During those years she helped develop and/or administered at least 11 nursing programs in seven states during their formative years.

Sanderson was born on July 5, 1911, in Cedarville, Ohio. Her father, William John Sanderson, was a minister, and her mother, Anna Mary (Adams) Sanderson, was a teacher and homemaker. She was the second of three children; her sister Esther was two years older and brother W. Kenneth was five years younger than she. Sanderson spent her childhood in Ohio and graduated from high school in Belle Center in 1927.

In 1932 she received a diploma in nursing from the Grant Hospital School of Nursing, Columbus, Ohio. She earned a bachelor of science degree in nursing education from Ohio State University in 1937 and a master of arts degree in nursing administration from Teachers College, Columbia University, New York, in 1943. In 1961, at the conclusion of her doctoral education at Teachers College, she was certified in both educational and agency administration and received a doctor of education degree. Her formal education in nursing was not terminated after receiving her doctorate. Between 1975 and 1977 she earned graduate credits in psychiatric nursing at the University of South Carolina and in 1986 completed one year of course work toward a master's degree in family counseling at the Reformed Theological Seminary, Jackson, Mississippi.

Although little is known about Sanderson's early years of practice as a professional nurse, she held numerous positions as a nurse educator after earning her bachelor's degree. Beginning in 1937, she served as educational director and an instructor of fundamentals of nursing and other clinical nursing courses at Bethany Hospital, Kansas City, Missouri for six years. Then, in 1943 she moved to Detroit, where she was educational director and instructor at the Henry Ford Hospital for two years. Sanderson returned to Kansas City and Bethany Hospital to become director of the School of Nursing and Nursing Service with a primary focus on nursing-service administration in 1945. She served on the Kansas State Board for Nursing as a member and officer from 1943 to 1948.

In 1948 Sanderson returned to her home state of Ohio, where she stayed until 1961. During this period she served as director of the School of Nursing, a diploma program, at the Miami Valley Hospital in Dayton and also as director of nursing service. In 1950 she collaborated with the local vocational-technical school to establish the first practical nursing program in Dayton. For four years (1952–56) she was a member of the Ohio State Board of Nursing.

After leaving Ohio, Sanderson moved to Baltimore and became assistant administrator for patient care and director of nursing services at University Hospital for 1961–64. Here she was influential in implementing experimental staffing patterns in the hospital, participated in and wrote the report for the Task Force on Nursing Services and Needs in Maryland, and lectured in the nursing administration graduate program at the University of Maryland School of Nursing. In 1964 she left the hospital to become associate professor and associate dean of the baccalaureate program at the School of Nursing, University of Maryland. She also held the position of director of the Walter Reed Army Institute of Nursing at the university concurrently with her other positions.

In 1968 she moved on to become director of the graduate program in nursing at the College of Nursing, Medical College of Georgia, Augusta. During her year in Georgia she developed and implemented the college's first graduate program in nursing and served as a consultant to develop an associate-degree program at Georgia State College, Atlanta.

Sanderson spent eight years at the University of South Carolina beginning in 1969. The first four years she was dean of the College of Nursing and the last four was professor of nursing administration and curriculum development. She developed and established the first graduate program in nursing in South Carolina at the university, and she implemented regional campus programs to facilitate the education of associate-degree and RN students in addition to serving on several state committee's for educational planning.

From 1977–80 she was professor and chair of the Department of Nursing at York College of Pennsylvania, York, where she guided the development of the baccalaureate program and a learning center for nursing students. She also consulted with Mercer College in Dayton, Ohio, in 1979 to assist in the establishment of a baccalaureate program. For one year, in 1980, she was professor in charge of continuing education at the Pennsylvania State University. Her final position was that of associate dean for nursing, the only position of its kind on campus, at East Stroudsburg State University, Pennsylvania; before her retirement in 1982, she assisted that program in obtaining initial National League for Nursing accreditation.

Few of her research studies were published. Sanderson did conduct eight unpublished studies on topics relevant to both educational and nursing-service administration, including a survey of faculty attitudes; assessment of educational programs; a community survey of needs; administration of in-service education programs; a historical review of administration; an analysis of charge nurse activities; planning, implementing, and evaluating an intensive-care unit; and nurses' attitudes toward using disposable syringes.

Involvement in professional organizations was a major part of Sanderson's life. She became a member of the American Nurses' Association in 1933 and held positions at all levels of the organization—local, state, and national. In 1964 she was on the ballot for treasurer of the national organization but, unfortunately, was defeated in that election. She was also an active member in the National League for Nursing, Sigma Theta Tau, and the American Association for Higher Education.

Sanderson also made ongoing contributions through community service and church organizations by volunteering for special projects and by serving on numerous committees and boards of directors.

Finally, Sanderson made sure that future students in nursing would be recognized. In 1979 she established and endowed the Anna M. Sanderson Award in honor of her mother at York College of Pennsylvania. This award recognized superior clinical competence of a sophomore nursing student and was later amended to recognize outstanding achievement of a junior nursing student in long-term care in the program at York College. At East Stroudsburg she established a monetary award, the Dr. Marjorie E. Sanderson Award, to recognize outstanding writing ability by a nursing student in that program.

During her professional career Sanderson's contributions were recognized. In 1955 she was the Isabelle Hampton Robb Fellow at Teachers College. At the University of South Carolina, she was named Distinguished Professor in 1973; also in 1973 she became one of 36 nationally prominent nurses selected for charter membership as a fellow in the American Academy of Nursing.

In 1987 her activities were thwarted by the onset of Parkinson's disease. At that time she entered a church-affiliated nursing home in Pittsburgh, where she continues to reside and where her medical condition has stabilized.

PUBLICATIONS BY
MARJORIE E. SANDERSON

CHAPTERS IN BOOKS

"Quality Patient Care." In *Blueprint for Action in Hospital Nursing.* Pp. 53–56. New York: National League for Nursing, 1964.

Chapter 3. In *Survey of Nursing Needs and Resources in Maryland.* Pp. 23–25. Annapolis: Planning Council for the Board of Health and Mental Hygiene, State of Maryland, 1966.

ARTICLES

"Is Nursing Education Meeting the Needs of Nursing Service?". *Maryland Nursing News* 32 (Summer 1963): 27–33.

"The Cooperative Venture of the Department of the Army and the University of Maryland School of Nursing (WRAIN Program)." *The Bulletin* (University of Maryland) 45 (1966–67): 13–14.

BIBLIOGRAPHY

"Candidates for ANA Elections." *American Journal of Nursing* 64 (Supplement April 1964): S6-S10.

"Charter Fellows Named to Academy of Nursing by ANA Board of Directors." *American Journal of Nursing* 73 (March 1973): 521–22.

Kilker, M. Personal reminiscences. Chairperson, Department of Nursing, East Stroudsburg State University, Pennsylvania, July 13, 1990.

Sanderson, M. E. Curriculum vitae. Personal correspondence by the author with members of Sanderson's family, 1989–90.

Sanderson, M. E. Papers. Files, York College of Pennsylvania, York.

Judith E. Hertz

Levi Bissell Sanford
1856–1908

Levi Bissell Sanford served on the first New York State Board of Nurse Examiners following its establishment on September 14, 1903. New York was one of the first states to recognize officially the need for licensure of nurses; as such, it was one of the first to establish a legislated means of registration and licensure based on examination. This legislation was passed into law on April 24, 1903, and the responsibility for regulating nursing licensure was placed under the auspices of the State Education Department. The law stipulated an all-nurse Board of Examiners with the authority to require licensure by examination and registration through the Board of Regents of New York State. Sanford was one of only five nurses to be appointed to the first Board of Nurse Examiners and served under Sophia F. Palmer, the board's first president.

Sanford was born in the town of Bergen, New York, in 1856. Members of the Sanford family had resided in the area since the mid 1700s. His father, Marcus Sanford, was a farmer and landowner. His mother, Charlotte, was a housewife. There were two children; Charlotte Elizabeth was 4 years older than Levi. Sanford's father died in 1897 at age 72. His mother, who was 9 years older than her husband, had died at least 17 years earlier, and Marcus Sanford had not remarried.

L. Bissell Sanford, as he preferred to be known, spent a number of years in a normal school before pursuing a career in nursing, and this early training as a teacher helped to make him a valuable member of the Board of Nurse Examiners in New York State in later years. He entered the Mills School of Nursing for Men, Bellevue Hospital, on September 1, 1893, and graduated in September 1895. He remained in New York City and held the positions of assistant and acting superintendent of the Mills School in the years following his graduation. He became well recognized in the nursing profession and, as already noted, was selected to serve a term on the first all-nurse Board of Nurse Examiners in New York State.

In addition, he served as secretary of the Mills School Alumni Association and as registrar of the Mills School Nurses Registry during the last three years of his life. He was also a charter member of the County Nurses Association, which later became the New York Counties Registered Nurses Association and is now District 13 of the New York State Nurses Association.

L. Bissell Sanford died on January 25, 1908, in New York City of double pneumonia, before his first term of office on the State Board of Nurse Examiners was completed. A misunderstanding regarding the appointment of a successor to his position on the board led to the withdrawal of the Mills School Alumnae Association from membership in district and state associations for a number of years following his demise.

Had Sanford survived to a more advanced age, his continued activism might have prevailed to influence the professional nursing organizations that were being established during those years. Perhaps, official provision for the membership of men nurses in the ANA would have not been overlooked and delayed until the by-laws were finally revised in 1930 allowing qualified male nurses to attain official membership in the ANA, which they had been seeking since the early 1900s.

Sanford's activism in district and state professional nursing organizations and his service on the Board of Nurse Examiners reflect his recognition of the importance of commitment to professional nursing organizations and to the establishment and enforcement of licensure laws governing the practice of nursing.

BIBLIOGRAPHY

Archives. Bellevue Hospital Center, New York City.

Archives. Genesee County History Department, Batavia, New York.

Nash, H.J. "Men Nurses in New York State: Historical Sketch With Notes on Present Problems." *Trained Nurse and Hospital Review* 97 (August 1936): 123–29.

"Official Reports." *American Journal of Nursing* 8 (March 1908): 487.

Roberts, M.M., *American Nursing: History and Interpretation.* P. 318. New York: Macmillan, 1954.

Karen L. Buchinger

Emilie Gleason Sargent

1894–1977

Emilie Gleason Sargent was best known for her efforts to expand the role and function of public-health nursing.

The daughter of Flora (Ranger) and Henry Curtis Sargent, Sargent was born on April 26, 1894, in St. Paul, Minnesota. She attended Tift College in Forsyth, Georgia, during the 1911–12 school year and then transferred to the University of Michigan in Ann Arbor, where she received her B.A. in 1916. She taught high school in Ypsilanti, Michigan, from 1916–18, at which time she enrolled in the Vassar Training Camp for Nurses in Poughkeepsie, New York. Upon graduation she was assigned to the Vassar Rainbow Division. She then attended the Mt. Sinai Hospital School of Nursing in New York City, from which she graduated in 1920. She joined the Detroit Visiting Nurse Association as a staff nurse in 1920 and then served as executive director (1924–64) of the renamed Visiting Nurse Association of Detroit.

During her 40 years as director, she became known for her innovative leadership. Other nursing associations adopted the techniques and procedures that she pioneered, such as physical and occupational therapy, nutritional services, mental-health screening, care and services in industrial health, and the utilization of practical nurses and home aides. Sargent initiated supervised field experience for students of public-health nursing in cooperation with the Wayne State University public-health nursing program. She took the leadership in upgrading her staff by requiring them not only to be graduates of a recognized nursing school, but to also have a high-school diploma or equivalency certificate.

A pioneer in recognizing the need to improve conditions for the chronically ill and aged, she was the moving force in the Home Care Demonstration Project for Detroit, in 1955, which was funded by the McGregor Fund. The object of the project was to demonstrate methods of providing more effective home care. Sargent was also a leader in demonstration projects showing the importance of coordinating home-care programs for recently discharged hospital patients, and her efforts preceded the U.S. Medicare program, which adopted many of the concepts she had instituted.

Sargent was active in numerous nursing and public-health organizations: president of the National Organization for Public Health Nursing (1950–52) during its merger with the National League for Nursing; president, the Michigan Public Health Association (1943); vice-president of the American Public Health Association (1948); president of the Michigan State Nurses Association (1934–36). She was also a member of the board of the American Journal of Nursing Company (1952–55) and the National League for Nursing (1954–55). Among the community service agencies in which she was active were the United Community Service of Detroit, the National Foundation for Infantile Paralysis, National Nursing Committee, American Red Cross, Public Health Service, Michigan Crippled Children Commission, McGregor Health Foundation. She was chairperson of Region 10 of the White House Conference on Aging, a fellow of the American Public Health Association, and a member of the National Commission on

Aging, of the National Advisory Committee on Chronic Disease of the Aged of the U.S. Public Health Service, and of the National Committee on Aging of the National Social Welfare Assembly.

Among her awards were life membership in the National Organization for Public Health Nursing (1935), an honorary doctorate of science in nursing from Wayne State University (1946), the Pearl McIver Award of the American Nurses' Association (1960), the outstanding achievement award for the University of Michigan (1960), and honorary membership in the Michigan Public Health Association (1962). When she retired in 1964, the University of Michigan School of Public Health created the Emilie Gleason Sargent Prize in her honor.

She died on April 17, 1977, in Detroit, Michigan.

PUBLICATIONS BY EMILIE GLEASON SARGENT

"Hourly Appointment Service." *Public Health Nurse* 22 (April 1930): 199–200.

"The Nursing Council—A Device to Balance Nursing Needs." *Modern Hospital* 39 (October 1932): 116, 118, 120.

"The Nursing Profession for Recovery." *American Journal of Nursing* 33 (December 1933): 1165–72.

"Detroit's Pneumonia Nursing Campaign." *Public Health Nurse* 27 (April 1935): 190–92.

"When the Patient Needs Further Care at Home." *Hospitals* 18 (January 1944): 38–40.

"Nursing—A Service to Humanity." *School and College Placement* 8 (December 1947): 5–10.

"VNA Considers Patients' Fees." *Public Health Nurse* 43 (September 1951): 479–80, 482.

"What It Means to Become a Charter Member in NLN Through Your 1952 Membership in NOPHN." *Public Health Nurse* 44 (June 1952): 307–08.

BIBLIOGRAPHY

Clappison, G.B. *Vassar's Rainbow Division.* Pp. 259–61. Ames, Iowa: (no publisher listed), 1964.

Emilie Sargent Papers. Nursing Archives, Mugar Memorial Library, Boston University, Boston.

Who's Who of American Women. Chicago: Marquis, 1961, and subsequent editions.

Vern L. Bullough

Frances Schervier

1819–1876

Frances Schervier was the foundress and first superior general of the religious Congregation of the Sisters of the Poor of St. Francis. She devoted her life to the care of the young, the sick, the elderly, the imprisoned, and those wounded in battle.

Born in Aachen, Germany, on January 3, 1819, Mother Frances was of German-French heritage. Her father, John Henry Caspar Schervier, was a proprietor of a large needle factory and also served as vice-burgomaster. Her mother, Marie Louise Migeon, whom her father married one year after the death of his first wife, was a native of Chouville, France. Of the six children, four girls and two boys, born of this marriage, Frances was the second youngest. At the age of 14 she was to take charge of the household, having lost her mother and two sisters. This new role accelerated her development, maturity, judgment, and sense of responsibility that became the foundation blocks for her career leadership and charity. It was during this very same period she began her life of devotion and service to her fellow man, guided by Christian principles fostered in her family home life and exposure to religious upbringing in the parish school. She early on established a pattern of charity to be followed throughout the remainder of her life by using personal savings, by knitting for the needy, and by giving away her family's household goods to the destitute.

Since nursing and social work were not recognized professions when Mother Frances was a young woman, the only way for an individual to perform works of mercy was to enter a religious order or congregation. Mother Frances began her career of tending to the sick at a hospital under the direction of the Borromean Sisters, from whom she acquired her first training and experience in nursing.

In 1840 she joined a small group of young women dedicated to serving the needy and soon assumed the leadership role of the group because of her zeal, leadership, and judgment and her ability to inspire others. In 1844, shortly before the death of her father, she joined the Third Order Secular of St. Francis, which was recognized as an aid and inspiration for the more perfect Christian life.

In 1845, with four other women, she founded the congregation known as the Sisters of the Poor of St. Francis. Their fearless example soon attracted other women until their group reached 22 members. All became deeply involved in community work, assisting the local area during a smallpox and cholera epidemic by establishing an infirmary in Aachen. In 1850 they took over an abandoned Dominican convent and converted it into a hospital for incurable diseases.

On August 25, 1852, "Mother" Frances, a title that had been bestowed on her by then, and her sisters took their perpetual vows of obedience, chastity, and poverty. In both the eyes of the world and the Catholic Church, the Mother Frances community was now firmly established and allowed to spread to other dioceses. The group quickly set up nursing homes throughout Germany.

In 1858, while Mother Frances was busily engaged in establishing and extending her congregation's work of charity in Europe, a request for a foundation came from the United States. Mrs. Sarah Peter of Cincinnati, Ohio, a recent convert to the Catholic faith and a woman of wealth, was eager to introduce sisters of various nationalities to care for the destitute and sick, especially among the immigrants in her home city.

As a result of this request, Mother Frances commissioned six sisters to travel from Germany to Cincinnati, and by 1861 there were four hospitals in Ohio, one in Cincinnati and one in Columbus, under the jurisdiction of the Sisters of the Poor of Saint Francis.

In 1861, as the sisterhood in the United States continued to grow, a novitiate became a critical need, and Mrs. Peter came to Mother Frances's assistance by turning over much of her own personal residence for this purpose. On Christmas Day 1861 the archbishop dedicated the novitiate, known as St. Clare's Convent.

The sisters were increasing their homes and hospitals in the United States at about the rate of one each year. Mother Frances was frequently reluctant to give her consent to this expansion because she feared the problems that might result from over-extension. But her primary concern for the poor and suffering generally overruled her expessed fears. In addition, she was planning to visit the United States and observe firsthand the works of her sisters.

In June 1862, to the mutual joy and consolation of Mother Frances and her sisters, her trip to the United States was realized. During her stay she visited many of her hospitals to interact with as many patients as possible. At this time she was also bombarded with numerous requests from various bishops to set up additional nursing centers, which she placed under cautious consideration. Mother Frances was in Cincinnati while the American Civil War was being waged. Because of the fear of Southern troops by the city's populace, the bishop requested Mother Frances and her sisters to pray for the city. She later attributed the city's preservation to these prayers. Because of the effects of the war, Mother Frances found it necessary to establish orphanages for babies deserted by mothers, many of whom had been deserted by the children's soldier fathers.

Events in Europe required Mother Frances to leave the United States. Soon after her return to Aachen, Germany, two other wars found her and her sisters serving as nurses, giving their aid impartially to the wounded of both sides.

In 1868 when Mother Frances had visited her communities in the United States for a second time, the number of institutions under her order had doubled. There were now hospitals a distance from the original one in Cincinnati, such as in Jersey City, New Jersey; Brooklyn, New York; Quincy, Illinois; and Newark, New Jersey.

For Mother Frances, herself in poor health, suffering from an asthmatic condition that predated her first visit to the United States, her second visit became a physically taxing journey. Despite her own condition, she was more affected by the hard and overburdened life of her sisters. She found the trials and crosses here to be greater and heavier than in Europe. Physically, the summer heat was intense, and mosquitoes were tormenting the patients and their care givers incessantly. In addition, the patients that filled the hospitals were for the most part the poor of the area. Surprisingly, Mother Frances found great happiness among her sisters who staffed the facilities.

Upon her return to Europe, Mother Frances's health was in a state of deterioration. Her asthmatic attacks grew worse, becoming a great hindrance to the performance of her duties. For a number of years she had requested that she not be reelected superior general because of her failing health. Despite her pleas, she continued to be elected. Her condition became so serious that a pilgrimage was made to Our Lady of Lourdes to implore recovery or death. On the second day after her arrival Mother Frances seemed to improve greatly, and this further intensified her devotion to the Mother of God.

Mother Frances then found herself and her sisters immersed in the suffering of the Franco-Prussian War. The victories of Prussia resulted in large numbers of French prisoners, and her congregation became involved with the care of the prisoners, their wives, their children, healing the physically wounded but never forgetting their spiritual well-being. Despite the sisters' services even to their own country in the time of war and receiving honors, including the Iron Cross, they were not exempt from the repressive laws affecting religious congregations.

Again in 1875 Mother Frances tried to refuse the office of Superior General because she did not believe she would outlive the term of office. The burdens of the office weighed heavily on her, and her health continued to deteriorate. On November 30, 1876, she was overcome with pain in the stomach and vomiting, and an alarming ruptured hernia was discovered. On December 4 an operation was performed, prior to which Mother Frances had informed the two attending physicians that if death would follow, she was totally resigned to it.

As knowledge of her condition spread, thousands of her devoted friends from throughout the Rhineland prayed for her recovery. On Thursday, December 14, 1976, she died, and her body laid in state until December 18, resulting in a pilgrimage never before witnessed by the city of Aachen.

Frances Schervier's body was first buried, in accordance with the law, in the general cemetery, but on May 26, 1880, permission was granted to transfer the body to the mother house. One source states her body was relocated a third time, but the location was unclear and not verifiable in other sources.

In 1912 the first steps began toward beatification by ecclesiastial authorities, and in 1934 the apostolic process was opened thereby allowing the possibility for Mother Frances to become a canonized saint of the Catholic Church.

BIBLIOGRAPHY

Dehey, E.T. *Religious Orders of Women in the United States* Pp. 421–24. Hammond, Ind.: Conkey, 1930.

Delaney, J.J. *Dictionary of Catholic Biography.* P. 1036. Garden City, N.Y.: Doubleday, 1961.

Jeiler, I. *The Venerable Mother Frances Schervier.* St. Louis: Herder, 1895. (Various editions in English and German, 1893–1912).

Jolly, E.R. *Nuns of the Battlefield.* Providence, R.I.: Providence Visitor Press, 1927.

Maynard, T. *Through My Gift.* New York: Kennedy, 1951.

McAllistister, A.S. *In Winter We Flourish.* New York: Longmans, Green, 1939.

Pauline, Sister. *Frances Schervier Mother of the Poor.* Paterson, N.J.: St. Anthony Guild Press, 1946.

Pennock, M.R. *Makers of Nursing History.* P. 22. New York: Lakeside, 1940.

Paul A. Zadner

Mathilda Scheuer

1890–1974

Mathilda Scheuer was a leader in public-health nursing in Pennsylvania and served as president of the American Nurses' Association.

Scheuer was born in Berryville, Clarke County, Virginia, on January 26, 1890, the fourth of seven children born to respected merchant Louis Scheuer and his wife. The father had emigrated from Germany at the age of 14. Scheuer received her primary education at Miss Virginia Washington's school and also attended Miss Mac-Donald's classes for young ladies in Berryville. She was later sent to finishing school at the Academy of Visitation in Baltimore, Maryland.

Throughout her childhood service to the less fortunate was stressed, and Scheuer always wanted to become a nurse. She applied to the Johns Hopkins Hospital Nursing School but was denied admittance because she was too young. She then applied to Mercy Hospital's School of Nursing in Baltimore, was accepted, and graduated in 1910. Like many others she started her nursing career as a private-duty nurse. She became active in professional organizations and attended her first national convention as a delegate of the Maryland Nurses Association.

With the advent of World War I, Scheuer tried to enlist for overseas duty but was turned down because of an infected tooth. Subsequently, she was invited to join the staff of the Philadelphia Visiting Nurse Society, and in 1920 she enrolled at the University of Pennsylvania, where she completed the required course in public-health nursing. She later received additional training at Teachers College, Columbia University.

By the time Scheuer retired from the Visiting Nurse Society in 1956, she had advanced to acting director of the society. Shortly after her retirement, she was asked by the Pennsylvania Department of Welfare to supervise the Bureau of Services for the Aging and later the Bureau of Convalescent and Nursing Homes. In 1958 and in 1960 she was elected president of the American Nurses' Association. Scheuer also served as president of the Pennsylvania State Nurses Association from 1949 to 1950 and as president of District One of the Pennsylvania State Nurses Association from 1951 to 1954. Other offices included president of the Pennsylvania Organization for Public Health Nursing in the 1940s.

Scheuer's leadership ability was widely recognized, and she was appointed to the State Board of Nurse Examiners in Pennsylvania in 1950 and to the health Subcommittee of the Governor's Committee for the White House Conference for Children and Youth. She also sat on the executive committee and overall committee of the U.S. Committee of the United Nations. She died in January, 1974.

BIBLIOGRAPHY

Benson, E. R. "Mathilda Scheuer (1890–1974): A Biographical Sketch." *Journal of Nursing History* 2 (November 1986): 36–42.

Schutt, E., "A Conversation with ANA Presidents." *American Journal of Nursing* 71 (September 1971): 1792–98.

Lilli Sentz

Rozella May Schlotfeldt

b. 1914

One of the most influential nurses during the second half of the twentieth century, Rozella May Schlotfeldt was the recipient of many nursing honors. She served as dean of the Frances Payne Bolton School of Nursing at Case Western Reserve University (Cleveland), was a member of various national task forces dealing with nursing issues, both private and governmental, and was one of the few nurses to be elected to the Institute of Medicine of the National Academy of Sciences.

Schlotfeldt was born in DeWitt, Iowa, on June 29, 1914, the daughter of John W. and Clara C. (Doering) Schlotfeldt. She was one of two daughters. She received her bachelor's degree in 1935 from the State University of Iowa at Iowa City. After her graduation she became a staff nurse, first at the University of Iowa hospital and then at the U.S. Veterans administration Hospital in Des Moines, positions she held from 1935–39, when she became an instructor and supervisor of maternity nursing at the University of Iowa. She left

to serve in the U.S. Army Nurse Corps, 1944–46, where she served in the European theater. In 1946 she entered the University of Chicago, receiving her M.S. in 1947, whereupon she joined the faculty of the University of Colorado School of Nursing.

In 1948 she joined the faculty at Wayne State College of Nursing in Detroit, and while there completed the requirements for her Ph.D. at the University of Chicago, receiving the degree in 1956. From 1957–60 she served as associate dean of nursing at Wayne State, and in 1960 she moved to Cleveland, where she became dean and professor of nursing at Case Western Reserve University. She stepped down as dean in 1972 but continued to serve as professor until her retirement in 1982.

Schlotfeldt's numerous national positions included special consultant to the surgeon general's Advisory Group on Nursing (1961–63); membership in the nursing research study section of the U.S. Public Health Service (1962–66); member of the Division of Nursing Advisory Committee of the W.K. Kellogg Foundation (1959–67); member of the National Health Service Research and Training Committee (1970–71); consultant to the Walter Reed Army Institute for Nursing Research (1967–74); member of the Department of Defense Advisory Committee on Women in the Services (1972–75); board member of the Nursing Home Advisory and Research Council (1975) and for several years afterward; member of the advisory panel to Health Services Research Council on Human Resources of the National Academy of Science (1977–80); and member of numerous other groups. She also served as president of the Ohio Board of Nursing Education and Nurse Registration (1971–72); on various health-oriented committees in Cleveland; as an interim director of the Midwest Alliance in Nursing; on the accrediting board for baccaleureate and higher-degree programs of the NLN; on the ANA Study Committee on Credentialing in Nursing; on the governing council of the American Academy of Nursing; on the board of visitors of Duke University Medical Center; on the council executive committee of the Institute of

Medicine of the National Academy of Sciences; and on many more committees.

Schlotfeldt has more than 100 publications to her credit, and these have appeared in a variety of scientific and professional journals, as chapters in books, as monographs, and as research reports. She was a member of the editorial board of *Advances in Nursing Science* and the *Journal of Nursing Education*, as well as on the review panel of *Nursing Research.*

Among her many honors are the Centennial Award from Wayne State University (1968); Honorary Recognition Award of the ANA (1970); election to the Institute of Medicine of the National Academy of Science (1971); honorary doctorates from Georgetown University (1971), Medical University of South Carolina (1976), Adelphi University (1979), Wayne State University (1983), University of Illinois (1985), Kent State University (1986), and University of Cincinnati (1989); distinguished service award of the University of Iowa (1973); elected fellow of the American Academy of Nursing (1974); merit award for distinguished service in nursing, Boston University (1975); merit award for distinguished service, University of San Diego, (1979); Copeland (Founders) Award for Creativity, Sigma Theta Tau, International (1985).

PUBLICATIONS BY ROZELLA M. SCHLOTFELDT

ARTICLES (Selected)

"Doctoral Study in Basic Disciplines—A Choice for Nurses." *Nursing Forum* 5 (1966): 68–74.

"Nurses and Physicians—Professional Associates and Assistants to Patients." *Ohio Nurses Review* 45 (March 1970): 6–12.

"Research in Nursing and Research Training for Nurses." *Nursing Research* 24 (May-June 1975): 177–83.

"Can We Bring Order out of Chaos." *American Journal of Nursing* 76 (January 1976): 105–07.

"Recruiting, Appointing, and Renewing Faculty." *Nursing Outlook* 24 (March 1976): 148–54.

"The Professional Doctorate: Rational and Characteristics." *Nursing Outlook* 26 (1978): 302–11.

"Nursing in the Future." *Nursing Outlook* 29 (May 1981): 295–301.

"Critical Issues in Nursing Practice, Education, and Research." *Occupational Health Nursing* 32 (January 1984): 11–16.

"A Brave New Nursing World." *Journal of Professional Nursing* 1 (1985): 244–51.

"Defining Research—A Historical Controversy." *Nursing Research* 36 (1987): 64–67.

CHAPTERS IN BOOKS (SELECTED)

"The Need for a Conceptual Framework." In *Nursing Research.* P. Verhonick, ed. No. 1, Pp. 3–23. Boston: Little Brown, 1975.

"Long-Term Care in Perspective." *Long-Term Care: Some Issues for Nursing.* Pp. 22–38. Kansas City: American Academy of Nursing, 1976.

"The Scholarly Nursing Practitioner." In *Alternative Conceptions of Work and Society: Implications for Professional Nursing.* C. Lindeman, ed. Pp. 15–29. Washington, D.C.: American Association of Colleges of Nursing, 1988.

BIBLIOGRAPHY

Personal Vita and checking by author with subject, 1990.

Who's Who in America, 1990–91. Chicago: Marquis Who's Who, 1990.

Who's Who of American Women, 1989–90. Chicago: Marquis Who's Who, 1989.

Vern L. Bullough

Barbara Gordon Schutt

1917–1986

As editor of the *American Journal of Nursing* (1958–71), Barbara Gordon Schutt influenced the development of nursing on the national level for more than a decade. She was particularly noted for her advocacy of the right to organize for collective bargaining and for her belief that nurses should control their own practice.

Schutt was born on March 25, 1917, in Ithaca, New York, the daughter of Warren Ellis and Clara Gordon Schutt. Her father was a Rhodes scholar at Cornell University. After graduating from Ithaca High School in 1935, she entered Jefferson Medical College Hospital School of Nursing in Philadelphia. She received her nursing diploma in 1938, her bachelor of arts degree in psychology from Bethany College, West Virginia, in 1942, and a master of science degree in nursing education from the University of Pennsylvania in 1949.

From 1938–44 Schutt worked as a general-duty nurse at her home hospital, as assistant in the Bethany College student health service, and as a camp nurse and assistant counselor. While earning her bachelor's degree she held a faculty position at the Jefferson School. During World War II in 1944 she entered the Army Nurse Corps, serving as a first lieutenant in Hawaii and Okinawa.

After the war Schutt joined the staff of the Pennsylvania Nurses Association, serving as assistant, associate, and executive director. The association numbered more than 17,000 members and was particularly active in nursing education and in working to improve the economic welfare of its members, utilizing such techniques as public relations and collective bargaining. Schutt also edited the *Pennsylvania Nurse* and served as member and chair of the Economic and General Welfare Committee of the American Nurses' Association (ANA), 1952–58.

In 1952 and 1954 the *Pennsylvania Nurse* in competition with other state nurses' association publications was honored by the American Journal of Nursing Company for general excellence. Schutt's reputation as editor led to her appointment in 1958 as editor of the *American Journal of Nursing*, a post she filled until 1971. She gained the respect of the entire nursing profession, and her editorials forcefully addressed nurses' rights to organize for collective bargaining and professional control. During her tenure she wrote more than 150 editorials, and after relinquishing her post as editor-in-chief, she continued to serve as contributing editor until 1974, when she became director of the nursing division at Mohegan Community College in Norwich, Connecticut. Upon her retirement five years later she received a presidential citation from the college.

Schutt was active in professional and community affairs and served on numerous local and national committees throughout her life, including a term as president of the Connecticut Nurses Association, 1977–79.

The recipient of many honors, she was elected by the ANA board of directors as a charter fellow of the Academy of Nursing in January 1973 and also received ANA's Honorary Recognition Award in 1968. The honorary doctor of science degree was conferred upon her by Bethany College, Bethany, West Virginia, in 1973.

She died on December 26, 1987, in Montville, Connecticut, after a long struggle with cancer. Upon her death the Connecticut Nurses Foundation established a nursing scholarship in her name.

PUBLICATIONS BY BARBARA GORDON SCHUTT (SELECTED)

"At Your Service." *American Journal of Nursing* 47 (September 1947): 592–95.

Editorials. *Pennsylvania Nurse* (1948–58).

"Confessions of a Committee Woman." *American Journal of Nursing* 49 (March 1949): 158–60.

"The Local Unit—A Place of Strength and Growth." *American Journal of Nursing* 53 (April 1953): 420–22.

"The ANA Economic Security Program . . . What It Is and Why." *American Journal of Nursing* 58 (April 1958): 520–24.

Editorials. *American Journal of Nursing* (1958–71).

"The ANA—Illustrious Past, Challenging Future—the Recent Past." *American Journal of Nursing* 71 (September 1971); 1785–91.

"A Conversation with A.N.A. Presidents." *American Journal of Nursing* 71 (September 1971): 1792–98.

"Frontier's Family Nurses." *American Journal of Nursing* 72 (May 1972): 903–09. Reprinted in the *Congressional Record* (May 1972).

"Spot Check on Primary Care Nursing." *American Journal of Nursing* 73 (November 1973): 1946–52.

BIBLIOGRAPHY

"Barbara Schutt to Become Journal Editor." *American Journal of Nursing* 58 (August 1958): 1114.

Haney, D.E. Correspondence with the author, 1989.

Kalisch, P., and B. Kalisch. *The Advance of American Nursing*. Boston: Little, Brown, 1978.

"New Journal Editor Arrives." *American Journal of Nursing* 59 (January 1959): 22.

"Nursing Profiles." *Canadian Nurse* 55 (July 1959): 637.

Obituary. *American Journal of Nursing* 87 (February 1987): 249.

Schutt, B. "The Care and Feeding of an Editorial Writer." *American Journal of Nursing* 71 (April 1971): 703.

Lilli Sentz

Jessie M. Scott

b. 1915

Jessie M. Scott was a nursing educator before her distinguished administrative tenure in the U.S. Public Health Service in the Division of Nursing Resources. Health-care systems were undergoing rapid changes when she had the responsibility of overseeing federal health programs that related to nursing. Scott's view of nursing as an entity—that is as a service, a field of practice, and a profession—shaped how she interpreted nursing to the federal government in terms of nursing needs. In the Division of Nursing intramural activities and extramural activities needed to complement each other in order to address the scope of nursing as an entity. Under Scott's guidance construction and curriculum grants and experimental short-term training were dovetailed with planned evaluation under research grants in order to accomplish this aim.

Scott was born on May 2, 1915, in Wilkes Barre, Pennsylvania, the third child of Chester A. and Eva M. Scott. She lived in Wilkes-Barre with her family until her affiliation with the University of Pennsylvania. She attended Wilkes-Barre General Hospital School of Nursing and graduated in 1936. Following this she worked in private-duty nursing for four years, until 1940. For the years 1941–43 she worked as an infirmary nurse and then as an assistant in biological sciences at the hospital affiliated with the University of Pennsylvania, Philadelphia, while obtaining a B.S. in education from the same institution. For the next four years (1943–47) she taught science, first at Mount Sinai Hospital and then Jefferson Medical College Hospital, both in Philadelphia. In her teaching she stressed the importance of knowledge in microbiology for student nurses as a tool for providing community health care.

After serving as general staff nurse and assistant science instructor at St. Luke's Hospital, New York City (1947–49), Scott became assistant executive secretary of the Pennsylvania Nurses Association, a post she held from 1949–55. During this period, in 1949, she received an M.A. in personnel administration from Teachers College, Columbia University. Scott developed a program of field training in counseling for graduate students which was the first program of its kind in the country.

Jessie M. Scott was commissioned in the Nurse Corps of the Public Health Service in 1955. Her assignment was with the Division of Nursing Resources, which subsequently became the Division of Nursing. She served first as a nurse consultant (1955–57) and in 1957, in recognition of her outstanding ability was selected to be deputy chief. In 1964 she became director of the division, the only government program where nursing is the primary concern. Scott was respected and admired for her integrity and ability to use the resources of government to improve nursing nationally. She organized the Division of Nursing staff and activities so that nursing practice, nursing service, nursing research, and nursing education were considered together. Under her direction the staff of consultants developed and provided a wide range of assistance in response to general and specific operative efforts with outside organizations and agencies.

In 1956 Scott had investigated the concept of "self-care" and reported her findings to Dr. L.T. Coggeshall, a medical advisor serving on an advisory committee appointed by Marion B. Folsom, then secretary of health, education and welfare. As a result of Scott's report, research was conducted of various patient-care units, including intensive care, intermediate care, long-term care, self-care, and home care.

While serving as a consultant with the Division of Nursing, Scott worked with nursing groups in several states, including Arkansas, Tennessee, Texas and Connecticut. Specifically, she consulted on statewide surveys that attempted to assist states in dealing with nurse shortages. Home visiting, preventative and therapeutic clinic services, health education, and personal hygiene were among the services that were assessed. Scott was also a consultant to nursing groups, hospitals, and schools of nursing on such issues as staffing problems and resources, and she conducted various training conferences.

According to Scott the mandate of the division of Nursing was "to advance health-care planning and knowledge about the characteristics, distribution, and utilization of nursing manpower and improvement of nursing education, practice, and research." The Division of Nursing Resources, established in 1949, at first focused on helping states assess nursing capabilities and conditions. In 1955 this role expanded to include support of nursing research projects and fellowships to prepare nurses for research careers, the first nursing research unit in the Federal Service. In 1956 the division was designated to administer traineeships for preparing nurses for teaching and other leadership assignments.

In 1960 the surgeon general of the Public Health Service appointed a Consultant group on Nursing in order to determine the federal role for nursing education. The Division of Nursing was the staff resource and manpower research arm for the group. This led to the first comprehensive legislation for aid to nursing education, the Nurse Training Act of 1964. The Division of Nursing was delegated to administer this legislation and the subsequent Health Manpower and Nurse Training Acts in 1964, 1968, 1971, and 1975.

Scott has been very active in international nursing. She did consulting with the directorate general of health of the Ministry of Health in India in 1960 for a study on nursing, was a member of a joint PHS and AHA team to study services for the chronically ill in Scotland (1961), participated with a team sent to Liberia to design a national medical center (1964), served as a United States delegate to the Seminar for Nurses of the King's Fund College of Hospital Management, London, (1972), and was an official participant in the First International Seminar of the National League for Nursing in Israel (1972). In 1973 she took part in the first Trans-Pacific Seminar in Nursing in New Zealand and Australia. For the five-year period 1975–80 Scott was a member of the Health Resources Administration four-person team invited to Egypt to evaluate Ministry of Health nurse training programs and recommend changes for effectiveness and efficiency. She was a participant in the ANA tour of the People's Republic of China in 1977 and the International Council of Nurses and World Health Organization Conference on Primary Care in Nairobi, Kenya, in 1979. From 1977–81 she chaired the Professional Services Committee of the International Council of Nurses, Geneva. She was a member of the board of directors of the Commission on Graduates of Foreign Nursing Schools from 1979–84 and served as president from 1980–82.

In the United States too Scott was an active member and leader in many professional organizations, including the American Nurses' Association, National League for Nursing, International Council of Nurses, American Public Health Association, Commissioned Officers Association, American Academy of Nursing, and History of Nursing Archives Associates.

Her honorary degrees and special awards include the Distinguished Service Medal of the Public Health Service, 1973; Meritorious Service Medal of the Public Health Service, 1970; honorary membership, Sigma Theta Tau National Honor Society of Nursing; the Mary Adelaide Nutting Award for Leadership in Nursing; Pennsylvania Nurses Association Award for Distinguished Service to Nursing; Sesquicentennial Award from Indiana University School of Nursing for Distinguished Service to Nursing; Florence

Nightingale Medal, State University of New York; honorary recognition, by the ANA (1972). University of Arizona Alumni Association Distinguished Citizen Award, 1978; and the Distinguished Service Award, University of San Diego, 1979. Scott gave the Seventh Anne Walker Sengbusch Distinguished Lecture at the State University of New York at Buffalo, 1971; and the Sybil Palmer Bellos Distinguished Lecture at Yale University, 1972.

Scott retired on July 1, 1979, from the Division of Nursing, National Institutes of Health and Health Resources Administration, Public Health Service. Since that time she has been a lecturer at George Mason University, Fairfax, Virginia, on international nursing issues, 1980; an associate professor at the University of Maryland Graduate Program for Nursing and Health Policy, 1980–82; and adjunct professor at the University of Texas, Austin, 1982. She continues to be an active consultant in international nursing issues and in projects concerning public-health policy.

PUBLICATIONS BY JESSIE M. SCOTT

ARTICLES (SELECTED)

"Seeing Nursing Activities as They Are." *American Journal of Nursing* 62 (November 1962): 70–71.

"Three Years with the Nurse Training Act." *American Journal of Nursing* 67 (October 1967): 2107–09.

"Federal Support for Nursing Education 1964 to 1972." *American Journal of Nursing* 72 (October 1972): 1855–61.

"The Changing Health Care Environment—It's Implications for Nursing." *American Journal of Public Health* 64 (April 1974): 364–69.

"Federal Support of Nursing Education, to Improve Quality of Practice." *Public Health Reports* 94 (January–February 1979): 31–35.

BIBLIOGRAPHY

Scott, J.M. Personal correspondence with the author, 1989.

Scott, J.M. Personal papers. Nursing Archives, Mugar Memorial Library, Boston University, Boston.

Valerie Hart-Smith

Gladys Sellew
1887–1977

Nurse, sociologist, educator, author, and humanitarian, Gladys Sellew advanced pediatric nursing care and promoted the social significance of nursing. Throughout her life she demonstrated an active concern for human welfare, both in her professional activities and in her personal life.

Sellew was born in Cincinnati, Ohio, on July 29, 1887, the daughter of Ralph and Rachel (Moore) Sellew. Inspired by the work of Jane Adams, she was drawn to social services and worked as a volunteer in the Cincinnati University Settlement and in the Cincinnati General Hospital Social Service Department. When the city took over the department, she matriculated at the University of Cincinnati. In 1917 the director of the School of Nursing appealed to university students to enter the school in order to alleviate the nursing shortage caused by World War I. Sellew responded and received her nursing diploma as well as a bachelor of arts degree in economics in 1918, a bachelor of science degree in nursing in 1919, and a master's degree in economics in 1921. In 1938 she received a Ph.D. in sociology from Catholic University.

In the early 1920s she specialized in pediatric nursing, working first as head nurse in the children's ward of the Cincinnati General Hospital and later as instructor in the School of Nursing at the University of Cincinnati and as supervisor in the Pediatric Division at the hospital. Following an address to the American Nurses' Association in 1924, she began assembling her data in written form, resulting in the publication of her first book *Pediatric Nursing* in 1926.

In 1925 she had been appointed superintendent of nursing service at the Babies' and Children's Hospital in Cleveland, and also served as professor of nursing at Western Reserve University. Three years later she became director of pediatric services at Cook County Hospital, Chicago, where she initiated the formation of a teaching unit. She also worked as assistant to the dean in charge of pediatric nursing service at Illinois Training School for Nurses and developed a course in the theory and practice of ward administration.

Sellew resigned in 1932 in order to complete her work on a Ph.D. in sociology at Catholic University in Washington, D.C. Her thesis investigated black families in Washington, and was one of the first if not the first nursing dissertation that was not focused on educational issues. From 1932 to 1942 she held the position of assistant professor of sociology and nursing at Catholic University, and in 1946 she became associate professor and later professor and chair of the Department of Sociology at Rosary College in addition to serving as visiting professor of pediatric nursing at the University of Maryland. After leaving Rosary College in 1956, she spent two years as professor of pediatric nursing at the University of Maryland until her retirement in 1958.

Following her retirement, she moved to her native state of Ohio and settled in Oberlin, where she began providing housing for families who could not afford to become houseowners. Using her own savings, she financed home loans for families without any credit rating. She believed that all individuals given the opportunity will meet their responsibilities, and no one ever defaulted on her loans. Each year Sellew also gave lodgings in her own home to a number of Oberlin College students who demonstrated financial need.

A prolific writer, Sellew authored or coauthored multiple editions of seven books, several of which have been translated into foreign languages, including Chinese and Japanese. Her work *Ward Administration* was the first book to apply time study to nursing. She was the recipient of many honors. In 1970 she received the Senior Citizen's Award from the Oberlin Health Commission and also the Man of the Year Award from the *Oberlin News-Tribune*. Three years later she received a special award from the Ohio Planning Conference, a professional organization of state, regional, and city planners. She was also recognized by President Richard Nixon in 1971 for her work in providing funds for housing of local residents, and

she was the recipient of the first Distinguished Community Service Award from Oberlin College in 1971.

An influential author and teacher of pediatric nursing, Sellew advocated better bedside nursing practice based on a firm theoretical foundation, and she applied the knowledge gained from many fields to the problems of pediatric nursing. Dedicated to furthering human welfare both professionally and in her private activities, Sellew was generous and modest, refusing to talk about herself or seek credit for her accomplishments. She died in Oberlin, on July 6, 1977.

PUBLICATIONS BY GLADYS SELLEW

BOOKS (FIRST EDITIONS)

Pediatric Nursing. Philadelphia: Saunders, 1926. Later editions entitled *The Child in Nursing* and *Nursing of Children*

A Textbook of Ward Administration. Philadelphia: Saunders, 1930.

Sociology and Social Problems in Nursing Service. Philadelphia: Saunders, 1941.

A History of Nursing. St. Louis: Mosby, 1946.

With P.H. Furfey and W.T. Gaughan. *An Introduction to Sociology.* New York: Harper, 1958.

THESIS AND DISSERTATION

"Theories and Forces Relating to the Determination of Wages." M.A. unpublished thesis. University of Cincinnati, 1921.

"A Deviant Social Situation, a Court." Unpublished Ph.D. Dissertation, Catholic University of America, 1938.

ARTICLES (SELECTED)

"Basic Care of Infants. Comments and Suggestions in Pediatric Nursing." *American Journal of Nursing* 26 (March 1926): 193–96.

"The Admission of Children to a General Hospital." *American Journal of Nursing* 26 (October 1926): 781–84.

"Some Time Studies. How Many Hours of Nursing Service Do Our Patients Require." *American Journal of Nursing* 27 (February 1927): 99–101.

"How to Harmonize Patients' Needs and Nurses' Educational Needs." *Modern Hospital* 29 (November 1927): 144, 146.

"Correlation of Theory and Practice in Pediatric Nursing." *American Journal of Nursing* 28 (December 1928): 1245–49.

"Correlation of Theory and Practice." *Hospital Progress* 13 (January 1932): 29–31.

"Occupational Therapy for Children." *Occupational Therapy Rehabilitation* 11 (October 1932): 379–81.

"Recruitment of Student Nurses." *Hospital Progress* 26 (November 1945): 347–50.

BIBLIOGRAPHY

American Men of Science. A Biographical Directory, 10th ed. Tempe, Ariz: Cattell, 1962.

Archives. Oberlin College, Oberlin, Ohio.

Editorials. *Oberlin News-Tribune*, January 1, 1970.

Gipe, F.M. "Courage of their Convictions." *Nursing Science* 2 (October 1964): 391–93.

Jennings, S.A. "Credit Risks? Service Award Winner Admires Their Reliability." *Oberlin Alumni Magazine* (July/August 1971): 18–19.

Logan, L.R. "Eminent Teachers. Gladys Sellew, A.B., B.S., A.M., R.N." *American Journal of Nursing* 29 (May 1929): 565–66.

Pennock, M.R. *Makers of Nursing History*. New York: Lakeside, 1928, 1940.

Schryver, G.F. *A History of the Illinois Training School for Nurses 1880–1929*. Chicago: Illinois Training School for Nurses, 1930.

Lilli Sentz

Anna Pearl Sherrick

b. 1899

Anna Pearl Sherrick established the baccalaureate nursing program at Montana State College in 1937 and served as director of the School of Nursing until her retirement in 1965. She believed that nurses needed liberal arts and sciences in addition to their nursing courses to qualify as professionals, so support for collegiate education for nurses was an important agenda for her life's work. A master's degree was initiated at the school in 1957, and it served not only Montana nurses but also nurses from surrounding states. Sherrick was a pioneer in the use of innovative educational and communications technology and an important leader in Montana nursing and community organizations.

Sherrick was born on November 26, 1899, on the "Old Sherrick Homestead" in Houston Township, Adams County, Illinois, to Joel D. Sherrick and Josephine Harris Sherrick. She was the youngest of eight children. She lived on the Homestead until she was 9 years old, attending a one-room school house for three years. In 1909 when she was in the fourth grade, the family moved to Bowen, which was a town about 8 miles from the farm, in order for the children to attend a larger school. She graduated from Bowen High School in 1918.

Sherrick entered Knox College in Galesburg for two years. Following a two-year illness, she enrolled in the Illinois Women's College (now McMurray College) in Jacksonville, Illinois, receiving her bachelors degree in 1924.

Nursing had always been Sherrick's career goal, so she went to the University of Michigan School of Nursing at Ann Arbor for a two-and-a-quarter-year program, earning a diploma and completing the Michigan State Board of Nursing licensing examination in 1927. She worked briefly as a private-duty nurse, then accepted a position at St. Lukes Hospital School of Nursing in Chicago teaching science. Before the end of the quarter, she was found to have tuberculosis, which kept her at home for three years.

Moving to Colorado because it was believed the high dry climate would keep her well, in 1930 she began working at the Park View School of Nursing in Pueblo, Colorado, instructing nursing students in the application of science. While she was in Colorado she was also able to complete a master in arts degree at Colorado State Teachers College in 1934.

She then moved to Montana, which she thought might be a healthier area for her, and accepted an instructor's position at the Montana Deaconess Hospital School of Nursing in Great Falls. The position was exciting, but she could not put aside her goal of initiating a baccalaureate nursing program. She was successful in this effort in 1937 when two small schools, Bozeman and Havre, joined forces with the Montana Deaconess Hospital School in Great Falls to establish a baccalaureate program affiliated with Montana State College. The school at Havre dropped out the next year because of financial problems related to the Depression. However, the program was further strengthened when the Deaconess Hospital program at Billings came into the network in 1943.

In 1943 Sherrick began a summer course for prenursing students. In 1943 the school was funded by the U.S. Public Health Service as a part of the Cadet Nurse Corps. Sherrick believed strongly in nursing organizations and established the Lambda Chapter of Alpha Tau Delta as an honor society for nursing students.

Sherrick ranged widely in securing good clinical sites for student experiences, establishing an affiliation for students at the State Mental Hospital in Warm Springs in 1940, the Tuberculosis Sanitarium of Galen in 1942, and various state and local health departments in 1954. She supported the concept of a career ladder, and a program for registered nurses was a part of the initial program established in 1937. A two-year associate degree program was initiated at the college in 1960, but it moved to a community college in 1965.

Sherrick was an innovative educator. In order to reach students on all of the scattered campuses that made up the program, she established a teleconference hook up. In 1964 she wrote a five-year grant proposal, which was funded by the Division of Nursing, U.S. Public Health Service, to develop further teaching technology using teleconferencing. She directed the project after her retirement in 1965 from her position as director of the school.

Sherrick was active in the Montana Nurses Association and was elected president of the local district several times. In 1946 she served as chair of the Bordeaux Memorial Fund to gather funds to build a memorial to World War I nurses. She served as vice-president and president of the Montana League for Nursing. In 1934 she joined the American Association of University Women and served on several committees. From 1937 to 1970 she was a member of the Bozeman Chamber of Commerce, and an officer at times. She founded the Gallatin County Chapter of the Montana Association for Mental Health. In 1938 she joined the Business and Professional Women's Club, and became a life member in the Montana Education Association. Appointed by the governor in 1935 to the State Board of Nursing, she was elected president of the board in 1936 and remained in that office until 1951.

Voted "Woman of the Year" by the Montana Federation of Business and Professional Women's Clubs in 1969, she also received the outstanding community service award in 1978. Upon her retirement from the university, the president presented her with the Distinguished Service Award. The Montana Public Health Association recognized her with a plaque in 1963 for her achievements and contributions to nursing. In 1965 she received a WICHE Education Award for her service in the cause of higher education in the west.

The nursing building of the university, completed in 1973, was named the Anna Pearl Sherrick Hall in tribute to her pioneering work in the field of nursing education and health care. A life-sized bronze bust by Ed Groenhout was finished in 1976 and mounted in the patio of Sherrick Hall.

Her later retirement years have been spent in travel, in efforts to improve the lives of senior citizens, and quietly at home in Bozeman.

PUBLICATIONS BY ANNA PEARL SHERRICK

BOOKS

Worldwide Events Influencing Nursing in Montana. Bozeman, Mont.: Art Craft, Printers, 1989.

With S.R. Davison and M. Munger. *Nursing in Montana.* Great Falls, Mont.: Tribune Printing, 1962.

With J.M. Claus and J.P. Parker. *The Montana State University School of Nursing: A Story of Professional Development.* Bozeman, Mont.: Big Sky Books, 1976.

With A. Sherrick. *A Pioneer Family in Illinois: Martin and Susannah Sherrick.* 1979.

ARTICLES (SELECTED)

"The Best in Nursing," Bozeman *Daily Chronicle,* February 29, 1984, 4.

"Reflections on My Career and Retirement." *Pulse* (Montana Nurses Association) 22 (June/July 1986): 8, 11.

"Nurturing Nursing." *Montana State Collegian* (Montana State University) 66 (December 1989): 2.

PAMPHLETS (SELECTED)

"The Department of Nursing Montana State College Announces Psychiatric Nursing Program." Warm Springs: Montana State Hospital, September 30, 1940.

With M.B. Ferguson. "Outline Showing the Relation of Nursing History in Montana to World History and to Montana History: 1749–1968." Bozeman: Montana State University, 1968.

BIBLIOGRAPHY

"B & PW Club Names Woman of the Year." *Bozeman Daily Chronicle*, March 16, 1964, 3.

Barkley, S. "1937—Fifty Years of Nursing Education Excellence—1987." In *Alumni Newsletter* (Montana State University College of Nursing) 1987.

Barkley, S. "Recognizing Dr. Anna Pearl Sherrick as a WCHEN Emeritus." Boulder, Colo.: WCHEN, 1985.

Barkley, S., and B. Rogers. "Historical and Social Contributions of MSU College of Nursing in the Development of Nursing in Montana: Roots, Roles and Responsibilities." Bozeman: MSU Telecommunications: Film and Television. 1987.

Barkley, S. "WICHE/WCHEN, Graduate Program and Research in the Development of the College of Nursing." *Alumni Newsletter* (Montana State University College of Nursing), 1986.

Burlingame, M.G. *A History: Montana State University*. Bozeman: Montana State University, 1968.

"Consolidated Deaconess School of Nursing: 1941–1943." Montana State College the Department of Nursing, Bozeman and Great Falls, January 1941.

"Council on Aging Honors Sherrick." *Bozeman Daily Chronicle*, March 14, 1984, 21.

"Dr. Sherrick is 'Woman of the Year'." *Great Falls Tribune*, June 15, 1969.

A History of the Montana Deaconess Hospital School of Nursing. Bozeman: White Caps Montana Deaconess Hospital School of Nursing, 1937.

Interview by J. Terreo with A.P. Sherrick, Bozeman, Montana, January 12, 1990.

Interviews by S. Barkley with various Montana nurses, 1980, 1985, 1987, 1988, 1990.

McCullough, R.S. "Development of Four Pioneer Deaconess Hospital Training Schools for Nurses in Montana—1902–1937." Unpublished master's thesis, Montana State University College of Nursing, 1968–70.

McDonnell, C. L. "Study of the Development of the Montana State College School of Nursing." Unpublished master's thesis, Montana State University College of Nursing, Bozeman, July 1961.

"Nursing Building Dedicated to Dr. Sherrick, Retired Teacher of '72." *Gallatin County Tribune and Belgrade Journal*, June 15, 1972. 12.

Sue Barkley

Cora E. Simpson
c. 1880–c. 1960

Cora E. Simpson was a missionary nurse who was the chief founder of the Nurses' Association of China (NAC) in 1909 and became its first executive secretary in 1922. The concept of nursing was so new to the Chinese when she arrived there in 1907 that there was not even a word in the language for nurse.

Little is known of Simpson's early life except that she was educated in public schools and a ladies' seminary and with private tutors. She entered nurse training at the Methodist Hospital in Omaha, Nebraska, in 1902 and was graduated in 1905 in a class of 11. After graduation, she took courses in theology, Bible, and social services. Later in her career, she added a four-year course in the Chinese language, a government certificate in pharmacy received on the field, and a course in public-health nursing taken at Simmons College in Boston while on furlough.

She traveled to China in 1907 as the first fully qualified nurse to be sent there by the Woman's Board of the Methodist Episcopal Mission of the United States. Motivated by her deep religious fervor, she got a brief introduction to Chinese medicine in a stop at the West Gate Hospital in Shanghai, later known as the Margaret Williamson Hospital.

Simpson continued on to Foochow, where she found no nurses of any kind. The hospital there was a typical one for China at the time: a mud house, with an operating room in the corner of the veranda. The patients wore their own clothes, and relatives came to care for them. Patients brought their own food, and it was commonplace to find a dried fish tied to the foot of a bed and delicacies hidden for security under the covers. Nursing work was regarded as disreputable, and foreign nurses such as Simpson often were told that they were not wanted.

Several weeks after arriving in Foochow, Simpson wrote to Dr. Phillip Cousland regarding the work of nurses in China. The letter and his response were published in the *China Medical Journal* in 1908, along with a call for organization. This was the genesis of the NAC, and Cousland became recognized as its founding father.

A preliminary meeting was held later that year at Kuling, and in 1909 the association was formally organized, with 13 full members and 4 associates. It prospered for a few years but then experienced a decline in members. In 1912 another conference was held at Kuling, with delegates from all over China attending. An education committee was formed to decide on procedures for nursing programs, such as registration, curricula, textbooks, examinations, and diplomas. From that point on, the NAC grew and strengthened, except for a brief period during World War I, when its ranks were depleted by demands elsewhere. It began receiving increasing support from the China Medical Missionary Association.

At NAC's first national conference in 1914 in Shanghai, the first nursing schools were formally established and given registration certificates. In that year a word for "nurse" was added to the Chinese language. In spite of the difficulties of translating text materials into Chinese and integrating procedures with Chinese customs, the first diplomas were awarded in 1915. In 1920 the association began publishing its *Quarterly Journal for Chinese Nurses.*

Meanwhile, Simpson established the Florence Nightingale School of Nursing at the Magaw Memorial Hospital in Foochow and served as superintendent of nurses. The hospital grew into a modern, four-story "hall of healing" and received the first registration certificate issued by the association in 1914.

Simpson adapted the services of her nursing corps to the needs of the community by organizing a special service for lepers, instituting district and school nursing, extending the work of her dispensary, and carrying out special projects, such as health campaigns, baby weeks, and relief work. In 1910 she was the first nurse delegate invited to attend the Medical Conference in China, held that year in Hankow. Her presence there strengthened medical support for the association and the nursing programs. Simpson was active in the Chinese Red Cross nursing committee, and in 1919 it chose her hospital as a center for cholera relief work.

Simpson obtained a release from the Board of Missions to become the first general secretary of the NAC in 1922, the year the association was recognized by the International Council of Nurses. She traveled the land, working out of headquarters in Shanghai, later Peking, and finally Nanking. The addition of a cosecretary soon after her appointment enabled Simpson to extend her services.

Simpson described her often colorful and harrowing adventures in a book, *A Joy Ride Through China for the N.A.C.*, which she published in 1927. The enthusiasm she expressed in it was instrumental in promoting the rapid growth in association membership and the number of schools registered. She donated all profits from the book toward building a new headquarters for the organization, which opened in Nanking with a formal ceremony on June 10, 1937.

Simpson attended the NAC national conference in Canton in 1923 and was a member of the delegation from China attending the International Congress of Nurses in Helsingfors, Finland, in July 1925. She was instrumental in getting the International Congress of Nurses to meet in Peking in 1929.

When political turmoil overtook China, Simpson was one of the last foreigners to leave Nanking. She went to Hong Kong and later Shanghai. Returning to Nanking, she assisted her Chinese cosecretary in helping nursing schools in occupied China give examinations and diplomas. After a six-month furlough in 1941, she was unable to return to Nanking. She proceeded to the Chungking headquarters of the NAC to serve as secretary until ordered by her consulate to return to the United States in December 1944. By the time peace was restored in China, her mission board refused to let her return because of her age.

Simpson remained in the United States, giving speeches about the NAC and her experiences in China. In October 1947 she was honored with the title of general secretary emeritus of the NAC.

In June 1957 she was awarded the Alumni Service Medal of Nebraska Methodist Hospital for her contributions to nursing but was too ill to attend the ceremony. Simpson was one of two graduates honored posthumously for their distinguished careers when the Nebraska Methodist College of Nursing & Applied Health celebrated its centennial in 1991.

PUBLICATIONS BY CORA E. SIMPSON

BOOKS

A Joy Ride Through China for the N.A.C. Shanghai: Kwang Hsueh, 1927.

ARTICLES

"Does China Need Nurses?" *American Journal of Nursing* 14 (December 1913): 191–214.

"A Wireless from China to You!" *American Journal of Nursing* 23 (March 1923): 504–05.

"Examination for Nurses in China." *International Nursing Review* 5 (May 1930): 236–42.

BIBLIOGRAPHY

"Cora E. Simpson, R.N." *British Journal of Nursing* 96 (June 1948): 71–72.

Goodnow, M. *Nursing History.* Philadelphia: Saunders, 1953.

Makers of Nursing History. M.R. Pennock, ed. New York: Lakeside, 1940.

"School Cites Alumnae." *American Journal of Nursing* 57 (August 1957): 984.

Stewart, I.M., and A.L. Austin. *A History of Nursing.* New York: Putnam, 1962.

Alice P. Stein

Margaret Elliot Francis Sirch
1867–1954

Superintendent of nurses at Buffalo General Hospital from 1887 to 1889, Margaret Elliot Francis Sirch established and edited the *Trained Nurse*, the first permanent nursing journal to serve the profession in the United States. After her move to California she helped develop public-health nursing and social services in that state.

Sirch was born at Owen Sound in the Georgian Bay region of Canada in 1867, the daughter of John G. and Catherine (Chisholm) Francis. A descendant of the Vikings, her grandfather was one of the colonists in Virginia who remained loyal to the king during the War of Independence. As a consequence he had to withdraw to Canada, where the family settled on the Niagara River. During her last year of high school Sirch's father died. Throughout her childhood she had shown an inclination to become a nurse, and her mother fully approved of her decision.

Sirch received her diploma from the Buffalo General Hospital School of Nursing in 1887 and served as acting superintendent of the school during her last six months of training. Upon graduation she was asked by the board of trustees to accept the position permanently. She recalled later the 12-hour shifts often lengthened by extra hours or night emergencies, but she was young and healthy and loved her work.

In 1888 she accepted the challenge of establishing and editing the *Trained Nurse*, the first permanent national nursing journal in the country. Sensing the scientific isolation felt by graduate nurses, she discussed the problem with Alfred E. Rose, a Buffalo businessman, who immediately offered to finance such a publication if Sirch would provide the professional content. The first volume of *Trained Nurse* appeared in August 1888, and the lead article gave a historic summary of nursing through the ages, taken from the *Woman's World* and written by Her Royal Highness Princess Christian of Schleswig—Holstein (the daughter of Queen Victoria). In subsequent issues Sirch addressed such issues as the need for pediatric affiliation, continuity of ward service through record keeping, and nursing psychology and education.

The pressure of holding two positions finally led to her resignation from both in 1889. During the next phase of her career she organized three new hospitals, two in New York and a third in Wisconsin. While visiting Chicago in 1894, she accepted an offer to accompany an ill patient abroad and spent a year in France, Germany, and other European countries. Upon her return she was offered another private position wintering in California. She left that position in 1899 to marry Charlemagne Sirch, an electrical engineer, and moved to Arizona.

In 1903 the couple relocated to California, where she continued to watch the progress of her brain child, the *Trained Nurse*. When the journal carried an article on visiting-nurse procedures in 1909, Sirch was stimulated to take a civil service examination to enter public-health nursing, and in 1910 when the state of California passed a law making married women eligible for public employment, she was appointed staff nurse with the Los Angeles City Department of Health. In 1913 she became the first chief nurse of the newly established Bureau of Nursing in the department, and in 1915 the California Board of Charities and Correction, later the Department of Social Welfare, offered her the position of agent. The department grew and expanded under her direction, and standards were set up for custodial institutions, children's hospitals and day nurseries. Her reports helped change unsanitary institutions into modern hospitals and also influenced state laws regulating children's institutions, schools, and homes.

To all her activities Sirch brought energy, efficiency, and organizational ability. When she retired in January 1937 at the compulsory age of 70, she was district supervisor of all the territory south of Tehachapi. In an interview after her retirement, she reflected upon an offer by Dr. Roswell Park, the Buffalo cancer specialist and founder of Roswell Park Institute, in 1887 to work in his bacteriological laboratory. The offer appealed to her, but she also liked her work as a nurse. The decision to be a nursing school superintendent was decided by the toss of a penny.

Sirch died on July 17, 1954, at the age of 91 after spending the last year of her life in a California nursing home.

PUBLICATIONS BY MARGARET ELLIOT FRANCIS SIRCH

Editorials. *Trained Nurse* (1888–89).

"Municipal Nursing—Some of Its Problems." *Public Health Nurse Quarterly* 8 (July 1916): 41–54.

BIBLIOGRAPHY

"In Memory of Our First Editor." *Nursing World* 128 (September 1954): 17.

Obituary. *American Journal of Nursing* 54 (October 1954): 1198.

Pennock, M.R. *Makers of Nursing History.* New York: Lakeside, 1940.

Potemkina, A. "Meet the First Editor." *Trained Nurse and Hospital Review* 100 (April 1938): 345–51.

Lilli Sentz

Jessie C. Sleet (Scales)

ca. 1875–1950

Jessie C. Sleet (Scales) was the first known graduate black nurse to be appointed as a district public-health nurse. The difficulties that she overcame, including racial prejudice and employment discrimination, reflect her personal resolution to pursue a career in a nursing specialty to which she felt especially committed but which had not previously been open to black nurses. By achieving this professional goal, which extended beyond the accepted social norm of the day, she expanded the opportunities for both her black contemporaries in nursing and for future generations of black nurses who succeeded her in district nursing.

Sleet was born in Stratford, Ontario, Canada, about 1875 and received her initial education there. She entered the nursing school at Provident Hospital in Chicago in 1893. Provident was one of the first hospitals to provide medical care for the black community in Chicago and gained further distinction when Dr. Daniel Hal Williams performed the first recorded operation on the human pericardium at this institution.

After graduating in 1895, in the fourth class to complete the nursing program at Provident Hospital School of Nursing, Jessie Sleet enrolled in a special course of instruction under Dr. Williams, who was teaching at Freedman's Hospital in Washington, D.C. She initially worked as a private-duty nurse for two seasons in a winter health resort located in Lakewood, New Jersey, but felt drawn to a career in public health and subsequently traveled to New York City and sought a position in public-health nursing there.

Sleet's appointment as a public-health nurse in 1900 was only achieved by her persistence in seeking such an employment opportunity. She initially discovered that not one of the existing public-health or district nursing organizations in New York City employed black nurses as district nurses. Undaunted by the employment discrimination she encountered during the numerous interviews for district nursing positions for which she applied, she continued her quest for such a position over the next several years. She was eventually able to elicit the support of Dr. Edward T. Devine, the general secretary of the Charity Organization Society in New York City. She was employed by the society on the personal recommendation of Devine, for an initial two-month trial basis, beginning on October 3, 1900.

Sleet's public-health assignment was under the auspices of the Tuberculosis Committee of the Charity Organization Society, which later was reorganized as the New York Tuberculosis Association. This special committee was especially concerned with the high morbidity and mortality rates in New York City's black population.

Sleet's responsibilities included home health visits to encourage members of the black community who were ill to seek recommended medical treatment. A brief self-authored account of her experiences as a district nurse was published by one of her supervisors in the *American Journal of Nursing* in 1901. In this report Sleet included several elucidative case studies and outlined the services that she had rendered during a two-month period of community outreach, which included house-to-house visits in the black community in New York City.

She provided such competent care as a district nurse that her temporary position was extended beyond the trial period, and she was offered a permanent position as a district nurse with the society a year later. Sleet continued in that position as a district nurse for the next nine years until she resigned to marry John R. Scales in 1910.

Jessie Sleet Scales died in November 1950, after spending the last fifteen years of her life bedridden. Despite her illness she continued to be an influential member of her family.

Additional details of her private life and involvement in nursing do not appear to be publically available after her marriage. She assisted in the training of her successor, Cecile Batey Anderson, at the request of Dr. Devine, before she resigned from her district nursing position; in so doing she assured that succeeding generations of black nurses would find that public-health nursing remained a viable career option.

PUBLICATIONS BY
JESSIE C. SLEET (SCALES)

"A Successful Experiment." *American Journal of Nursing* 1 (1901): 729–31.

BIBLIOGRAPHY

"Breaking the Barrier." *New York State Nurses Association Report* 21 (January/February 1990): 5.

Carnegie, M.E. *The Path We Tread: Blacks in Nursing 1854–1984* Philadelphia: Lippincott, 1986.

Colon, J.D. "Letters to the Editor." *New York State Nurses Association Report* 21 (March 1990): 5.

Elmore, J.A. "Black Nurses: Their Service and Their Struggle." *American Journal of Nursing* 76 (March 1976): 435–37.

Morais, H.M. *The History of the Negro in Medicine.* New York: Publishers Co., 1969.

Staupers, M.K. "The Negro Nurse in America." *Opportunity: Journal of Negro Life* 15 (November 1937): 339–41, 349.

Staupers, M.K. *No Time for Prejudice: A Story of Negroes in Nursing in the United States.* New York: Macmillan, 1961.

Thoms, A.B. *Pathfinders: A History of the Progress of the Colored Graduate Nurse.* New York: Kay, 1929.

Karen L. Buchinger

Sarah E. Sly

1870–1944

Sarah E. Sly was the first interstate secretary of the American Nurses' Association (ANA) and served as its president from 1911–13. She was president of the Michigan State Nurses Association during the time it was campaigning for the establishment of state registration for nurses. She also was an outspoken advocate of a sliding pay scale for nurses.

Sly was born in Bloomfield Township, Michigan, on March 24, 1870, the daughter of George and Jane Clendenning Sly. Her father was a Bloomfield native and a fruit farmer; her mother an Irish immigrant.

After graduating from the Farrand Training School, Harper Hospital, Detroit, in 1898, Sly spent several years on the staff of Pennsylvania Hospital, Philadelphia, and a short period as a private-duty nurse. When health problems prevented her from continuing in nursing practice, she entered organization work.

She helped smooth the transition of the Nurses' Associated Alumnae of the United States to become the ANA in 1911. During her tenure as interstate secretary she unified the organizational structure so that the state group became the membership unit. She also served for 15 years on the board of directors of the *American Journal of Nursing*, part of that time as its president.

Sly was general secretary of the Michigan State Nurses Association in 1923, during its biennial celebration. Later, in addition to being president, she also served it as a councillor. She was a member of the committee to write by-laws for the International Council of Nurses.

Suffering from nephritis, diabetes, and arteriosclerosis, she retired to the family fruit farm near Bloomfield to live with her sister, Addie Sly, in 1943. She died there on May 27, 1944, of multiple disorders.

BIBLIOGRAPHY

American Nurses' Association Collection. Untitled typescript, Mugar Memorial Library, Boston University, Boston.

Flanagan, L. *One Strong Voice.* Kansas City, MO.: American Nurses' Association, 1976.

Obituary. *American Journal of Nursing.* 44 (July 1944); 718.

Alice P. Stein

Martha Ruth Smith

1894–1960

Martha Ruth Smith was founding director of the Boston University's Division of Nursing Education, established in 1939, and the first dean of the Boston University School of Nursing, established in 1946. She was an early advocate of integrating theory and practice into nursing programs and was coauthor of an influential nursing text.

The daughter of Frank A. and (Wanen?) S. Smith, Smith was born on November 14, 1894, in Lebanon, New Hampshire. Her father was a physician. She graduated from Lebanon High School in 1913 and went on to attend the University of Wisconsin in the 1914–15 year. She then entered the Peter Bent Brigham Hospital School of Nursing in Boston, from which she graduated in 1919. At graduation she was appointed a head nurse at her alma mater, and in 1920 she served briefly as a superintendent there before leaving to become resident school nurse at the Kimball Union Academy in Meriden, New Hampshire, a position she held for about a year. From 1921–23 she was an instructor at the Samaritan Hospital School of Nursing in Troy, New York. In 1924 she received her B.A. from Teachers College, Columbia University, after which she became an instructor at the Massachusetts General Hospital School of Nursing in Boston. For seven years (1929–35) she served as an instructor of nursing education at Teachers College, Columbia University, and in 1931 she received her M.A. from that institution. She returned to Boston in 1935 as instructor in the School of Nursing at Simmons College as well as assistant principal of Massachusetts General Hospital School of Nursing. In 1939 she was appointed professor of nursing education at the Boston University School of Education and director of the Division of Nursing Education. When the division was established as a separate School of Nursing, Smith was appointed dean, a position she held from 1946–63.

Smith seized upon the recommendation of the *Goldmark Report* (1923) emphasizing that nurses have an understanding of nursing theory as well as practice, and as supervisor of instruction at Massachusetts General Hospital School of Nursing, she encouraged the adoption of such ideas. While at Teachers College she and her colleagues integrated theory and practices into a textbook, *An Introduction to the Principles of Nursing Care*, for which she served as general editor. The text was widely used. She also developed a procedure manual and a system for evaluating student practice and attempted to provide students with a coherent rotation through the various clinical specialties in order to ensure students a reasonable amount of classroom time.

Under her leadership the Boston University School of Nursing moved to a position of leadership in nursing. In the school's first class of 170 were 125 veterans of World War II on the G.I. Bill. Continually seeking to update her skills, Smith periodically enrolled in special courses. Among them was a four-month course with the Visiting Nurse Association of Boston and a special program in mental hygiene and psychiatric nursing at Butler Hospital in Providence, Rhode Island.

Smith held various offices and assignments in the National League of Nursing Education, the American Nurses' Association, and the American Red Cross Nursing Service and was active in Pi Lambda Theta and Sigma Theta Tau. Upon her retirement from Boston University in 1955, she was named dean emeritus. She died August 21, 1960.

PUBLICATIONS BY MARTHA RUTH SMITH

BOOKS

Suggested Teaching Outline for Use with An Introduction. Philadelphia: Lippincott, 1937. 2nd ed., 1939; 2nd ed. rev., 1946.

Editor. *An Introduction to the Principles of Nursing Care.* Philadelphia: Lippincott, 1937.

ARTICLES

With M.E. Newman. "The Nursing School Goes to the Community." *Public Health Nurse* 35 (February 1943): 107–09.

BIBLIOGRAPHY

"Boston University Establishes School of Nursing." *American Journal of Nursing* 46 (September 1946): 420.

"Boston University Opens School of Nursing." *American Journal of Nursing* 47 (June 1947): 420.

"Dean Emeritus of Boston University Dies." *Nursing Outlook* 8 (November 1960): 583.

Martha Smith Collection. Nursing Archives, Mugar Memorial Library, Boston University, Boston.

Vern L. Bullough

Brother Camillus Snyder

1897–1984

Brother Camillus Snyder was dedicated to helping the Alexian Brothers care for the sick and poor. His thorough and diverse education allowed him to work in many areas, and his leadership qualities brought him positions as a nursing educator, assistant superior, and provincial.

Brother Camillus was born in Fremont, Ohio, on March 17, 1897, to John Franklin Snyder and Ellen House Snyder. There were five children in the family—three boys and two girls. Brother Camillus entered the order of Alexian Brothers on September 1, 1917. He took his first vows on March 19, 1918, and his final professional vows on March 19, 1925. He had the rare distinction of serving in every province of the Alexian Brothers order.

Brother Camillus began his medical education at the Dr. Kirk School of Laboratory Technology in 1921. He then studied nursing at the Alexian Brothers School of Nurses in Chicago. He passed the Illinois Nursing State Board Examination in May 1925 and became a registered nurse. In addition, he took special courses in biological science at St. Louis University. His diverse education allowed him to work as a registered nurse, a laboratory and x-ray technician, and an apprentice pharmacist. More importantly, his education allowed him to gain experience in all facets of health care, and thus he was an asset to the Alexian Brothers and to the nursing profession.

Brother Camillus began his career as a laboratory technician at the Alexian Brothers Hospital in Elizabeth, New Jersey. He then spent nine years at the order's hospital in St. Louis, where he was the first director of the School of Nursing. From 1932–35, Brother Camillus was sent to Germany to serve the order in its province there as a Laboratory Technician and a supervisor of the pharmacy at the Maria Hilf Hospital. He later stated, concerning that time period, that Hitler "received a vote of confidence from the German people" and he realized that "the handwriting was on the wall and that World War II was inevitable." He was allowed to return to the United States and worked as a laboratory technician in Chicago. After World War II the hospital of the Alexian Brothers in London underwent reconstruction, and Brother Camillus was asked to help. He was given the position of superior, and he helped reorganize many programs within the hospital. He returned to the United States in 1948 and spent the next 18 years working in Elizabeth, New Jersey, Chicago, and Elk Grove Village, Illinois. In 1966 he was appointed to the administrative board of the order in Chicago. His final assignment was in San Jose, California, on the central service staff. He retired in 1970, and in 1978 he moved to the Alexian Brothers Resort at Signal Mountain, Tennessee.

Brother Camillus Snyder died of diabetes mellites and an acute myocardial infarction at the Alexian Brothers Health Center, at Signal Mountain, on March 15, 1984. He has been described as a "keen cultured man who had an appreciation for good reading and good music. . . . He nurtured his talent for learning and was interested in furthering the work of the congregation in their care and concern for the sick."

BIBLIOGRAPHY

Archives. PRO-7.B, SS 134.4. Alexian Brothers Immaculate Conception Province, Elk Grove Village, Illinois.

Brother Roy Godwin

Eugenia Kennedy Spalding

1896–1978

Eugenia Kennedy Spalding is best remembered by her book *Professional Adjustments in Nursing*, which oriented several generations of American nurses to the roles and standards of the profession in the 1940s and early 1950s. She was the first lay teacher and the second member of the faculty at the Catholic University of America School of Nursing.

Spalding was the fourth of six children born to John B. and Anastasia (Hickey) Kennedy. She was born on October 19, 1896, in Lawrenceburg, Indiana. Her parents had immigrated to the United States from Ireland in 1877. She and her siblings (Margaret, John, Emmerett, Flora, and Daniel) were raised on the family farm and attended the local schools in Lawrenceburg.

The summer of 1915 after graduating from high school Spalding entered Moores Hill College, Moores Hill, Indiana, for teacher training. Upon completion, she taught elementary school in Bonnell, Indiana, for the school year 1915–16, after which she entered St. Vincent's Hospital School of Nursing, (Indianapolis) which was a three-year program. During her nursing school years she earned six credits in histology from Indiana University at Bloomington and eight credits in pathology from the Indiana University School of Medicine, Indianapolis.

When she graduated in 1919, she worked at St. Vincent's Hospital as a librarian and lab technician. In 1921, she became an assistant director and teacher of nursing at St. Vincent's School of Nursing. She remained in this position until 1929, when she was appointed as the education director of the Indiana State Board of Examination and Registration of Nurses. She also held the office of executive secretary for the Indiana State Nurses Association during 1929–31.

Spalding entered Teachers College, Columbia University, in 1931, to begin work on her bachelor of science degree. Upon graduation in 1932, she began work on a master of arts degree, which she completed in 1934. During this time she was contacted by Sister Olivia Gowan to assist with the establishment of the Catholic University of America's School of Nursing. Not only did she develop a curriculum for the school, but she became the school's first lay instructor.

On January 7, 1932, she married Dr. George Spalding; they had no children. Spalding taught at the Catholic University of America until 1941, at which time she was granted a leave of absence to serve as a member of the U.S. Public Health Service

(USPHS) during World War II. She was a senior nursing education consultant for the service from 1941–42. In 1942 she became the associate director in charge of standards for the U.S. Cadet Nurse Corps program. In this position she directed many studies. One of these consisted of a survey of the marine hospitals of the USPHS. She also served as coordinator of staff education for the Office of Nursing, USPHS, from 1943–45.

In February 1946 she returned to Catholic University of America as an associate professor until she left in October 1946 to be professor of nursing and director of nursing education at the School of Nursing Education at Indiana University, Bloomington. Spalding returned to Teachers College, Columbia University, in 1950, first as an associate professor and later professor until her retirement in August 1959 as professor emeritus.

Following her retirement, Spalding spent several months in Istanbul, Turkey, directing an educational survey that led to the establishment of higher education programs for nursing. This survey was sponsored by the International Cooperation Administration of the United States and Teachers College, Columbia University.

The years 1960–62 Spalding was very active in numerous professional organizations and served on many committees. Her positions included secretary for the District of Columbia League for Nursing; national member of the National League for Nursing; secretary for the District of Columbia Graduate Nurses Association; national member of the American Nurses' Association; national member of Sigma Theta Tau; national member of Pi Gamma Mu; and national member of Pi Lambda Theta. Spalding served as a consultant to the American Nurses' Association on federal aid to nursing education and as a consultant for curriculum on the committee for state boards for flexible standards for nursing education. She chaired the Joint Committee of the Graduate Nurses Association (D.C.) and the League for Nurses (D.C.) to prepare suggestions for D.C. commissioners to launch a program provided through the D.C. Practical

Nurses Licensing Act. She was also a member of the Committee on Legislation for the Graduate Nurses Association (D.C.); member of the Woman's Joint Congressional Committee; member of the Committee on Practical Nurses Education for the League for Nurses (D.C.); chair of the subcommittee on Professional Adjustments and the Committee on Programs for the League for Nursing Education (D.C.); chaired the Working and Advisory Committee on Ethical Standards for the American Nurses' Association; a member of the board of directors of the *American Journal of Nursing*; member of the Central Curriculum Committee and its subcommittee on program of studies; and chair of the Production Committee on Ethics and Professional Problems Subcommittee for the (D.C.) National League of Nursing Education. She was also a member of the American Association of University Professors, the International Council of Catholic Nurses, and the editorial board of the Teachers College *Record*.

During these same years Spalding was a visiting professor at the Catholic University of America and was involved with several committees for the School of Nursing. She was a member of the Advanced Committee on Curriculum Study; chairperson of the Committee on General Studies and Criteria for Improving the Curriculum Design of the Graduate Instruction Program; chairperson of the Committee on Beliefs about Curriculum Design and Curriculum Improvement of the Graduate Instruction Program; and member of the Committee on Beliefs about Consultation in Nursing.

Spalding was the recipient of an honorary doctor of humane letters by Keuka College (New York) in 1944 for her contributions towards outstanding work in the development of regional nursing education programs in New York during World War II. She also received a special citation from the Indiana State Nurses Association in recognition of her contributions to nursing in Indiana. In addition, she was an honorary member of the International Mark Twain Society in recognition of her writings and an honorary member of the nursing and writer's association. Her bi-ography appears in several *Who's Who*, including the first edition of *Who's Who of American Women*.

During her career Spalding wrote many books and publications on nursing education. In addition, she traveled extensively in Europe, and in 1957 she was educational leader for a travel tour during which the health services were studied in Italy, Switzerland, Germany, Belgium, and England.

Spalding retired from the Catholic University of America in 1962 and remained in Washington, D.C., until her death on December 17, 1978. Spalding was truly a national leader in nursing education.

PUBLICATIONS BY EUGENIA KENNEDY SPALDING

BOOKS

A Suggested Vocational Guidance Program for Schools of Nursing. New York: National League of Nursing Education, 1935.

Professional Adjustments in Nursing; Being Professional. Philadelphia: Lippincott, 1939.

Professional Adjustments in Nursing; For Senior Students and Graduates. Philadelphia: Lippincott, 2nd ed. 1941; 3rd ed. 1946, 4th ed. 1950.

Professional Nursing; Trends and Adjustments. Philadelphia: Lippincott, 1950.

Professional Nursing; Trends and Relationships, 5th ed. Philadelphia: Lippincott, 1954.

Professional Nursing; Trends, Responsibilities, and Relationships. Philadelphia: Lippincott, 1959.

Nursing Legislation and Education; a Study of the Role of National Governments and Voluntary Nursing Associations. Washington, D.C.: Catholic University of America, 1963.

Professional Nursing; Foundations, Perspectives, and Relationships. Philadelphia: Lippincott, 1965.

With L.E. Notter. *Professional Nursing; Foundations, Perspectives, and Relationships*, 9th ed. Philadelphia: Lippincott, 1976.

MONOGRAPHS

A Suggested Vocational Guidance Program for Schools of Nursing. New York: National League of Nursing Education, 1935.

Symposium on Clinical Experience in Medical and Surgical Nursing in the Providence Division of the School of Nursing Education. The Catholic University of America, School of Nursing Education. Washington, D.C.: University of America Press, 1940.

The Public Health Nursing Curriculum Guide.
New York: National Organization for Public
Health Nursing, 1942.

*Faculty Positions in Schools of Nursing and
How to Prepare Them.* New York: National
League of Nursing Education, 1946.

Guidance Program for Schools of Nursing. New
York: National League of Nursing Education,
1946.

*Survey Methods Applied to Schools of Nursing
and Hospital Nursing Services.* Nursing Education Monograph No. 2. Bloomington: Indiana University Bookstore, 1948.

Editor. *What Should Indiana Plan in Relation
to Recommendations in Nursing for the Future.* Nursing Education Monograph No. 4.
Bloomington: Indiana University Bookstore,
1949.

*Financial Problems in Schools of Nursing,
Hospital Nursing Services and Public
Health Nursing Agencies.* Nursing Education Monograph No. 3. Bloomington: Indiana University Bookstore, 1949.

*Nursing Organization Curriculum Conference:
Report of Proceedings of Conference De-
cember 3, 4, 5, 1949.* Curriculum Bulletin
No. 1. New York: National League of Nursing
Education, 1950.

*A Checklist on Abilities Needed by Nurses:
With Suggestions for Continued Curricu-
lum Study.* New York; National League of
Nursing Education, December 1951.

*Joint Nursing Curriculum Conference: Curricu-
lum Bulletin No. 2.* New York: National
League of Nursing Education, 1951.

Problems of Graduate Nurse Education. Working Conference Report No. 2. New York: Bureau of Publications, Teachers College, Columbia University, 1952.

*Work Conference on the Basic Nursing Curric-
ulum in Transition.* Work Conference Report No. 3. New York: Bureau of Publications,
Teachers College, Columbia University,
1953.

Education for Nursing in Wisconsin. New York:
Institute of Research and Service in Nursing
Education, Teachers College, Columbia Uni-
versity, 1955.

*A Look at Education for Nursing: Past, Present,
and Future.* New York, National League for
Nursing, 1959.

With M. Bridgman, et al. *Report of the Survey of
Education in Nursing at Louisiana State
University, May 18–28, 1952.* New Orleans:
Department of Nursing Education, Louisi-
ana State University, 1952.

With E. Kum, K. Sehl, R. Tuzun, and P. Velioglu.
*Report of the Educational Survey Prelimi-
nary to Establishment of the Florence
Nightingale Higher Educational Program
for Nursing: Istanbul, Turkey.* New York:

Teachers College, Columbia University,
1960.

ARTICLES (SELECTED)

"Bedside Nursing." *American Journal of Nursing* 30, No. 3 (A30): 289.

"Discussion: Education Preparation for Supervision." *Hospital Progress* 27, No. 12 (1936):
437.

"How to Secure a Position." *American Journal
of Nursing* 37, No. 5 (1937): 499–502.

"The Bolton Act Provides Federal Funds for
Post Graduate Programs." *American Journal of Nursing* 43, No. 9 (1943): 833–35.

"The College and Centralization of Nursing Instruction." *American Journal of Nursing* 43,
No. 2 (1943): 195–201.

"The Senior Cadet Nurse." *American Journal of
Nursing* 43, No. 8 (1943): 749–51.

"Contractual Agreements." *American Journal
of Nursing* 44, No. 4 (1944): 385–87.

"What do Shortages Mean?" *American Journal
of Nursing* 44, No. 4 (1944): 379–80.

"Your Problems as a Nurse and a Woman and
Their Solution." *American Journal of Nursing* 44, No. 10 (1944): 945–49.

"Orientation of Nursing Students." *American
Journal of Nursing* 45, No. 12 (1945): 1047–
50.

"The Student Nurse in this Postwar Period and
Her Guidance." *Report of Institute for Directors and Nurses.* Emmitsburg, Md.: St. Joseph's Central House, April 1946.

"Trends and Problems in Advanced Nursing
Education." *American Journal of Nursing*
47, No. 2 (1947): 113–15.

"Appraising Basic Collegiate Programs in Nursing." *American Journal of Nursing* 50, No.
12 (1950): 796–98.

"Current Problems of Nurse Educators."
Teachers College Record 57: 38–46.

"Progress Reports: Joint Committee of Graduate Nurses' Association (D.C.) and League
for Nursing to Prepare Preliminary Suggestions for the Commissioners Relating to
Rules & Regulations to Launch Operation of
the D.C. Practical Nurses Act, Public Law
(86–708, S1870)." *Quarterly Review* (1960).

"Comprehensive Evaluation of an Educational
Program in a Hospital School of Nursing."
Hospital Progress 42, No. 1 (1961): 72–73,
112–14.

"New Directions in Preservice Education for
Nursing." *Nursing Outlook* 10, No. 8 (1962):
239–42.

With J. Bartsch. "Nursing-Problem Clinic: Handling the Problems that Violate Ethics."
Registered Nurse 25, No. 5 (1962): 42–46,
100–05.

With S.M. Sturtevant. "A Suggestion Toward Vocational Guidance Within the School of Nursing." *American Journal of Nursing* 35, No. 1 (1935): 67–69

BIBLIOGRAPHY

Defferrari, R.J., *Memoirs of The Catholic University of America, 1918–1960.* Boston: Daughters of St. Paul, 1961.

Faculty File of Mrs. Eugenia Kennedy Spalding (1934). Archives, Catholic University of America, Washington, D.C.

Gowan, O., and R. Bergeron. *The Development of Professional Nursing at The Catholic University of America, 1932–1958.* Duluth, Minn.: College of St. Scholastica, 1967.

Obituary. *Washington Post,* December 21, 1978.

Obituary. *Washington Star,* December 21, 1978.

Who's Who of American Women, 1958/1959. Wilmette, Ill.: Marquis, 1958.

Sandra A. Nagy
Rosemary T. McCarthy

Marietta Burtis Squire

1868–1933

Known as the "Mother of Nursing in New Jersey," Marietta Burtis Squire was one of the state's pioneer professional nurses.

Squire was born in Rahway, New Jersey, on October 20, 1868, the first of four children of Benjamin and Maria L. (Crowell) Squire. Her father, a tea merchant, and her mother were descendants of some of New Jersey's original settlers.

Her family valued education, and she attended the Friend's Select School, Rahway High School, and Miss William's School for Young Ladies. This education was interrupted by the death of her father, which profoundly affected the family, forcing them to move from Rahway to Newark. Unable to afford college, Squire entered the training school at Orange Memorial Hospital (Orange, N.J.) in 1885, graduating from the two-year program at the age of 19 in November 1887. She was to return to Orange Memorial briefly, 1906–07,

to serve as the superintendent during a reorganization period.

Squire said that she never regretted the interruption to her education that carried her into nursing instead of Vassar. Like most other trained graduate nurses she sought private-duty cases immediately following graduation. She spent 24 of her 41 years of nursing practice as a private-duty nurse. But from 1893 until 1901 she was employed as a faculty member and nurse at Miss Dana's School in Morristown. Thus Marietta B. Squire is considered the first school nurse in New Jersey.

A charter member of the New Jersey State Nurses Association (NJSNA) in 1901, she was very active in that organization's formative years. She served as a delegate to several early American Nurses' Association conventions. Squire was also involved in the Private Duty Section, which was created in 1925. She was also a charter member of the New Jersey League of Nursing Education, and she actively pursued higher educational standards for nursing schools.

Squire was appointed by Governor Woodrow Wilson to the first New Jersey Board of Nurse Examiners in 1912. Her application was the very first for licensure as a registered nurse in New Jersey. She was elected as the president of the Board of Nurse Examiners and served in that role for seven years. Under her guidance the board developed New Jersey's first curriculum guidelines, for which requests were received from across the country.

She addressed the American Nurses' Association convention in 1913 on nursing registration laws. Noting that 30 of 39 states with registration laws had permissive (rather than mandatory) licensure laws, she felt that more statistical studies needed to be done on the effects of such laws before conclusions could be drawn.

Because of her long-term involvement in NJSNA, she was asked to compile the history of the association for the twentieth and twenty-fifth anniversaries. She had planned to expand the organization's history into the history of nursing in New Jersey, but it was unfinished when she died and her manuscript was never recovered.

Squire's last nursing position was as the welfare director and nurse at Gimbels department store in New York City. She held this position from 1920–28; the store's employees referred to her as "our nurse."

In May 1932 Squire was placed on the Endowment Fund Honor List of the New Jersey State Federation of Women's Clubs in recognition of her many years of service to that organization, for which she served as the first delegate from the NJSNA. She was also active in the Guild of St. Barnabas for Nurses and was a contributing member of the New Jersey Historical Society.

Squire died of cancer on December 21, 1933, at Orange Memorial Hospital at the age of 65. The *New York Times* obituary called her the "Mother of Nursing in New Jersey," a tribute to her influence on professional nursing in the state.

PUBLICATIONS BY MARIETTA BURTIS SQUIRE

"Is compulsory registration desirable and how may it be obtained?" *American Journal of Nursing* 13 (September 1913): 955–57.

BIBLIOGRAPHY

Archives. New Jersey Board of Nursing, New Jersey State Archives, Trenton.

Archives. New Jersey State Nurses Association, Trenton.

"Marietta B. Squire." Obituary. *American Journal of Nursing* 34 (February 1934): 199–200.

"Marietta B. Squire." Obituary. *East Orange Record,* December 29, 1933.

"Marietta B. Squire." Obituary. *New York Times,* December 23, 1933.

Some Account of The Orange Training School. Orange, N.J., 1899.

Janet L. Fickeissen

Mabel Keaton Staupers

1890–1989

(See *Volume 1, pp. 295–97.*)

Mabel Keaton Staupers, a leader in racially integrating the nursing profession in the United States, died on September 30, 1989, of pneumonia at her home in Washington, D.C. She was 99.

Staupers was the first executive secretary of the National Association of Colored Graduate Nurses and helped to found the National Council of Negro Women in 1935.

BIBLIOGRAPHY

"Mabel Staupers, 99, Who Led Black Nurses." Obituary. *New York Times* October 6, 1989.

Beatrice Van Homrigh Stevenson

1874–1948

Beatrice Van Homrigh Stevenson, a hospital administrator and crusader for higher professional status for nurses, lobbied for over 40 years in Albany, New York, on behalf of bills favorable to the nursing profession in the state. She was instrumental in gaining passage of the New York State Nurse Practice Act. She supported establishment of the Army Nurse Corps and, after serving in the Spanish-American War, sought admission of Red Cross nurses into the United States Spanish-American War Veterans Organization. At the national convention of the National League of Nursing Education in 1914, she delivered a landmark address, "Organization of Nurses for a Landmark Campaign." She held several offices including that of president in the New York State Nurses Association and designed its seal.

Educated also in the law, Stevenson was a leading suffragist, a Republican Party leader, and a highly vocal advocate for many other causes. She spent the last 13 years of her administrative career as superintendent of nurses at Welfare Island Hospital in New York City.

(Marie) Beatrice Van Homrigh was born in Killashee, Ireland, on November 19, 1874, to Lt. Col. Alexander P. and Bessie Dundas Van Homrigh. During her childhood her father served in Malta, Gibralter, and other places, but she attended private schools in England. Her father died when she was 11 and her mother three years later.

At age 15 Stevenson expressed a desire to enter nursing but was too young to be admitted to a training program. She worked as a companion to invalids and came to the United States in 1892 in the employ of the William Bennet family of Blacksburg, Virginia.

In 1896 she graduated from the City Hospital School of Nursing on Blackwell's Island (later Welfare Island), New York City. She did private-duty nursing until the outbreak of the Spanish-American War, when she applied for U.S. citizenship and was accepted as a Red Cross nurse. She served on the hospital ship *Lampasas* off Puerto Rico from April through early August 1898, when her service was cut short by typhoid fever.

Recovered from her illness, she did private-duty nursing again until February 2, 1902, when she became the bride of another Spanish-American War veteran, Charles G. Stevenson. He was a New York attorney, and the couple moved to Brooklyn, where they lived the rest of their lives.

Stevenson worked with Jane Delano in the early years of the American Red Cross Nursing Service. She taught Red Cross home nursing in Brooklyn, beginning in 1908, and later sponsored the introduction of Red Cross courses on the subject in the public schools.

She served on the New York State Red Cross Committee and was a charter member of the Brooklyn committee, organized in 1910. Over the next seven years she spoke and wrote widely on behalf of the recruitment of Red Cross nurses. During World War I she became known as "Mrs. Red Cross." At that time she was chairperson of the advisory committee of the Red Cross Center of the New York County Chapter of the ARC.

She was president of the New York State Nurses Association from 1913–14 and vice-president and chair of the legislative committee from 1916–17. She chaired the legislative committees of District 13 of the New York State Nurses Association and the Alumnae Association of the City

Hospital School of Nursing during World War II. She had a special fondness for the City Hospital group, was active in many of its committees, and wrote for its journal throughout her career.

In 1915–16 she attended the New York University women's law class and specialized in constitutional law. She was a charter member of its alumnae association.

Stevenson was named superintendent of nurses of the correction hospital on Welfare Island (later moved to Rikers Island) in 1935 and received a letter of commendation from the commissioner of correction. Beginning in 1944, she served on the Civil Service Committee of the New York State Nurses Association and crusaded for improved pay and working conditions for nurses in public hospitals. During World War II she perceived a growing role for unions in promoting improved conditions for nurses and became active in the Nurses Guild of the American Federation of Labor.

She died at her Brooklyn home on March 12, 1948, the 86th birthday of her old friend, Jane Delano. She was buried in Oakwood Cemetery, Troy, New York, beside her husband, who had died in 1934. The September 1948 issue of the *Alumnae Journal* of the City Hospital School of Nursing was dedicated to her memory and contains a memoir written by her son, Charles G. Stevenson, and daughter, Cornelia Stevenson Clark.

PUBLICATIONS BY BEATRICE VAN HOMRIGH STEVENSON

"The Red Cross Nurse Corps." *Trained Nurse* 38 (February 1907): 73–75.

"A Visit to the *Solace*, the Hospital Ship of the United States Navy." *American Journal of Nursing* 10 (December 1910): 84–87.

"Organization of Nurses for a Legislative Campaign." *NLNE: Annual Report, 1914, and Proceedings of the 20th Convention.* Baltimore: Williams and Wilkins, 1914.

"American Prison Hospitals." *Trained Nurse* 98 (April 1937): 351–54.

BIBLIOGRAPHY

"Mrs. Beatrice Van Homrigh Stevenson." *American Journal of Nursing* 48 (May 1948): 48 adv.

"Mrs. C. Stevenson, Suffragist, Dies." *New York Times*, March 14, 1948.

Stevenson, C.G., and C.S. Clark. "Beatrice Van Homrigh Stevenson." *Alumnae Journal, City Hospital School of Nursing* (September 1948): 5–20.

Alice P. Stein

Anne Hervey Strong

1876–1925

An early leader in public-health nursing, Anne Hervey Strong was the first director of the School of Public Health Nursing at Simmons College, Boston, where she gave special attention to the correlation of practical and theoretical learning in the education of nurses.

Strong was born on January 1876 in Wakefield, Massachusetts, to Rear Admiral Edward T. and Anna G. Hervey Strong. The family was among the first settlers of the area. During her early schooling Strong became proficient in the classics, French, astronomy, and navigation. She also showed an interest in caring for the sick and considered a career as a physician. She graduated from Bryn Mawr College in 1898. During convalescence from a back injury at Albany (New York) Hospital and a later period of invalidism, Strong decided to become a nurse. She entered the Albany Hospital Training School for Nurses in 1903 and at graduation in 1906 became an instructor and supervisor there. However, the work proved too strenuous, and she was forced to resign.

She accepted a post as an instructor in mathematics at the Mary C. Wheeler School in Providence, Rhode Island, in 1907 and served as assistant principal from 1913–14. During the summers she worked as a volunteer and staff nurse at the Henry Street Settlement Nursing Service in New York City.

In 1913 she began studies in the Department of Nursing Education at Teachers College, Columbia University, choosing public-health nursing as her specialty. The following year, under the patronage of Mary Adelaide Nutting, she became an instructor in public-health nursing there.

In 1916 she was appointed assistant professor in a program cosponsored by Simmons College and the Instructive District Nursing Association of Boston. During that year she divided her professional time between New York and Boston.

When the School of Public Health Nursing was started at Simmons in 1918, Strong was named director and professor. During a tenure that lasted until 1925, she organized a five-year bachelor of science program in connection with Children's, Massachusetts General, and Peter Bent Brigham hospitals. To help unify instruction, she also began an instructors' club that later extended to other schools. She worked to attract college women to careers in public-health nursing because she felt that they had been preselected by the colleges and had the maturity and educational background that the profession required.

During 1919 and 1920 Strong was assistant secretary and consultant to the committee for the study of nursing education supported by the Rockefeller Foundation. On that committee she worked with Josephine Goldmark.

She served for several years as chair of the Educational Committee of the National Organization of Public Health Nursing (NOPHN) and was a member of the National League of Nursing Education, the American Child Health Association, and the Massachusetts Nurses Association. She also published several articles on public-health nursing in professional journals.

Strong suffered from a menopausal heart condition and died June 17, 1925, of a cerebral hemorrhage and bronchopneumonia. At the time she was a resident of Boston.

Following her death, the NOPHN adopted a resolution that read, in part: "Anne Hervey Strong, through her rare personality, keen insight, scholarly mind, and lofty vision, has stimulated careful thinking in others and has been one of those largely responsible for sound progress in public health nursing."

PUBLICATIONS BY
ANNE HERVEY STRONG

"Teaching Problems of Public Health Nursing Instructors." *American Journal of Nursing* 17 (July 1917): 1188–92.

"Recent Developments in Preparation for Public Health Nursing." *Public Health Nurse Quarterly* 10 (July 1918): 284–90.

"The Nursing Situation from the Public Health Point of View." *Transactions of the Twenty-first Annual Conference of the American Hospital Association, 1919.* Pp. 302–09. Chicago: American Hospital Association, 1919.

"The Education of Public Health Nurses." *Public Health Nurse* 13 (May 1921): 226–30.

BIBLIOGRAPHY

"Anne Hervey Strong." *American Nurses' Association Hall of Fame.* Publication G-123 8M. Kansas City, Mo.: American Nurses' Association, 1984.

"Miss Anne Hervey Strong." *New York Times*, June 20, 1925, 13.

Weston, A.A. "Anne Hervey Strong." *Trained Nurse and Hospital Review* 85 (August 1930): 187–90.

Alice P. Stein

Elizabeth Eleanor Sullivan

1890–1941

Elizabeth Eleanor Sullivan was one of the first nurses to hold an earned doctorate and yet remain committed to nursing.

Daughter of Maurice J. and Ann Mansfield Sullivan, she was born on May 17, 1890, in Newburyport, Massachusetts. Her father was a hatter. She attended high school in Newburyport and Haverhill, Massachusetts, and went from there to Massachusetts General Hospital Training School for Nurses, Boston, from which she graduated with honors in 1913. She then went to work as head nurse on Ward H, the hospital's children's ward. To encourage her interest in pediatric nursing, she was given a scholarship by Dr. Fritz Talbot. This enabled her to travel and observe nursing in children's hospitals in New York, Philadelphia, and Baltimore. After working briefly in the years 1914–15 as a supervisor at Huntington Hospital in Boston, she moved to Children's Hospital in Boston, first as instructor and first assistant (from March to August 1915), and then as superintendent of nurses.

Sullivan resigned as superintendent in 1919 in order to attend Teachers College, Columbia University, New York City. On her return to Boston in 1920, she taught as a nonresident instructor at a number of nursing schools in the greater Boston area, principally Faulkner Hospital in Jamaica Plain and Anna Jacques in Newburyport. She also attended Boston College on a part-time basis. After 1933 she also taught sociology part time at Boston College. She earned her B.Ed. in 1932 and an M.Ed. in 1933, and in 1938 she received a PH.D. in sociology from Boston College. Her doctoral dissertation focused on the ethical and social implications of modern nursing.

In 1936 she had been appointed the first supervisor of schools of nursing for the Massachusetts State Board of Registration, a position modeled on a similar one in New York and one for which nurses had long lobbied. She viewed her position as state supervisor of nursing schools as supportive and educational rather than supervisory or punitive, and she worked hard to improve the quality of training programs.

Sullivan's career was cut short by illness, and she died of cancer on October 17, 1941, in West Roxbury, Massachusetts.

PUBLICATIONS BY
ELIZABETH ELEANOR SULLIVAN

Problems in Solutions. Boston: Barrows, 1932.

Ethical and Sociological Implications in the Ideology of Modern Nursing. Boston: Boston College, 1938.

BIBLIOGRAPHY

Goostray, S. *Fifty Years; A History of the School of Nursing.* Boston: Alumnae Associates of the Children's Hospital, 1940.

Hawkins, J.W. "Elizabeth Eleanor Sullivan," *Dictionary of American Nursing Biography.* M. Kaufman, ed. Pp. 358–59. Westport, Conn.: Greenwood, 1988.

Nursing Archives. Mugar Memorial Library, Boston University, Boston.

Obituary. *Boston Globe*, October 18, 1941.

Vern L. Bullough

Irene H. Sutliffe

1850–1936

Irene H. Sutliffe was one of the pioneer nursing administrators in the United States. She was among the nurses who participated in the nursing subsection of the International Congress of Charities and Corrections held in conjunction with the World's Fair in Chicago in 1893. It was this group that set the agenda for much of early American nursing.

Born in Albany, New York, on November 12, 1850, Sutliffe was the daughter of George Washington and Charlotte (Ramsey) Sutliffe. She attended Cathedral School in Albany and in 1878 entered the New York Hospital School of Nursing in New York City, from which she graduated in 1880. After graduation she moved to Erie, Pennsylvania, where she became superintendent of the Hamot Hospital and established a school of nursing there. In 1886 she returned to New York to develop the Long Island College Hospital School of Nursing in Brooklyn. Shortly after she was appointed director of the New York Hospital School of Nursing, a position she held for the years 1886–1903.

During the Spanish-American War she also served for a brief period in 1898 as head of the nursing service at Camp Black, Hempstead, Long Island, New York. In 1908 she established a similar unit at New York Hospital, and in 1916 she organized an emergency hospital for the treatment of polio.

Both of her younger twin sisters and several of her nieces became nurses, and one of her twin sisters, Ida, succeeded her at the Long Island College Hospital School. Several of the early leaders of nursing were her pupils in New York, including Mary Beard, Lillian Wald, and Lydia Anderson. Although not always in good health, Sutliffe ran New York Hospital with only one assistant. Among her accomplishments was establishing an affiliation with Sloane Maternity Hospital. In 1890 she set up one of the first, if not the first, diet kitchen in the country.

In 1890 she was appointed honorary vice-chairperson of the committee of five nurses designated to plan the subsection on nursing of the International Congress of Charities and Correction. At that meeting in 1893, the first meeting of nurses from different countries, she read a paper in which she emphasized the importance of organizing the profession to maintain high ideals and standards. She also participated in the meeting that led to the development of the Superintendents Society, which in 1912 became the National League of Nursing Education. In New York she supported the organization of an alumnae group that joined with others to help form the American Nurses' Association.

Sutliffe was given the title of dean emeritus in 1932 and given quarters in the nurses residence of the New York Hospital, where she spent her last years. Two of her graduates helped nurse her as her health declined. Though she had never married, in 1887 she had adopted a baby girl who had been abandoned in a vacant lot near the hospital. The girl died some three years later. Upon her death, on December 30, 1936, in New York City, Sutliffe was buried next to the child.

BIBLIOGRAPHY

M. Adelaide Nutting Collection. Teachers College, Columbia University, New York. Microfiche number 0934.

Mottus, J.E. "New York Nightingales: The Emergence of the Nursing Profession at Bellevue and New York Hospital." Unpublished Ph.D. dissertation, New York University, 1980. University microfilms 801 7582.

Obituary. *American Journal of Nursing* 37 (February 1937): 215–18; 37 (April 1937): 451.

Pennock, M.R., ed. *Makers of Nursing History*, 2nd ed. P. 34. New York: Lakeside, 1940.

Vern L. Bullough

Ethel Swope
1885–1937

Ethel Swope was known in her time as the "Apostle of the Eight-Hour Day for Nurses." She was a 1912 graduate of the Connecticut Training School for Nurses at New Haven. After graduation, she directed nursing in the communicable-disease department of the Cincinnati General Hospital.

In World War I she enrolled in the American Red Cross Nursing Service and in 1918 went to France to care for soldiers who had communicable diseases. She moved to the Army Nurse Corps and was released in July 1919. She did public-health work at veterans' bureaus in Pennsylvania and Arizona until 1921. Moving to Los Angeles, she became superintendent of the Golden State Hospital and then director of nursing at the Methodist Hospital.

In 1927 she began seven years as executive secretary of the Fifth District of California State Nurses Association, the first district in California to have this office.

Swope believed that the exhaustion suffered by private-duty nurses during long hours of work interfered dangerously in their ability to serve the needs of their patients. During her tenure with the state association, many California hospitals agreed and shortened work periods to a maximum of 10 and then 8 hours. The action was largely the result of Swope's efforts. Swope also sought to bring the schools of nursing, the graduate nurses, and the community into closer cooperation by developing a registry of nurses.

In 1933 Swope became assistant director of the American Nurses' Association, then headquartered in New York City. She traveled throughout the country, giving lectures, attending meetings, and granting interviews.

She was a member of the American Red Cross Nursing Service, the American Hospital Association, the National Organization of Public Health Nurses, the National League of Nursing Education, the Western Hospital Association, the American League, and the Women's Overseas League.

Stricken with leukemia, she collapsed during a field assignment in Greenville, Mississippi, and died at the home of a brother, Dr. Chester D. Swope, in Washington, D.C., on May 27, 1937. She was buried at Arlington National Cemetery.

PUBLICATIONS BY ETHEL SWOPE
"The Need for Public Library Service for Nurses at the Hospitals." *Trained Nurse* 85 (October 1930): 471–72, 506.

"The Eight-Hour Day Makes Progress." *American Journal of Nursing* 33 (December 1933): 1147–52.

"The CWS Program and the American Nurses' Association." *American Journal of Nursing* 34 (April 1934): 356–60.

BIBLIOGRAPHY
Jamme, A.C. "Ethel Swope, Apostle of the Eight-Hour Day." *Trained Nurse and Hospital Review* 98 (August 1937): 130–31.

Pennock, M.R., ed. *Makers of Nursing History.* New York: Lakeside, 1940.

Alice P. Stein

Susie (Baker) King Taylor
1848–1912

Susie Baker King Taylor served as a nurse to the first official black regiment formed to fight in the Civil War as Union Army volunteers. Although she was initially employed as a laundress to the company, she demonstrated great capability in providing nursing care to the sick and wounded. She had critical knowledge about medicinal plants, was immune through vaccination to smallpox, and demonstrated such empathy for the soldiers in the regiment that she was permitted to attend to those in the company requiring nursing care.

Taylor was born on August 6, 1848, on the Grest Farm, on the Isle of Wight, located off the coast of Georgia. She was the eldest of the nine children of Raymond and Hagar Ann (Reed) Baker. Three of her siblings died in infancy. She was born into slavery, as her mother was a slave on the Grest Farm. Baker was able to trace back her family for six generations. She recollected that her great-grandmother lived to be 100 years old; gave birth to 24 children, of which 23 were female; and was a noted midwife of her day.

When Taylor was 7 years old, she and a younger brother and sister were allowed to leave the Grest Farm to live with their grandmother, an active tradeswoman and landowner in Savannah. While living with her grandmother, Taylor was surreptitiously educated to read and write by attending a clandestine school for black children, run by a freed black woman. Providing and obtaining such an education was extremely dangerous at that time, as it was illegal for blacks, whether slave or freemen, to learn to read and write. She received further secret private tutoring from Mary Beasley, a black nun, and later from several young white friends.

In early 1862 she fled with her uncle's family to St. Catherine's Island, off the coast of Georgia, which was under Union Army control. She traveled to St. Simon's Island, where she established and ran a school. She also married Sergeant Edward King, a black noncommissioned officer in Company E of the First South Carolina Volunteers, when she was only 14, and subsequently accompanied her husband's regiment during the succeeding four difficult years of fighting at the battlefronts of the southeastern United States. During the summer of 1862 she met Clara Barton and frequently accompanied her on nursing rounds at the battlefronts in South Carolina and the Sea Islands.

She was officially employed in the regiment as a laundress but was almost immediately recognized for her skill as a nurse and teacher, and she quickly assumed nursing and teaching responsibilities in the company. Her ability to read and write, a rarity for blacks in those times, proved to be an additional highly valued asset. When time and circumstances allowed, Taylor willingly taught many in the regiment who were eager to learn, and often read or wrote letters for those who were illiterate.

She was only 17 years old at the end of the Civil War when she accompanied her husband to Savannah, where she opened a school for black children. Although her husband was an excellent carpenter, he was unable to find work in that trade because of racial discrimination. His subsequent employment on the harbor docks as a loader ended with his accidental death on the docks in December 1866. Taylor was expecting their first child at the time. She resourcefully supported herself and her newborn son by opening a night school for adults. When she found it necessary to close the school because of competition from other free schools, she found employment in 1872 as a laundress with a wealthy white family and eventually traveled north with them as their cook. In 1874 she traveled to Boston, where she found domestic employment with another family. She was remarried in 1879, at age 31, to Russell L. Taylor. After her second marriage she no longer found it necessary to work outside her home and continued to live in Boston with her husband. Her second husband, Russell Taylor, died in May 1889.

Taylor became involved in organizing Corps 67 of the Boston Branch of the Woman's Relief Corps, a relief auxiliary to the Union veterans. In this capacity she helped to identify many Civil War veterans who were entitled to receive benefits in recognition of their war service. She held a number of official positions in this organization, including guard, secretary, and treasurer. In 1893 she was made president of the corps.

She was informed in February 1898 that her son, an actor in a traveling acting company, was gravely ill. Taylor traveled by train to Shreveport, Louisiana, to be at his bedside, enduring several incidents of racial prejudice and segregation as she traveled south by train.

It was apparent that her son was mortally ill, and in an effort to grant his wish that he might be able to return to his home in Boston to die, she attempted to reserve a train berth for him to travel home. Again she was faced with further evidence of racial discrimination when the train agent refused to sell her a berth ticket. Taylor remained in Shreveport to care for her son until his death. She then returned to Boston, where she continued to reside until her death in 1912.

Susie Taylor was never able to obtain remuneration for the four years of army nursing service that she rendered as a volunteer during the Civil War. She never received more than the $100 allotted by the government to her as a veteran's widow, six years after the death of her first husband. Although her wartime service was thoroughly documented, she was denied any benefits, pension, or official recognition of her service as a nurse due to a technicality—she had never signed official papers to work as a contract nurse.

Her retrospective anecdotal narrative of her experiences as a Civil War nurse continues to be recognized as an insightful, unique account of the conditions that prevailed in military camps during the Civil War. This account, which Taylor privately published in 1902, reflects the sympathetic commitment of this young nurse, who intimately knew the pain and suffering that accompanied each skirmish and battle of the war. Her intelligence, her compassion, and her commitment to the soldiers she cared for are clearly documented in the volume that she wrote. Her book continues to raise relevant, haunting questions about racial prejudice and racial equality in the post-Civil War years in the United States.

PUBLICATIONS BY SUSIE KING TAYLOR

Reminiscences of My Life in Camp with the 33rd United States Colored Troops, Late 1st S.C. Volunteers Boston: Privately published by the author, 1902.

BIBLIOGRAPHY

Carnegie, M.E. "Black Nurses At the Front." *American Journal of Nursing* 84 (October 1984): 1250–52.

Carnegie, M.E. *The Path We Tread: Blacks in Nursing 1854–1984.* Philadelphia: Lippincott, 1986.

Dannett, S.G. *Profiles of Negro Womanhood.* Vol. I, Pp. 166–73. Negro Heritage Library. Yonkers: Educational Heritage, 1964.

Davis, M., ed. *Contributions of Black Women to America.* P. 369. Columbia, S.C.: Kenday Press, 1982.

Elmore, J.A. "Black Nurses: Their Service and Their Struggle." *American Journal of Nursing* 76 (March 1976): 435–37.

Fleming, J.E. "Susie King Taylor." In *Dictionary of American Negro Biography.* R.W. Logan and M.R. Winston, eds. Pp. 581–82. New York: Norton, 1982.

Hine, D.C. *Black Women in White.* P. 4. Bloomington, Ind.: Indiana University Press, 1989.

Jackson, G.F., *Black Women Makers of History: A Portrait.* Pp. 47–48. Oakland, Calif.: GRT Book, 1975.

Romero, P.W., ed. *A Black Woman's Civil War Memoirs: Reminiscences of My Life In Camp With the 33rd Colored Troops, Late 1st South Carolina Volunteers.* Reprint of book originally published by Susie King Taylor. New York: Markus Weiner, 1988.

Tomes, E.K., and E. Shaw-Nickerson. "Predecessors of Modern Black Nurses: An Honored Role." *Journal of National Black Nurses Association* 1 (Fall 1986–Winter 1987): 72–78.

Karen L. Buchinger

Julie Chamberlain Tebo

1882–1966

A native New Orleanian, Julie C. Tebo was a nurse from the Deep South who became instrumental in formulating the national nursing agenda during the first half of the twentieth century.

On February 9, 1882, in New Orleans, Tebo was born, one of the five daughters and one son of Jessie Robertson (Wing) Tebo and Albert Gallitin Tebo, affluent and prominent members of New Orleans society.

Perhaps influenced by an illness that interrupted her early education, Tebo, a debutante, attended St. Luke's Hospital Training School for Nurses in Richmond, Virginia, the native state of her paternal grandmother. She graduated in 1910, one of only two non-Virginians in the class.

A private-duty nurse in the mountains of Virginia and North Carolina, an operating-room supervisor at Watts Hospital in Durham, North Carolina, and a resident nurse in a girls' boarding school were all a part of Tebo's activities following her graduation.

American Red Cross nursing was of particular importance to Tebo, who enrolled in the service in 1916 and received badge 12005. She served as a volunteer while in Richmond and following her return to Louisiana. Agnes Daspit, director of the Gulf Division of the American Red Cross and a friend of the Tebo family, recruited the young Tebo to the New Orleans Red Cross Nursing Committee. A 1919 New Orleans newspaper photograph caption referred to Tebo as "Instructor of Elementary Hygiene and Home Care of the Sick."

Tebo was active in the legislative arena as evidenced by her 1920 motion to assess individual members of the Louisiana State Nurses Association to fund the amendment to the 1912 Nurse Practice Act. The Suffrage Bill made it possible for the nurses themselves to serve on the Board of Nursing. In 1922 Julie Tebo was the first nurse appointed to the state board, and she became secretary and the first employee of the board. In 1930 she served as president of the Louisian section of the National League of Nursing Education. At the 1933 special conference of the State Boards of Nurse Examiners, following the Chicago Convention of the National League of Nursing Education, Tebo contributed the fact that the Louisiana board's five physicians had made it possible for the secretary of the board (Tebo) to inspect nursing schools before such inspection was made a requirement by law. By the time the requirement was written into the law, board inspection was well established.

Mary M. Roberts, editor of the *American Journal of Nursing* wrote Tebo to suggest that the Louisiana experience be a part of the journal's state and nursing education series. The series, "The State and Nursing Education," included only one southern state, Virginia, before the 1934 September focus on Louisiana.

Tebo was elected second vice-president of the National League of Nursing Education and served as a member of the board of directors of the American Journal of Nursing Company, a member of the American Red Cross National Nursing Committee, and a member of the advisory group that selected Blanche Pfefferkorn as director of studies of the National League of Nursing Education. In 1939 Tebo was very active in the National League of Nursing Education convention held in New Orleans. During the 1940s Louisiana was one of the states to be selected for a study of nursing needs and resources, and Tebo assisted in this study.

The 1949 retirement of Julie Tebo from the Louisiana State Board of Nurse Examiners was announced in the May issue of the *American Journal of Nursing*. The article includes the description of Tebo as being "a gentle but potent force." A framed "Resolution of Appreciation to Miss Julie C. Tebo," including numerous whereas clauses referring to efficiency and loyalty, adopted and signed by the five members of the State Board of Nurse Examiners, can still be found hanging in various New Orleans nursing sites.

In 1953 the New Orleans chapter of the American Red Cross presented her with a service bar marking her 35 years of service. In that same year the Louisiana League for Nursing presented her with life membership in the National League for Nursing. In 1954 at the golden anniversary celebration of the Louisiana State Nurses Association Tebo received a Certificate of Merit.

A year before her death, in 1965, Tebo received the Anne Medcalf Estabrook Award from the American Red Cross.

Julie Tebo died on October 28, 1966.

BIBLIOGRAPHY

Biographical and Historical Memoirs of Mississippi. Vol. I, p. 177; Vol. II., p. 212. Chicago: Goodspeed, 1891.

Celestine, S. "The State and Nursing Education: Julie C. Tebo, R.N." *American Journal of Nursing* 34 (September 1934): 887–888.

Louisiana State Nurses Association Archives. Hill Memorial Library, Louisiana State University, Baton Rouge.

Metzler, S. "Our Miss Julie." *Pelican News*, July 9, 1965.

"Miss Tebo Retires." *American Journal of Nursing* 49 (May 1949): 16.

"Special Conference, State Board of Nurse Examiners." *American Journal of Nursing* 33 (August 1933): 809–810.

Tebo, J.C. Papers. Special Collections, Hill Memorial Library, Louisiana State University, Baton Rouge.

Tebo, J.C. Scrapbook. Personal property of Mrs. Charles Sinnott (niece of Julie Tebo), New Orleans.

P.J. Ledbetter

Elnore Elvira Thomson

1878–1957

Elnore Elvira Thomson was a nursing educator and leader in the fields of mental hygiene and public health. From 1925–44 she was director of the School of Nursing Education of the University of Oregon Medical School, Portland.

The daughter of John Calvin and Mary Eliza Edwards Thomson, she was born in Illinois on November 4, 1878. The family moved to Massachusetts and then Colorado in search of a climate more favorable to her ill mother. She received her early education with tutors and continued working with them to complete the curriculum of Wellesley College. Interested in psychology, she also took a two-year independent-study program with a Harvard professor.

Incidents in her personal life convinced her of the value of skilled nurses to society, and she began nursing studies. In 1909 she received an RN from the Presbyterian Hospital School of Nursing in Chicago, where she was a member of Zeta Tau Alpha, Alpha Tau Delta, and Alpha Kappa Delta. Because of her background in psychology, she was granted an affiliation in psychiatric nursing with the nearby Elgin State Mental Hospital. She did postgraduate work at the Chicago School of Civics and Philanthropy.

After completing her studies in 1910, she became chief nurse at the Elgin State Hospital. There, she worked closely with Julia Lathrop, who was then doing social work in Chicago and later was named chief of the United States Children's Bureau. Lathrop invited Thomson to become director and executive secretary of the newly organized Illinois Society for Mental Hygiene, and she held the post from 1911–18. In the summer of 1917 Thomson also was part-time director of the public-health nursing curriculum at the Chicago School of Civics and Philanthropy.

During World War I she served as director of public-health nursing education for the American Red Cross Tuberculosis Commission in Italy in 1918–19. Upon her return, she directed the public-health course at the Chicago School of Civics and Philanthropy for one year.

Moving to the West Coast, she inaugurated and became director of the public-health nursing program at the University of Oregon School of Social Work in 1920. In 1923 she left the school for two years to serve as eastern representative of the American Child Health Association in San Francisco. In 1925 she was named director of public-health nursing activities for a Commonwealth Fund demonstration project in Marion County, Oregon. Simultaneously, she returned to the University of Oregon to work part time as a professor of applied sociology and director of health and nursing education at the School of Applied Social Science. She was named director in 1928. Four years later, she became director of the Department of Nursing Education of the University of Oregon Medical School.

After her retirement in 1944, Thomson remained active, teaching courses in public-health nursing and nursing history at the University of California at Los Angeles, where she previously had taught summer school.

Throughout her career Thomson was active in professional organizations at the local, state, national, and international levels. She was president of the Illinois State Nurses Association in 1917 and of its First District in 1919. In 1922 she was on the boards of directors of both the National League of Nursing Education and the National Organization of Public Health Nurses. She also served on the National Committee on Nursing Service of the American Red Cross. She was vice-president of the American Nurses' Association, 1922–30, and then president, 1930–34. As president, she represented American nurses at the International

Council of Nurses (ICN). She served on the ICN executive committee in 1933 and chaired its program committee for meetings held in the United States in 1941. In Oregon she served as the president of the Oregon Organization for Public Health Nursing, 1923, and as president of the state chapter of the American Social Workers Association, 1935. In addition, she was on the board of directors of the Oregon Society for Mental Hygiene.

Thomson also found time to be active in numerous other professional and civic groups. Her hobbies were opera and theater.

She died at age 88 of cardiovascular disease and bronchial pneumonia at Garden Hospital in San Francisco on April 24, 1957.

PUBLICATIONS BY ELNORE ELVIRA THOMSON

"The Frenocomio of Reggio-Emilia" [It.]. *Public Health Nurse* 12 (January 1920): 74–76.

BIBLIOGRAPHY

American Women 1935–1940: A Composite Biographical Dictionary. D. Howes, ed. Detroit: Gale Research, 1981.

"Elnore E. Thomson, Led Nursing Group." Obituary. *New York Times,* April 27, 1957, 19.

Flanagan, L. *One Strong Voice.* Kansas City, Mo.: American Nurses' Association. 1976.

"Obituary: Elnore E. Thomson." *American Journal of Nursing* (June 1957): 718, 782.

Soule, E.S. "Elnora Thomson." New York: National League of Nursing Education, undated biographical sketch.

"Thomson, Elnore E." *American Journal of Nursing* 34 (March 1934): 288.

"Who's Who in the Nursing World." *American Journal of Nursing* 28 (June 1928): 592.

Alice P. Stein

Margaret Anthony Tracy

1893–1959

An early advocate for and one of the pioneers of collegiate education for nurses, Margaret Anthony Tracy was a highly respected nursing leader who made enduring contributions to the profession. Under her direction the University of California became the first state-supported institution to establish an autonomous school of nursing.

Tracy was born on January 1, 1893, in Danville, Kentucky. Her parents were of English and Irish descent.

She was awarded an A.B. degree from the University of Cincinnati in 1915 and taught school before entering the Army School of Nursing in Washington, D.C. Her clinical practice was done at Walter Reed Army Hospital. After receiving her diploma in 1921, Tracy was employed for the next two years by the Henry Street Visiting Nurse Service in New York City, first as a staff nurse and then as supervisor. She left to become an instructor and director of nurses at the Glen Falls, New York, Hospital School of Nursing.

In 1925 she accepted a joint position as instructor in the newly established School of Nursing at Yale University and supervisor of surgical nursing at the New Haven Hospital. While in New Haven, she completed requirements for her master of science degree in 1929.

The Rockefeller Foundation awarded Tracy a fellowship in 1931 to study schools of nursing and public-health nursing in Europe. There she visited schools and agencies in 12 different countries. Later she directed a series of institutes under the auspices of the Rockefeller Foundation for visiting instructors from 24 schools in the United States.

Tracy went to California in 1934. Three years earlier friction between the director of the Training School of the University of California Hospital in San Francisco and the person in charge of the Division of Nursing Education in the Department of Hygiene on the Berkeley campus led university officials to search for a qualified person to head both positions. Tracy was selected, and she accepted with the encouragement of Annie Goodrich, dean of the School of Nursing at Yale University, who felt she would be able to cope with the challenges. She arrived on January 1, 1934, and by July of that year she worked out a consolidation of all the special nursing programs offered by various university departments, such as hygiene, public health, and education. The consolidation of these various programs led to greater uniformity and relevance of the credentials of the graduates of the baccalaureate program. She soon proposed the creation of a five-year curriculum (the acceptable length for a baccalaureate nursing program at the time) to replace the three-year diploma program that had existed since 1907.

With the merger of the nursing programs, Tracy carried the triple title of director for the Division of Nursing Education, for the Training School for Nursing, and for nursing. Eventually, she was given the title of dean; in the third edition of her book, *Nursing, an Art and a Science*, published in 1949, she is listed as "Dean, University of California School of Nursing, San Francisco and Berkeley."

The challenges Tracy faced were formidable, complicated by the fact that she had to travel between the Berkeley campus and the University Hospital in San Francisco. Yet she found time to write for nursing publications and work on a book. The first edition of the nursing text that bears her name was published in 1938, only four years after she arrived in California. It was unusual in the number of collaborators, written at a time when most nursing books had only one or two authors. Her collaborators were her colleagues at the University of California: Pearl Castile, M. Olwen Davies, Virginia Dunbar, Alice Ingmire, Agnes Moffat, Barbara Munson, and Mildred Newton. Several of these nurses themselves became well-known nursing leaders.

After the bombing of Pearl Harbor, Tracy was concerned for the welfare of the Japanese students and staff in her programs, even before relocation was suggested. She made arrangements for advantageous transfer of credits and supplied necessary references for these nurses to appropriate locations; this action was career saving for many.

During World War II she went to Hawaii to establish nursing services in two hospitals for emergency care of the wounded. While she was there, the Hawaii Nurses Association requested her to make a survey of nursing facilities throughout the islands. As a member of the Nursing Education Advisory Committee of the U.S. Public Health Service, she contributed to the development of the Cadet Nurse Corps, designed to help alleviate the nation's growing demand for nursing services during wartime.

As a school of nursing administrator, Tracy did not have much time for nursing research, but she undoubtedly would have made a good researcher. Certainly she was interested in nursing research. Before going to California, she completed a highly acclaimed time study of surgical nursing procedures. As dean, she was involved in several nursing investigations. She spoke on "The Need for Research in Our Schools of Nursing" at the 1947 National League for Nursing Education Convention, held in Seattle. She served for four years on the editorial board of *Nursing Research*, from its inception in 1952.

Tracy's career at the University of California has been described as a stormy one, in part because of the low academic status of nursing at the time, associated with a lack of precedent for the task she was undertaking. But another factor was her uncompromising personality; she did not deviate one iota from her intent to establish a school of nursing worthy of a place in an institution of higher learning and did not tolerate opposition to her plans.

Tracy has been described as brilliant, dedicated, determined, analytical, creative, and perceptive, but also as frank, blunt, and outspoken. A workaholic, she had a flair for problem solving. Her foremost interest was in students and their education, instilling in them the value of excellent care for patients. She prodded faculty to broaden their educational backgrounds and expand their concepts of nursing care, and she supported them as they pioneered new ways of looking at nursing and explored innovative approaches to teaching. She was not very tolerant of slow thinking or of any one with pretentious airs. She had unusual ability to recognize and attract talented faculty. Students were in awe of her, but they appreciated her concern for their welfare.

She was a large woman, made seemingly larger by her outstanding leadership attributes. She wore her straight, long hair in a knot at the back of her head. As director of nursing, she wore a uniform, but not a white one—hers was navy silk with a white collar, and she wore no cap.

She was well informed, not only about academic and professional affairs, but also about social, economic, and political trends. She spoke well and easily and was often sought as a speaker for national nursing meetings. She served on a number of national committees, though she did not devote much time to appointments that were more honorary than substantive.

Tracy was not well the last two years before her retirement in 1956. Many of her responsibilities were carried out by her associate and friend Pearl Castile, with whom she shared a home in Atherton, California. She died in the Julia Convalescent Home in Mountain View, California, on July 19, 1959.

PUBLICATIONS BY MARGARET TRACY

BOOKS

With seven collaborators. Nursing, an Art and a Science. St. Louis: Mosby 1st ed 1938; 2nd ed 1942; 3rd ed 1949.

MONOGRAPHS

Time Study of Nursing Procedures Used in the Care of a Variety of Surgical Cases. Bulletin No. 1. New Haven: Yale University School of Nursing, 1928.

ARTICLES

"Supervision and the Teaching of Surgical Nursing." *American Journal of Nursing* 26 (October 1926): 793–97.

"Making a Bed Around Traction Apparatus." *American Journal of Nursing* 27 (May 1927): 336.

"A Heliotherapy Tent." *American Journal of Nursing* 27 (June 1927): 451–52.

"What Background of Education and Experience Should We Expect for Members of Faculties of Schools of Nursing?" In *Transactions of the American Hospital Association,* Thirty-first Annual Convention. Pp. 645–50. Chicago: The Association, (1929).

"The Eight-Hour Day for Special Nurses at the University of California Hospital." *American*

Journal of Nursing 35 (January 1935): 29–32.

"The Growth of an Idea." *Pacific Coast Journal of Nursing* 33 (September 1937): 365–71.

"Florence Nightingale and Her Influence on Hospitals." *Pacific Coast Journal of Nursing* 36 (July 1940): 406–07.

"Speeding Up Production of Nurses." *American Journal of Nursing* 42 (February 1942): 193–95.

"Nursing 'Round the World'." *California Monthly* 15 (February 1953): 58–60.

With J. Nicholson. "Integration of Public Health Nursing in the Nursing Curriculum." *Pacific Coast Journal of Nursing* 31 (April 1935): 181–85.

BIBLIOGRAPHY

Carroll, M.C. Letter to the author, April 22, 1990.

Flood, M. "The White Mortarboard: Continuity with Change." Unpublished paper.

"Former UC Dean Tracy Dies." *San Francisco Chronicle,* August 20, 1959.

Harms, M. Letter to the author, May 9, 1990.

Hiller, J.S., H.E. Nahm, and F.S. Smyth. Margaret Anthony Tracy 1893–1959. In Memoriam, University of California, April 1960.

Incerti, W. Letter to the author, May 12, 1990.

"Margaret A. Tracy." *Pacific Coast Journal of Nursing.* 30 (January 1934): 13.

Phelps, H. Letter to the author, May 15, 1990.

Tracy, M.A. Papers. Archives, University of California, San Francisco.

Signe S. Cooper

Susan Edith Tracy

1864–1928

Susan Edith Tracy was a pioneer in recognizing the link between mind and body and in advocating the teaching of occupations as therapy for sick persons. She was also the first person in the United States to provide systematic training in occupational therapy to nurses. In the 1920s she established departments of occupational therapy in hospitals in New England and the Midwest, thus propagating her ideas and laying the foundations of occupational therapy as it is known today.

Born on January 22, 1864, in Lynn, Massachusetts, Tracy was the daughter of Caroline Mary (Needham) Tracy and Cyrus Mason Tracy, who was well-known in Lynn as a writer, a poet, a professor of botany, and an environmentalist. Tracy had two sisters, Laura Caroline and Julia Mason, as well as a brother George L., who later became a composer and musician. According to newspaper accounts, the Tracy home was a happy one. Mary Barrows, Tracy's friend and publisher, wrote that for economic and educational reasons, the family made their own toys and gifts, and were often occupied doing paper cutting and drawing. Barrows speculates that Tracy's interest in prescribing occupations for invalids may have stemmed from these family activities.

Tracy attended the Massachusetts Homeopathic Hospital School of Nursing, Boston, and was graduated in 1895. Following graduation, she worked as a private-duty nurse for several years and also took the course in hospital economics at Teachers College, Columbia University. While at Teachers College she observed in the Manual Arts Department and in the College's kindergarten.

In 1905, immediately after finishing at Teachers College, Tracy joined the nursing staff at the Adams Nervine Asylum, a hospital for the mentally ill in Jamaica Plain, Massachusetts. At Adams Nervine Tracy soon began a course in occupation therapy (bookbinding) for her patients. The next year, in 1906 when she became director of the Training School for Nurses at Adams Nervine, Tracy offered the first systematic training course in occupations to student nurses to prepare them to teach patient activities. The course included ten case studies for which each student was to prescribe an appropriate occupation and make a sample of the product to be made. Previously, craftsmen had been hired to teach crafts to patients. Tracy advocated that nurses should be trained to teach them. She believed that the object of the activity was to heal the patient rather than to produce a product. Tracy felt that work in occupations helped patients maintain social relationships with others and that the product linked them to other people and their needs. Tracy was staunch in her belief that only nurses, or possibly kindergarten teachers who had become nurses, should teach occupations to the sick.

Tracy's textbook, *Studies in Invalid Occupations, A Manual for Nurse and Attendants*, considered a classic, was published in 1910. The book was composed of her ten lectures for her course and included an illustrated guide for teaching occupations to students as well as teaching methods and explanations for the use of specific activities to treat various illnesses in different settings.

Following the initiation of her course, Tracy began to expand her teaching to other hospitals. In 1911 she taught occupational therapy at the Massachusetts General Hospital Training School for Nurses. It was the first course taught at a general rather than a mental hospital. In February 1912 Tracy left Adams Nervine, and in March became director of her own workshop called Experiment Station for the Study of Invalid Occupations in Jamaica Plain, Massachusetts. There she continued to lecture and teach occupations. Her students included those both inside and outside institutions: invalids, student nurses, and graduate nurses.

In addition to teaching, Tracy was a prolific writer who wrote not only about occupations, but also about care of kidney and obstetrical patients. During the Jamaica Plain period, Tracy taught nursing students at the School of Nursing, Teachers College, Columbia University, New York City; at Newton Hospital and Children's Hospital in the Boston area, as well as other hospitals throughout New England; and at Michael Reese Hospital and Presbyterian Hospital in Chicago. Her goal was to train the personnel to staff occupational therapy departments, set up a model program, and then move on.

Little is known about Tracy's private life. According to friend and colleague Eleanor C. Slagel, Tracy had an enthusiastic and magnetic personality and was dedicated to helping others. In July 1928 Tracy returned to her father's house in Lynn, Massachusetts. She suffered a stroke on September 9 of that year and died in Lynn on September 12, at the age of 64.

In 1917 the Maryland Psychiatric Quarterly named its January issue the "Susan E. Tracy Number" in her honor. In the issue Dr. George E. Barton states that although occupational therapy was not a new idea, it was Tracy who revived and organized the training and teaching of the discipline. Thus Susan E. Tracy is credited with establishing the foundations of occupational therapy in America.

PUBLICATIONS BY SUSAN E. TRACY

BOOKS

Studies in Invalid Occupation, A Manual for Nurse and Attendants. Boston: Whitcomb & Barrows, 1910.

Rake Knitting and its Special Adaption to Invalid Workers. Boston: Whitcomb & Barrows, 1916.

ARTICLES (SELECTED)

"Some Profitable Occupations for Invalids." *American Journal of Nursing* 8 (December 1907): 172–77.

"Occupation Treatment for Sick Children." *Pedagogical Seminary* 19 (1909): 457–58.

"The Place of Invalid Occupation in the General Hospital." *Modern Hospital* 2 (1914): 386–87.

"The Influence of Hospital Architecture on Methods of Occupational Teaching." *Proceedings of the First Annual Meeting of the National Society for the Promotion of Occupational Therapy, New York* 1 (1917): 42–44.

"A Three Months' Test of Invalid Occupations in a Large General Hospital." *Maryland Psychiatric Quarterly* 6 (January 1917): 54–56.

"Twenty-five Suggested Mental Tests Derived From Invalid Occupations." *Maryland Psychiatric Quarterly* 8 (1918): 15–18.

"Power Versus Money in Occupational Therapy." *Trained Nurse and Hospital Review* 66 (1921): 120–22.

"Getting Started in Occupational Therapy." *Trained Nurse and Hospital Review* 67 (1921): 397–99.

"Development of Occupational Therapy in the Grace Hospital, Detroit, Michigan." *Trained Nurse and Hospital Review* 66 (1921): 401–03.

"Treatment of Disease by Employment at St. Elizabeth's Hospital." *Modern Hospital* 20 (1923): 190–200.

"Two Practical Suggestions for Occupying Desperate Cases." *Occupational Therapy and Rehabilitation* 4 (June 1925): 181–83.

BIBLIOGRAPHY

Barrows, M., "Susan E. Tracy, R.N." *Maryland Psychiatric Quarterly* 6 (January 1917): 57–62.

Barton, G.E. "The Susan E. Tracy Number: An Appreciation." Editorial. *Maryland Psychiatric Quarterly* 6 (January 1917): 51–52.

Brainerd, W. "The Evolution of an Occupational Therapy Department in a General Hospital." *Occupational Therapy and Rehabilitation* 11 (1932): 33–50.

Cameron, R.G. "An Interview With Miss Susan Tracy." *Maryland Psychiatric Quarterly* 6 (January 1917): 65–66.

Dunton, W.R., Jr. "Susan E. Tracy." Editorial. *Occupational Therapy and Rehabilitation* 8 (1929): 63–65.

Hopkins, H.L., and H.D. Smith, eds. *Willard and Sparkman's Occupational Therapy,* 6th ed. Pp. 6–7. Philadelphia: Lippincott, 1983.

Parson, S.E. "Miss Tracy's Work in General Hospitals," *Maryland Psychiatric Quarterly* 6 (January 1917): 63–64.

Pennock, M.R., ed. *Makers of Nursing History.* P. 118. New York: Lakeside, 1940.

"Personalities From the Past." *Trained Nurse and Hospital Review* 81 (November 1928): 582.

Reed, K.L., and S.R. Sanderson, *Concepts of Occupational Therapy,* Pp. 199–200. Baltimore: Williams & Wilkins, 1983.

Slagle, E.C. "Occupational Therapy." *Trained Nurse and Hospital Review* 100 (1928): 375–82.

"Tracy, Susan E." In *Dictionary of American Nursing Biography.* M. Kaufman, ed. Westport, Conn.: Greenwood, 1988.

Dorothy Tao

Joyce E. Travelbee

1925–1972

Joyce E. Travelbee was recognized nationally as a nursing theorist and for her works in psychiatric nursing. During her 27 years of nursing practice, her activities as an author, nurse theorist, and educator had a significant impact upon nursing thought and practice, especially in the field of psychiatric nursing.

Travelbee was born on December 14, 1925, in New Orleans. She was one of two children of Charles R.T. Travelbee, and Marie Combel Travelbee. She attended the Crossman School in New Orleans and graduated from Joseph Kohn High School there in 1943. In 1946 she graduated from the Charity Hospital School of Nursing diploma program, which was operated by the Sisters of Charity. She was a member of the Cadet Corps while attending Louisiana State University Medical Center School of Nursing, from which she received her B.S.N. in education in 1956. She earned an M.S.N. in 1959 from Yale University, where her study concentration had been psychiatric nursing. The title of her thesis was "A Comparative Analysis of Certain Aspects of the Admission Procedure." At the time of her death she was working by correspondence on a Ph.D.

From 1946–52 Travelbee was a staff nurse in hospitals in New Orleans, Minneapolis, Washington, D.C., and New York City. She returned to New Orleans in 1952 to work as a staff nurse, head nurse, and instructor in psychiatric nursing at De Paul Hospital. From 1954–56 she taught psychiatric nursing at Charity Hospital and then until 1965 was an associate professor of psychiatric nursing at Louisiana State University in New Orleans. She then was appointed instructor in psychiatric nursing in the master's program at New York University, and in 1966 became a professor of psychiatric nursing at the University of Mississippi in Jackson. In 1969 Travelbee was appointed project director to teach psychiatric nursing and direct a curriculum project at the Hotel Dieu School of Nursing. She remained there until 1971, when she accepted a position as associate professor and director of graduate education in nursing at Louisiana State University.

Joyce Travelbee was a lay nun of the Order of Discalced Carmelites, founded by St. Teresa of Avila in 1567. The order is a contemplative order, devoted to the exercises of spiritual life, particularly mental prayer. The writings of St. Teresa and her religious faith influenced Travelbee's work on the human-to-human relationship and nurse-patient relationship model. The works of Victor Frankel and Ida Jean Orlando are perhaps the other major influences on her theoretical development, particularly on her concept of finding meaning in illness and suffering. Her other chief concerns included caring, empathy, sympathy, and rapport.

Travelbee was a member of Kappa Delta Pi, an honorary education society, and was listed in *Who's Who in American Education: Leaders in American Science Education.* She received the Teacher of the Year award from the University of Mississippi in 1969 and the Outstanding Alumni Award from Louisiana State University in 1970.

Travelbee died at Touro Hospital in New Orleans, at age 47, three days after being diagnosed with cancer. The cause of death was respiratory complications.

PUBLICATIONS BY JOYCE E. TRAVELBEE

BOOKS

Interpersonal Aspects of Nursing. Philadelphia: Davis, 1st ed. 1966; 2nd ed. 1971.

Intervention in Psychiatric Nursing, Process in the One-to-One Relationship. Philadelphia: Davis, 1971.

ARTICLES AND PAMPHLETS

"Concepts of Behavior." In *Institute on Behavioral Concepts in Basic Curriculum.* Pp. 1–15. New Orleans: De Paul Hospital, February 1962.

"Concepts of Communication." In *Institute on Behavioral Concepts in Basic Curriculum.* Pp. 32–49. New Orleans: De Paul Hospital, February 1962.

"Concepts of Observation." In *Institute on Behavioral Concepts in Basic Curriculum.* Pp. 16–31. New Orleans: De Paul Hospital, February 1962.

"The concept of rapport." In *Institute on Behavioral Concepts in Basic Curriculum.* Pp. 49–64. New Orleans: De Paul Hospital, February 1962.

"What Do We Mean by Rapport?" *American Journal of Nursing* 63 (February 1963): 70–72.

"Humor Survives the Test of Time." *Nursing Outlook* 11 (February 1963).

"Notes by a 19th-Century Nurse." *Nursing Mirror* 116 (May 1963): 3.

"What's Wrong with Sympathy?" *American Journal of Nursing* 64 (January 1964): 68–71.

"The concept of behavior." In *Communication in the Helping Process in Nursing.* Pp. 9–16. Proceedings of a Nursing Conference sponsored by the Louisiana State Board of Health, the Louisiana Department of Hospitals, and the National Institute of Mental Health, New Orleans, February 15–18, 1965.

"The Concept of Observation." In *Communication in the Helping Process in Nursing.* Pp. 17–22. Proceedings of a Nursing Conference sponsored by the Louisiana State Board of Health, the Louisiana Department of Hospitals, and the National Institute of Mental Health, New Orleans, February 15–18, 1965.

"The Concept of Envy." In *Conference on Teaching Psychiatric Nursing in Baccalaureate Programs.* Atlanta: Southern Regional Education Board, 1967.

"*Involvement.*" Keynote address, Louisiana Association Student Nurses' Convention, New Orleans, Touro Infirmary, November 21–23, 1969.

"Consultant's Opinion on Finding Meaning in Illness." *Nursing '71* 1 (1971).

"Consultant's Opinion on Suicide." *Nursing '71* (1971).

BIBLIOGRAPHY

Aggleton, P., and H. Chalmers. "Models of Nursing, Nursing Practice and Nursing Education." *Journal of Advanced Nursing* 12 (1987): 573–81.

Chinn, P. "The Utility of System Models and Development Models for Practitioners." In *Conceptual Models for Nursing Practice.* J. Riehl and C. Roy, eds. Pp. 46–53. New York: Appleton-Century-Crofts, 1974.

Chinn, P., and M. Jacobs. *Theory and Nursing: A Systematic Approach.* Pp. 188–89. St. Louis: Mosby, 1987.

Cook, L. "Nurses in Crisis: A Support Group Based on Travelbee's Nursing Theory." *Nursing & Health Care* 10 (1989): 203–05.

Fenton, M.V. "Development of the Scale of Humanistic Nursing Behaviors." *Nursing Research* 36 (1987): 82–87.

Gadow, S. "Introduction." In *Nursing: Images and Ideals—Opening Dialogue with the Humanities.* S. Spicker and S. Gadow, eds. New York: Springer-Verlag, 1980.

Hinds, P.S. "Introducing a Definition of Hope Through the Use of Grounded Theory Methodology." *Journal of Advanced Nursing* 9 (1984): 357–62.

Hobble, W. and T. Lansinger. "Joyce Travelbee: Human-to-Human Relationship Model." In *Nursing Theorists and their Works.* A. Marriner ed. Pp. 196–204. St. Louis: Mosby, 1986.

Meleis, A.I. "Joyce Travelbee." *Theoretical Nursing: Development and Progress.* Pp. 254–62. Philadelphia: Lippincott, 1985.

Pallikkalharyel, L, and A.B. McBride. "Suicide Attempts. The Search for Meaning." *Journal of Psychosocial Nursing Mental Health* 24, No. 8 (1986): 13–18.

Roy, C. "Travelbee's Developmental Approach. In *Conceptual Models for Nursing Practice.* J.P. Riehl and C. Roy eds. Pp. 267–68. New York: Appleton-Century-Crofts, 1974.

Sarter, B. "Evolutionary Idealism: A Philosophical Foundation for Holistic Nursing Theory." *Advances in Nursing Science* 9 No. 2 (1987): 1–9.

Sloane, A. Review of *Interpersonal Aspects of Nursing* by J. Travelbee. *American Journal of Nursing* 66 (June 1966): 77.

Spratlen, L.P. "Introducing Ethnic-Cultural Factors in Models of Nursing: Some Mental Health Applications." *Journal of Nursing Education* 15 (March 1976): 23–29.

Thibodeau, J.A. "An Interaction Model: The Travelbee Model." *Nursing Models: Analysis and Evaluation.* Pp. 89–104. Belmont, Calif.: Wadsworth, 1983.

Who's Who in American Education. Vol. 23. Hattiesburg, Miss: 1968.

Lee Kraft

Sojourner Truth

ca. 1797–1883?

Abolitionist, lecturer, women's rights advocate, Civil War nurse, Sojourner Truth was noted for all of these activities in spite of having been born a slave and remaining illiterate her entire life.

Details of her early life are incomplete. She was born in Hurley, Ulster County, New York, most likely in 1797, to Elizabeth and James, slaves owned by Charles Hardenbergh. Her given name at birth was Isabella, and she was the next to the youngest of her parent's 12 children. Her last name varied: she was known by her father's surname (Baumfree or Bomefree) or by the names of her owners, Hardenbergh, Neely, and Dumont among them.

Since her owners at birth were Dutch settlers, her first language was most likely Dutch rather than English.

After she had been sold three times, Truth was married to Thomas, also a slave, and bore at least five children, some of whom may have been fathered by one of her owners. She escaped from her last owner after he reneged on his promise to free her a year before the New York State law emancipating all slaves was to take effect. The family with whom she found refuge purchased her freedom for $20; she took their name and was known as Isabella Von Wagener. Shortly thereafter, she sued for the return of one of her sons who had been sold out of state illegally. Her victory was one of the first in which a black woman won a suit against a white man.

For the next 15 years Isabella worked as a maid, cook, and laundress and was affiliated with various religious groups. She had claimed that she heard the voice of God her whole life, and in 1843, following His instructions, she took the name of Sojourner Truth and began preaching. Her travels took her to New England, and she became a famous abolitionist, widely acclaimed for her powerful speeches and often sharing the platform with orator Frederick Douglass. She raised money for her causes and her living expenses by selling pictures of herself. In 1850, with the help of a friend, Olive Gilbert, she published and sold copies of the story of her life to further supplement her income.

In 1851 Truth addressed the National Women's Suffrage Convention in Akron, Ohio, where she delivered her famous "And Ar'n't [ain't] I a Woman?" speech. She continued to lecture and travel from her home in Battle Creek, Michigan, for many years. William Wetmore Story heard of her from Harriet Beecher Stowe and was inspired to sculpt a statue of her, which he called Sibilla Libica and exhibited it at the World's Exhibition in London.

When black regiments were formed during the Civil War, Truth began to solicit food and clothing for them. In the spring of 1864, at about 77 years of age, she left home once again. After speaking in New York City and its environs, she traveled to Washington, D.C., where she was received by President Abraham Lincoln in October of that year. Following that visit, she was appointed a counselor by the National Freedman's Relief Association and worked in Freedman's Village, a camp in Arlington Heights, Virginia. There she instructed the women in the need to maintain cleanliness amidst the deplorable conditions. She showed them how to fight to protect their children from being stolen from them in raids by Marylanders, and she had her grandson read newspapers to them.

On September 13, 1865, Truth was appointed by the War Department's Bureau of Refugees, Freedmen, and Abandoned Lands to work with Surgeon Gluman, the head of the Freedmen's Hospital in Washington, D.C. Although detailed information about her nursing activities is incomplete, it is known that for over two years she nursed the black soldiers at the severly understaffed hospital. In addition, she taught the inexperienced nurses how to change bandages, wash wounds, and make beds. She organized a group of women to clean the dirty hospital and brought order to the chaotic conditions. She also went to Congress and urged them to provide funds for the training of nurses and doctors.

While in Washington Truth continued her attacks on other fronts. She forced streetcar conductors to allow her to ride on public transportation, as was supported by a law President Lincoln had signed, and successfully sued the railway when she was injured in an altercation. She continued to preach and to solicit clothing and supplies for the destitute former slaves, all the while working tirelessly to find jobs for them.

Following her years in Washington, Truth embarked on another journey. She began a campaign to have land in the West given to the newly freed slaves so that they could become independent and self-supporting. Her first speech on the subject was delivered in 1870 in Providence, Rhode Island, and she traveled throughout the Northeast and as far as Kansas to spread her message. Although she was not successful, a large number of former slaves did move to Kansas and obtained land under the Homestead Law.

After a number of years, Truth returned home to Battle Creek, Michigan. She died November 26, 1883(?), at about age 86, survived by three of her daughters. Memorabilia relating to her life are in the Kimball House Historical Museum in Battle Creek. She was inducted into the Michigan Women's Hall of Fame and the National Women's Hall of Fame, Seneca Falls, New York.

PUBLICATIONS BY SOJOURNER TRUTH

Narrative of Sojourner Truth. Boston. Printed for the author. 1850. Reprint, Salem, New Hampshire: Ayer, 1987.

BIBLIOGRAPHY

Bernard, J. *Journey Toward Freedom: The Story of Sojourner Truth.* New York: Dell, 1969.

Carnegie, M.E. *The Path We Tread: Blacks in Nursing, 1854–1984.* Philadelphia: Lippincott, 1988.

Fauset, A.H. *Sojourner Truth: God's Faithful Pilgrim.* Chapel Hill: University of North Carolina Press, 1938, Reprint, New York: Russell & Russell, 1971.

Pauli, H. *Her Name Was Sojourner Truth.* New York: Appleton-Century Crofts, 1962. Reprint, New York: Avon, 1976.

Redding, S. "Truth, Sojourner." In *Notable American Women 1607–1950: A Biographical Dictionary.* E.T. James, ed. Vol. 3, Pp. 479–81. Cambridge: Belknap Press of Harvard University Press, 1971.

Truth, S. Papers, ca. 1850–1976, Willard Library, Battle Creek, Michigan.

Truth, S. Research Collection, 1830–1986, State University of New York, College at New Paltz. Sojourner Truth Library, New Paltz, New York.

Wrench, S.B. "Truth, Sojourner." In *American Reformers: An H.W. Wilson Biographical Dictionary.* Alden Whitman, ed. Pp. 814–16. New York: Wilson, 1985.

Gayle J. Hardy

Stella Boothe Vail
1890–1926

Stella Boothe Vail used her artistic and dramatic talents to promote health education to a variety of audiences.

Vail was born in Illinois in 1890. Her mother died at an early age. Soon thereafter the family moved to Spokane, Washington, and became prosperous enough to send Vail to an exclusive Boston finishing school. She graduated from Children's Hospital School of Nursing, Columbus, Ohio, in 1913, and after working with the mentally ill for two years, she became a social worker at the Music School Settlement in New York City in 1915. One year later she began organizing community health work at the Cheney Silk Mills, a program that preceded by several years similar industrial programs elsewhere.

During World War I she joined the Army Nurse Corps and was in charge of the pneumonia ward of 100 patients at Camp Lewis, Washington. In recognition of her administrative ability, the medical staff asked her to make a statistical study of the cases. After being released from military service she investigated the Seattle canneries, impersonating the fictitious Susie Brown looking for a job as ward maid in a children's hospital. She later became Red Cross home hygiene instructor in Idaho and worked closely with the Nez-Perc Indian tribe.

While working as a hygiene instructor, Vail conceived the idea of health marionettes and the suitcase theater. She planned traveling exhibits that explained the role of the visiting nurse and conveyed basic health messages to a variety of audiences. Interested in the advancement of nursing education, she originated the Museum of Hygiene connected with the Medical School of New York University in New York City in order to teach students simple facts and details frequently omitted in formal courses. She planned and executed the nursing exhibit at the Atlantic City (N.J.) convention in 1926 which portrayed nursing at the Sesquicentennial in Philadelphia. While working on the exhibit in early August, she was suddenly stricken with appendicitis. She was rushed to the hospital for an operation but died of shock three days later.

The creator of Mary Gay, Kimmie, and the Junior Safety Council, a series of imaginative books providing health information for children, Vail approached health education with enthusiasm and energy to audiences of all ages and backgrounds.

PUBLICATIONS BY STELLA BOOTHE VAIL

"Let's Go to the County Fair." *Public Health Nursing* 15 (August 1923); 387–92.

BIBLIOGRAPHY

Pennock, M. *Makers of Nursing History.* New York: Lakeside, 1928, 1940.

"Stella Boothe." *American Journal of Nursing* 26 (October 1926): 789.

Van Ness, E. "Telling the World About Nursing." *American Journal of Nursing* 26 (October 1926): 775–79.

Lilli Sentz

Jane Van de Vrede

1880–1972

Jane Van de Vrede was a leader in nursing in Georgia during the first half of the twentieth century. Her life and work made significant contributions to the status of women in the South, to improved educational and practice standards for nursing, and to more comprehensive approaches to public-health needs in the South. She was particularly adept at promoting collaboration between nurses and physicians and between black and white nurses in a traditional South with prescribed sex roles and institutionalized segregation.

Jennie Van de Vrede was born on August 12, 1880, of Dutch parents in Wausau, Wisconsin. Her parents died during her childhood, and she and her four sisters were separated, being reared by different relatives. In spite of, and perhaps because of this separation, the sisters remained close in their adult lives. She worked in a family friend's home in "town" in exchange for three years of room and board in high school. At some point, she decided to change her name to *Jane*, telling friends later that she believed Jennie to be childish. She received teacher certification at the County Teacher Training School in Wausau in 1899 and taught in the public-school system there for several years.

At age 23, Van der Vrede was hospitalized in Chicago for surgery, and postoperatively she developed hemorrhage and infection. Negative conditions in the hospital, such as bug infestation and the poor quality of the nursing care that she received, affected her profoundly and influenced her decision to nursing as a career. A letter to Charlotte Burgess in 1926, relative to State Board business, mentions this experience:

> Are you the Miss Burgess that back in 1903 was in the Ill. Training School and came into the room of a girl on the corner of the then new part of the Presbyterian Hospital, Room 208 and said one noon as you put on your cap: "It's a weary world and none of us gets out alive." That made a great impression of me about to go to operation and has had a great influence on my nursing work.

She applied to the Milwaukee General Hospital School of Nursing and was refused admission because her hair was short. Her long hair had been braided and cut during her extended hospitalization and illness. Finally, after promising the director that she would wear braids and appear respectable, she was accepted into the school. She graduated in 1907, at 27 years of age. Following graduation, she worked as laboratory assistant in bacteriology with Dr. V.H. Bassett, at Milwaukee General Hospital. She went to Savannah, Georgia, in 1908 after a typhoid epidemic there, working with Bassett to establish a bacteriology laboratory. She taught bacteriology classes in schools of nursing in Savannah and began involvement with the Red Cross and the newly formed Georgia Nurses Association. She remained in Savannah working with Bassett until 1917, when, at age 37, she moved to

Atlanta to assume her position as director of nursing service, Southern Division, American Red Cross. She retained this position until 1925, when the Southern Division united with the national headquarters in the Washington, D.C., office. She was offered a position in this office at this time, but decided to remain in Georgia.

During World War I, in an attempt to recruit nurses for military service she visited hospital schools of nursing and found many nurses unqualified for Red Cross service because of the limited education and clinical experiences offered by these small schools. These experiences sparked her motivation later to provide leadership in accreditation efforts through the Georgia State Board and the Georgia Hospital Association.

Van der Vrede believed that prevention of illness and disability, particularly tuberculosis, infant mortality, and defective and malnourished children, was the unique contribution of the public-health nurse, both because of the acceptance of the nurse by the population and the ability of the nurse to teach prevention "with the least presumptuousness and fear of being misunderstood. To this phase of health work the nurse, and in the immediate future the nurse only, can make the greatest contribution." Few nurses were prepared by training and experience for preventive aspects of public health. She summarized the problem in 1921:

> [T]he knowledge of the training school was not broad enough. There the patient was considered only for the period of acute illness in home or hospital, disassociated from his past and his family; in a new environment with only the nurse in charge. All this is changed in the public health field. The nurse keeps constantly in mind the family environment, the previous conditions and social causes which bear upon the illnesses.

In order to utilize Red Cross scholarships for study of public-health theory, southern nurses were required to go North to Columbia University or Boston University. Neither program addressed the particular problems of public health

in the South, especially the rural South. To overcome this problem, Van der Vrede collaborated with Peabody College, the Nashville chapter of the Red Cross, and the American Red Cross to establish a program in public-health nursing at Peabody College in Nashville, Tennessee. Abbie Roberts Weaver, later the first director of the State Department of Public Health Nursing in Georgia, was appointed director of the Peabody program, which provided public-health theory as well as clinical practice in surrounding rural areas. A similar program was set up at Medical College of Virginia (Richmond) for black nurses with Lillian Bischoff as the first director.

As the Red Cross Southern Division director of nursing for the Red Cross, Van de Vrede was involved in a variety of issues. She was a member, in 1919, of the Red Cross committee to decide a memorial for Jane Delano. The committee decided on a trust fund to implement a visiting-nurse service in remote areas such as Alaska. Van der Vrede exercised influence to guarantee health insurance eligibility and treatment of nurses under the Bureau of War Risk Insurance. These efforts were successful in securing coverage for Red Cross nurses. Her interest in insurance benefits for nurses continued, and in 1931 she advocated a retirement insurance plan for all nurses in the Harmon Plan.

For her service to the Red Cross, at the twenty-eighth annual meeting of the Georgia State Nurses Association, on October 25, 1934, she was awarded lifetime membership. She was awarded a 40-year service pin in 1955 and a 50-year pin in 1967

She was a charter member of the Atlanta Business and Professional Women's Association, serving on the board of directors at its inception and as president in 1922–23.

Van de Vrede was one of 16 persons who organized the Georgia Hospital Association on January 17, 1929, and served as its first president. As president, she sought cooperation from affiliate hospitals to insure quality nursing care and nursing education in the 54 hospital-owned and -operated schools of nursing in Georgia. Since standards were so varied Van der Vrede, who was also executive director of the Georgia State Board of Examiners of Nurses, sought such minimum standards for nursing schools as an organized nursing-service department in the hospital; qualified teaching faculty; entrance requirements including minimum entrance age of 17 and high school graduation; adequate range and variety of clinical experiences and laboratory and classroom facilities; recordkeeping for both hospital and school of nursing; and quality control measures like defined nurse-patient ratios, specific assignments for student nurses, and competent supervision of student nurses in all nursing procedures.

She had been appointed to the Board of Examiners of Nurses in 1925 and served continuously until 1933, at which time political pressure was exercised to prevent her reappointment by the governor. She succeeded in establishing mandatory registration of all nurses, annual re-registration, licensing of nurses, and examination of nurses for licensure. She also closed substandard schools. By 1933, 41 of 54 schools of nursing in Georgia had been closed, and it was in large part due to opposition from the hospitals where schools had been closed that she was not reappointed.

Van der Vrede was active in the Georgia State Association of Graduate Nurses almost as soon as she arrived in the state. She served as president of GSNA in 1922. In 1925 the state convention of GSNA voted to establish headquarters in Atlanta, and Van de Vrede was appointed executive secretary, and she assumed office in 1926. She served the GSNA in other offices in the 1924–50 period, as secretary, vice-president, parliamentarian, chaplain, and treasurer. She, at 90, presided over the installation of officers at the GSNA's sixty-fourth convention in 1971.

In 1972 the Georgia State Nurses Association adopted a resolution in memory of Van de Vrede summarizing her contributions. The GSNA dedicated and named the board room at GSNA headquarters in her honor. Her portrait hangs in this room.

Van de Vrede was also active in the Georgia State League for Nursing (GSLN), the Georgia chapter of the National League for Nursing, the body that accredits schools of nursing and constructs the test pool from which licensing examinations are drawn. Van de Vrede continued work with the Georgia league during her retirement, going daily to the league office and doing volunteer work in the 1960s. The GSLN established the Jane Van de Vrede Award in 1973 to honor her. The purposes of the award are:

> Recognition of outstanding service to the people of Georgia in improving the delivery of health care.
> Recognition of unusual support in improving the delivery of health care to the people of Georgia.

Because of her effectiveness in collaborating with physicians, in establishing nursing-defined legislation, and in promoting standards for schools of nursing, she was spokeswoman to various medical groups including the Southern Medical Association, Medical Association of Georgia, and the American College of Surgeons.

Van de Vrede's leadership in facilitating interracial communication and planning among black and white nursing organizations in the segregated South in the 1920s and 1930s is documented in letters held in her personal papers. While secretary of the state board, she worked with local and national leaders of black and white groups to promote joint planning, participation, standard setting, and employment. At that time, black nurses were ineligible for membership in many southern state nurses' associations, but they were eligible for membership in such national groups as the American Nurses' Association, the American Red Cross, and the National Association of Public Health Nursing. Both black and white nurses were licensed by the same process.

During the 1930s and early 1940s, Van de Vrede, then in her fifties, was active in the Work Projects Administration (WPA). She assumed the position of director of women's work, under the Bureau of Professional and Women's Services in Georgia. Under WPA jurisdiction, the Department of Public Health Nursing was developed in the State Department, and organization of visiting nurse and public-health nursing efforts were coordinated on a state level. Van de Vrede retired from the WPA in 1942.

Jane Van de Vrede spent the years prior to her death in Smyrna, Georgia, in a home that she had designed. Blind for the last years of her life, she lived with her friend and supporter, Lillian Bischoff, herself a nurse and educator, who not only loved her and cared for her, but was sensitive to her need to exercise an alert mind. After Van de Vrede's death in 1972, Bischoff donated Jane's personal papers to the American Nurses' Association archives at Boston University, with copies in Georgia at the State Department of Archives and History.

PUBLICATIONS BY
JANE VAN DE VREDE

"Bacteriology in the Curriculum of the Training School." Read before the National League for Nursing Education, May 2, 1916. Van de Vrede personal papers.

"The Value of the Nurse in Public Health Work in the South." *Southern Medical Journal* 14 (1921): 463–69.

"Cooperation Between the Medical and Nursing Professions." Paper presented before the American College of Surgeons, 17th Annual Session, Detroit, October 3–7, 1927. Program documented in *American College of Surgeons Yearbook 1928*. Van de Vrede papers.

"Georgia's Headquarters." *American Journal of Nursing* 27 (1927): 89–91.

"The Future of the Small School of Nursing in Georgia." *Journal of the Medical Association of Georgia* 19, No. 1 (1930).

"Some of the Particular Problems That Face Us in Georgia." Speech January 19, 1930. Van de Vrede papers.

"The Harmon Plan, Why I Am A Participant." *American Journal of Nursing* 31 (1931); 1285–86.

"The Preparatory and Technical Education of the Nurse." *Southern Medical Journal* 24 (1931): 907–12.

"What's the Matter With Nursing?" Paper presented before the House of Delegates of the Medical Association of Georgia, May 18, 1932. Van de Vrede papers.

BIBLIOGRAPHY

Bischoff, L. "Jane Van de Vrede (1880–1972), Pioneer, Humanitarian, Leader, Friend." Eulogy at memorial service at GSNA headquarters, at the dedication of the Jane Van de Vrede Board Room, 1973. Van de Vrede papers, American Nurses' Association (ANA) Archives, Boston University, Boston.

Bischoff, L. "Our Jane." Biographic sketch. Van de Vrede papers, ANA Archives, Boston University, Boston.

Bischoff, L. Taped interview with the author, April 30, 1977.

Dock, L. *History of American Red Cross Nursing.* New York: Macmillan, 1922.

Georgia Nursing, 1929–1946. Vol. 1, *Year Book and Roster.* Atlanta: Georgia State Nurses Association, 1946.

"Georgia State League for Nursing Awards Brochure: Jane Van de Vrede Award, 1973." Atlanta: Georgia State League for Nursing, 1973.

Georgia State Nurses Association, Executive Board. "Resolution in Memory of Miss Jane Van de Vrede, February 18, 1972." Atlanta: The Association, 1972.

Henley, R. *One Boundless Reach.* Atlanta: Georgia State League for Nursing, Historical Committee, 1967.

Hogan, G. Letter from the executive director, Georgia Hospital Association, to A. Ditchfield, January 17, 1972. Van de Vrede papers, ANA Archives, Boston University, Boston.

"Jane Van de Vrede." Obituary. *Atlanta Constitution,* January 5, 1972.

"Red Cross Awarding of Fifty-Year Service Pin." *Atlanta Constitution.* July 13, 1967.

"Red Cross Awarding of Forty-Year Service Pin." *Atlanta Constitution,* October 20, 1955.

Van de Vrede, J. Letter to C. Burgess, University Hospital, Omaha, Nebraska, August 11, 1926. Van de Vrede papers, ANA Archives, Boston University, Boston.

Van de Vrede, J. "Summary Statement on Retirement from State Board," 1933. Van de Vrede papers, ANA Archives, Boston University, Boston.

Wescott, E.C. Letter conferring lifetime membership in the American Red Cross to Van de Vrede, October 25, 1934. Van de Vrede papers, ANA Archives, Boston University, Boston.

Jacqueline C. Zalumas

Phyllis Jean Verhonick

1922-1977

Army nurse, university professor, charter member, and later vice-president of the American Academy of Nursing, Phyllis Jean Verhonick was an early advocate of clinical-nursing research and champion of research education at the baccalaureate level. Her service to the profession, nationally and internationally, won her the gratitude of many and the respect of all she taught.

Verhonick was born to Leona Louise (Kolbeck) and Peter James Verhonick on May 26, 1922, in Enumclaw, Washington. The second of three girls (Bethel, Phyllis, and Verda), she grew up in Missoula, Montana, where she attended the public schools. Intent on becoming a nurse, she was very concerned about finding a school that would accept her. Her sister Verda remembers her spending time in the basement trying to stretch herself to the five feet needed for admission to the schools. Fortunately, she found a school, the College of Nursing, University of Portland, Oregon, that accepted her as a student, and she graduated in 1944 with a bachelor of science in nursing.

Following graduation from nursing school, she was an instructor for a year at Columbus Hospital, Great Falls, Montana, and then joined the Army Nurse Corps in 1945. She served at the Army Hospital at Fort Ord, California, as staff nurse and later head nurse, 1945-48. She returned to civilian life and spent one year as nursing instructor at Seattle University, returning to the Army in 1949. Her army career was characterized by a succession of key clinical, administrative, and educational positions. She served as staff nurse, head nurse, educational coordinator, nursing methods analyst, and clinical supervisor in army hospitals in the United States and Japan.

The army sent her for schooling at Teachers College, Columbia University, where she met and worked with many who were to encourage and help her achieve the professional status and recognition that she acquired in her career. Although her original aim at Teachers College was to get a master's degree in nursing, she instead concentrated on preparing herself for research, studying under Dr. Elizabeth Hagen and developing her research skills through learning experiences with Dr. Helen Bunge in the Institute for Research and Service in Nursing Education at Teachers College.

In three years she completed the work required for a master of arts (1956) and a doctor of education (1958). Thereafter she devoted her professional life to nursing or patient-care research and assisted in the development of the research talents of others.

On return to the U.S. Army after completing her doctorate, she joined Lt. Col. Harriet H. Werley in the Department of Nursing at the Walter Reed Army Institute of Research (WRAIR) as assistant chief for research. During these years (1958-62) Phyllis helped establish the international reputation of the Department of Nursing, WRAIR, as a leader in clinical-nursing research. In 1962 she became the chief of the department, a position she held until her retirement as a lieutenant colonel in 1968. Upon retirement, Verhonick joined the faculty of the School of Nursing, University of Virginia, Charlottesville, where she was a professor and the director of research until her death, except for the years 1972-74, when she was acting dean.

Verhonick was a great teacher and one of the first to recognize the need to introduce research emphasis at the baccalaureate level. She wanted young nursing students to develop a research awareness. She assisted them in developing this awareness through a course on introduction to research, and then she was their mentor as each developed a small project and worked through the experience of conducting a study. That she was effective in this endeavor is attested to by the fact that her students can now be found among the most productive nursing researchers in this country.

Verhonick was known nationally and internationally for her research in the area of decubitus ulcers and skin care. She persevered in her efforts to conduct in-depth research in this area and moved along from descriptive studies to sophisticated multidisciplinary research involving bioengineering quantitative measures. Her studies were designed to gain greater understanding of phenomena and then to develop predictive studies.

Phyllis Verhonick was an original thinker who willingly shared her research expertise. She did this primarily through her service on local and national research committees, such as the American Nurses' Foundation (ANF) the Planning Committee for Nursing Research Based on the National Sciences (1962–64); the American Nurses' Association (ANA), Standing Committee on Research and Studies (1963–68); ANF Research Advisory Committee (1967–75); and the Walter Reed Army Institute of Nursing (WRAIR) Planning Committee for Research Activities. She served as a member of many review groups including the Presidential Technical Committee—Office of Science and Technology, Presidential Technical and Advisory Board to Study Operations of the National Institutes of Health (1964); and as a liaison member of the Nursing Research Study Section, Department of Health, Education and Welfare, Grants Research Branch (1962–67). In addition, she found time to act as reviewer for the professional journals *Nursing Forum* and *Nursing Research.*

She was research consultant to the Veterans Administration Central Office Committee to Develop Clinical Nursing research (1964–68) and to the Pan American Health Organization, World Health Organization for Nursing Studies in British West Indies and South America (1968–70). The warmth of the relationships she was able to establish with students and research colleagues always brought out the best in individuals and contributed to advancing research. She also possessed a great sense of humor, which was invaluable in helping to overcome the frustrations and obstacles so frequently encountered in research endeavors.

Throughout her career, Verhonick had the respect of her peers and was selected as a charter member of the American Academy of Nursing in 1973, one of 36 so honored. She served as vice-president of the academy in 1975. Her military honors include the Legion of Merit, the highest noncombat award for exceptionally meritorious service.

Following her death on October 1, 1977, at the age of 55, she has been remembered by her associates in several ways. At Walter Reed Army Medical Center on July 10, 1980, the presidential suite of the Dwight D. Eisenhower Executive Nursing Suite was named in her honor. In 1982 the Army Nurse Corps dedicated one of its continuing-education courses to her with the purpose of providing a forum for Army Nurse Corps officers to present and discuss nursing research. Papers concerned with clinical practice, administration and management in the military, and the maintenance of the highest standards of professional nursing practice for the care of soldiers and their families are solicited and reviewed. Two recognition awards have been given: one to the author of the most outstanding report by an experienced researcher and one to the author of the study accomplished while in a student status. The sixth Phyllis J. Verhonick Nursing Research Courses sponsored by the Army Nurse Corps was held in April 1990. Similarly, the University of Virginia School of Nursing started the annual Phyllis J. Verhonick Nursing Research Conferences in 1986 at which outstanding students are selected to receive the Verhonick Research Award. These expressions of respect and admiration are made not only for Verhonick's contribution to the science and art of nursing, but also in thanks for her kindness and encouragement. Through these memorials her influence continues.

PUBLICATIONS BY PHYLLIS JEAN VERHONICK

BOOKS

Descriptive Study Methods in Nursing. Washington, D.C.: Pan American Health Organization, Regional Office of the World Health Organization, 1971.

Nursing Research I. Boston: Little Brown, 1975.

Nursing Research II. Boston: Little Brown, 1975.

With C.C. Seaman. *Research Methods for Undergraduate Students in Nursing.* New York: Appleton-Century-Crofts, 1978.

DISSERTATION

"A Plan for Field Experience in Nursing Service and Administration for Army Nurse Corps Officers." Unpublished doctoral dissertation, Teachers College, Columbia University, (1958).

ARTICLES (SELECTED)

"Decubitus Ulcer Observations Measured Objectively." *Nursing Research* (1961): 211-14.

"Note Taking and Organizing Materials for Writing." In *Report on Nursing Research Conference* (February 24 to 7 March 1959). Pp. 278-86. Washington, D.C.: Walter Reed Army Institute of Research, 1962.

"Nursing Care of Traumatic Injuries." *American Association of Industrial Nurses Journal* (May 1963): 7-10.

"Natural Science Basis for Nursing Research, Education and Practice." In *The Continuing Search for Meaning* (June 18, 1964), Pp. 15-18. American Nurses' Association 44th Convention. Kansas City, Mo.: American Nurses' Association, 1964.

"Research in Nursing Practice." *The Quarterly Review* (December 1966): 21-22.

"Critique of Research: The Nurse-mentor in a Patient Care System." In *Third Nursing Research Conference* (February 27 to March 1, 1967). Pp. 32-38. (Nu-00132-03). Seattle: American Nurses' Association, 1967.

"The Nurse's Responses to Human Suffering Today: Teaching and Research in Nursing." *Bulletin des Infirmieres Catholique du Canada* (June 24, 1967): 217-24.

With G.A. Nichols. "Time and Temperature." *American Journal of Nursing* (November 1967): 2304-06.

With G.A. Nichols, B.A. Glor, & R.T. McCarthy. "I Came, I Saw, I Responded: Nursing Observation and Action Survey." *Nursing Research* (January-February 1968): 38-44.

With G.A. Nichols. "Temperature Measurement in Nursing Practice and Research." *Canadian Nurse* (June 1968): 41-48.

"Introduction to Research in Nursing." In *Methodology of Nursing Studies: Course Report.* Pp. 13-36. Washington, D.C.: Pan American Health Organization, Reports on Nursing, December 1968.

"The Nurse Monitor in the Patient-Care System." *Southern Medical Bulletin* (December 1968): 24-28.

"Teaching and Research in Nursing." *Catholic Nurse* (June 1969): 34-39.

"A Preliminary Report of a Study of Decubitus Ulcer Care." *American Journal of Nursing* 69 (August 1969): 68-69.

"Clinical Investigations in Nursing." *Nursing Forum* (1971): 80-88.

"Nursing Research: Its Implications for Nursing Practice and Nursing Education." *Virginia Nurse Quarterly* (1971): 31-38.

"Research Awareness at the Undergraduate Level." *Nursing Research* (May-June 1971): 261-65.

"Problem Forum on Development of Criterion Measures: Nursing Measures in Prophylaxis of Pressure Sores." In *Eighth Nursing Research Conference* (March 5-17, 1972). Pp. 221-26. Albuquerque, N.M.: American Nurses' Association, 1972.

"Clinical Studies in Nursing: Models, Methods, and Madness." *Nursing Research* (November-December 1972): 490-93.

"Clinical Studies in Nursing: Models, Methods and Madness." *Japanese Journal of Nursing Research* (1973): 24-28.

"Creativity through Research at the Undergraduate Level." *Image* (1973): 19-23.

With M.A. Rowland. "Problem-solving Approach to a Nursing Situation. *Military Medicine* (October 1960): 685-88.

With D.J. Dennis, J.G. Zimmer, and P.M. Catalano. "The Pharmacology of Human Skin: I. Epinephrine and Norepinephrine; Catecholamine-serotonin Combinations." *Journal of Investigative Dermatology* (November 1962): 419-29.

With H.H. Werley. "Experimentation in Nursing Practice in the Army." *Nursing Outlook* (March 1963): 7-10.

With D.T. Resio. "On the Measurement and Analysis of Clinical Data in Nursing." *Nursing Research* (September-October 1973): 388-93.

With R.S. Trandel and D.W. Lewis. "Thermographical Investigation of Decubitus Ulcers." *Bulletin of Prosthetics Research* (1975): 137-55.

With D.W. Lewis and H.O. Groller. "Thermography in the Study of Decubitus Ulcers: Preliminary Report." *Nursing Research* (1982): 233-37.

BIBLIOGRAPHY

Engert, R.M. "A Concise Biography of Lieutenant Colonel Phyllis J. Verhonick, ANC." Historical Reference Branch, U.S. Army Center of Military History, Washington, D.C., January 1979.

Francis, G. "Remembering (Dr. Phyllis J. Verhonick." *VA Nurse* 46 (Spring 1978): 6.

"Memorialization Program Ceremony. Dwight D. Eisenhower Executive Nursing Suite, Walter Reed Army Medical Center, Washington, D.C., July 10, 1980.

Parsons, L.C. "Eulogy for Phyllis J. Verhonick." *VA Nurse* 45 (Winter 1977): 47.

Rummel, V. (Mrs. J.C.). Telephone conversation with the author, June 21, 1990.

Werley, H.H., and R.T. McCarthy, "IN MEMO-
RIAM. Phyllis J. Verhonick: Practitioner, Researcher, Teacher, and Scholar." *Research
in Nursing and Health* 2 (June 1979).

Rosemary T. McCarthy

Eugenia Helma Waechter

1925–1982

Eugenia Helma Waechter was best known
as a researcher in pediatric nursing
issues and for her textbook on nursing
care of children.

She was born in Crespo, Argentina, on
March 29, 1925, while her parents were
serving as missionaries in Argentina. The
family later moved to Bunker Hill, Illinois,
where she graduated from Meissner High
School in 1942. She attended St. John's
College in Winfield, Kansas, from which
she received an associate degree with high
honors in 1944. She then entered the
Lutheran Hospital School of Nursing in
St. Louis, Missouri, graduating in August
1947. Next she enrolled in the University
of Chicago, from which she received a
bachelor's degree in 1948.

Waechter began her nursing career in
Hillsboro, Illinois, in November 1948 as a
public-health nurse in the Montgomery
County Health Department, a position she
held until 1954, when she was appointed
a supervising nurse. In March 1955 she
was appointed a nursing consultant to
the University of Illinois Division of Services for Crippled Children in Olney. She
took a leave of absence from this position
in June 1958 to attend graduate school at
the University of Chicago, from which she
received an M.A. in 1959. She returned to
the position in Olney and worked there
from September 1959 to August 1963.
From September 1963 to September
1964, she was enrolled in the School of
Nursing at the University of California
(UC), San Francisco, specializing in advanced maternal–child nursing. She left to
enroll in a program in child development
and education at Stanford University and
received her Ph.D. from that program in
1968. For most of the time she was enrolled in Stanford, she held the position of
lecturer in the School of Nursing at UC,
San Francisco, with a break between June
1966 and September 1967. Upon receiving her Ph.D. in 1968, she was appointed
an assistant professor at UC, San Francisco; she was promoted to associate professor in July 1973, and at the time of her
death she was professor and acting chair
of the family-health nursing department.

Her doctoral dissertation was on death
anxiety in children with fatal illness, and
it was this topic that continued to hold
her interest after completing her Ph.D.
Generally, her research program focused
on problems of children with chronic and
life-threatening illnesses as well as the
concerns of their family. She served as
coauthor with Florence Blake of the
eighth and ninth editions of *Nursing
Care of the Children*, a popular text in
pediatric nursing. At the time of her death
she was completing the tenth edition of
the book.

Waechter made numerous presentations, speeches, and papers on her research not only in the United States, but
also in Canada, Nigeria, Turkey, and Yu-
goslavia. She contributed to three widely
used audiovisual presentations concerned
with pediatric nursing, the death of a child,
and fear and pain as experienced by children. She was a member of a review panel
for *Nursing Research* from 1973 and on
the editorial board of *Hospitals* from
1976–78. At the time of her death she was
involved in a federally funded investigation of the responses of children who were
found to have cancer. She was elected as a
fellow of the American Academy of Nursing in 1978.

She died January 12, 1982, in Redwood
City, California, of the effects of smoke in-
halation from a fire in her home.

PUBLICATIONS BY EUGENIA HELMA WAECHTER

DISSERTATION

Death Anxiety in Children with Fatal Illness.
Unpublished Ph.D. dissertation, Stanford
University, 1968. Available on microfilm
from University Microfilms.

BOOKS

With F. Blake. *Nursing Care of Children.* Philadelphia: Lippincott, 8th ed. 1970; 9th ed. 1976.

Nursing Care of Children. Philadelphia: Lippincott, 10th ed. 1985.

ARTICLES

"Death Anxiety in Children with Fatal Illness." In *Fifth Nursing Research Conference.* Pub. #NU-00322-01R. Pp. 83–101. New York: American Nurses' Association, 1969.

"Developmental Correlates of Physical Disability." *Nursing Forum* 9 (1970): 90.

"Children's Awareness of Fatal Illness." *American Journal of Nursing* 71 (June 1971): 1168–72.

"Developmental Consequences of Congenital Abnormalities." *Nursing Forum* 14 (1975): 108–29.

"Bonding Problems of Infants with Congenital Abnormalities." *Nursing Forum* 16 (1977): 298–317.

"The Birth of an Exceptional Child." *Nursing Forum* 9 (1978): 202.

BIBLIOGRAPHY

"Eugenia Helma Waechter," *American Journal of Nursing* 82 (May 1982): 863.

Krulik, T., B. Holaday, and I. Martinson. *The Child and Family Facing Life Threatening Illness: A Tribute to Eugenia Waechter.* Philadelphia: Lippincott, 1987. Articles by Waechter are included.

Vern L. Bullogh

Lena Angevin Warner

1869–1948

Much of Lena Angevin Warner's life can be measured in firsts and lasts. She was the first nurse to graduate from a nursing school south of the Mason-Dixon Line and the first nurse to be registered in Tennessee. Later she helped found and became the first president of both her district and state nursing associations. She was the first Tennessee nurse to enroll in the Red Cross and the first chairperson of the first Tennessee State Board of Nurse Examiners. And in the closing years of her life, she was the last survivor of the Walter Reed Committee that discovered the cause of yellow fever. However, she is best remembered by the people of Tennessee for the 30 years she spent as health specialist for the University of Tennessee College of Agriculture Extension Service.

A devastating childhood experience with yellow fever left her with no doubt that she would become a nurse. Her parents were Saxton Smith, a lawyer, and Jean Mayhew Angevin. They lived in Grenada, Mississippi, but moved to Memphis, Tennessee, soon after their daughter's birth in 1869. Both parents and five siblings died when a yellow fever epidemic swept the city in 1877. Warner survived and was sent back to Grenada to live with grandparents. She soon returned to Memphis to attend St. Mary's Episcopal Boarding School for Girls.

The Memphis Training School for Nurses was chartered on December 28, 1887, as an affiliate of the Maury Clinic, a private hospital operated by two local physicians. It was the first in Tennessee, perhaps the first in the South. After she and three other nurses were graduated in 1889, Warner took further training at Cook County Hospital in Chicago, under Isabel Hampton.

After a brief time as a nursing supervisor, Warner accepted an invitation to return to the Maury Clinic as a surgical nurse. Five years later, she left to marry Charles Edward Warner, of St. Louis. Within five months, he was dead of a heart attack, and she was back at the Maury Clinic. In 1896 she helped Memphis General Hospital establish a nursing school.

When the Spanish-American War broke out in 1898, she volunteered for service through the Daughters of the American Revolution. Sent to Cuba, she became a chief nurse in charge of yellow fever tents at Mataugas. She assisted Dr. Walter Reed and his team in discovering that the bite of the stegomyia mosquito causes yellow fever. In 1901 she became one of the first chief nurses in the newly established Army Nurse Corps.

During this period, Warner designed a uniform for Red Cross nurses serving with the U.S. Army. It featured a blue Zoave jacket, long navy skirt, white linen shirt, a red sash five yards long, and a feminine version of the hat worn by Roosevelt's Rough Riders.

Warner returned from the war determined to specialize in preventive nursing for the rest of her career. Concerned about the lack of public-health nursing in Memphis, she convinced the Metropolitan Life Insurance Company to establish a visiting-nurse service, then organized and directed it for several years in both Memphis and Nashville. She drew up a plan for a city-county cooperative tuberculosis hospital in the Memphis area in 1908.

In 1915 she was appointed to the position that she later said gave her the greatest satisfaction—that of specialist for health in the University of Tennessee College of Agriculture Extension Service. For 30 years she traveled through East Tennessee, advising the people on health care. During World War I she also directed the enrollment of nurses for the Memphis General Hospital Unit, which served overseas. On a leave of absence in 1919 she helped the Knox County Red Cross chapter organize city and county demonstrations of public-health nursing. She retired in 1946.

Throughout her career Warner was active in nursing-related groups of various sorts. She was chair of the Tennessee State Board of Nurse Examiners from its inception in 1911 until it was revised in 1915. As such, she was the first nurse to be registered in the state. During her tenure she met opposition from many physicians to her efforts to raise the education standards of nurses and reduce the menial tasks to which they often were assigned.

The first nurse to enroll in the Red Cross in Tennessee, Warner served as its state chair of nursing from 1910–22. She helped to revitalize the inactive Memphis Graduate Nurses Association to form the West Tennessee Graduate Nurses Association in 1905. From that year until 1918, she also was president of the Tennessee State Nurses Association.

During her career Warner was named an honorary member of three alumnae associations and a life member of the state group. She received the U.S. medal for her service in Cuba and the Saunders Medal.

A portrait of her was unveiled at the John Gaston Hospital in Memphis on April 12, 1948.

Warner died August 19, 1948, in Knoxville.

PUBLICATIONS BY LENA ANGEVIN WARNER

What to Do to Keep Well. Knoxville: University of Tennessee College of Agriculture Extension Division, 1916.

BIBLIOGRAPHY

"Bouquets to Nurses." *American Journal of Nursing* 48 (August 1948): 20 adv.
"Lena Angevin Warner." Undated typescript, University of Tennessee College of Nursing, Knoxville, Tn.
"Mrs. Lena A Warner." Obituary. *American Journal of Nursing* 48 (October 1948): 32 adv.
"Mrs. Lena Warner of Reed Mission, 79." Obituary. *New York Times*, August 20, 1948.

Alice P. Stein

Emma Louise Warr

1847–1937

Emma Louise Warr received many accolades in her long career in nursing but none that surpassed her title as the "Florence Nightingale of Missouri." She was the first superintendent of nursing for the St. Louis Training School of Nurses at the City Hospital, the first training school for nurses west of the Mississippi River.

There are questions concerning the birthplace of Warr. Most biographies list Brooklyn, New York, in 1847. Her death certificate lists her birthplace as England. At a memorial service held in St. Louis on June 6, 1937, a friend of hers gave a short address on her life. According to this account, Warr was the sole survivor of a shipwreck on the Atlantic Ocean near New York City. She was placed in a foundling home in New York City and a short time later adopted by Jesse and Helen Warr of Jamestown, New York. Her father was a florist who was born in England.

Her early education was in Jamestown. As a young girl, she served as a nurse to Frances Bailey, the child of Mr. and Mrs. Edward Bailey. The Baileys recognized her abilities for nursing and encouraged her to seek formal training. Warr entered the New York Hospital School of Nursing (New York City) in 1880 and received her diploma on October 5, 1882.

She served one year as superintendent of nursing at Hamot Hospital in Erie, Pennsylvania, and traveled for several months in Europe visiting European hospitals. In 1884 she was invited to St. Louis to become the superintendent of its new school of nursing.

When Warr came to St. Louis, the state of nurse's training in Missouri was in its infancy. St. Louis was ten years behind the development of nurses' training as it existed on the East Coast. Nursing in the mid-nineteenth century could be categorized as the pioneer Nightingale period. After the Civil War interest in nursing education was high, and in 1873 three nursing schools were established. Others soon followed, mostly in the Eastern states.

The unsanitary health conditions experienced by soldiers in military hospitals during the Civil War gave rise to members of organizations in Missouri, such as the Western Sanitary Commission, to campaign for the establishment of nursing schools in the state. In order to establish such a school in St. Louis, a society was formed of prominent community people with Mrs. William H. Pulsifer as president of the board. On December 7, 1883, the St. Louis Training School for Nurses was established.

The school was part of the City Hospital. The St. Louis Board of Aldermen passed an ordinance making the school official and made provisions for monthly allowances for the students: $10 for the first year and $12 a month for the second year. This sum was for dress, textbooks, and any other personal expenses. Other benefits included free board, laundry, and medical care.

On April 7, 1884, a superintendent and two students were enrolled as hospital employees. Within a month the superintendent, Abbie Hunt, was forced to leave on account of family illness. In August 1884 Emma Louise Warr took over the position and is listed as the first superintendent of the school.

All accounts describe Warr as having a sweet dignified personality, frail in physical appearance, but steel-like in determination, all of which helped her in building the nursing program in St. Louis.

When she arrived, the nurses had been given one ward at the hospital. By 1891 Warr supervised all but two wards. Warr described the conditions of the hospital when she first came as follows:

> The patients laid on ticks stuffed with straw [and] often had no sheets. Dysentery in the summer and frost-bite in the winter were the common ailments. ... All the nursing was done by middle-aged women accustomed to menial tasks. No St. Louis young woman of education or character would have thought of entering nursing service.

Warr not only managed the school, but she was the only instructor. With only one textbook she began teaching the methods and professional ethics of nursing. At times she met resistance from physicians and politicians who looked askance at the "trained nurse," regarding her as a curiosity. Money to sustain the school had to be raised by private subscription. Seeing the need for more extensive nurses' training, Warr planned to implement a three-year curriculum. In her 1897 annual report to the Society of the St. Louis Training School for Nurses, she wrote of the reasons for the adoption of such a curriculum: for "the work of nursing is difficult and exacting, and demands much practical knowledge. The almost lack of such knowledge or home training of any kind, ... renders it impossible for us to teach them in two years all that they should know."

On May 27, 1896, her plans for the new curriculum were delayed when the hospital was destroyed by a cyclone. During this catastrophe she led the nurses in saving the lives of many of the patients. In characteristic style, she took charge of the prisoners' ward and unlocked their cells. She told them if the Lord saved their lives to report to her the next day. These men assisted in clearing the debris and to a man reported to her the next morning. Of the 403 patients in the hospital on that day, only one was killed. The nurses immediately began turning the cloistered hall of an old convent into cheery hospital wards. The convent served as the city hospital until a new facility was completed in 1905. Finally, in 1907 Warr began the implementation of a three-year nursing curriculum.

Nursing in the early 1900s was demanding. Warr described the nursing loads in her 1898 annual report to her sponsoring society. In 1897 30 nurses, including 6 in the nurses' training program, and 5 night nurses, took care of 570 patients. These nurses worked in the operating room, which had operations any hour, day or night, and in the gynecological and obstetrical wards. In the 1908 annual report many changes were reported in the hospital. The departments of nursing then included medical, surgical, obstetrical, contagious, and out-clinic wards; this last gave the nurses experience in emergency work. In this report Warr also emphasized her demand for excellence by her nurses and wrote of the need to discharge two nurses for inefficiency. After 25 years of hard work and labor of love, Emma Warr retired in 1909 as superintendent of nurses. She continued her interests in nursing affairs and the organizational activities of Missouri nurses in establishing a statewide association. She also served as state secretary for the American Red Cross.

Many tributes came her way. The quarterly bulletin of the St. Louis Training School Nurses Alumnae, entitled *The Warr-ior*, was named after her. In 1933 as one of the events in the golden jubilee celebration of the founding of the school, members of the original Society of St. Louis Training School, under whose auspices the school was started, honored Emma Warr with a bronze plaque for her achievements in nursing.

Warr spent her entire life caring for the sick. From her first days at the St. Louis Training School for Nurses, having well-educated nurses administering wards and taking care of the patients was her goal. Her work at the school in making her goal a reality gave credence to the nursing movement in the first two decades of the twentieth century for the adoption of standard credentials through the registration of nurses by the states.

Agitation for state registration of nurses began in the East. In 1906 Warr received a registered nurse certificate from the University of the State of New York, the state in which she had received her nursing education. She then began using RN after her name.

In 1909 the Missouri law was passed to register nurses. Warr did not apply under this law for RN status. Although she had earned the RN designation as described in the requirements set forth in the state law, she was cited in 1912 by the Missouri Nurses Association for placing RN after her name without officially applying to the Missouri state board. Most thought the indictment to be out of place for the pioneering nurse who was given credit for establishing the first nursing school in Missouri. Finally, in 1921 the Missouri State Board of Examiners awarded her a registered nurse certificate. Emma Louise Warr remained a spirited fighter until the end.

During her retirement years she also served as house mother for a group of nurses that had moved into quarters in City Hospital. Retiring from that position, she lived out her years quietly.

After a brief illness, Emma Warr passed away on Monday, April 19, 1937, at the age of 90. The cause of death was listed as bronchopneumonia. Although she spent most of her years in St. Louis and called it her home, her remains were sent to Jamestown, New York, for interment.

Emma Louise Warr's life spanned the times during which great changes occurred in nursing, and she was one of the important innovators in making nursing a profession.

BIBLIOGRAPHY

"Annual Reports of the St. Louis Training School for Nurses." St. Louis: Missouri Historical Society Archives, 1896, 1897, 1898, 1908.

Christ, E.A. *Missouri's Nurses, The Development of the Profession, Its Associations, and Its Institutions.* Jefferson City: Missouri State Nurses Association, 1957.

"Emma Louise Warr." Obituary. *American Journal of Nursing* 37 (June 1937): 705.

"Emma Louise Warr." Collection of Obituaries (1937), Missouri Historical Society Archives, St. Louis.

Flanagan, J.G. *Makers of Nursing History.* M.R. Pennock, ed. New York: Lakeside, 1940.

Green, E. *History of the St. Louis (Mo.) Training School for Nurses.* St. Louis: The School Alumnae, 1941.

Plunkett, M.M. "History of Nursing West of the Mississippi." *American Journal of Nursing* 33 (October 1933); 929–30.

Robinson, V. *White Caps: The Story of Nursing.* Philadelphia: Lippincott Company, 1946.

Trenholme, L.I. *History of Nursing in Missouri.* Columbia: Missouri State Nurses Association, 1926.

The Warr-ior. St. Louis: St. Louis Training School for Nurses Alumnae, memorial edition, 1937.

Mary K. Delmont

Yssabella Gertrude Waters

1862–1938

Yssabella Gertrude Waters worked closely with Lillian Wald at the Henry Street Settlement in New York City, served as a nurse in the Spanish-American War, was an author of an early study of public health, and was a pioneer in applying statistical methods to nursing.

Born on February 22, 1862, in Groton, Massachusetts, Waters was the daughter of Mary Farnsworth and Charles E. Waters. She did marry, but her husband left her. She obtained a divorce, and the court allowed her to resume her maiden name. In 1895 she entered the Johns Hopkins Hospital Training School for Nurses in Baltimore, from which she graduated in 1897. She almost immediately became associated with Lillian Wald at the Henry Street Settlement in New York City and except for serving in the Spanish-American War for approximately a year during 1898–99, she remained there until 1912.

While at the Henry Street Settlement, beginning in 1902, Waters collected (at her own expense) statistics on public-health nursing and nurses that were published and distributed through the National Organization for Public Health Nursing (NOPHN). Her data included the activities of nurses in visiting-nurse associations, the Red Cross, public-health agencies, and nurses working for hospitals, counties, and other local government bodies. In 1905 at the International Conference of Charities and Corrections she presented a paper on the status of organizations and nurses based upon her work.

Her informal activities became more formalized in 1912 when she moved to the newly opened office of the NOPHN in New York City, serving as statistician, mostly on a volunteer basis. When the NOPHN moved to larger quarters in 1915, she rented an office in the organization's suite in order to continue her work. The data she collected were summarized annually in a compilation dealing with public-health agencies. In 1919 she published a description of nursing in industry as well as a description of the qualifications and responsibilities of industrial nurses. In addition, she responded to numerous requests for information about public-health nursing addressed to NOPHN.

Among her other volunteer activities were serving on the Endowment Committee of the Johns Hopkins Nursing School (1915–26), a term as vice-president of the Society of Spanish-American War Nurses, and in 1916 as president of the Nurses' Club of the New York City area. During World War I she organized the placement efforts of the public-health division of the American Red Cross. She also served as a member of the committee on Home Nursing in the welfare section of the Committee on Labor, Council of Defense. Her book *Visiting Nursing*, first published in 1909, was a major source reference.

Waters retired in 1920 to her home in Groton, Massachusetts, where she was active in various clubs and church groups. Her hobby was gardening. She died on August 16, 1938, in Groton.

PUBLICATIONS BY YSSABELLA GERTRUDE WATERS

BOOKS

Visiting Nursing in the United States. New York: Charities Publication Committee, 1st ed. 1909; 2nd ed. 1912. This work contained a directory of organizations employing trained visiting nurses with chapters on principles, organization, and methods of administration of such work.

ARTICLES

"Statistical Table of Visiting Nursing in the United States." *American Journal of Nursing* 6 (October 1905): 26–31.

"Report of the Statistical Department." *Public Health Nursing* (June 1920): 473–75.

"Industrial Nursing." *Public Health Nursing* 11 (1919): 728–31 [a history]; 12 (1920): 886–87; 14 (1922): 491.

BIBLIOGRAPHY

Alan Mason Chesney Medical Archives. Johns Hopkins Medical Institutions, Baltimore.

Dock, L., et al. *History of American Red Cross Nursing, 1912–1952.* New York: National League for Nursing, 1975.

Johns Hopkins Nurses Alumni Association. Biographical information. Baltimore, Maryland.

Public Health Nursing (1919): 658–59; (1920): 886–87; (1922): 491.

Woman's Who's Who of America, 1914–15. J.W. Leonard, ed. New York: American Commonwealth, 1914.

Vern L. Bullough

Harriet Helen Werley

b. 1914

Major Harriet Helen Werley established the Department of Nursing Research at Walter Reed Army Institute in Washington, D.C., and served as director of the Center for Health Research at Wayne State University, Detroit, the first research center for nursing in the country. Concerned with the communication of nursing research, Werley founded the journal *Research in Nursing and Health* and developed the *Annual Review of Nursing Research* series. Throughout her career she has served as an inspirational role model and has encouraged nurses to become active in research.

Werley was born on October 12, 1914, in Berks County, Pennsylvania, the daughter of Thomas G. and Cora M. (Hein) Werley. She grew up during the Great Depression and attended a one-room country school in Berks County. Her father died when she was 12 years old. After graduating from high school, she found full-time employment and at times was the only employed member of her family. Motivated to become a nurse by the death of her father, she saved enough money to enter nursing school.

Werley received her diploma in nursing from Jefferson Medical College Hospital, Philadelphia, in 1941, a B.S. in nursing education from the University of California at Berkeley in 1948, an M.A. in nursing administration from Columbia University in 1951, and a Ph.D. in psychology from the University of Utah in 1969. After receiving her diploma in 1941 during World War II, she joined the Army Nurse Corps and served in the Mediterranean theater for 37 months. After the war she completed her bachelor's degree under the GI Bill of Rights and again returned to active duty, this time at the U.S. Army Hospital, Camp Stoneman in Pittsburg, California. Invited to attend Teachers College under army sponsorship, she spent the year 1950–51 pursuing a master's degree in nursing administration and was subsequently assigned to the Office of the Surgeon General in the Personnel Division. In 1957 Werley became the first full-time director of the Department of Nursing, Walter Reed Army Institute of Research, a post she retained until September 1962, when she joined the U.S. Eighth Army as chief nurse, stationed in Seoul, Korea.

Stimulated by the research activities she had witnessed during her years in Washington, Werley decided to end her army career in 1964 and enrolled as a doctoral student at the University of Utah. Upon completing her degree, she took a position as the first director of the Center for Health Research at Wayne State University, and in 1974 she became associate dean of research at the College of Nursing, University of Illinois Medical Center in Chicago and then at the University of Missouri School of Nursing, Columbia. She is currently distinguished professor at the University of Wisconsin-Milwaukee School of Nursing.

Werley's major research interests include social-psychological aspects of health, family planning and population concerns, health services and nursing. She has written and edited numerous books and articles. In 1978 she founded the influential journal *Research in Nursing and Health* and served as its editor. She also developed the *Annual Review of Nursing Research* series, which has been published since 1983. After joining the University of Missouri School of Nursing, Werley began work on the development of a nursing minimum data set to facilitate information processing and compare research data, and in 1988 her book *Identification of the Nursing Minimum Data Set* was published.

Werley has received many awards in recognition of her commitment to health care, including the U.S. Legion of Merit in 1964, the Alumni Special Achievement Award from Thomas Jefferson University, Philadelphia, in 1978, and the American Nurses' Foundation Award for Distinguished Contribution to Nursing Science in 1980. She was the recipient of a National Institute of Health Research Fellowship from 1964–69 and a charter fellow of the American Academy of Nursing in 1973. The book award of the *American Journal of Nursing* was given to her twice, first for her book *Nursing Information Systems* and later for the *Annual Review of Nursing Research.*

Her primary contribution has been directed toward research and research development, the quality of nursing doctoral programs, and concern about scholarly publications in nursing. The incumbent of many newly created positions, Werley has had a major impact on nursing research in this country.

PUBLICATIONS BY HARRIET HELEN WERLEY

BOOKS

Report on Nursing Research Conferences. Washington, D.C.: Walter Reed Army Institute of Research, 1962.

Survey of Health Professionals Regarding Family Planning. Detroit: Wayne State University College of Nursing; Springfield, Va.: NTIS, 1975.

Health Research, the Systems Approach. New York: Springer, 1976.

Nursing Information Systems. New York: Springer, 1981.

Identification of the Nursing Minimum Data Set. New York: Springer, 1988.

DISSERTATION

"Sex Differences in Cognitive Consistency and Persuasibility with Respect to Real Life Issues." Ph.D. dissertation, University of Utah, Salt Lake City, 1969.

ARTICLES (SELECTED)

"The ANC's Career Guidance Program." *American Journal of Nursing* 54 (January 1954): 60–62.

"Care of Casualties Caused by Nuclear Weapons. 2. The Nurse's Role in Nuclear Disaster." *American Journal of Nursing* 56 (December 1956): 1580–83.

"Research in Nursing as Input to Education Programs." *Journal of Nursing Education* 11 (November 1972): 29–38.

"This I Believe—About Clinical Nursing Research." *Nursing Outlook* 20 (November 1972): 718–22.

"Medicine, Nursing, Social Work. Professionals and Birth Control: Student and Faculty Attitudes." *Family Planning Perspectives* 5 (Winter 1973): 42–49.

"Nursing Research in Perspective." *International Nursing Review* 24 (May–June 1977): 75–83.

"Research Publication Credit Assignment: Nurses' Views." *Research in Nursing and Health* 4 (June 1981): 261–79.

BIBLIOGRAPHY

American Men and Women of Science, 12th ed. New York: Bowker, 1972.

Making Choices Taking Chances. Nurse Leaders Tell Their Stories. T.M. Schorr and A. Zimmerman, eds. St. Louis: Mosby, 1988.

"Nursing Research Department at Walter Reed Has Full-Time Director." *American Journal of Nursing* 58 (June 1958): 784.

Who's Who of American Women, 10th ed. Chicago: Marquis, 1977–78.

Lilli Sentz

Myrtle Viola Werth

b. 1907

Myrtle Viola Werth played an important role in the development of nursing in a small northwestern Wisconsin community. Her contribution was so great that when a new community hospital was built in 1980, the hospital was named after her.

Werth was born on November 25, 1907, in Menomonie, Wisconsin to Henry and Emily Micheels Werth. As the oldest of five children, she attended St. Paul Lutheran School and Menomonie High School, graduating in 1926. She then attended Luther Hospital's nursing program in Eau Claire, Wisconsin, graduating in 1931. During her enrollment in the diploma program, she also took further training at Milwaukee Children's Hospital in Milwaukee.

After graduation, Werth did private-duty nursing for about one year in the Menomonie area and was then hired by Memorial Hospital in Menomonie in 1932. Her primary area of interest was surgery, although she did work on general nursing units. During the time she was employed by the hospital (1930–74) she pursued additional training in the area of administration at John Hopkins Hospital in Baltimore, Maryland. Her roles within the Menomonie Memorial Hospital changed over the years of her tenure. Prior to 1949 she was superintendent of the hospital. During reorganization of hospital ownership in 1948, Werth was appointed director of nursing and served in that capacity until 1972, and then until 1974, when she retired, the assistant administrator of nursing. Her dedication to the profession is evidenced by her 12–14 hour days as

well as taking only two vacations during the time of her employment.

In 1980, when a new 63-bed community hospital was built and dedicated, it was named the Myrtle Werth Medical Center in recognition of her long-standing devotion to nursing in the community. Werth is very humble about the medical center being named after her, and in her retirement remains active and committed to nursing in the Menomonie area.

She has been instrumental in developing and operating the Telecare program sponsored by the hospital auxiliary since its inception in 1972. This program involves contacting elderly individuals living alone to confirm their safety and well being. Werth personally has been responsible for saving several lives through the program. When possible, Werth goes with the police officer or sheriff to an individual's home if he or she does not respond to her daily call.

In addition to her work with the Telecare program, Werth also works at Memorial Hospital's information desk. Since her "retirement" she has put in thousands of hours of volunteer time at the hospital. In 1973 she was honored by the Menomonie Area Chamber of Commerce as "Citizen of the Year." The hospital auxiliary has established a scholarship in her name to be awarded to a junior or senior student enrolled in a four-year nursing program.

Myrtle Werth, a very spry, small-built individual, is very warm, humble, and gracious, yet a little shy. She has no immediate family in the Menomie area, but her many friends keep her involved and take her places since she does not drive. Her memories of working so many years at one hospital include the very many long hours at her stations, especially during bad weather, high census, and nursing shortages as well as "working with wonderful interesting people." Her "people-focused" orientation is very evident in her accomplishments.

Halsey Douglas, a retired hospital administrator from New Jersey, now residing in Menomonie and a personal friend of Werth, had the following to say about her: "Myrtle Werth is a very dedicated person. Not only has she devoted her entire working lifetime to her profession as a nurse, but in her retirement she has continued to give of herself by caring about many people who are home bound and live alone through the Telecare program sponsored by the Myrtle Werth Medical Center named for her."

BIBLIOGRAPHY

Bjork, V. Interview with Myrtle Werth, November 22, 1988, Menomonie, Wisconsin.

"Ground Broken for 63-Bed Hospital." *Dunn County News*, August 2, 1978.

"A Health Security Program for Those Who Live Alone." *Dunn County News*, November 25, 1981.

"Medical Center Auxiliary Awards Scholarships." *Dunn County News*, May 14, 1980.

"Memorial Hospital News." *Dunn County News*, January 8, 1975.

"Miss Werth, Langmack Receive Chamber Awards." *Dunn County News*, December 12, 1973.

"Myrtle Werth Medical Center Opens Thursday." *Dunn County News*, January 9, 1980.

"Myrtle Werth Scholars." *Dunn County News*, May 16, 1984.

"Volunteers Honored by Hospital." *Dunn County News*, February 14, 1979.

"Volunteers Recognized." *Dunn County News*, February 24, 1982.

"Volunteers Recognized." *Dunn County News*, April 27, 1983.

Michaeline P. Mirr

Claribel Augusta Wheeler

1881–1965

Nurse educator and administrator, Claribel Augusta Wheeler directed the Mount Sinai Hospital School of Nursing in Cleveland and the Washington University School of Nursing in St. Louis and served as executive secretary at the National League of Nursing Education. She provided nursing education effective and far-sighted leadership both on a regional and a national level.

Wheeler was born in Prospect, New York, on August 13, 1881, the daughter of Schuyler Van Rensselaer and Lucia (Kellogg) Wheeler. Her father was a druggist.

Wheeler spent most of her childhood at her mother's ancestral home north of Utica and attended Utica Academy. When she was in her late teens, the family moved to Poughkeepsie. Wanting initially to become a librarian because of her love of books, her interest was diverted to nursing, which she felt offered greater possibility for self-expression and usefulness. She entered Vassar Brothers Hospital School of Nursing in 1904. After a postgraduate course at Sloane Maternity Hospital in New York City in 1907, she returned to her alma mater and worked first as a night supervisor, then as assistant superintendent of nurses, and finally as superintendent and principal of the school.

Feeling the need for further preparation, Wheeler enrolled at Teachers College, Columbia University, in 1912, taking the course in hospital and training-school administration. She then became superintendent at the United Hospital, Portchester, New York, and in 1916 accepted the invitation to organize the school of nursing at Mount Sinai, Cleveland, Ohio, which continued under her leadership for seven years. In 1923 she moved to St. Louis to direct the Washington University School of Nursing. There she established a combined degree program with the university, offering students college courses in addition to their professional education. She also organized the first course in public-health nursing available to graduate nurses and to degree-course students interested in this specialty. She was a member of numerous professional committees both in Ohio and Missouri and served as president of the Cleveland League of Nursing Education, the Ohio State Nurses Association, and the Missouri National League of Nursing Education.

On February 1, 1932, Wheeler became executive secretary of the National League of Nursing Education, a post she held for 10 years. During the first year of her tenure, the league became the Department of Education of the American Nurses' Association; but due to Wheeler's foresight and planning it did not lose its autonomy, and the two associations worked closely together in order to achieve common objectives. Under her leadership the league completed the *Curriculum Guide for Schools of Nursing* as well as many other studies and publications. Wheeler also initiated the accreditation program for nursing schools and promoted advanced nursing courses for public-health nurses. A skilled administrator, she was often dependent on the work of volunteer committees. She broadened the influence of the league by encouraging the development of cooperative relationships with other organizations and lay groups.

After her retirement, she moved to Richmond, Virginia, to be near her sister. Wheeler possessed a great capacity for friendship, a quality noted by her associates throughout her career. An accomplished horseback rider, swimmer, and oarswoman, she was also an amateur photographer and painter and knowledgeable about wild flowers and birds. She died on December 8, 1965.

PUBLICATIONS BY CLARIBEL AUGUSTA WHEELER

"The Educational Problem of the Small Hospital." *American Journal of Nursing* 17 (July 1917): 928–32.

"Nursing Preparatory Courses in Schools and Colleges." In *Annual Report, 1919 and Proceedings of 35th Convention.* National League of Nursing Education. Pp. 270–78. Baltimore: Williams & Wilkins, 1919.

"Value of Public Health Nursing Affiliation of Student Nurses." *Public Health Nursing* 11 (December 1919): 958–59.

"Use of Ward Helpers in Hospitals." In *Transactions of the Twenty-Second Annual Conference of the American Hospital Association.* Pp. 158–62. Chicago: The Association, 1920.

"The Profession of Nursing." *Public Health Nursing* 13 (April 1921); 201–06.

"The Function of the Private Duty Nurse in the Community." *American Journal of Nursing* 25 (March 1925): 199–203.

"The Role of the Nurse in the Social Hygiene Movement." *Journal of Social Hygiene* 11 (October 1925): 402–06.

"Equipping a Nurses' Residence." *American Journal of Nursing* 28 (August 1928): 787–92.

"The Status of the Special Duty Nurse." *Bulletin of the American Hospital Association* 3 (October 1929): 768–71.

"The Selection of Students for Schools of Nursing and Problems of Adjustment." *American Journal of Nursing* 30 (September 1930): 1169–76.

"Are Nursing Schools Improving?" *Modern Hospitals* (January 1936): 47–49.

BIBLIOGRAPHY

Archives. Vassar College, Poughkeepsie, N.Y.

Archives. Washington University School of Medicine, Library and Biomedical Communications Center. St. Louis.

Deming, D. "Claribel A. Wheeler Retires." *Public Health Nursing* 34 (September 1942): 519.

Goostray, S. "Report of the President." *American Journal of Nursing* 42 (July 1942): 800.

Manuscripts Collection. National Library of Medicine, History of Medicine Division, Bethesda, Md.

Munson, H.W. *The Story of the National League of Nursing Education.* Philadelphia: Saunders, 1934.

National League for Nursing Archives. New York City.

Robson, E.G. "Claribel A. Wheeler, R.N." *American Journal of Nursing* 36 (March 1936): 226–29.

Who's Who in the East. A Biographical Dictionary of Leading Men and Women of the Eastern United States. Boston: Larkin, Roosevelt & Larkin, 1943.

Lilli Sentz

Carolyn Ladd Widmer

b. 1902

Carolyn Ladd Widmer was founder of the University of Connecticut School of Nursing and its dean for 25 years. She contributed to international nursing as a public-health nursing organizer in Bogota, Colombia, and as dean of the nursing school and supervisor of nurses at the American University in Beirut, Lebanon. Widmer promoted scholarship in nursing through leadership positions in Sigma Theta Tau. A leader in community affairs, she held offices in a variety of local and state organizations in Connecticut.

Widmer was born on January 19, 1902, in Randolph, Vermont. Her only sibling, Alice, was 15 months her senior. Her parents were George Ladd and Mary Hamlin. George Ladd was a clergyman, a graduate of Williams College and Yale University Divinity School. Widmer's maternal grandfather was Cyrus Hamlin, the founder of Robert College in Istanbul, Turkey. Earlier, as a missionary there, he started a bakery to employ Christians. This bakery provided bread for British soldiers during the Crimean War. Widmer wrote a story about this entitled, "Grandfather and Florence Nightingale."

Election to Phi Beta Kappa at Wellesley College was Widmer's entrance into a scholastic honor society, an association that remained lifelong. She graduated in 1923 and her interest in science led her to a job in biological research in Boston, where she assisted in the pioneering work of Drs. Minot and Murphy in pernicious anemia. For a short period after this, she was a laboratory instructor at the University of Vermont.

Yale University School of Nursing had been open only a few years when Widmer entered in the class of 1929. Here she was taught by the case method of patient care similar to the modern concept of primary-care nursing. Widmer formed a close personal relationship with Dean Annie W. Goodrich. This friendship had a great influence on her career and the nursing school she would establish. After graduation Widmer became a head nurse on the West I wing of Yale New Haven Hospital.

Widmer's first experience in international nursing came as a response to a request by the government of Colombia to organize public-health nursing in Bogota. Widmer and another Yale nurse arrived there in late 1929.

In an article, "Nursing on Top of the World," Widmer describes the primitive conditions encountered there, where even the basic nursing supplies—such as pure water, newspaper, and safety pins—were hard to find. Even locating the home of a patient was difficult. The local health visitors from the United States were really only health visitors, but invaluable, and Widmer's example was a beginning in showing what could be done in basic sanitation and health teaching.

As a result of this experience, Widmer was recommended by Mary Beard, then director of Nursing Services with the Rockefeller Foundation, to become direc-

tor of nursing and dean of the School of Nursing at the American University in Beirut, in what was then called Syria. This school had been started in 1905 by Jane Van Zandt, who remained director for 20 years. In 1932 at the time Widmer was appointed, the school was seeking to have its course upgraded. As it was the major qualified nursing school in the Middle East, the student body came from a large area, diversified in nationality, religion, and language. Widmer's aims at the school were to raise the status of nursing, to attract more Muslim girls, particularly Syrians, to create nurses who could become nursing leaders in their own countries, and to give more public information about nursing and the need for government regulation of the profession.

One of Widmer's first innovations was to raise the entrance requirement to high-school graduation. She created a three-year course with 600 hours of classroom work and clinical experience at the American University of Beirut Hospital with rotation on all services except mental health. The course also included public-health experience in the health center and the outpatient clinic. Midwifery was a popular course, and there was much demand for the graduates, especially in Persia.

In Beirut Widmer met Robert Widmer, whom she married on April 27, 1934. She continued to serve as supervisor of nurses and dean of the nursing school until 1938. Two years later the threat of World War II led her to return to the United States for the safety of her two young sons. Widmer recalled her experience in Beirut as fulfilling.

After the United States declared war and the nursing shortage became acute, Widmer became director of a nurse refresher course at Yale New Haven Hospital, implemented so that housewives could reenter nursing to serve on the home front. Having two small children of her own at the time, she could understand the problems of the young wife entering the work force. She found that bedside care came back naturally but that the technology had to be newly learned. She exhorted hospital employers to give on-the-job training and flexible hours.

At this time a committee of health and education leaders in Connecticut were drawing up a report for the new University of Connecticut (formerly Connecticut State College) entitled, "A School of Nursing for Connecticut." The report outlined a program for registered nurses leading to a bachelor of science degree. Toward the end of the report, consideration was given to a five-year program in nursing as a second step. However, because of the war emergency, the university administration decided that a basic school of nursing was imminently needed. Another committee formed by the university, chaired by Dean Charles B. Gentry and including Annie W. Goodrich, called for a basic program of five years including three of university courses and two of clinical experience in a hospital setting leading to a bachelor of science degree. This program was announced in the catalogue of February 1942, although a nursing school dean and faculty had not yet been found.

President Albert Nels Jorgenson approached Widmer to be dean on the recommendation of Annie Goodrich. At first Widmer refused to accept because she knew of the difficulty in finding housing for herself and two sons. Later, when the president phoned to say he had a home for her, she accepted and arrived in Storrs on August 6, 1942, just a few weeks before the school was scheduled to open. Hurriedly, Widmer met with the Board of Consultants to work out policies and curricula. The stated purpose of the school was to offer opportunity to incorporate a general college education with professional preparation in nursing, to offer collegiate work to graduate nurses, and to aid in research and study for the advancement of nursing education.

Thirteen students entered the school in September 1942 to begin the basic program. The whole university campus was in the early stages of development in a distinctly rural area. The nursing school was first installed in the Home Economics Department and later in the old infirmary building. The first full-time faculty member appointed by Widmer was Josephine Dolan.

The most pressing problem for the new dean was to arrange clinical experience for the students. Jorgenson had originally assumed that Hartford Hospital would welcome the students, but after a campus visit the nursing personnel decided not to make that commitment. After much negotiation and consultation with Agnes Ohlson, then chief nursing examiner for the state of Connecticut, Widmer was able to arrange for 12 months of medical and surgical nursing at the William W. Backus Hospital in Norwich, pediatric and communicable disease at the Yale New Haven Hospital, psychiatric experience at the Norwich State Hospital, and public-health nursing at the Hartford Visiting Nurse Association. In 1944 to accomodate the Cadet Nurse Corps the course was made a four-and-a-half-year one and in 1953 finally a four-year program.

During the early years the school was a small, friendly place. Widmer took a personal interest in the progress of each student, each of whom she knew by name. The freshman-sophomore picnics were held at her home. There was a White Caps Club and an RN Club. Students were permitted to live at home and to marry, unusual liberties for the time.

To provide herself with a better understanding of modern educational concepts, Widmer commuted to Trinity College, Hartford, part time, earning enough credits to receive an M.A. in education in 1951.

From the beginning there was a cooperative relationship between the nursing school and the rest of the university, although as Widmer stated the nursing school was not expected to cost much or have a large faculty.

As ideas regarding nursing education were changing rapidly during Widmer's tenure, the curriculum underwent constant revision. These changes were subject to review by the State Board of Nurse Examiners, which Widmer believed was sometimes a barrier to progress as it measured "clock hours" rather than college credits. In 1949 the National Committee for the Improvement of Nursing Services placed the University of Connecticut School of Nursing in the top 25 percent of schools in the nation. In the 1950s and 60s when the National League for Nursing reviewed the school for accreditation, differences sometimes arose about the aims of nursing education. In 1966, under advice from the league, the program in general nursing that enabled registered nurses to earn a degree was discontinued. Although Widmer was concerned about giving up this opportunity to the backlog of diploma graduates, the National League for Nursing did not favor any type of special program for registered nurses.

In the 1960s much planning went into inaugurating a master's program, but it was not implemented under Widmer's deanship because of the difficulty in obtaining qualified faculty and the demands of the growing baccalaureate program. By September 1967, when Widmer retired after 25 years as dean, the school had 483 students and a faculty of 38. Widmer had started a school under emergency wartime conditions and left a thriving modern university nursing school. She was succeeded by Eleanor K. Gill, also a Yale School of Nursing graduate.

After retirement, Widmer was able to devote more time to honor societies. She believed that these societies were important in recognizing and encouraging scholarship and that this was particularly important to the concept of nursing. In 1954 the Mu chapter of the nursing national honor society Sigma Theta Tau was established in Storrs. In 1965 Widmer was elected its national second vice-president in charge of admission and new members. After retirement as dean, she became its executive secretary, traveling widely around the country establishing new chapters and visiting old ones. She held this position for six years, during which time the national headquarters was at her home.

Also after retirement Widmer was able to devote more time to the numerous state and local organizations in which she had always been active. She was president of the Mansfield Historical Society, the Heart Association Fund Drive, the Windham Hospital Auxiliary, later the Storrs Golden Age Club, and held countless positions of leadership on boards of Connecticut health organizations.

Honors bestowed on this woman of achievement include Honorary Recogni-

tion by the Connecticut Nurses Association in 1967 and the Distinguished Alumna Award, Yale University School of Nursing, 1975. Scholarships were established in her name by the University of Connecticut Alumnae Association and the Storrs-Willimantic Branch of the American Association of University Women. A Carolyn Ladd Reading Room is dedicated to her at the School of Nursing. Her portrait hangs in this room.

Widmer lives in Storrs, Connecticut, in her home of many years. Known to all her friends of whatever age or position as "Laddie," she projects a friendly and unpretentious manner. She is full of humorous stories and is famous for playing jokes. Her seriousness about scholarship and dedication to nursing has always been lightened by her warm and gregarious personality. In a tribute to her at the Sigma Theta Tau convention in Indianapolis in 1973, Josephine Dolan stated, "In reflecting upon my close association with Laddie, the things that pop into my mind are her humanness, her scholarship, and her humanitarian endeavors."

PUBLICATIONS BY CAROLYN LADD WIDMER

BOOKS

With M.S. Infante, J.E. Hayes, and M. Kramer. *Heritage of Accomplishment. The History of the University of Connecticut School of Nursing, 1942–1981.* Storrs: University of Connecticut School of Nursing Alumnae Association, 1982.

ARTICLES

"Nursing on Top of the World." *Public Health Nursing* 24 (April 1932): 187–91.

"Nursing in Syria." Personal manuscript of the subject, May 1934.

"The Housewife Reenters Nursing." *American Journal of Nursing* 43 (January 1943): 10–14

"The Brown Report and Its Relation to Nursing in Connecticut." *Connecticut State Medical Journal* 49 (September 1949): 864–67.

"Sigma Theta Tau: Golden Anniversary." *Nursing Outlook* 20 (December 1972): 786–88.

BIBLIOGRAPHY

Dolan, J. "A Tribute to Carolyn Ladd Widmer." Sigma Theta Tau Convention, Indianapolis, October, 1973.

Goodnow, M. and J. Dolan *History of Nursing*, 10th ed. P. 369. Philadelphia: Saunders, 1958.

"News of Nursing." *American Journal of Nursing* 43 (August 1943): 772.

Widmer, C.L. Interview with the author, April 19–21, 1989; June 1, 1989.

Who's Who in America, Vol. 35, p. 2344. Chicago: Marquis, 1968.

Stephanie Cleveland

Mary Bristow Willeford

1900–1941

Mary B. Willeford was a pioneer midwife with the Frontier Nursing Service in Kentucky, where her exceptional ability to ride horses made her a great asset. An early nurse researcher, she conducted studies of infant and maternal mortality rates in rural areas of the United States, demonstrating the success of the approach that Mary Breckinridge had developed at the Frontier Nursing Service. Her knowledge and advanced degree standing (she was one of the first to have a Ph.D. in nursing) led to her appointment as a consultant to the California State Department of Health and to the U.S. Children's Bureau.

Born in Flatonia, Texas, on February 4, 1900, she graduated from the University of Texas at Austin and then went on to attend the Army School of Nursing at Walter Reed Hospital in Washington, D.C. In 1926 she completed a midwifery course at York Lying-in Hospital in London and received a certificate from the English Central Midwive's Board in London. In August 1926 she became a member of the Frontier Nursing Service (then known as the Kentucky Committee for Mothers and Baby) as a nurse midwife. Breckenridge refers to her as "Tex" in her book. In 1929 Willeford took leave to return to England, where she received a certificate as teacher of midwifery. From 1930 to 1938 she was assistant director of the Frontier Nursing

Service. While serving in this capacity, she took periodic leaves to complete studies at Columbia University, from which institution she received her Ph.D. in 1932. Her dissertation, "Income and Health in Remote Rural Areas," was based on residents of Leslie County, Kentucky, one of the areas covered by the Frontier Nursing Service. She emphasized that poverty had a great impact on public health.

While still with Frontier Nursing Service, she did a study of nursing needs in the Ozark region at the request of an interested group in St. Louis, Missouri, and in 1935 she made a survey of the health on Indian reservations. In 1938 she left the Frontier Nursing Service to become a consultant to the California State Department of Health on maternal and child health, and in 1940 she was appointed as a public-health nursing consultant to the U.S. Children's Bureau in Washington, D.C.

Among other things, Willeford assisted with the establishment of a school of midwifery at Tuskegee Institute in Alabama and other schools of midwifery that requested appropriations under the nursing education section of the Social Security Act. She helped organize the Kentucky State Association of Nurse-Midwives, which later became the American Association of Nurse-Midwives, founded in 1928, with Willeford as a charter member. She died on December 24, 1941, at Presbyterian Hospital in New York City.

PUBLICATIONS BY MARY BRISTOW WILLEFORD

MONOGRAPHS

Income and Health in Remote Rural Areas. A Study of 400 Families in Leslie County, Kentucky. Ph.D. dissertation, Columbia University, New York, 1932. Two editions, one with thesis notes and one without.

ARTICLES

"Frontier Nursing Service." *Public Health Nursing* 25 (1933): 6–10.

BIBLIOGRAPHY

Breckinridge, M. *Wide Neighborhoods: A Story of the Frontier Nursing Service.* New York: Harper, 1952.

Dammann, N. *A Social History of the Frontier Nursing Service.* Sun City, Ariz.: Social Change Press, 1982.

"Mary B. Willeford." *American Journal of Nursing* 42 (1942): 231.

Nursing Archives. Mugar Memorial Library, Boston University, Boston.

Poole, E. *Nurses on Horseback.* New York: Macmillan, 1933.

Vern L. Bullough

Anne A. Williamson
1868–1955

Anne A. Williamson was a nursing educator and author. She spent 48 years as an administrator of the California Hospital in Los Angeles, the longest service record in that hospital's history. During the Spanish-American War, she helped lay the groundwork for the later victory of the American Nurses' Association in gaining military rank for the Army Nurse Corps. In 1898 she was in the first contingent of women nurses ever to be allowed to serve officially in a U.S. Army camp.

Williamson was the daughter of Charles and Martha Allen Williamson, both New Yorkers of Irish descent. She was born on May 3, 1868, in Palmyra, New York, and had one sister, Katherine, two years older. During her early childhood the family moved to New York City and later to a town 10 miles outside the city. Williamson attended several schools, including St. Agnes Episcopal Girls' School. At age 15, she also took Saturday classes at Miss Parloa's Cooking School and won a county fair prize for her bread. She was named class poetess when she graduated from high school in 1886.

Joining her sister, Williamson entered Mt. Holyoke College, South Hadley, Massachusetts. After two years, she transferred to Wilson College, Chambersburg, Pennsylvania, and was nearing graduation when called home by her father's loss of employment. She did not finish at Wilson.

She took secretarial studies near home and soon became engaged to a young banker, Robert Stevens. Shortly before the wedding, Stevens died, and she never married.

As a young teen, Williamson had met Clara Barton, a friend of her mother. Barton told her, "Some day your help will be needed. Try to be ready when the time comes." For the rest of her life, Williamson looked to Barton as a primary role model, and after her fiancé died, she dedicated her life to nursing.

She entered New York Hospital School of Nursing as a probationer and within weeks was accepted for the two-year program. During those years, she served as night cook, worked in the children's ward, and spent three months on the staff of the Sloan Maternity Hospital. While at Sloan, she was successful in convincing the administration to pass a regulation that barred them from disturbing the rest periods of off-duty nurses.

Before graduating in October 1896, she also worked at the Hudson Street Hospital, an emergency facility, and finally as head nurse of the men's surgical Ward G at New York Hospital. When she received her diploma in 1896, Barton sent her flowers.

Taking rooms across the street from New York Hospital, she began a career as private-duty nurse. She had numerous well-known patients, including Rudyard Kipling; Harry K. Thaw, a poker player; and Joe Jefferson, an actor.

When the battleship *Maine* was attacked in February 1898, Williamson immediately volunteered her services to Barton. On July 23 she was ordered to duty with Red Cross Auxiliary No. 3. The nurses were paid $25 a month plus transportation, but they had to supply their own uniforms and equipment. Each was allowed only one suitcase for all that.

Arriving at City Hospital in Charleston on July 27, Williamson was put in charge of a typhoid ward and the next day also became night superintendent. Beginning August 17, she served at Sternberg Hospital, Chicamuga Park. There, she defied military orders if necessary to get the supplies she needed for her wounded.

Discharged at the end of the war, she spent three more years in private duty. On a visit to her mother in California in 1907, Williamson decided to change to institutional nursing. She began her record-breaking affiliation with the California Hospital on November 1, 1907, as night supervisor. She rose rapidly through the ranks to assistant superintendent, superintendent in charge of nurses' training, and finally director of nurses.

Always concerned for the welfare of her nurses, Williamson reorganized their schedule, rearranged classes so they could get more rest, and saw that their health and recreational needs were met more adequately. She made arrangements that expanded through the years to send student nurses for additional class work at area high schools, junior colleges, and universities. However, she also spoke out against the eight-hour law, saying nurses would be "running around . . . tiring themselves out before they begin their work."

When the first aviation meet in U.S. history was held in Los Angeles in January 1910, Williamson supervised a field hospital that treated 54 patients, only one an aviator. She was awarded a gold medal by the meet's organizing committee.

In her late 40s when the United States entered World War I, she was not accepted for overseas nursing. Instead, she recruited nurses for the Navy Base 3 nursing unit and Army Unit 512 in 1917 and 1918. Three evenings a week she gave speeches to promote the sale of war bonds.

In 1918 she saw the hospital through a major crisis when it was swept by the national flu epidemic. On another occasion, she did detective work that resulted in the apprehension of a nurse who had nearly killed several infants in the hospital nursery with heroin. Her father and mother died in 1918 and 1920, respectively.

The privately owned hospital was sold to the Lutheran Hospital Association of Southern California in 1921, and Williamson loaned the association funds to build a new nurses' residence across the street. When the building was opened on February 14, 1924, she was given an apartment there.

In May 1925, as she neared age 60, Williamson was placed on a year's leave at half salary and given a testimonial dinner. She became secretary of the hospital's women's auxiliary and of the local nursing committee of the Red Cross Committee on Nursing Service. After the leave, she worked three days a week as the hospital's director of social services. In that capacity she continued for 22 years to serve the women's auxiliary, assist the hospital auditor, and represent the hospital in small-claims court cases.

Beginning in 1927, Williamson served for a decade as an administrator of the California State Nurses Association, the first two years as president, then four years each as a director and parliamentarian. In 1931 the association presented her with a gold gavel engraved with the dates of her presidency. She also served as president of District Five of the association in 1912 and again in 1930.

For eight years, beginning in 1925, she was secretary of the local Red Cross Nursing Service. She also was a member of the National Relief Fund Committee of the American Nurses' Association.

During the later years of her career, Williamson was honored at several other testimonial events. In October 1936 a dinner commemorating her 40 years of nursing service was attended by hospital staff and members of professional organizations. In 1942 she was cited for 35 years of service to the California Hospital. On her seventy-fifth birthday in 1943 she received a diamond-set award for the longest service record in the hospital's history.

50 Years in Starch, her autobiography written in the third person, was published in 1948. In October 1950 her historical article, "A Backward Glimpse," appeared in the *American Journal of Nursing*. In it, she recalled her private-duty nursing days when she assisted at major operations performed on the patients' kitchen tables and wrapped new mothers in bindings that required 150 carefully spaced safety pins.

Williamson succumbed to a long-standing heart ailment on August 11, 1955, at the home she shared with her sister in South Pasadena.

PUBLICATIONS BY
ANNE A. WILLIAMSON

BOOK

50 Years in Starch. Culver City, Calif.: Murray and Gee, 1948.

ARTICLES

"Emergency Hospital Service of Aviation Week." *Nurses' Journal of the Pacific Coast* 6 (March 1910): 114–17.

"California and the Eight-Hour Law." *Modern Hospital* 3 (September 1914): 183–87.

"The Eight-Hour Law, Its Present and Its Future." *Transactions of the Seventeenth Annual Conference of the American Hospital Association, 1915, Northfield, Minnesota.* Pp. 132–38. Chicago: American Hospital Association. 1915.

"Evolution of the Training School." *Pacific Coast Journal of Nursing* 23 (April 1927): 207–08.

"A Backward Glimpse." *American Journal of Nursing* 50 (October 1950): 637–38.

BIBLIOGRAPHY

"News about Nursing." *American Journal of Nursing* 37 (January 1937): 97.

"Obituaries." *American Journal of Nursing* 55 (October 1955): 1178.

"Well-earned Honors." *American Journal of Nursing* 43 (July 1943): 688.

Private papers. Sophia F. Palmer Historical Library Collection, Mugar Memorial Library, Boston University, Boston.

Alice P. Stein

Maud H. Mellish Wilson

1862–1933

Maud H. Mellish Wilson combined health care and language skills to become one of the great medical editors of the twentieth century. She personally edited or oversaw the editing of thousands of medical publications prepared by the staff of the Mayo Clinic and Foundation and founded and administered its library from 1907 until her death in 1933.

Annie Maud Headline was born near Faribault, Minnesota, in 1862, the youngest of seven children of Swedish parents. She attended rural schools, where she gained a love of literature by reading extensively in the classics.

Lacking funds to attend medical school, she was attracted to the training school for nurses of Presbyterian Hospital, Chicago, because it adjoined Rush Medical College. The leader in her nursing class, she attended as many lectures as possible at Rush and soon became a protégée of distinguished faculty members of both institutions. Moses Gunn became a special mentor, and she nursed him through his terminal illness.

She graduated from Presbyterian on May 10, 1887, and did private-duty nursing in and out of that hospital until September, when she was named superintendent of Maurice Porter Memorial Hospital for Children in Chicago.

At Rush and Presbyterian Hospital, she became acquainted with Dr. Ernest J. Mellish, a young surgeon, whom she married on September 28, 1889. At his request, she dropped "Annie" from her name. Mellish's tuberculosis forced the couple to seek more favorable climates. They lived in Ishpeming, Michigan, back in Chicago, and then in El Paso, Texas, where he died in April 1905. Maud Mellish had edited his many medical papers and also those of Dr. A.J. Ochsner. On her husband's death, she continued to work with Ochsner and worked for two years as librarian for Augustana Hospital in Chicago.

At the beginning of 1907, staff at the Mayo Clinic were expressing concern that the facility had no central library. Ochsner recommended Mellish to Dr. William J. Mayo, and he hired her to develop a library and edit publications. In 1914 a division of publications was organized with library, editorial, and art sections. Mellish was named division director and head of the editorial section. Thereafter, she did mostly editing, leaving the library to a professional librarian. Beside more than 5,000 papers, she and her staff edited the weekly Proceedings of the staff meetings of the Mayo Clinic, which began publication in 1926.

She worked closely with each staff writer to produce publications that were accurate, truthful, clear, and concisely written. Her style was to subordinate the self-interests of the writer to the overall interests of the institution. Absorbed in promoting the work of others, she wrote little for publication under her own by-line.

She married a long-time associate, Dr. Louis B. Wilson, head of the division of laboratories of the Mayo Clinic and director of the Mayo Foundation, in 1924. She was found to have a widespread abdominal malignancy in October 1932 and died the following year.

PUBLICATIONS BY
MAUD H. MELLISH WILSON

A Collection of Papers Published Previous to 1909 by William J. Mayo and Charles H. Mayo. Philadelphia and London: Saunders, 1942.

The Writing of Medical Papers. Philadelphia and London: Saunders, 1942.

BIBLIOGRAPHY

"Maud H. Mellish Wilson." *Supplement to the Proceedings of the Staff Meetings of the Mayo Clinic.* Rochester, Minn.: Mayo Clinic, November 8, 1933.

Mayo, W.J. "Maud H. Mellish Wilson and the Mayo Clinic." *Supplement to the Proceedings of the Staff Meetings of the Mayo Clinic.* Rochester, Minn.: Mayo Clinic, December 20, 1933.

Wilson, L.B. "A Woman Pioneer in a New Profession, Medical Editing." *Supplement to the Proceedings of the Staff Meetings of the Mayo Clinic.* Rochester, Minn.: Mayo Clinic, December 15, 1933.

Pennock, M.R. *Makers of Nursing History.* New York: Lakeside, 1940.

Alice P. Stein

Sophie Gran Jevne Winton
1887–1989

World War I was the first time the army and navy trained nurses as anesthetists for war service. American nurse anesthetists established an enviable record and won the admiration of some of the most celebrated surgeons and medical practi-

tioners in the Western world. Their performance helped solidify the position of the nurse in the field of anesthesia. One of the most distinguished and highly decorated of these nurses was Sophie Winton. She was also one of the first nurse anesthetists to establish herself as an independent practitioner and was a force in the early professional organization of nurse anesthetists in California.

Born Sophie Christina Gran on a Minnesota farm, on April 24, 1887, she received her nurse's training at Swedish Hospital, Minneapolis. She and her fellow graduates of 1911 were the first to take the state nursing board examination, making Winton one of the first registered nurses in Minnesota. Two years later, at the urging of hospital superintendant Gustaf W. Olson, she returned to Swedish Hospital to begin training as a nurse anesthetist. Her education in anesthesia was furthered by frequent visits to the Mayo Clinic in Rochester, Minnesota, where nurse anesthetists had been practicing with distinction since the clinic's opening in 1889. She also benefited from the proximity of the Ohio Chemical Company. When Dr. J.A. Heidbrink introduced his new anesthesia machines, he employed Winton to demonstrate them. By 1918 she had five years of anesthesia experience and a record of more than 10,000 cases without a fatality. She then joined the Army Nurse Corps (through the Red Cross) because "it was the patriotic thing to do."

Winton and nine other nurses from Minneapolis Hospital Unit No. 26 were assigned to Mobile Hospital No. 1 in the Chateau-Thierry area in France with the pioneering physician anesthetist James T. Gwathmey. She later reported to her former mentor, Olson, that she:

gave anesthetics from the first of June [1918] to November after the Armistice. How many anesthetics I gave during the World War, I cannot determine, except that when the big drives were on, lasting from a week to ten days, I averaged twenty-five to thirty a day. The first three months I gave chloroform entirely, after which a ruling came that we were to use ether because there had been too many deaths from chloroform in inexperienced hands. Many a night I had to pour ether or chloroform on my finger to determine the amount I was giving, because we had no lights except the surgeon had a searchlight for his work, so the only sign I had to go by was respiration.

Elsewhere, she recalled that "during the drives, patients came in so fast that all the surgeons could do was to remove bullets and shrapnel, stop hemorrhages, and put iodoform packs in the wound and bandage it. As soon as they were through operating on one patient, I would have to have the next patient anesthetized." She frequently gave anesthesia as shells fell close to the hospital. For Winton, "the most pitiful thing of the work overseas was to step outside the hospital tents and see hundreds of stretchers on the ground, each bearing a man who must wait probably for hours before he could be taken care of. We had 17 operating tables working day and night and yet we could not keep up with the work."

Mobile Hospital No. 1, under the command of Lt. Col. Donald Macrae, Jr., was cited twice for its brave service. According to Major General C.P. Summerall, commanding general of the Fifth Army Corps, American Expeditionary Forces in France, Macrae had "requested that his hospital be moved further forward in order to receive the wounded more promptly, and explained that his officers and nurses had no fear of shells and were only anxious to do all that was possible for the care of the wounded. To the noble women nurses of this hospital, the corps is especially indebted. They brought comfort and assistance to our wounded which none but women of such high attainments and ideals could administer. Their labors were an inspiration and they have written a new chapter in the annals of womanhood which in future will be cherished by our people."

All the nurses in Winton's unit were awarded the Croix de Guerre. Winton herself was also awarded six overseas service bars as well as honors from the Overseas Nurses Association, the American Legion, and the Veterans of Foreign Wars. It is important to note that Winton and her fellow nurses in this war, though serving in military organizations, came under the auspices of the Red Cross. They did not receive full military rank or the pay and allowances equal to male military personnel. Nor did they receive veterans' compensation.

The expertise of American nurse anesthetists led to the British decision to train their own nurses in the work. As the history of the Pennsylvania Hospital Unit (Base Hospital No. 10) recorded: "Throughout the British Army anesthetics had hitherto only been administered by doctors and when shortly after our arrival our women began their work, they were greatly astonished. The skill and care which was displayed soon caused their amazement to yield to admiration. The idea was soon adopted by the British authorities, and in the early spring of 1918 classes were formed of British nurses who received instruction at our hospital and at several others, and before the end of the war a number of British nursing sisters were performing the duties in various hospitals throughout the BEF." Years later, Dr. George W. Crile observed that "if the Great War had gone on another year, the British army would have adopted the nurse anesthetists right in the middle of the war." But, as Daryl Pearce has shown in her study of the professional anesthetist in Britain, a British nurse anesthetist "might (barely) be acceptable in times of war but definitely not in peacetime." Though the Royal College of Nursing took the position in 1919 that the British nurses should be given "a chance for success" in anesthesia, the field remained the province of the British physician.

After World War I American nurse anesthetists also continued to face legal challenges from some physicians, but they were ultimately successful in securing their position in the field.

After the war Winton (now married to George W. Jevne) moved to California because the climate was more healthful for her ailing husband. Welcomed by her former mentor, G.W. Olson, then assistant superintendent of Los Angeles County

General Hospital, she nevertheless encountered the significant anti-nurse anesthetist activity in that area and never practiced in a hospital. She became a partner in a private dental clinic, did research on dental anesthesia, and was honored by the Mexican Dental Society in association with the International Dental Association for her work in advancing that field. She later opened the Jevne Minor Surgery Hospital in Hollywood, which specialized in cosmetic surgery, and attended some of the most notable film celebrities of the era.

Winton also played a significant part in supporting the rights of other nurse anesthetists by helping form the first California Association of Nurse Anesthetists. In February 1930 the first meeting was held in Los Angeles. Thirteen members were present at the second meeting, held in Anaheim, and Winton was elected president. The group became an affiliate of the National Association of Nurse Anesthetists in 1935.

The economic pressures of the Great Depression intensified anti-nurse anesthetist activities. More physicians were looking to anesthesia practice as a supplemental source of income. In the fall of 1933 the Anesthetic Section of the Los Angeles County Medical Association asked a physician, Dr. William V. Chalmers-Francis, to test legally the right of nurse anesthetists to administer anesthetics. On July 12, 1934, nurse anesthetist Dagmar Nelson went on trial in Los Angeles. The prosecution sought to establish that "the giving of anesthetics and the employment of nurses or any other person who is not a registered physician and surgeon, is in violation of the California Medical Practice Act." Winton not only testified for the defense but contributed to its financial support. The court found that Nelson's activities were part of "established and uniformly accepted practice followed by surgeons and nurses." The legality of nurse anesthetists was thus definitively established.

For her lifelong contribution to the art and science of nurse anesthesia, Winton was honored in 1984 by the American Association of Nurse Anesthetists with its Agatha Hodgins Award for Outstanding Accomplishment. Her first marriage had ended in divorce; she was widowed by her second husband. She died in Hollywood on April 24, 1989—her 102nd birthday.

BIBLIOGRAPHY

Bankert, M. *Watchful Care, A History of America's Nurse Anesthetists.* New York: Continuum, 1989.

"Sophie Winton Presented with AANA Hodgins Award." *AANA News Bulletin* (November 1984).

"Sophie Winton's Scrapbook." Archives, American Association of Nurse Anesthetists, Park Ridge, Illinois.

Marianne Bankert

Annie Turner Wittenmyer
1827–1900

Throughout the Civil War Annie Turner Wittenmyer untiringly offered her services to the Union Army in a variety of roles: nurse, sanitary agent, pioneer dietician, and relief worker. Afterward she was instrumental in obtaining federal pensions for Civil War nurses and in establishing retirement homes for them as well as for the widows and mothers of veterans.

Born Sarah Anne Turner on August 26, 1827, in Sandy Springs, Ohio, she was the eldest daughter of six children born to Elizabeth Cathelia (Smith) and John G. Turner. Her mother's family traced their roots back to the legendary John Smith of Jamestown, Virginia. Nicknamed "Annie" by her family, she attended school in Kentucky and finished at a seminary in Ohio. She was well educated for a woman of the period and became an avid writer, publishing her first poem at the age of 12.

In 1847 she married William Wittenmyer, a prosperous Ohio merchant several years her senior. Only one of their five children, Charles Albert, survived infancy. The small family moved to Keokuk, Iowa, in 1850, where Wittenmyer later opened a free school for poor children. Her husband's death shortly before the outbreak of the Civil War left her comfortably situated and freed her to do charitable work for the remainder of her life.

During the Civil War Wittenmyer increasingly became involved in relief work, visiting troop encampments and helping to establish a statewide system of soldiers' aid societies in Iowa to collect much needed supplies. Her volunteer work in this area led to her eventual appointment by the Iowa State Legislature as one of several paid state sanitary agents.

Throughout her many visits to the front lines in this capacity, Wittenmyer often doubled as a nurse in the field hospitals, ministering to the needs of the sick and wounded soldiers. Her generous and diligent efforts in these roles, as sanitary agent, as nurse, and as relief worker, led the soldiers to nickname her "God's Angel." The government also rewarded her with special privileges. Secretary of War Edwin Stanton supplied her with authorization to move freely within the battlefields, and, later, President Abraham Lincoln issued her a pass entitling her to free transportation and special privileges. Additionally, the United Telegraph Association awarded her unlimited free access to telegraph facilities and messages until the end of the Civil War.

Wittenmyer often came under enemy fire while performing her duties in the battle zones. While riding to a field hospital near Vicksburg, she was fired upon and nearly drowned after falling from her horse. At the Battle of Shiloh the hospital ship on which she was working came under fire. Another time Confederate sharpshooters shot at an ambulance in which she was tending to the injured. These and other incidents are detailed in Wittenmyer's autobiographical account of her wartime experiences, *Under the Guns*.

In 1864 Wittenmyer began implementing a plan to open special dietary kitchens at army hospitals. She felt that the poor nutritional value of the food served to the convalescing soldiers contributed to their deaths almost as much as the unsanitary conditions of the hospitals and that proper diets were as important as medication in saving lives in the battlefields. The first kitchen was established at the Cumberland Hospital in Nashville, Tennessee, with support from the United States Christian Commission. Similar kitchens rapidly emerged throughout the front lines, eventually developing into an integral part of the military hospital system.

Wittenmyer's next endeavor, the establishment of homes for war orphans, stemmed directly from the many pleas she had received from dying soldiers to care for their families. She was successful in obtaining both private and federal backing in establishing several orphanages in Iowa and spent the years immediately following the Civil War as the matron of the Iowa Soldiers' Orphan's Home in Davenport.

After leaving her position in 1867, Wittenmyer became involved in Christian charity work, founding the Ladies' and Pastors' Christian Union, a Methodist organization that catered to the needy. She later moved to Philadelphia and in 1871 founded the journal *Christian Woman*, which she edited for 11 years.

In 1873 Wittenmyer joined the "Woman's Crusade" against the evils of liquor, and by November 1874 she was elected the first president of the National Woman's Christian Temperance Union (WCTU) at its inaugural convention, a position to which she was continuously reelected until 1879. Throughout her term she traveled extensively across the country organizing local WCTU branches to join in the Gospel Temperance Movement.

In 1879 the conservative Wittenmyer lost her bid for reelection to the WCTU presidency to a more progressive candidate, Frances E. Willard. While Wittenmyer preferred to view the temperance movement as a single-issue, religiously motivated movement, Willard wanted to politicize the movement, advocating massive societal reforms, especially women's suffrage, to accomplish the goals of the temperance movement. Though Wittenmyer remained active in the WCTU, she was nevertheless unsuccessful in opposing Willard's many reforms, and in 1890, she supported formation of the Non-Partisan Woman's Christian Temperance Union, a conservative group that opposed women's suffrage, serving as president from 1896–98.

During the 1880s and 1890s Wittenmyer became increasingly involved with the Woman's Relief Corps, the women's auxiliary of the Grand Army of the Republic, serving as its national chaplain in 1883 and as its president from 1889–90. She successfully campaigned for the establishment of National Woman's Relief Corps Homes for Civil War nurses and the widows and mothers of Civil War veterans and lobbied Congress for pensions for Civil War nurses. Wittenmyer later served as director of the National Woman's Relief Corps Homes in Ohio and Pennsylvania. In April 1898 she received a special pension from Congress in recognition of her contributions throughout the Civil War.

On February 2, 1900, Wittenmyer died of cardiac asthma at the age of 72 at her son's home in Sanatoga, Pennsylvania, only a few hours after presenting a lecture in nearby Pottstown.

PUBLICATIONS BY ANNIE TURNER WITTENMYER

A Collection of Recipes for the Use of Special Diet Kitchens in Military Hospitals. St. Louis: Prepared and published under the auspices of the U.S. Christian Commission by R. P. Studley, 1864.

Women's Work for Jesus. New York: Nelson & Phillips, *Christian Woman*, 1873. Reprint, New York: Garland, 1987.

The Women of the Reformation. New York: Phillips & Hunt; Cincinnati: Cranston & Stowe, 1885.

Under the Guns: A Woman's Reminiscences of the Civil War. Boston: Stillings, 1895.

BIBLIOGRAPHY

Brockett, L.P., and M.C. Vaughan. *Woman's Work in the Civil War: A Record of Heroism, Patriotism and Patience.* Philadelphia: Zeigler, McCurdy, 1865.

Davies, W.E. *Patriotism on Parade: The Story of Veterans' and Hereditary Organizations in America, 1783–1900.* Cambridge: Harvard University Press, 1955.

Newberry, J.S. *The U.S. Sanitary Commission in the Valley of the Mississippi, During the War of the Rebellion, 1861–1866.* Cleveland: Fairbanks, Benedict, 1871.

Willard, F.E. *Woman and Temperance, or, The Work and Workers of the Woman's Christian Temperance Union.* Hartford, Conn.: Park; Chicago: Goodman, 1883. Reprint, New York: Arno, 1972.

Woman's Christian Temperance Union. Records. Woman's Christian Temperance Union National Headquarters, Frances Willard Memorial Library, Evanston, Illinois.

Wood, A.D. "The War Within a War: Women Nurses in the Union Army." *Civil War History* 18 (1972): 197–212.

Wittenmyer, A. Papers. Iowa State Historical Library, Des Moines, Iowa.

Wittenmyer, A. Papers. Library of Congress, Washington, D.C.

Ellen Greenblatt

Helen Wood
1882–1974

Helen Wood was a nurse educator who headed several schools of nursing. She was an organizer and the first director of the Strong Memorial Hospital School of Nursing and also was director of schools of nursing at Simmons College, Boston, and Washington University, St. Louis.

Wood lived most of her life in the Boston area. She was born in suburban Newton on May 13, 1882, to William B. and Amelia Adelaide Pott Wood. Her father had been born in Newton and her mother in Pottsville, Pennsylvania.

She received an A.B. degree from Mt. Holyoke College in 1904 and was graduated from the Massachusetts General Hospital Training School for Nurses, Boston, in 1909. She received an M.A. from Columbia University in 1924. She was a recipient of the Isabel Hampton Robb Scholarship, and in 1927 Mt. Holyoke College named her an alumnae member of Phi Beta Kappa.

Wood was assistant superintendent of Faulkner Hospital, Boston, and then superintendent of nurses at Children's Hospital, Boston. She also served on the staff of the Grenfell Mission on the Labrador coast. From 1919–23 she directed the Washington University School of Nursing, St. Louis.

During the summer of 1923 she directed a summer school for nurse instructors at Stanford University, California.

From 1924–31 she was an organizer and the first director of the Strong Memorial Hospital School of Nursing at the University of Rochester Medical Center, Rochester, New York. The school became a college of the university in 1972. In 1929 alumnae of the school named the residence hall of the medical center in Wood's honor, and that building became the center of the school's activities. In 1970 the university presented Wood with a plaque honoring her lifetime of contributions to nursing.

She returned in 1931 to her home state to become assistant superintendent and then acting superintendent of nurses at Massachusetts General Hospital. In 1933, she conducted classes in ward administration and teaching for the Brown University extension department and Simmons College.

She became director at Simmons in 1934 at a time when the nursing program was replacing its undergraduate focus on public-health nursing with a more liberal education. The students continued to train at Massachusetts General, Peter Bent Brigham, and Children's hospitals and to take classes at Simmons. Upon successful completion of the five-year program, they received both a B.S. degree and a nursing diploma. Public-health nursing became a graduate concentration.

Wood served on two state boards of nurse examiners: Massachusetts (1917–20) and Missouri (1920–23). From 1920–23 she was a member of the Winslow-Goldmark Committee, formerly the Committee for the Study of Public Health Nursing Education, created by the Rockefeller Foundation in 1919.

She represented the American Nurses' Association on the Committee on Grading Nursing Schools from 1926–34. She also was a director of the National League of Nursing Educators and president of the New York Chapter.

Wood died on September 23, 1974, of a cerebral thrombosis and hypostatic pneumonia, at age 92. At the time, she was living in Newton Center.

PUBLICATIONS BY HELEN WOOD

ARTICLES

"The Value of the Clinical Method of Teaching and How It Can Be Organized." *National League of Nursing Education Annual Report, 1919,* and *Proceedings of the 25th Convention.* Baltimore: Williams and Wilkins, 1919.

"Constructive Facts Regarding Schools." *National League of Nursing Annual Report, 1921,* and *Proceedings of the 27th Convention.* Baltimore: Williams and Wilkins. 1922.

"The Place of the Student Nurse in the Nursing Service of the Hospital." *American Journal of Nursing* 25 (March 1925): 183–88.

With H.I.P. Friend. "Value of Institutes, Summer Schools and Extension Courses to Instructors and Superintendents." *National League of Nursing Education Annual Report, 1923,* and *Proceedings of the 29th Convention.* Baltimore: Williams and Wilkins. 1923.

BIBLIOGRAPHY

American Women, 1935–1940: A Composite Biographical Dictionary. D. Howes, ed. Detroit: Gale, 1981.

News Releases. History of Medicine Collection, Edward G. Miner Library, University of Rochester Medical Center, Rochester, N.Y.

"Reorganization at Simmons College." *American Journal of Nursing* 34 (July 1934): 656.

To Each His Farthest Star, University of Rochester Medical Center, 1925–1975. Rochester, N.Y: University of Rochester Medical Center, undated.

"Wood, Helen." *American Journal of Nursing,* 39 (March 1939): 330.

Alice P. Stein

Lucia E. Woodward
1843–1934

Lucia E. Woodward, a pioneer in mental-health nursing, served as superintendent of McLean Hospital School of Nursing, Belmont, Massachusetts, for 28 years.

Woodward was born on a farm near the village of Plainfield, New Hampshire, on February 2, 1843, the daughter of Frederick and Lucy (Fay) Woodward. Her parents were of New England heritage and raised their children in a strict religious atmosphere. Little is known about her early education, but Woodward probably attended the academy in the neighboring town of Cornish. On September 5, 1864, she became an attendant at McLean Asylum and after six years was promoted to supervisor. During her first 15 years at McLean there was practically no change in the working routine. Patients were called boarders, and the attendants worked 12 to 16 hours per day, serving as caretakers and companions as well as doing all the housework.

In 1879 Dr. Edward A. Cowles came to McLean and began planning for the conversion of the asylum into a hospital. He wanted to establish a school of nursing, and three years later he hired Mary Palmer as superintendent of nurses. The beginning of McLean Training School for Nurses traditionally dates from 1882, although classes did not start until a year later. The reorganization under Cowles involved the replacement of attendants by professional nurses and the introduction of student nurses. Cowles and Palmer, who had graduated from the Massachusetts General Hospital Training School and spent 12 years as an attendant and then matron at the Vermont Asylum, worked with Linda Richards at Boston City Hospital to design a curriculum for training nurses to work with mental patients. Due to Palmer's poor health, much of the work of introducing the training program fell to Woodward, who was sent to the Boston City Training School in 1882 for six months to gain experience in general medical nursing under Linda Richards. When Palmer resigned, Woodward was appointed superintendent of nurses on November 1, 1884. Formal lectures were given by members of the medical staff, and Woodward held classes that she based on available nursing texts. She also acquainted the students with the history of nursing. Her most effective teaching method, however, was through personal interviews with the students and through the example she set.

Woodward was shy and reserved and seemed austere and unapproachable to many. Tall and bony with piercing blue eyes and a stern mouth, she reminded one student nurse of the Statue of Liberty. But upon further acquaintance she became much less formidable; she always showed a personal interest in the welfare, careers and personal lives of her nurses. To the medical officers, she was dependable, resourceful, and always of good judgment; to the patients, she was kind, patient, and considerate.

Woodward retired on August 3, 1912, and lived with two friends for 15 years. After fracturing her hip in 1927, she was invited to spend the rest of her days as guest of McLean Hospital.

She died on June 29, 1934, at the age of 91 of arteriosclerosis and senility.

BIBLIOGRAPHY

Abbott, E. Stanley. "A Pioneer in Mental Nursing." *American Journal of Nursing* 36 (February 1936): 147–48.

Archives. McLean Hospital, Belmont, Massachusetts.

Bragg, T.A. *Guide to the Archives of the McLean Hospital Corporation.* Belmont, Mass.: The Hospital, 1984.

Sutton, S.B. *Crossroads in Psychiatry: A History of the McLean Hospital.* Washington, D.C. American Psychiatric Press, 1986.

Lilli Sentz

Jane Stuart Woolsey

1830–1891

Jane Stuart Woolsey was one of four sisters in a prominent New England family who became noted for their nursing and philanthropic efforts during the Civil War and later contributed richly to the nursing profession. Jane Woolsey chronicled some of her experiences in a privately printed book, *Hospital Days*, which has been valued by historians as a sensitive, insider's view of a military hospital of the time. After the war she was resident directress of the Presbyterian Hospital in New York City, playing a strong role in its organization.

Woolsey was the second of seven daughters plus one son born to Charles William and Jane Eliza (Newton) Woolsey. Her father was head of a sugar-refining business and a staunch Presbyterian and abolitionist. Woolsey was born aboard the ship *Fanny* as it sailed between Norwich, Connecticut, and New York City. She began her education at the fashionable Miss Murdoch's School, near the family home in East Boston, Massachusetts. After Charles Woolsey died in a fire in 1840, his wife moved with her children to New York City to be near a supportive uncle. Woolsey attended the Rutgers Female Institute in New York and then finished secondary school at Bolton Priory, New Rochelle. While she was at Rutgers, her interest in public affairs was stimulated by constant exposure to lectures by nationally known speakers. After graduation she and other members of her family traveled in Europe. In 1853 they moved to a new home in New York City on Brevoort Place, which was to become the headquarters of their Civil War efforts.

At the onset of the war Woolsey, her mother, and her sisters Abby and George Anna all began gathering and distributing supplies for war relief. Jane and Abby Woolsey joined the Woman's Central Association of Relief and visited and nursed wounded and ill soldiers at several New York City hospitals, including Bellevue. When the New England Soldiers Relief Association organized a temporary hospital known as the New England Rooms in 1862, Jane Woolsey became a nurse in regular rotation. Newspapers of the time often carried notes about the beauty, grace, and devotion with which she went about her duties. Later in the year, she visited the City Hospital on Broadway and was so impressed that she signed on as a volunteer nurse, working every day from 7 A.M. to 7 P.M. After a short time she moved on again, this time to become an assistant superintendent of a hospital camp at Portsmouth Grove, Rhode Island, near Newport. She supervised female nurses and the diets of the patients. This was the most responsible position she had held to date in a U.S. government hospital. In 1863 she and her sister George Anna served as paid nurses at Hammond General Hospital, Point Lookout, Maryland. Each month, they returned their $12 in wages to the surgeon-in-charge to use for items for the soldiers.

The two sisters went to the Fairfax Theological Seminary Hospital, near Alexandria, Virginia, in the fall of 1863. The seminary had been deserted on the spur of the moment, with the belongings of its staff and students left behind. These had to be packed away carefully before the building could be converted for hospital use. Jane took charge of the diet kitchen and endeared herself to the patients by giving attention to their personal food preferences. Though George Anna soon left, Jane stayed on until the end of the war. The Fairfax Hospital was the setting for her book, *Hospital Days*, first published in 1868. She also wrote letters that appeared in several newspapers and some finely crafted poetry, which is preserved in collections of family papers and biographical writings.

After the war, Jane Woolsey's friend, General Samuel Chapman Armstrong, established Hampton Normal and Agricultural Institute in Virginia and asked her to become director of girls' industries. She held this post between 1869 and 1872 and established a scholarship there when she left.

Her last professional position was as directress of the Presbyterian Hospital in New York City. She assisted in organizing the hospital and organized its nurses, kitchen, supply and other departments. Together with Abby, who served as hospital clerk, she set the high standards of nursing for which the hospital became noted. Plagued by ill health, she resigned in March 1876, and her sister joined her.

The two sisters both were active in the New York State Charities Aid Association from the time of its organization in 1872 for the rest of their lives. After retirement from Presbyterian Hospital, Jane Woolsey participated regularly, serving on the centennial committee and the committee for the insane and making generous donations.

After many years as an invalid, Woolsey died of septicemia in 1891 at the home of her sister, Eliza Woolsey Howland, in Matteawan, New York.

PUBLICATIONS BY
JANE STUART WOOLSEY

Hospital Days. New York: Van Nostrand, 1868, 1870. Printed for private use.

BIBLIOGRAPHY

Austin, A.L. "Abby Howard, Jane Stuart and George Anna Muirson." In *Notable American Women 1607–1950.* Vol. 3. E.T. James, ed. Cambridge: Belknap Press of Harvard University Press, 1971.

Austin, A.L. *The Woolsey Sisters of New York 1860–1900.* Philadelphia: American Philosophical Society, 1971.

Alice P. Stein

Mary Lewis Wyche
1858–1936

Known for her organizational leadership and administrative skills, Mary Lewis Wyche is credited with establishing the Raleigh Nurses Association in 1901, helping to found the North Carolina State Nurses Association (NCSNA) in 1902, and initiating the movement toward state registration for nurses in North Carolina in 1903.

Born on February 26, 1858 in Henderson, North Carolina, Wyche was the second of ten children of Benjamin and Sara (Hunter) Wyche. Her early education was conducted first by governesses and later in private schools. After graduating from Henderson College in 1889, she taught school for several years and then chose to pursue a career in nursing. Although Wyche provided the means whereby some of her younger brothers could attend college, further information about the Wyche family is unknown.

Wyche graduated from the Philadelphia General Hospital School for Nurses in 1894 and soon after accepted the position of superintendent of Rex Hospital in Raleigh, North Carolina, where she organized the first training school for nurses in the state. Following her resignation from Rex Hospital, Wyche practiced briefly as a private-duty nurse and in 1899 became the head nurse of the infirmary at the State College for Women in Greensboro. From 1903–13, she was superintendent of Watts Hospital and Training School in Durham and from 1915–17 held the position of superintendent of Sarah Elizabeth Hospital and Training School in Henderson. In the later years of her career Wyche returned to private-duty nursing until her retirement in 1925.

Wyche was strongly committed to the development of a professional nursing association in North Carolina. In 1901 she attended the meeting of the International Council of Nurses held in Buffalo in conjunction with the World Pan-American Exposition. There she heard nursing leaders discuss the need for organization as the means to unite nursing and the need for a system of registration whereby educational and practice standards could be upgraded.

On her return to North Carolina, Wyche established the Raleigh Nurses Association, which became the North Carolina State Nurses Association (NCSNA) in 1902. Although modest in number (only 14 nurses attended the first meeting), the association's members formulated its purposes in keeping with those of the existing larger nursing bodies, that is, the improvement of nursing, the development of reciprocal agreements with other states, and the attainment of registration. Wyche was elected first president of NCSNA (a position she held for six years) as well as chair of the association's legislative committee. The committee's task was the framing of a nurse-registration bill that could be put before the North Carolina General Assembly.

Although the bill presented required compulsory registration for anyone practicing as a nurse, the legislation finally enacted in March, 1903 was permissive and protected only those nurses who qualified for the RN title. Disappointed by the revisions that had substantially weakened the law, Wyche continued to work for stronger legislation. In 1907 amendments to the existing law generated considerable improvement. Mandatory registration, however, was still unattainable. Irrespective of its flaws, the North Carolina registration law, by initiating the RN credential, was the first of its kind in this country and was considered a major achievement by organized nursing.

The Board of Examiners of Trained Nurses of North Carolina provided for in the law was organized on December 16, 1903, and Wyche was elected secretary-treasurer, a post she held until 1909. During this period her other activities included participation as a North Carolina delegate in the proceedings of the tenth annual convention of the Nurses Associated Alumnae of the United States and as a member of the Associated Alumnae's Pension and Insurance Fund Committee.

Among the first Red Cross nurses in North Carolina, Wyche was a member of the group that developed the first state Red Cross Nursing Committee, on which she served from 1912 to 1922. In 1913 Wyche and another nurse, Birdie Dunn, collaborated in the establishment of a residence for nurses who were ill or disabled. Called Dunnwyche, the home was opened for residents the same year. Wyche was secretary-treasurer of the board of directors and took an active role in the early management of the facility. In 1919 the residence was sold, and its proceeds used to found a permanent state relief fund for nurses in need.

Wyche envisioned university education as most appropriate for nurses. In 1907 she spearheaded the movement to implement a prenursing course at North Carolina College for Women (Greensboro) and later influenced the establishment of a school of nursing at Duke University in Durham.

Following her retirement, Wyche compiled the *History of Nursing in North Carolina*, which was published after her death. She died on August 22, 1936 at Wychewood, her childhood home in Henderson.

PUBLICATIONS BY MARY LEWIS WYCHE

BOOKS

The History of Nursing in North Carolina. Chapel Hill: University of North Carolina Press, 1938.

ARTICLES

"Nursing Conditions in the South." *American Journal of Nursing* 7 (August 1907): 866–72.

"A Pre-Nursing Course Outlined." *American Journal of Nursing* 19 (June 1919): 715.

BIBLIOGRAPHY

Birnbach, N. "The Genesis of the Nurse Registration Movement in the United States, 1893–1903." Unpublished doctoral dissertation, Teachers College, Columbia University, 1982.

Historical Collection of the North Carolina Board of Nurse Registration and Nursing Education. North Carolina State Department of History and Archives, Raleigh.

"In the Nursing World." *Trained Nurse and Hospital Review* 32 (February 1904): 118.

"Individual Histories." Folder in the American Journal of Nursing/Sophia F. Palmer Historical Library Collection, Mugar Memorial Library, Boston University, Boston.

"Mary L. Wyche." *American Journal of Nursing* 36 (October 1936): 1064.

Minutes of the North Carolina State Nurses Association, 1902–04, Raleigh.

Public Laws and Resolutions of the State of North Carolina, c. 359, secs. 1–11, 1903.

Robinson, V. *White Caps.* Philadelphia: Lippincott, 1946.

"Who's Who in the Nursing World." *American Journal of Nursing* 24 (April 1924): 552.

Nettie Birnbach

Susie Yellowtail

1903–1981

Susie Yellowtail was one of the first Native American registered nurses. She is remembered by her people as a strong and effective advocate for better health and education on reservations in the United States.

Born Susie Walking Bear on Crow Agency in southeastern Montana, she attended the reservation school during the primary grades, then went to boarding school in Pryor, Montana, for high school. Baptist missionaries sponsored her college education at Bacone College in Oklahoma and then her training to become a nurse at East Northville Hospital Training School in Springfield, Mass. After an internship at Boston Hospital, she became a registered nurse in 1926.

For the next two years she worked as a nurse for the U.S. Public Health Service at reservations in Minnesota and Montana. In 1928 she returned to her own people at Crow Agency. For the next three decades (until 1960) she continued to work as a nurse for the Public Health Service (PHS) but also provided midwife services to women—Indian and non-Indian—in the Little Horn Valley. During that era many women still birthed at home, since the nearest hospital was in Sheridan, Wyoming, 45 miles away, and the nearest big hospital was in Billings, Montana, 100 miles away.

Meanwhile, she married Tom Yellowtail, who would later become the Crow medicine man and would revive the "Sundance," a traditional healing ceremony among the Crow. During the 1950s, the couple toured Europe and Israel with the Native American Indian Dance Troop. They had three children, raised two adopted sons, and three of their grandchildren, as well.

By 1960 Yellowtail had stopped practicing nursing and midwifery on the reservation, and her national career began. President John Kennedy appointed her to the Public Health, Education and Welfare Board in 1961. This federal agency administered services to Indian reservations in the United States. She served on the board through the Johnson and Nixon administrations. In 1962 she received the President's award for Outstanding Nursing and Health Care.

Her 30 years of working for the PHS, and now her travel in conjunction with her board appointment, convinced her that the health and education systems, as administered by the federal government, were badly in need of reform. In particular, she suspected that Native American women were being sterilized without their knowledge or consent. More generally, she deplored the ill treatment she felt Native Americans received at the PHS clinics. Privately, she thought the ill treatment was because health practitioners were not trained to practice "bedside nursing," and the result was cold, distant treatment of patients. Now that she was no longer working for the PHS, and from her position on the board, she could speak out about the problems and suggest reforms. In the early 1960s she helped found the Native American Nurses Association, an organization of Native American nurses who had become concerned about sterilization abuse and poor treatment of clients by the PHS. One solution was to acquire more scholarship funds to train Native Americans as doctors and nurses. Perhaps if they had greater control over PHS operation, they could effect reforms.

Meanwhile, she and her husband successfully reintroduced the traditional healing ceremony of the "Sundance" (to supplement the shortcomings in the modern, white-dominated system of health care?). It became very popular, and the Sundance movement spread to many other tribes as well during the 1960s and 1970s. Yellowtail always maintained that the traditions of her people should be welded with modern science and technology. Thus she was a proponent of better health care and education for her people, at the same time that she subscribed to their traditional ways.

By the 1970s, she was traveling throughout the United States again, this time as official chaperon for the Miss Indian America winner. She herself was selected Mrs. Indian America in 1970.

Susie Yellowtail's activism for better health and education on reservations in the United States has emboldened younger generations of Native Americans—both health-care practitioners and patients—to demand reform in the PHS system, as well as greater control over its operation. She died in 1981. She is buried at Crow Agency.

BIBLIOGRAPHY

Weatherly, M.B. Personal communication of Yellowtail's biographer with the author, Stephensville, Montana, 1990.

Wyles, V. Personal communication of Yellowtail's daughter with the author, Wiola, Montana, 1990.

Susan M. Davis

Helen Young
1874–1966

As director of the Presbyterian Hospital School of Nursing in New York City for over 30 years, Helen Young helped many hospitals throughout the world to improve their nursing education programs. She was instrumental in passage of the New York State Nurse Practice Act of 1938, which defined the duties of graduate nurses. Under the influence of Anna Maxwell, she worked throughout her career to make nursing a more socially accepted career for the young women of her time. In 1933 she was the first editor of *Lippincott's Quick Reference Book for Nurses*, which was used by over 100,000 English-speaking graduate nurses.

A native of Canada, Young was born on November 17, 1874, in Chatham, Ontario, to parents of Scottish descent. She attended public schools in Chatham and graduated from the Collegiate Institute in 1893.

She finished a normal-school course in 1895 and was awarded a teacher's diploma the next year by the Toronto School of Pedagogy. For the next three years she divided her time between substitute teaching and home responsibilities. In 1899 she began a decade as a permanent teacher in a Chatham public school.

She entered the Presbyterian Hospital School of Nursing in New York in September 1909 and became a protégée of Anna C. Maxwell, its first director. She graduated in 1912 with the intention of doing private-duty nursing but was asked by Maxwell to stay on as head nurse on the women's surgical ward and later the women's medical service. In June 1915 she took three months' leave to work in Mrs. Harry Payne Whitney's wartime hospital in Juilly, France. In 1917 she organized nurses of Unit No. 2 of the British Expeditionary Forces.

As acting assistant to Maxwell from 1917–19, Young helped the school establish a five-year course leading to a B.S. degree in cooperation with the department of nursing and health of Teachers College, Columbia University. When Maxwell retired in 1921, Young replaced her, first as acting director and then as director of the Nursing Service and the School of Nursing.

The opening of the Columbia-Presbyterian Medical Center in 1929 enabled Young to expand the school's program in clinical teaching. In 1937 the school became the nursing department of the Columbia University Faculty of Medicine. In that year Young received a Columbia University medal for excellence. In 1953 she was the only female among 25 recipients of the center's Distinguished Service Award.

Throughout her career Young was active in professional organizations. She became Red Cross chairperson of her alma mater's alumnae association in 1915 and treasurer in 1917, serving in both posts for many years. She was a delegate to the American Nurses' Association convention in Philadelphia in April 1917. In the 1930s she was a member of the National Committee on Red Cross Nursing Service, encouraging nursing graduates to enter the service. She was president of the New York State League of Nursing Education from 1930–34 and of the New York City League of Nursing Education from 1936–40.

Young died November 23, 1966, in the Harkness Pavilion of the Columbia-Presbyterian Medical Center. She was 92 and lived in New York City at the time.

PUBLICATIONS BY HELEN YOUNG

BOOKS

Lippincott's Quick Reference Book for Nurses. Philadelphia: Lippincott, 1933. Six further editions to 1955.

Essentials of Nursing. New York: Putnam, 1942. Further editions with E. Lee, 1948, 1953.

ARTICLES

"Responsibility of the Hospitals and Nursing Agencies for the Care of Their Sick Nurses." *American Nurses' Association: Proceedings of the 28th Convention, 1932.* New York: American Nurses' Association. 1932.

BIBLIOGRAPHY

"Award to Nursing Service Administrator." *Nursing Outlook* 1 (November 1953): 649.

"Helen Young Dies; Nursing Official." *New York Times.* November 25, 1966, 37.

Lee, E. "Helen Young." New York: National League of Nursing Education, undated or paged.

"Obituaries." *American Journal of Nursing* 67 (January 1967): 141.

Alice P. Stein

Anne Larson Zimmerman

b. 1914

Anne Larson Zimmerman has been a major voice in nursing through her service as administrator of various state nursing organizations, as president of the American Nurses' Association (ANA), and particularly for her advocacy of the Economic and General Welfare Program of the ANA.

She was born on September 1, 1914, the eldest of five children of Theresa Betor and George Larson, in Marysville, Montana, a small gold mining town about 20 miles from Helena. During much of her childhood her mother was in ill health, and much of the responsibility for her brothers and sisters fell on her shoulders. It was her contact with nurses during this period as well as her own hospitalization for a fractured femur that aroused her interest in nursing.

In fact, she attended nursing school at the same hospital where she had been hospitalized, the St. John's Hospital in Helena run by the Sisters of Charity of Leavenworth. After graduating in 1935,

she worked as a staff nurse in pediatrics at St. John's until her marriage to Kenneth Zimmerman in 1936. In 1939 her daughter Nancy was born. Eighteen months later she was divorced, a single parent looking for a job in Butte, where she had moved. Hospitals at that time were reluctant to hire a woman with a child, and even the jobs offered to her made it difficult to support a child. This experience influenced her to become active in the Montana State Nurses Association, first as a volunteer and then in 1945 as executive secretary. At the same time she was elected vice-chair of the ANA General Duty Association, and in 1946 she became chair when the current chair resigned. This position automatically made her a member of the ANA board of directors.

It was here that she met Shirley C. Titus, executive director of the California Nurses Association (CNA) and the prime mover within the ANA for the establishment of an economic and general welfare program for nurses.

In 1947 Titus offered her the position of assistant executive director of the CNA, and Zimmerman and her daughter moved to San Francisco to promote CNA's economic security program. In 1951 Zimmerman took a leave of absence to become director of the ANA's economic and general welfare program. Though the ANA wanted her to remain in the position, she returned to California in 1952 with the title of deputy executive director of CNA and with the assumption that she would succeed Titus on her retirement. Titus, however, changed her mind about retiring, and in 1954 Zimmerman was offered the position of executive administrator of the Illinois Nurses Association (INA), which she accepted, and in September 1954 she moved to Illinois. Since the INA had already decided by referendum to take up the economic security issue, Zimmerman was in a position to build upon her California experience.

Zimmerman remained as executive administrator of the INA for 26 years, retiring in 1981. During those years she developed a strong economic and general welfare program, established a branch office in Springfield to lobby for the INA, and established the first continuing-education program to be certified by the ANA.

In 1976 she ran for president of the ANA, the candidate of a coalition of executive directors and presidents of state nurses' associations. One of her platform planks was to establish a salary for the president instead of following the traditional pattern of having the president's employer pay her. The implementation of this change opened up the presidency to a wider group of nurses. During her presidency the ANA House of Delegates voted to move forward in implementing its resolution calling for two levels of nursing education—baccalaureate and associate degree.

Zimmerman retired from the position of executive administrator of INA in 1980. From 1981–85 she held the Marcella Niehoff Chair in the Niehoff School of Loyola University in Chicago.

Among her international activities in nursing was serving as the ANA delegate to the International Council of Nurses in 1961, and in 1975 participated in a conference called by the World Health Organization and the International Labor Organization to develop a document on the work and life of health-care workers. This later became a covenant of the ILO. In 1975 Zimmerman was invited by the Medical Workers Union of the USSR to present a paper on the life and work of the nurse in the United States, and in 1972 she led the first delegation of nurses to the Peoples Republic of China.

Zimmerman also served as a member and later chair of the board of directors of the American Journal of Nursing Company, as a member and vice-chair of the board of directors for the Commission on Graduates of Foreign Nursing Schools, and on a variety of other committees of the ANA. She continues to remain active as a lecturer and consultant in nursing organizations. She also enjoys her role as grandmother for five children of Nancy Zimmerman and Edward Burke. Her daughter Nancy holds a master's degree in nursing.

PUBLICATIONS BY ANNE LARSON ZIMMERMAN

BOOKS

"Collective Bargaining in the Hospital." In *Current Issues in Nursing.* J.C. McCloskey, ed. Boston: Blackwell Scientific, 1981.

With T. Schorr. *Making Choices, Taking Chances—Nurse Leaders Tell Their Stories,* St. Louis: Mosby, 1988.

ARTICLES

"Economic Security in the Decade Ahead." *American Journal of Nursing* 62 (December 1962): 98–101.

"The ANA Economic Security Program in Retrospect." *Nursing Forum* 10, (1971): 312–21.

"Taft-Hartley Amended: Implications for Nursing." *American Journal of Nursing* 75 (February 1975): 284–87.

"ANA: Its Record on Social Issues." *American Journal of Nursing* 76 (April 1976): 588–90.

"A Look Toward the Future." *American Nurse* 8 (November 1976): 4.

"Collective Actions by Professional Employees." *The Impact of Collective Actions on Hospitals.* A report of the 1976 Forum on Hospital and Health Affairs, Duke University, Durham, North Carolina, 1977.

"Nursing's Concerns: Credentialing Proposal," *AORN Journal* 25 (June 1977): 1356–72.

"The American Nurses' Association: Its Relevance to the Membership of the American Association of Nurse Anesthetists." *AANA Journal* 45 (October 1977): 478–84.

"Power and Politics in Nursing," *Nursing Administration Quarterly* 20 (Spring 1978): 68–70.

"AJN Interviews the ANA President." *American Journal of Nursing* 78 (June 1978): 1018–21.

"Toward a Unified Voice–Individual and Collective Responsibility of Nurses." *Journal of Advanced Nursing* 3 (September 1978): 475–83.

BIBLIOGRAPHY

Zimmerman, A. Interview with the author, October 23, 1990, Chicago.

JoAnn Appleyard

INDEXES

DECADES OF BIRTH

BEFORE 1800
Evans, M., Seton, Truth, d'Youville

1801-1820
Bickerdyke, Dix, Gonazaga, Phillips, H.N., Ropes, Schervier, Tubman, Whitman

1821-1840
Alcott, Angela, Barton, Blackwell, Browne, Cumming, Davis, M.E., Fisher, Harvey, Livermore, Mills, Molokai, Pelchin, Pember, Schuyler, Tompkins, Trader, Wittenmyer, Woolsey, G.A.M., Woolsey, J.S.

1841-1860
Batterham, Boardman, Chase, Cushman, Damer, Darche, Dempsey, Dewey, Dock, Drown, Fedde, Glenn, Gretter, Hibbard, Jenkins, Kessel, Kinney, Lathrop, Lounsbery, Loveridge, MacLeod, Mahoney, Maxwell, McIssac, Meyer, Nathoy, Nutting, Nye, Palmer, Reid, Richards, Riddle, Robb, Sanborn, Sanford, Seelye, Shaw, Sutliffe, Taylor, S.B., Warr, Woodward, Wyche

1861-1880
Aikens, Alline, Amy Margaret, Anderson, Ariss, Ayers, Bailey, Baker, Banfield, Belmont, Braunard, Brockway, Burgess, C., Burgess, E.C., Butler, Cabrini, Cannon, Clayton, Cooke, Crandall, Crowell, Curtis, Dakin, Deans, Delano, De Witt, Dietrich, Eldredge, Erdmann, Fallon, Fitzgerald, Foley, Francis, Franklin, Fuller, Fulmer, Gabriel, Gardner, B.J., Gardner, M.S., Gladwin, Goldman, Goodnow, Goodrich, Gray, Hall, C.M., Hansen, Hasson, Hay, Hickey, Higbee, Hitchcock, Hodgkins, Holman, Jean, Johns, Johnson, J.M., Johnson, S.M., Jones, E.R., Kelly, H.W., Knapp, Lamotte, Lamping, Leete, Lent, Logan, Lowman, Maass, Mansfield, Markol, Mathews, McCarron, McCrae, McGee, McMillan, McMillen, Mellichamp, Minnigerode, Minor, Noyes, Parsons, S.E., Parsons, M.G., Pope, Powell, Purtell, Rinehart, Roberts, Russell, Sanger, Sirch, Skenadore, Sleet, Sly, Squire, Stevenson, B.V., Stewart, Strong, Taylor, E.J., Thompson, D.E., Thomson, Thoms, Tracy, Urch, Van Blarcom, Vrede, Wald, Warner, Waters, Wheeler, M.C., Williamson, Wilson, Young

1881-1900
Austin, Beard, Beck, Beeby, Behrnes, Best, Blanchfield, Bolton, Bowman, Breckinridge, Brink, Brinton, Brogan, Burgess, M.A., Carr, Carter, Collins, Corbin, Craig, Dauser, Davis, F.E., Deming,

Dennison, Deutsch, Deves, Domitilla, Essig, Faddis, Faville, Flikke, Fox, France, Gage, Gault, Geister, Given, Goff, Goostray, Gowan, Grant, Gregg, Harmer, Haupt, Havey, Hawkins, Hawkinson, Henderson, Hoffman, Hogan, Howell, Hubbard, Jensen, Johnson, J.M., Jones, F.W., Kasmeier, Keaton, Kennedy, Kenny, Kuehn, Lee, Lynch, McClelland, McGarrah, McIver, Magnussen, Mary Claudia, Matthews, Morse, Nelson, Northam, Odegard, Olmsted, Pfefferkorn, Prochazka, Render, Sargent, Scheuer, Schulte, Scott, A.H, Sellew, Sherrick, Smith, Snyder, Soule, Spalding, Staupers, Stevenson (West), J.L., Stimson, Sullivan, Swope, Tebo, Thompson, B.A., Titus, Tracy, Tucker, Utinsky, Vail, Van Kooy, Wheeler, C.A., Willeford, Willms, Winton, Wolf, Wood, Zabriskie

1901–1920

Ainsworth, Alford, Armiger, Arnstein, Austin, Aynes, Beckwith, Black, Blake, Boyle, Brown, A.F., Brown, M.M., Brown, S.J., Browne, H.E., Bunge, Christman, Cole, Coulter, Day, Dolan, J.A., Dolan, M.B., Dorr, Ellis, Errickson, Fife, Frank, Freeman, Garrett, Garrigan, Germain, Greenough, Hall, L.E., Hassenplug, Ingles, Kain, Kelly, D., Kemble, Kiniery, Leone, Lewis, Maher, Manfreda, Marshall, McQuillen, Miller, Montag, Mullane, Myers, Nahm, Newton, Notter, Ohlson, A.K., Ohlson, V.M., Osborne, Peplau, Phaneuf, Phillips, M.G., Reiter, Robinson, Rogers, Sanderson, Schlotfeldt, Schutt, Scott, J.M., Stahl, Thielbar, Thompson, J.C., Vreeland, Wandelt, Werley, Werth, Widmer, Yellowtail, Zimmerman

1921–1940

Berthold, Christy, Evans, B.L., Heide, Hornback, Johnson, F.L., Lytle, Novello, Olsen, Pate, Poole, Travelbee, Verhonick, Waechter

FIRST NURSING SCHOOL ATTENDED

ALBANY HOSPITAL,
ALBANY, N.Y.
   Strong

ALEXIAN BROTHERS HOSPITAL,
CHICAGO
   Brogan, Snyder

ALLGEMEINES KRANKENHAUS,
VIENNA, AUSTRIA
   Goldman

ARMY SCHOOL OF NURSING
   Hassenplug, Henderson, Hubbard,
   Phillips, M.G., Tracy, Willeford

AUGUSTANA HOSPITAL,
CHICAGO
   Flikke

BOLTON SCHOOL OF NURSING,
WESTERN RESERVE UNIVERSITY,
CLEVELAND, OHIO
   Lewis, Stahl

BELLEVUE HOSPITAL TRAINING
SCHOOL,
NEW YORK CITY
   Darche, Delano, Dewey, Dock, Draper,
   Jones, F.W., Kimber, Loveridge, Min-
   nigerode, O'Donnell, Robb, Sanford

BOSTON CITY HOSPITAL,
BOSTON
   Drown, Gladwin, Hodgkins, Maxwell,
   Palmer, Parsons, M.G., Parsons, S.E.,
   Riddle

BROOKLYN CITY HOSPITAL,
BROOKLYN, N.Y.
   Batterham, Corbin, Lounsbery

BROOKLYN STATE HOSPITAL,
BROOKLYN, N.Y.
   Heide

BUFFALO CHILDREN'S HOSPITAL,
BUFFALO, N.Y.
   Hansen

BUFFALO GENERAL HOSPITAL,
BUFFALO, N.Y.
   Gretter, Sirch

BUFFALO HOMEOPATHIC HOSPITAL
(MILLARD FILLMORE),
BUFFALO, N.Y.
   Austin

CALIFORNIA, UNIVERSITY OF,
SAN FRANCISCO
   Alford, Ellis

377

CALIFORNIA HOSPITAL,
LOS ANGELES
  Dauser

CALIFORNIA WOMEN'S HOSPITAL,
SAN FRANCISCO
  Cooke

CATHOLIC UNIVERSITY,
WASHINGTON, D.C.
  Armiger, Str.

CENTRAL MAINE GENERAL HOSPITAL,
LEWISTON, ME.
  Render

CHARITY HOSPITAL,
NEW ORLEANS
  Travelbee

CHILDREN'S HOSPITAL,
BOSTON
  Goostray

CHILDREN'S HOSPITAL,
COLUMBUS, OHIO
  Vail

CHILDREN'S MEMORIAL HOSPITAL,
CHICAGO
  Kuehn

CINCINNATI, UNIVERSITY OF,
CINCINNATI, OHIO
  Dreves, Kemble, Sellew

COLORADO, UNIVERSITY OF,
BOULDER, COLO.
  Coulter

COLUMBIA-PRESBYTERIAN,
NEW YORK CITY
  Greenough, Hogan

COLUMBUS HOSPITAL,
GREAT FALLS, MONT.
  Gabriel

CONNECTICUT TRAINING SCHOOL,
NEW HAVEN, CONN.
  Ayers, Hasson

COOPER HOSPITAL,
CAMDEN, N.J.
  Fallon

COTTAGE HOSPITAL,
CRESTON, IOWA
  Given

DR. RAVN'S HOSPITAL,
MERRILL, WIS.
  Odegard

DUKE UNIVERSITY,
DURHAM, N.C.
  Robinson

EAST NORTHVILLE HOSPITAL,
SPRINGFIELD, MASS.
  Yellowtail

EASTERN MAINE GENERAL HOSPITAL,
BANGOR, ME.
  Mansfield

EITEL HOSPITAL,
MINNEAPOLIS
  Ainsworth

EVANSTON HOSPITAL,
EVANSTON, ILL.
  Newton

FAIRVIEW GENERAL HOSPITAL,
CLEVELAND, OHIO
  Lytle

FANNY ALLEN HOSPITAL,
WINOOSKI, VT.
  Fife

FARRAND TRAINING SCHOOL,
HARPER HOSPITAL,
DETROIT
  Deans, Germain, McGarvah, Sly

FAXTON SCHOOL OF NURSING,
UTICA, N.Y.
  Grant

FRAMINGHAM HOSPITAL SCHOOL,
FRAMINGHAM, MASS.
  Hawkinson

FRANKLIN HOSPITAL,
SAN FRANCISCO
  Behrens

FREEDMAN'S HOSPITAL,
WASHINGTON, D.C.
  Damer, Davis, Staupers

GEORGETOWN UNIVERSITY,
WASHINGTON, D.C.
  Dolan

GOOD SAMARITAN HOSPITAL,
PORTLAND, OREG.
  Miller

GRACE HOSPITAL,
NEW HAVEN, CONN.
  Phaneuf

GRADY MEMORIAL HOSPITAL,
ATLANTA, GA.
 Carter

GRANT HOSPITAL,
COLUMBUS, OHIO
 Sanderson

GUELPH GENERAL HOSPITAL,
GUELPH, ONTARIO, CANADA
 Ariss

HARTFORD HOSPITAL TRAINING
SCHOOL,
HARTFORD, CONN.
 Butler, Foley, Manfreda, Skenadore

HOLY NAME HOSPITAL,
TEANECK, N.J.
 Kelly, D., Mullane

HOMEOPATHIC HOSPITAL,
BROOKLYN, N.Y.
 Alline

HOMEOPATHIC HOSPITAL,
ESSEX COUNTY,
NEWARK, N.J.
 Willms

ILLINOIS TRAINING SCHOOL,
CHICAGO
 Burgess, C., DeWitt, Glenn, Havey,
 Hawkins, Hay, Kelly, H.W., Lamping,
 McIssac, McMillan, Prochazka, Thomp-
 son, J.C., Urch, Wheeler

INDIANAPOLIS CITY HOSPITAL,
INDIANAPOLIS
 Nye

IOWA, UNIVERSITY OF,
IOWA CITY
 Austin, L.M., Brown, A.F., Schlotfeldt

JEFFERSON MEDICAL COLLEGE,
PHILADELPHIA
 Schutt, Werley

JEWISH HOSPITAL,
CINCINNATI, OHIO
 Deutsch, Roberts

JOHNS HOPKINS HOSPITAL,
SCHOOL OF NURSING,
BALTIMORE, MD.
 Bailey, Baker, Beckwith, Brockway,
 Carr, Fitzgerald, Fox, Jammé, Jensen,
 LaMotte, Lent, Leone, Northam, Noyes,
 Nutting, Olmsted, Pfefferkorn, Reiter,
 Taylor, Van Blarcom, Waters, Wolf

KNOWLTON (COLUMBIA)
HOSPITAL,
MILWAUKEE, WIS.
 Mathews

LA CROSSE HOSPITAL,
LA CROSSE, WIS.
 Magnussen

LAKESIDE HOSPITAL,
CLEVELAND, OHIO
 Howell, Leete

LAS VEGAS HOT SPRINGS
SANITARIUM, N.M.
 Goodnow

LINCOLN HOSPITAL,
NEW YORK CITY
 Thoms

LUTHER HOSPITAL,
EAU CLAIRE, WIS.
 Werth

LUTHERAN HOSPITAL,
ST. LOUIS
 Waechter

MACK TRAINING SCHOOL,
MARINE HOSPITAL,
ST. CATHERINES, ONTARIO, CANADA
 Hibbard

McLEARN HOSPITAL,
WAVERLY, MASS.
 Craig

MacVICAR HOSPITAL,
ATLANTA, GA.
 Collins

MALDEN HOSPITAL,
MALDEN, MASS.
 Soule

MANHATTANVILLE COLLEGE OF THE
SACRED HEART,
PURCHASE, N.Y.
 Christy, Ingles

MARYLAND HOMEOPATHIC HOSPITAL
TRAINING SCHOOL,
BALTIMORE, MD.
 Jean

MASSACHUSETTS GENERAL
HOSPITAL,
BOSTON
 Davis, Dennison, Faville, Goff, Hall,
 C.M., Johnson, S.M., Kinney, Sullivan,
 Vreeland, Wood

MASSACHUSETTS HOMEOPATHIC
HOSPITAL,
BOSTON
  Tracy

MEDFIELD SCHOOL FOR NURSING,
MEDFIELD, MASS.
  Dowling

MEDICO-CHIRURGICAL HOSPITAL,
PHILADELPHIA
  Bowman

MEMPHIS CITY HOSPITAL,
MEMPHIS, TENN.
  Trader

MEMPHIS TRAINING SCHOOL,
MEMPHIS, TENN.
  Warner

MERCY HOSPITAL,
BALTIMORE, MD.
  Scheuer

MERCY HOSPITAL,
JANESVILLE, WIS.
  Kiniery

METHODIST HOSPITAL,
BROOKLYN, N.Y.
  Olsen

METHODIST HOSPITAL,
OMAHA, NEBR.
  Simpson

METHODIST HOSPITAL,
PEORIA, ILL.
  Boyle

MEYER MEMORIAL HOSPITAL,
BUFFALO, N.Y.
  Dorr

MICHAEL REESE HOSPITAL,
CHICAGO
  Blake, Myers, Wandelt

MICHIGAN, UNIVERSITY OF,
ANN ARBOR, MICH.
  Brown, M.M., Knapp, Sherrick

MILWAUKEE COUNTY HOSPITAL,
MILWAUKEE, WIS.
  Fuller

MILWAUKEE GENERAL HOSPITAL,
MILWAUKEE, WIS.
  Vrede

MINNESOTA, UNIVERSITY OF,
SCHOOL OF NURSING,
MINNEAPOLIS
  Haupt, McIver, McQuillen, Marshall,
  Montag, Thompson (Sharpless)

MISSOURI, UNIVERSITY OF,
COLUMBIA, MO.
  Nahm

MONMOUTH MEMORIAL HOSPITAL,
LONG BRANCH, N.J.
  Errickson

MT. SINAI HOSPITAL,
NEW YORK CITY
  Freeman, Logan, Sargent

NEBRASKA, UNIVERSITY OF,
OMAHA, NEBR.
  Johnson, F.L.P.

NEWARK GERMAN HOSPITAL
CHRISTIANA TREFZ TRAINING
SCHOOL,
NEWARK, N.J.
  Maass

NEW ENGLAND HOSPITAL
FOR WOMEN AND CHILDREN,
BOSTON
  Mahoney, Richards

NEW JERSEY GENERAL HOSPITAL,
PATERSON, N.J.
  Cushman

NEWPORT HOSPITAL,
NEWPORT, R.I.
  Gardner, M.S.

NEWTON HOSPITAL,
NEWTON, MASS.
  Tucker

NEW YORK CITY HOSPITAL,
BLACKWELL'S ISLAND
(WELFARE ISLAND), N.Y.
  Gray, Stevenson

NEW YORK HOSPITAL,
NEW YORK CITY
  Anderson, Beard, Dakin, Goodrich,
  Hall, L., Higbee, Hitchcock, Johnson,
  F.M., Russell, Sanborn, Shaw, Stimson,
  Sutliffe, Thompson, D.E., Wald, Warr,
  Williamson, Woolsey, G.A.M., Zabriskie

NORTHERN LOUISIANA SANITARIUM,
SHREVEPORT, LA.
  Pate

NORTHWEST TEXAS HOSPITAL,
AMARILLO, TEXAS
  Garrett

OHIO VALLEY SCHOOL OF NURSING,
STEUBENVILLE, OHIO
  Evans, B.L.

OLD DOMINION HOSPITAL,
RICHMOND, VA.
  Minor

ONTARIO HOSPITAL,
WHITLEY, ONTARIO, CANADA
  Black

ORANGE MEMORIAL HOSPITAL,
ORANGE, N.J.
  Gardner, B.J., Squire

PASSAVANT MEMORIAL HOSPITAL,
CHICAGO
  Essig

PEABODY COLLEGE
(GEORGE PEABODY COLLEGE),
NASHVILLE, TENN.
  Rogers

PENNSYLVANIA, UNIVERSITY OF,
PHILADELPHIA
  Lynch

PENNSYLVANIA HOSPITAL,
PHILADELPHIA
  Christman, Day, McClelland

PETER BENT BRIGHAM HOSPITAL,
BOSTON
  Ohlson, A.K., Smith, M.R.

PETERSON TRAINING SCHOOL,
ANN ARBOR, MICH.
  Morse

PHILADELPHIA GENERAL HOSPITAL,
PHILADELPHIA
  Brink, Clayton, Crandall, Gault, Holman, Jones, E.R.K., Kennedy, Price, Wyche

PITTSBURGH TRAINING SCHOOL,
PITTSBURGH, PA.
  Rinehart

PORTLAND, UNIVERSITY OF,
PORTLAND, OREG.
  Verhonick

POTTSTOWN HOSPITAL,
POTTSTOWN, PA.
  Peplau

PRESBYTERIAN HOSPITAL,
CHICAGO
  Schulte, Scott, A.H., Thomson, West, Wilson

PRESBYTERIAN HOSPITAL,
DENVER
  Aynes

PRESBYTERIAN HOSPITAL,
NEW YORK CITY
  Arnstein, Davies, Deming, Lee, Pope, Young

PRESBYTERIAN HOSPITAL,
PHILADELPHIA
  Brinton

PROVIDENT HOSPITAL,
CHICAGO
  Sleet

READING HOSPITAL,
READING, PA.
  Francis

RHODE ISLAND HOSPITAL,
PROVIDENCE, R.I.
  Maher

ROOSEVELT HOSPITAL SCHOOL OF
NURSING,
NEW YORK CITY
  Burgess, C., Gage

ST. ANTHONY'S HOSPITAL,
ST. LOUIS
  Beck

ST. BARNABAS HOSPITAL,
MINNEAPOLIS
  Erdman

ST. BARTHOLOMEW'S HOSPITAL,
LONDON, ENGLAND
  Banfield, Browne, H.E.

ST. JOHN'S HOSPITAL,
HELENA, MONT.
  Zimmerman

ST. JOHN'S HOSPITAL,
LOWELL, MASS.
Dolan

ST. JOHN'S HOSPITAL,
SAN ANGELO, TEXAS
Brown, S.

ST. JOHN'S RIVERSIDE HOSPITAL,
YONKERS, N.Y.
Dietrich

ST. JOSEPH'S HOSPITAL,
CHICAGO
Crowell

ST. JOSEPH'S HOSPITAL,
DENVER
Hoffman

ST. JOSEPH'S HOSPITAL,
MILWAUKEE, WIS.
Van Kooy

ST. JOSEPH'S HOSPITAL,
PARIS, TEXAS
Frank

ST. JOSEPH'S HOSPITAL,
PITTSBURGH, PA.
Novello

ST. LOUIS CITY HOSPITAL NO. 2,
ST. LOUIS
Osborne

ST. LUKE'S HOSPITAL,
CHICAGO
Beeby, Best, Eldredge, Fulmer, Keller,
McMillen

ST. LUKE'S HOSPITAL,
NEW YORK CITY
Breckinridge

ST. LUKE'S HOSPITAL,
RICHMOND, VA.
Powell, Tebo, Thielbar

ST. LUKE'S HOSPITAL,
SAN FRANCISCO
Titus

ST. MARY'S HOSPITAL,
BROOKLYN, N.Y.
Hickey

ST. MARY'S HOSPITAL,
DULUTH, MINN.
Gowan

ST. MARY'S HOSPITAL,
MILWAUKEE, WIS.
Kain

ST. MARY'S HOSPITAL,
ROCHESTER, MINN.
Domitilla, Johnson, J.M.

ST. MARY'S AND ELIZABETH
HOSPITAL,
LOUISVILLE, KY.
Notter

ST. PAUL CITY AND COUNTRY
HOSPITAL,
ST. PAUL, MINN.
Cannon

ST. PETER'S HOSPITAL,
OLYMPIA, WASH.
Keaton

ST. ROSA'S HOSPITAL,
SAN ANTONIO, TEXAS
Kasmeier

ST. THOMAS' HOSPITAL,
LONDON, ENGLAND
Fisher

ST. URSULA'S COLLEGE,
NEW SOUTH WALES, AUSTRALIA
Kenny

ST. VINCENT'S HOSPITAL,
INDIANAPOLIS
Spalding

SAMARITAN HOSPITAL,
TROY, N.Y.
McPherson

SARAH LEIGH HOSPITAL,
NORFOLK, VA.
Mellichamp

SCOTT AND WHITE HOSPITAL,
TEMPLE, TEXAS
Cole

SHERMAN HOSPITAL,
ELGIN, ILL.
Geister

SLOANE HOSPITAL FOR WOMEN,
NEW YORK CITY
France

SOUTHERN ILLINOIS HOSPITAL,
ANNA, ILL.
Clement

SOUTHSIDE HOSPITAL TRAINING
SCHOOL,
PITTSBURGH, PA.
  Blanchfield

SPRINGFIELD TRAINING SCHOOL,
SPRINGFIELD, MASS.
  Matthews

STRATFORD HOSPITAL,
STRATFORD, ONTARIO, CANADA
  Aikens

SWEDISH CONVENANT HOSPITAL,
CHICAGO
  Ohlson, V.M.

SWEDISH HOSPITAL,
MINNEAPOLIS
  Winton

TORONTO GENERAL HOSPITAL,
TORONTO, ONTARIO, CANADA
  Harmer

VASSAR BROTHERS HOSPITAL,
POUGHKEEPSIE, N.Y.
  Wheeler

WALTHAM TRAINING SCHOOL,
WALTHAM, MASS.
  Gregg, MacLeod, Markolf, Nelson

WESLEY MEMORIAL HOSPITAL,
CHICAGO
  McCleery

WESTCHESTER SCHOOL OF NURSING,
VALHALLA, N.Y.
  Garrigan

WHITE PLAINS HOSPITAL,
WHITE PLAINS, N.Y.
  Sanger

WILKES-BARRE GENERAL HOSPITAL,
WILKES-BARRE, PA.
  Scott, J.M.

WILLIAMSBURG HOSPITAL,
NEW YORK CITY
  McCarron

WINNIPEG GENERAL HOSPITAL,
WINNIPEG, MANITOBA, CANADA
  Johns, Stewart

WISCONSIN, UNIVERSITY OF,
MADISON
  Hornback

WOMAN'S HOSPITAL,
CHICAGO
  Kessel

WOMAN'S HOSPITAL,
PHILADELPHIA
  Franklin, Phillips, H.N.

YALE UNIVERSITY,
NEW HAVEN, CONN.
  Poole, Widmer

AREA OF SPECIAL INTEREST OR ACCOMPLISHMENT

ADMINISTRATION
Angela, Ariss, Beard, Cole, Darche, Davies, Dempsey, Fedde, Fisher, Loveridge, McClelland, McPherson, Stevenson, Trader, Werth, Wheeler, Williamson

CLINICAL PRACTICE
Blake, Dorr, Evans, Hall, Hodgkins, Keaton, Kenny, Kessel, Mary Claudia, Str., Molokai, Myers, Nathoy, Prochazka, Reiter, Robinson, Taylor, Tracy, Travelbee, Winton

EDUCATION
Alline, Amy Margaret, Str., Anderson, Armiger, Str., Austin, Baker, Banfield, Berthold, Boyle, Brogan, Brown, A.F., Brown, M.M., Bunge, Burgess, C., Burgess, E.C., Christman, Dakin, Dennison, Dewey, Dolan, Domitilla, Str., Dreves, Drown, Ellis, Erdmann, Faddis, Frank, Gabriel, Str., Gage, Garrigan, Germain, Given, Glenn, Goodrich, Goostray, Gowan, Gray, Gretter, Hall, Hassenplug, Hawkinson, Hay, Hibbard, Hornback, Ingles, Johnson, F.L.P., Johnson, S.M., Jones, Kasmeier, Kemble, Kiniery, Knapp, Kuehn, Lee, Logan, Lynch, MacLeod, McMillan,

Meyer, Mills, Montag, Mullane, Nahm, Newton, Nutting, O'Donnell, Odegard, Parsons, Pfefferkorn, Poole, Powell, Richards, Robb, Rogers, Sanborn, Sanderson, Schlotfeldt, Schulte, Scott, Sherrick, Smith, Snyder, Soule, Spalding, Stewart, Sullivan, Thielbar, Thompson, Tracy, Urch, Warr, Wheeler, Widmer, Willms, Wolf, Wood, Woolsey, Young

NURSING ORGANIZATION
Alford, Ayers, Batterham, Beck, Str., Beckwith, Behrens, Best, Boardman, Brown, Browne, Clayton, Damer, Davis, Deans, Delano, Dietrich, Draper, Eldredge, Errickson, Fife, Francis, Franklin, Fulmer, Gardner, Greenough, Hickey, Jammé, Kain, Kelly, Kennedy, Magnussen, Mansfield, Mathews, Maxwell, McCleery, McGee, McIssac, McQuillen, Mellichamp, Noyes, Nye, Ohlson, Osborne, Riddle, Russell, Sanford, Scott, Simpson, Sly, Squire, Stahl, Staupers, Sutliffe, Tebo, Thoms, Vrede, Wyche, Zimmerman

PUBLIC ACTIVITY
Barton, Belmont, Bolton, Butler, Cabrini, Cannon, Carr, Carter, Craig,

Cushman, Dix, Dolan, Fallon, Goff, Goldman, Harvey, Jenkins, Lytle, McIver, McMillen, Pate, Reid, Ropes, Sanger, Schuyler, Swope, Thompson, Truth, Wittenmyer, Yellowtail, d'Youville

WRITING

Aikens, Alcott, Austin, Bailey, Beeby, Black, Brinton, Burgess, M.A., Christy, Cooke, Day, Deming, France, De Witt, Geister, Goodnow, Harmer, Heide, Henderson, Jensen, Johns, Keller, Kelly, Kimber, LaMotte, Lewis, Livermore, Manfreda, McCrae, Miller, Morehead, Northam, Notter, Novello, Palmer, Pember, Peplau, Pope, Price, Render, Rinehart, Roberts, Schutt, Sellew, Shaw, Sirch, Van Blarcom, Verhonick, Vreeland, Wandelt, Waters, Waechter, Werley, Whitman, Wilson, Woolsey, Zabriskie

MILITARY

Ainsworth, Aynes, Bickerdyke, Blanchfield, Bowman, Browne, Mother, Clement, Cumming, Curtis, Dauser, Dita, Essig, Flikke, Gladwin, Hasson, Higbee, Hoffman, Jones, Kinney, Olsen, Parsons, Phillips, Purtell, Seelye, Stimson, Taylor, Thompson, Tompkins, Tubman, Utinsky

PUBLIC HEALTH NURSING AND PUBLIC NURSING

Arnstein, Beard, Brainard, Breckinridge, Brink, Brockway, Browne, H.E., Collins, Corbin, Coulter, Crandall, Crowell, Deutsch, Dock, Dowling, Evans, Faville, Fitzgerald, Foley, Fox, Freeman, Fuller, Gardner, Garrett, Gonzaga, Grant, Gregg, Hansen, Haupt, Havey, Hawkins, Hitchcock, Hogan, Holman, Howell, Hubbard, Jean, Johnson, F.M., Johnson, J.M., LaMotte, Lamping, Leete, Lent, Leone, Lounsbery, Lowman, Maher, Markolf, Matthews, McCarron, Minnigerode, Minor, Morse, Nelson, Ohlson, Olmsted, Pelchin, Sargent, Scheuer, Seton, Sleet, Stevenson (West), Strong, Thomson, Tucker, Vail, Van Kooy, Wald, Warner, Willeford

OTHER

Blackwell, Chase, Davis, Gault, Lathrop, Maass, Mahoney, Marshall, McGarvah, Pate, Phaneuf, Phillips, Schervier, Skenador, Titus, Woodward

STATE AND COUNTRIES OF BIRTH

UNKNOWN

Bailey, H., Berthold, J.S., Corbin, H., Curtis, N.G., Dakin, F., Fox, E.G., Harvey, G.P., Jamme, A.C., Jenkins, H.H., Jones, F.W., McCleery, A.B., McPherson, M.G., Morehead, W.C., Phillips, M.N., Price, L.D., Reiter, F., Shaw, C.S.W., Simpson, C.E., Staupers, M.K., Stevenson (West), J.L., Swope, E., Tucker, K.

UNITED STATES

ALABAMA

Kasmeier, J.C.

ARKANSAS

Coulter, P.P.

CALIFORNIA

Alford, M., Behrens, E., Cooke, G., Dauser, S.S., Ellis, R., Titus, S.C.

COLORADO

Gregg, E.D.

CONNECTICUT

Deming, D., Foley, E.L., France, B.S., Franklin, M.M., Johnson, S.M., Manfreda, M.L., Ohlson, A.K., Woolsey, J.S., Zabriskie, L.M.

GEORGIA

Carter, L.B., Collins, C.E., Taylor, S.K.

ILLINOIS

Austin, L.M., Best, E., Boyle, R.E., Brown, A.F., Brown, S., Clement, M.J., Geister, J.M., Glenn, E.C., Hay, H.S., Hoffman, M.M., Mathews, S., Ohlson, V.M., Sherrick, A.P., Thielbar, F., Thomson, E.E., Vail, S.B., Van Blarcom, C.C.

INDIANA

Brown, M.M., Deves, K.D., Essig, M.F., Lounsbery, H.C., Scott, A.H., Spalding, E.K.

IOWA

Bowman, J.B., Given, L.I., McIssac, I., Magnussen, A.K., Marshall, E.E.C., Montag, M.L., Myers, T.V., Newton, M.E., Olmsted, K.M., Schlotfeldt, R.M.

KANSAS

Aynes, E.A.

KENTUCKY

Hawkins, S.C., Keaton, M., Lamotte, E.N., Notter, L.E., Tracy, M.A.

LOUISIANA

Pate, M.O., Tebo, J.C., Travelbee, J.E.

MAINE

Alline, A.L., Burgess, E.C., Craig, L., Dix, D.L., Mansfield, B.D., Parsons, M.G., Ropes, H.A.

MARYLAND

Armiger, STR., Baker, B., Brockway, M.T., Clayton, S.L., Gonzaga, A.G., Hasson, E.V., Jean, S.L., McGee, A.N., Noyes, C.D., Pfefferkorn, B., Tubman, H.R.

MASSACHUSETTS

Barton, C., Burgess, M.A., Crowell, F.E., Dowling, M.T., Freeman, R.B., Gardner, M.S., Goostray, S., Hawkinson, N.X., Hitchcock, J.E., Lathrop, R.W., Lee, E., Livermore, M.A.R., Mahoney, M.E., Markolf, A.M.S., Palmer, S.F., Parsons, S.F., Russell, M.M., Soule, E.S., Stimson, J., Strong, A.H., Sullivan, E.E., Tracy, S.E., Vreeland, E.M., Waters, Y.G., Wood, H.

MICHIGAN

Domitilla, STR., Knapp, B.L., Matthews, M.L.W., Morse, E.L., Roberts, M.M., Sly, S.E., Thompson, B.A., Urch, D.D., Wamdele, M.E.

MINNESOTA

Gowan, STR., Haupt, A.C., Kessel, A.M., McIver, P.L., McQuillen, F.A., Sargent, E.G., Wilson, M.H., Winton, S.G.J.

MISSISSIPPI

Johnson, F.L.P., Trader, E.K.N.

MISSOURI

Beck, STR., Frank, C.M., Henderson, V., Nahm, H., Utinsky, M.D.

MONTANA

Beckwith, A.T., Yellowtail, Zimmerman, A.L.

NEW HAMPSHIRE

Ayers, L.C., Beard, M., Hall, C.M., Maher, M.A., Smith, M.R., Woodward, L.E.

NEW JERSEY

Brogan, B.S., Errickson, S.M., Falon, I.T., Gardner, B.J., Goodrich, A.W., Johnson, F.M., Maass, C.L., Squire, M.B.

NEW YORK

Anderson, L.E., Arnstein, M.G., Austin, A.L., Butler, I.D.F., Christy, T.E., Crandall, E.P., Cushman, E.D., Delano, J.A., Dempsey, STR., Dewey, M.E.B., DeWittik, K., Dietrich, A.L., Gage, N.D., Garrigan, M.A., Goodnow, M., Grant, A.H., Gray, C.E., Greenough, K., Hall, L., Hubbard, R.W., Kelly, D., Kinney, D.H., Lent, M.E., Loveridge, E.L., McCarron, S.A., Maxwell, A.C., Mills, D.O., Mullane, M.K., Nye, S.V., O'Donnel, M.A., Reid, E.M., Richards, L., Robinson, A.M., Sanford, L.B., Sanger, M., Schutt, B.G., Schuyler, L.L., Seton, E.A.B., Sutliffe, I.H., Thompson, D.E., Truth, S., Warr, E.L., Wheeler, C.A., Wheeler, M.C., Whitman, W., Williamson, A.A., Woolsey, G.A.M.

NORTH CAROLINA

Davis, F.E., Dolan, M.B., Wyche, M.L.

OHIO

Bickerdyke, M.A.B., Boardman, M.T., Bolton, F.P.B., Brainard, A.M., Carr, A.G., Faddis, M.O., Gault, A.E., Howell, M.G., Keller, M.W., Kemble, E.L., Leete, H.L., Leone, L.P., Lowman, I.W., Lytle, N.A., McClelland, H.G., McMillen, C.B., Sanderson, M.E., Sellew, G., Snyder, B.C., Stahl, A.D., Wald, L.D., Wittenmyer, A.T.

OREGON

Miller, M.A.

PENNSYLVANIA

Alcott, L.M., Angela, M., Brinton, M.W., Browne, Mother, Christman, L.P., Dock, L.L., Dorr, A.D., Francis, S.C.,

Fulmer, H., Hassenplug, L.K.W., Heide, W.S., Holman, L., Jones, E.R.K., Kennedy, C.R., Lewis, E.P., Novello, D.J., Peplau, H.E., Riddle, M.M., Rinehart, M.R., Scott, J.M., Werley, H.H.

RHODE ISLAND

Chase, M.J.W., Dolan, J.A., Drown, L.L., Gabriel, STR.

SOUTH CAROLINA

Evans, M., Mellichamp, J.L., Pember, P.Y.

SOUTH DAKOTA

Brink, F.V., Burgess, C., Ingles, T.M.

TENNESSEE

Breckinridge, M., Poole, D.R., Warner, L.A.

TEXAS

Cole, A.L., Garrett, M., Osborne, E.M.R., Rogers, M.E., Willeford, M.B.

VERMONT

Day, P.E., Fife, G.L., Meyer, L.J.R., Phaneuf, M.C., Sanborn, K.A.A., Widmer, C.L.

VIRGINIA

Lynch, T.I., Minnigerode, L., Minor, N.J., Northam, E., Powell, L.M., Scheuer, M., Thoms, A.D.S., Tompkins, S.

WASHINGTON

Hornback, M.S., Verhonick, P.J.

WEST VIRGINIA

Blanchfield, F.A., Evans, B.L.

WISCONSIN

Ainsworth, E.G., Black, F.G., Bunge, H.L., Cannon, I.M., Eldredge, A., Erd-

mann, B., Flikke, J.O., Fuller, S.L., Havey, I.M., Johnson, J.M., Kain, C.M., Kelly, H.W., Kiniery, G., Kuehn, R.P., Lamping, M.K., Odegard, E.J., Phillips, M.G., Purtell, STR., Skenadore, N.C., Thompson, J.C., Vrede, J.V., Werth, M.V.

COUNTRIES

CANADA

Aikens, C.A., Ariss, E.A., Blackwell, E., Damer, A., Darche, L.M., Davis, M.E., Deans, A.G., Dennison, C., Draper, E.A., Germain, L.D., Goff, H.A., Gretter, L., Harmer, B., Hibbard, M.E., Higbee, L.S., Hodgins, A.C., Hogan, A.I., Logan, L.R., MacLeod, C., McCrae, A., McGarrah, M.E., McMillan, M.H., Nutting, M.A., Pope, A.E., Render, H.W., Robb, I.A.H., Schulte, H.D., Seelye, E.E., Sirch, M.E.F., Sleet, J.C., Stewart, I.M., Taylor, E.J., Young, H., d'Youville, M.M.

BRITISH ISLES

Amy Margaret, STR., Banfield, E.M., Batterham, M.R., Belmont, B.R., Browne, H.E., Davies, M., Fisher, A., Hansen, A.L., Johns, E.M.I., Mary Caroline, STR.

OTHER

Beeby, N.V., Black, STR., Cabrini, M., Cumming, K., Deutsch, N., Fedde, E., Fitzgerald, A.L., Gladwin, M.E., Goldman, E., Hickey, M.A., Jensen, D.M.L., Kenny, STR., Kimber, D.E.C., Nathoy, L., Nelson, S.C., Olsen, B.A., Pelchin, K.P., Prochazka, A., Schervier, F., Staupers, M.K., Stevenson, B.V., Van Kooy, C., Waechter, E.H., Willms, E., Wolf, A.D.